*Edited by*

KENNETH DAVISON
ALAN KERR

# Contemporary Themes in Psychiatry

A Tribute to Sir Martin Roth

GASKELL

ISBN 0 902241 28 1

Gaskell is an imprint of the Royal College of Psychiatrists,
17 Belgrave Square, London SW1

Distributed in North America
by American Psychiatric Press, Inc.

**Acknowledgement**

Publication of this book was made possible by the kind help of a loan from
E. Merck Limited, Alton, Hampshire.

Phototypeset by Dobbie Typesetting Limited, Plymouth, Devon
Printed in Great Britain at the Alden Press, Oxford

# Contents

## Part V. Schizophrenia: Organic aspects and problems of drug treatment

## Part VI. Aspects of ethology

## Part VII. Miscellaneous

# List of Contributors

**Hagop S. Akiskal**, Professor and Director of the Section of Affective Disorders, University of Tennessee, Memphis, USA

**Nancy C. Andreasen**, Professor of Psychiatry, University of Iowa, USA

**Gavin Andrews**, University of New South Wales, Australia

**Tom Arie**, Professor, Department of Health Care of the Elderly, University of Nottingham, UK

**Thomas R. E. Barnes**, Consultant/Senior Lecturer, Department of Psychiatry, Charing Cross and Westminster Medical School, University of London, UK

**Klaus Bergmann**, Consultant Psychogeriatrician, The Maudsley Hospital, London, UK

**German E. Berrios**, Consultant/Lecturer, Department of Psychiatry, University of Cambridge, UK

**Garry Blessed**, Emeritus Consultant/Lecturer in Psychogeriatrics, University of Newcastle-upon-Tyne, UK

**William Bondareff**, Professor of Psychiatry and Gerontology, University of Southern California, Los Angeles, USA

**Sydney Brandon**, Professor of Psychiatry, University of Leicester, UK

**Walter M. Braude**, Consultant Psychiatrist, Cheadle Royal Hospital, Cheshire, UK

**Peter G. Britton**, Senior Lecturer in Applied Psychology, University of Newcastle-upon-Tyne, UK

**Michael W. P. Carney**, Consultant Psychiatrist, Northwick Park Hospital, Harrow, London, UK

**Giovanni B. Cassano**, Professor of Psychiatry, University of Pisa, Italy

**Alexander F. Cooper**, Consultant Psychiatrist, Leverndale Hospital, Glasgow, Scotland, UK

**Kenneth Davison**, Consultant/Lecturer, Department of Psychiatry, University of Newcastle-upon-Tyne, UK

**Kenneth Day**, Consultant/Senior Lecturer in Mental Handicap, University of Newcastle-upon-Tyne, UK

**Jonathan H. Dowson**, Consultant/Lecturer, Department of Psychiatry, University of Cambridge, UK

**Erik Essen-Möller**, Emeritus Professor of Psychiatry, Sweden

**Thomas J. Fahy**, Professor of Psychiatry, Regional Hospital, Galway, Irish Republic

**Daniel X. Freedman**, Professor of Psychiatry and Pharmacology, UCLA School of Medicine, USA

**Michael G. Gelder**, Professor of Psychiatry, University of Oxford, UK

**Elliot S. Gershon**, Chief, Clinical Neurogenetics Branch, NIMH, Bethesda, USA

**Max Harper**, Senior Lecturer, Department of Psychological Medicine, University of Wales College of Medicine, Cardiff, Wales, UK

**Fuad Hassanyeh**, Consultant Psychiatrist, Newcastle-upon-Tyne, UK

**Hugh C. Hendrie**, Professor of Psychiatry, Indiana University, USA

**Stephen J. Hucker**, Head, Forensic Division, Clarke Institute of Psychiatry; Associate Professor, University of Toronto, Canada

**Cornelius L. E. Katona**, Senior Lecturer in Psychiatry with Special Interest in the Elderly, Whittington Hospital, London, UK

**David W. K. Kay**, Honorary Consultant, Newcastle-upon-Tyne; Emeritus Professor of Psychiatry, Tasmania, Australia

**Alan Kerr**, Consultant Psychiatrist, Newcastle-upon-Tyne, UK

**Leslie G. Kiloh**, Emeritus Professor of Psychiatry, University of New South Wales, Australia

**Israel Kolvin**, Professor of Child Psychiatry, University of Newcastle-upon-Tyne, UK

**Gerald L. Klerman**, Cornell Medical Center, New York, USA

**J. C. Little**, Formerly Director of Clinical Research and Consultant Psychiatrist, Crichton Royal Hospital, Dumfries, Scotland, UK

**Juan-José López-Ibor, Jnr**, Professor of Psychiatry, University of Alcalá de Henares; Chief, Psychiatric Unit, Ramón y Cajal Hospital, Madrid, Spain

**Hamish McClelland**, Consultant/Lecturer, Department of Psychiatry, University of Newcastle-upon-Tyne, UK

**Alasdair A. McKechnie**, Physician Superintendent, Bangour Village Hospital, West Lothian, Scotland, UK

**Nathaniel D. Minton**, Consultant Psychiatrist, St Peter's Hospital, Chertsey, UK

**Christopher Q. Mountjoy**, Consultant Psychiatrist, St Andrew's Hospital, Northampton, UK

**James A. Mullaney**, Consultant Psychiatrist, Eastern Health Board, Dublin, Irish Republic

**Max F. Perutz, OM**, MRC Scientist, Laboratory of Molecular Biology, Cambridge, UK

**Detlev Ploog**, Director, Max-Planck Psychiatric Institute, Munich, Federal Republic of Germany

**John S. Price**, Consultant Psychiatrist, Milton Keynes Hospital, UK

**John R. Roy**, Professor, Psychiatry; Director, Geriatric Psychiatry Program, Chedoke-McMaster Hospitals, Hamilton, Ontario, Canada

**Melvin Sabshin**, Medical Director, American Psychiatric Association, Washington, DC, USA

**Kurt Schapira**, Consultant/Lecturer, Department of Psychiatry, University of Newcastle-upon-Tyne, UK

**David A. Shaw, CBE**, Professor of Neurology and Dean of Medicine, University of Newcastle-upon-Tyne, UK

**Pamela J. Shaw**, First Assistant in Neurology, University of Newcastle-upon-Tyne, UK

**J. Sydney Smith**, Neuropsychiatric Institute, Prince of Wales Hospital, Randwick, New South Wales, Australia

**Erik Strömgren**, Professor, Institute of Psychiatric Demography, Risskov, Denmark

**A. Arthur Sugerman**, Carrier Foundation, New Jersey, USA

**Malcolm P. I. Weller**, Consultant Psychiatrist/Senior Lecturer, Friern Hospital, London, UK

**F. Anthony Whitlock**, Emeritus Professor of Psychiatry, University of Brisbane, Australia

# Editorial foreword

For this 70th birthday tribute to Professor Sir Martin Roth former students and colleagues have been invited to write on a subject in which they had been influenced by him. Most of the contributors to this volume have worked with him at some time between 1956 and 1984 during which he held successively the Chairs of Psychiatry at Newcastle and Cambridge, but distinguished colleagues from elsewhere in the UK and overseas have also been eager to participate. Of the 49 chapters, 28 emanate from the UK, 11 from North America, five from mainland Europe and Scandinavia, three from Australia and two from the Irish Republic, demonstrating his truly international impact.

The chapters are organised into sections by theme, often reflecting Martin's own interests. In the spirit of a Festschrift, contributors have been encouraged to include personal references, where appropriate, but many have also produced authoritative topical reviews, of intrinsic scientific and educational interest, of many important areas of psychiatry.

For those with no personal acquaintance with Martin Roth we hope that the scientific tradition and standards he embodies are reflected in this tribute by his friends and colleagues which is presented in affection and admiration for his enormous contribution to psychiatry over 40 years.

KENNETH DAVISON
ALAN KERR

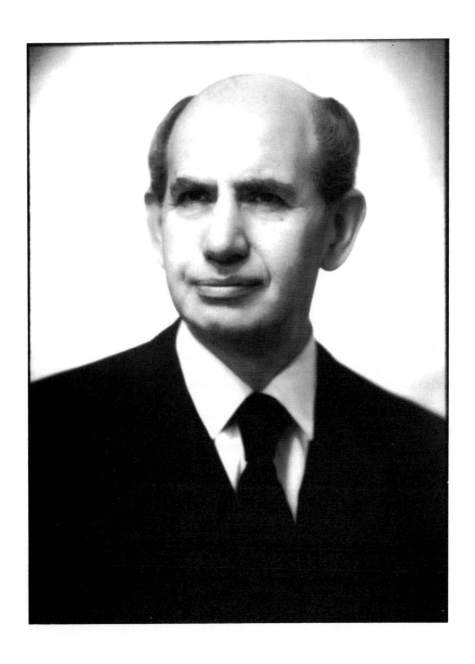

*Sir Martin Roth*

# Martin Roth

## A biographical note

Martin Roth was born on 6 November 1917 in Budapest and moved with his family to England five years later. He received his medical education at St Mary's Hospital and after qualification trained in neurology under Lord Brain. Brain's concern with the psychological aspects of illness and interest in psychoanalysis and philosophy stimulated Martin to think about the many psychiatric problems presenting in the neurological clinic and it was with Brain's encouragement that he decided to enter psychiatry.

At the Maudsley Hospital three men exerted a profound influence. Aubrey Lewis instilled a critical and incisive awareness of the difficulties inherent in the subject. Eliot Slater gave his enduring friendship and encouragement, was his single greatest intellectual influence and brought home to him how scientific methodology could illuminate clinical problems. Erich Guttman demonstrated the potential of the psychiatric interview and showed how the information could be distilled into a precise formulation based on reasoned evidence. Later, at the Crichton Royal Hospital, Willy Mayer-Gross conveyed a boundless enthusiasm for psychiatry and made a profound personal impression by his warmth and benevolence, and also instilled an awareness of the rich phenomenology of the German literature.

In 1950 Martin Roth was appointed Director of the Clinical Research Unit at Graylingwell Hospital, Chichester. Here his work on the differentiation of the mental disorders of old age, already begun at the Crichton Royal, rapidly expanded and included his first excursion into neuropathology. His success in the field foreshadowed the later, more difficult task, of differentiating the affective disorders. During this time, there came also a series of papers on the quantification of electroencephalographic phenomena and the changes associated with the response to electroconvulsive therapy. This was the period, too, when the first edition of the enormously influential *Clinical Psychiatry*, written with Mayer-Gross and Slater, was published. His achievements at Graylingwell led to an invitation in 1955 to become Director of a Medical Research Council Unit to be established in place of the existing Research Unit.

In 1956 he was appointed to the Chair of Psychological Medicine at the Newcastle Medical School, then a branch of the University of Durham, where the department became one of the main centres of clinical research in Britain and units devoted to child and geriatric psychiatry were established. In 1962 he became Honorary Director of the Medical Research Council Group for

Research into the Relation between Organic and Functional Mental Illness. In 1977 he became the first Professor of Psychiatry in Cambridge until his retirement in 1984. He is currently Fellow of Trinity College and Professor Emeritus of Psychiatry at the University of Cambridge.

Many distinctions and honours have been conferred upon him. He has served the World Health Organization in various capacities, recently as consultant for the development of its studies into mental health disorders of the aged, was a member of the Medical Research Council (1964–68), President of the Section of Psychological Medicine of the Royal Society of Medicine (1968–69), the Foreign Guest Lecturer of the Society of Biological Psychiatry (1971) and the Adolf Meyer Lecturer of the American Psychiatric Association (1971). He received the Paul Hoch Award of the American Psychopathological Association, the Strömgren Medal for investigations into problems of old age and the Anna Monika International Foundation Prize for enquiries into depressive illness and related disorders. In 1980 he received the Gold Medal of the Society of Biological Psychiatry and in 1986 the Kraepelin Gold Medal of the Max Planck Institute, Munich. He holds Honorary Fellowships in a number of national and international organisations and a Doctorate of Science (*honoris causa*) was conferred on him by the University of Dublin in 1976.

Martin Roth was elected first President of the Royal College of Psychiatrists in 1971 and played a crucial part in its early development. He forged close links with the Department of Health, played a central role in the negotiations and fund-raising activities which led to the establishment of the College's permanent home in Belgrave Square and took an active part in the establishment of the Membership Examination and approval system for assessing training standards. He has been Associate Editor of the *British Journal of Psychiatry* for over 20 years, is joint editor of *Psychiatric Developments* and serves on the editorial board of a number of other psychiatric journals.

Since his retirement Martin's productivity and energy have been undiminished. He continues to lecture on a wide international scene, has co-authored and co-edited further books, and his interest in research continues unabated as his outstanding output nears 300 papers. He also gives medico-legal advice to the Medical Defence Union on the burgeoning number of cases of litigation which has recently begun to afflict psychiatry.

Martin's own experience of serious illness while still a medical student gave him a strong sympathy for the predicament of individual patients and imparted a sharp sense of the impermanence of life and a desire to live it to the full. His great productivity stems from a formidable blend of intellectual power, imaginative and creative thinking, drive and sheer stamina. He is able to draw together many facets of a problem, is intrigued and attracted by paradoxes, and likes to arrive at constructive generalisations. His command of the English language and his multilingual background have made him an outstanding writer, teacher and speaker. His relaxations are predominantly literature and music, playing Bach on the piano being a cherished if occasional relaxation. He is supported by the devotion of a closely-knit family and his wife Constance leads a busy life in public service, in particular as a magistrate, and many have reason to be grateful for her warmth, friendship and hospitality. Of their three daughters, one is a doctor and another a psychologist.

The preparation of this tribute has been a privilege and pleasure and the task has been very much eased by the ready willingness and enthusiasm of the contributors to take part. It gave Martin particular pleasure to be able to honour Eliot Slater in a similar way and we feel privileged to play a part in this honour for Martin from his many friends and colleagues.

# I. General considerations and historical aspects

# 1 Science, pragmatism and the progress of psychiatry

## MELVIN SABSHIN

I am very pleased to participate in the tribute to Sir Martin Roth. In selecting my contribution I decided to present an overview topic which has a personal connection to Sir Martin. Indeed, an earlier version of this paper had been presented at Brisbane, Australia at the 22nd Congress of the Royal Australian and New Zealand College of Psychiatrists. Sir Martin was an active participant at the meeting and his scholarly comments broadened my thinking about my own paper.

In addition to the Australian setting and Sir Martin's presence, my paper was deeply influenced by the impact of the preceding week's massive annual meeting of the American Psychiatric Association. It had been an exciting, tumultuous panorama with well over 12,000 people in attendance. There were hundreds of presentations, symposia, workshops, case conferences, films, videotapes, ceremonial occasions, business meetings, exhibits, and social functions. What clearly predominated, however, was the extensive clinical impact of the neurosciences, neuropsychopharmacology and biological psychiatry. The meeting exemplified a remarkable scientific surge that has engulfed a significant segment of American psychiatry. Michael Shepherd's (1965) description of the dominance of psychoanalysis in the American psychiatry of the 1950s would not be relevant to the American psychiatry of the late 1980s. The scene, on the whole, has shifted significantly, perhaps dramatically. At the same time, however, psychiatry in the United States has become influenced even more intensely by an even more powerful force—namely a near revolutionary change in the economics of medical and health care. Our *laissez-faire* medical system dominated 30 years ago by the solo private practitioner is being swiftly replaced by a *managed* health care system (Sharfstein & Beigel, 1985). The rate of change is accelerating and it is especially bewildering to an older generation of psychiatrists who perceive themselves as being swept away in the currents of change.

The simultaneous impact of new science and new socio-economic political forces is the key dynamic to predict and to interpret the next stage in the history of psychiatry in the United States; I would submit that these forces and their accoutrements will have a major impact in most countries in the world—with each nation having special patterns and sub-patterns within the overall theme. From my perspective, efforts to find practical methods to cope with the new economic climate will absorb much of our future energy. Practical solutions will predominate and pragmatic functions will be emphasised in that we, and the

3

legions glancing over our shoulders, will ask more frequently: What works most efficiently? What treatments are genuinely cost-effective? and—very importantly—How can we demonstrate the empirical basis upon which we postulate cost-effectiveness? In some ways the scientific developments interdigitate very well with the pragmatic decisions. Science facilitates practice directly and indirectly, and practice helps to shape the contours of science. From other vantage points, however, there are sharp differences between economic forces and science. The resolution of these interdigitations and conflicts will play a key role in determining psychiatry's progress and for this reason I chose 'Science, Pragmatism and Progress in Psychiatry' for the title of this paper.

## The beginning of adulthood in American psychiatry

Psychiatry has moved into the third century of its life span in the United States. Indeed we are all very proud that a signer of our national Declaration of Independence was a psychiatrist—Benjamin Rush! But American psychiatry was relatively slow growing until after the second World War when it began a spurt of growth that is still manifest today. While brilliant leaders were active before the war, I would characterise our history up to the middle 1950s as one of child-like dependency on the beneficence of certain key leaders and institutions. We did not have to be very accountable for the quality of our dreams or fantasies or ideas; many varying but often conflicting flowers began to bloom. Psychoanalysis found a marvellous soil in post World War II America. An impressive array of European emigrés and their native counterparts assumed increasingly powerful functions in our medical schools and hospitals. Confident of their ideas—brilliant as teachers and supervisors—and not constrained by insurance carriers, congressional committees, or a sceptical public, they changed the shape of American psychiatry. Simultaneously social psychiatry began to take root as a developing area of concentration; charismatic leaders developed there also—as was true in child psychiatry, milieu therapy, community mental health and many other derivative fields.

Biological psychiatry had an American constituency which had taken root in the latter part of the 19th century. The optimism, idealism and vitality of the pioneers of American psychiatry (the American Psychiatric Association [APA] was founded in 1844) was replaced by the stolid pessimism that dominated clinical practice from about 1880 to 1955. The inexorable clinical course of dementia praecox became the symbol and the substance of a system in which chronicity, large hospitals and custodialism prevailed. Of course, some treatment was given; my early training was dominated by the use of insulin, paraldehyde, barbiturates, electric shock and malaria (for central nervous system syphilis). The biological psychiatrists had a strong ideology of biological aetiology and treatment but they lacked a theory and a convincing method of practice. Furthermore, they were not nearly as scintillating or charismatic as the psychoanalysts or the social psychiatrists. Nevertheless the latter two groups, whatever their protestations, had a relatively weak empirical base also and were, in fact, dominated by ideologies rather than science. With several colleagues I have documented the scope, extent and criteria for understanding and measuring psychotherapeutic, sociotherapeutic and somatotherapeutic ideologies (unsubstantiated belief systems about aetiology, treatment and the nature of psychiatric illnesses) (Strauss *et al*, 1981).

These ideologies (or as some say, 'schools of thought')—separate, disparate and in continuous conflict—taken *en masse*, formed the nuclear image of psychiatry as perceived in the media, in decision-making bodies and in the eyes of our colleagues in the rest of medicine. By the early 1960s this movement had achieved an enormous impact—but then it spawned another effect that had even larger ripples. During the 1960s up until the middle of the 1970s, American psychiatry expanded its boundaries further than in any other period of psychiatric history and far beyond any other country in the world. Indeed I doubt that there will be such a boundary expansion again![1] The expansiveness of American psychiatry took two major directions. In the first place, the role-functions of psychiatrists broadened dramatically like a mushroom cloud until there were no boundaries, no limits, and ultimately our perceived expertise began to lose any meaning. We became 'experts' in war and peace, in major moral issues, in crime and delinquency, in poverty and its consequences, in organisational structure and function at macro and micro-levels, in education, in religion, in arts and humanities, in psycho-biography and in epistemology and most other branches of philosophy. What an exciting period this became! It was attractive to many students and affected the career lines of many of us as well as dominating the field as a whole. Nevertheless its consequences were deleterious and I will return to that shortly.

The second direction of this expansiveness involved the boundaries of psychopathology which reached a stage in the early 1970s wherein a widely prevailing but implicit assumption of the universality of psychopathology dominated the field. Five major forces contributed significantly to this trend, and I will outline them briefly. Psychoanalytic theory and practice was perhaps the chief contributor. Freud's (1901/1960) genius and his prolific essays included assumptions about "the psychopathology of everyday life." Indeed all behaviour had at least some psychopathological roots. Normality or health were implicitly regarded as Platonic ideals never fully realisable. Since all of us experienced some painful affect and all of us had some neurotic analogues, anyone who sought help (and was sufficiently healthy) might be a candidate for psychoanalytic treatment. While many psychoanalysts were aware of some of the remarkable implications of these assumptions, they were never tested empirically nor, more precisely, did psychoanalysts have any interest in epidemiological research. Even more importantly, psychoanalysts never wrote about the broad policy implications of these concepts (Sabshin, 1985).

Child psychiatrists (whether or not they were psychoanalysts) also contributed to this *mélange*. It was frequently pointed out that relatively few children fully achieved the goals of each successive stage of development. Deficits were almost universal (of course many of the children's deficits were micro rather than macro), and in this sense an implicit assumption evolved which approximated a universality of psychopathology model. This model veered quite far from a medical model and, in fact, was quite close to an educational paradigm. All of

1. Nevertheless the phenomena were also manifested, at least in part, in many other countries— and the implications of this boundary expansion have great theoretical and practical significance in all countries.

us fail to achieve *optimal* educational objectives and could (if we or others are so motivated) be trained to learn more. If these deficits are viewed as illnesses and if all children manifest some deficits, the policy implications are enormous.

Adolescent psychiatry contributed to this broadening of the boundaries of psychopathology by dint of its heavy emphasis on the expectancy of tumultuous crisis periods during adolescent growth and development. Erikson's vivid descriptions of identity crises came to be perceived as an inexorable normative phase. Indeed, the teenager who failed to experience such a crisis was thought to be more vulnerable than one who went through the phase. When an insurance claims manager read the following prototypic case synopsis he (or she) could be understandably confused. "This 17 year old male high school student was too well defended to experience an identity 'crisis.' After one year of treatment his defences were weakened and a full-blown identity crisis has emerged. I anticipate that in two or three years he will reintegrate at a superior level." It is understandable that insurance managers blanched when they read such reports. Many came to the conclusion that psychiatry was in fact a *bottomless pit* without shape or limits or common-sense. The fourth and fifth contributions to the erosion of the boundaries of psychopathology were social and community psychiatry. The emphasis on sociological and economic factors as aetiological agents opened up another vista of uncharted (non-empirically derived) boundaries for our field. In fact, this too represented a strong ideological (and even moral) perspective. Furthermore, social and community psychiatry (and their accompanying arenas of work) also became extremely difficult to distinguish from social and community psychology; the overlapping roles of the psychologists and the psychiatrists were much broader than the separate functions. Emerging ineluctably from the developments described above is the conclusion that the broader the boundaries of psychiatry the greater the difficulty in distinguishing psychiatrists from other mental health professionals.

As a corollary, the broader the boundaries of psychiatry the more distant and remote it appears to the rest of medicine. By the 1960s the structural de-medicalisation of American psychiatry reached its peak (or nadir). We not only shed our white coats but we also underemphasised aetiology, nosology, principles and standards of treatment, and systematic studies of prevention. Kubie's (1949) proposal to merge clinical psychology and psychiatry reflected how far away we had moved from medicine. When the decision was made (in 1970) to terminate the requirements for a medical internship prior to psychiatric residency training it symbolised that a divorce had taken place.

Thus confluence of trends had occurred by 1970 in which boundary expansion, de-medicalisation, and the predominance of ideology over science exerted a powerful force. There were attractive aspects of this confluence and by the middle 1960s psychiatry was riding happily [not madly as Grinker (1964) stated] in all directions. There were plenty of patients; research funds were attainable as were training dollars. The need for professional accountability was not especially high. But this was a system that was much more vulnerable than many perceived. By the late 1970s events changed dramatically. Economic pressures, political events and new social values altered the American milieu and psychiatry was caught in this vortex. By 1977 events had changed so radically that the medical internship model was reinstated (with a different name but the same intent). Funding became more difficult to obtain. Competition with other mental health practitioners began to replace the prior pattern of relationships. We had encouraged the growth of these mental health workers and now they wished to become autonomous. Indeed, the large number of clinical psychologists and psychiatric social workers caused a massive wave of anxiety and to some extent elicited anger at organised psychiatry for permitting this to happen. Furthermore, research in neuropsychopharmacology had begun to accelerate and was exerting an ever-strengthening influence. Simultaneously the torrid affair between psychoanalysis and psychiatry began to cool and both disciplines began to seek new relationships. Decision-makers and the media did not know how to deal with us; the bottomless pit was sucking us in and we began to experience a genuine identity crisis. When I assumed the Medical Directorship of the APA these models predominated and most of my efforts and attention during these past 13 years have been devoted to attempts at coping with this professional dilemma.

Indeed my own assessment (shared by many leaders in the APA) was that it was time for a genuine **coming of age for psychiatry in the USA.** As a corollary, I believed that we were finally moving towards a termination of psychiatry's adolescence. From my perspective, adulthood is definitely present (and adolescence is over) when a profession manifests the following:

    (a) clear boundaries and priorities of its goals and objectives

    (b) a capacity to form stable relationships and alliances (with other organisations and institutions)

    (c) the means to earn and to compete for income

    (d) a capacity to cope with reality—even if somewhat unpleasant at times—and

    (e) an ability to achieve compromises which balance the objectives with the realities—an important corollary is the capacity to avoid the wishes for a perfect solution to interfere with a good solution.

These capacities apply to many countries besides the United States. It must be acknowledged, however, that American psychiatry has demonstrated greater oscillations and ideological variance than almost any other country in the world.

## Pragmatism and coping with the problems

The keys for coping by psychiatry (at least in the next decade) involve the interaction of scientific advances and effective pragmatic actions. Each nation will have its own admixture in this interaction; clearly the availability of technology, personnel, and other resources will make a substantial difference. For the United States it is essential that scientific developments be recognised as the keystone to the progress of psychiatry at every level. We have advanced beyond simplistic humanism, ideological dogma and loosely formulated judgements; this advance must continue, be widely publicised, and understood by decision-makers. In pointing out the limits of 'simple humanism', I am certainly not arguing against the value of humanistic principles. Indeed, I fear that there is a danger in an overbearing logical positivism that clinical skills and humanistic approaches to clinical practice may become somewhat atrophied. But humanism is not enough—not nearly enough—to be the central focus for the role of the psychiatrist, even though this approach has had some positive impact in various clinical settings.

The hegemony of ideology systems within psychiatry must be ended and I believe that we are well under way to accomplish that in the United States. In the past, psychiatry has been hurt by public perceptions that the field is characterised by warring parties, each advocating unsubstantiated theories and practices. These perceptions still carry a heavy weight and each week I read newspaper stories featuring this unfortunate characterisation of our field.

Indeed, a recent national television programme featured a debate in which a British psychiatrist author enunciated that most psychiatry is a hodge-podge of ideologies; he cautioned people to eschew seeing a psychiatrist as compared to a friend, a bartender, or pulling themselves up by their bootstraps. Significantly, however, his opinion was counteracted by a vigorous new breed type psychiatrist who pointed out the anachronisms in his argument. On the other hand, newspaper stories featuring scientific advances convey the imagery of a more empirically grounded field . . . and the reinforcement of this imagery has significant impact. Each year in the United States we have a congressionally authorised **mental illness awareness week** and we have used those occasions to make presentations before the public and key decision makers. For the last four years, as part of this week, we have had presentations before the staff of our national legislative bodies and these were very well received. The staff have, in turn, been helpful in supporting important legislation which, for example, has produced increasing support for psychiatric research while many other non-psychiatric programmes have been reduced in funding. Note that I have emphasised the pragmatic utilisation of science, research, and empiricism. I do indeed recognise that the research has been of extraordinary value and help to patients directly. That is being appreciated by families of the mentally ill and by patients—in a host of new ways including the proliferation of new national groups such as NAMI (National Alliance for the Mentally Ill—families of the mentally ill) and separate groups involved with schizophrenia, manic-depressive illness and phobias. The yields have been promising and are very important for psychiatry.

Another basic principle in the efforts to cope with the accountability requirements for psychiatric practice in the late 1980s and 1990s will be the continuing need for objectification in our field. All of those who make decisions about reimbursement for psychiatric treatment (government officials, insurance companies, industries, etc.) have been affected by the fear that providing reimbursement for psychiatric treatment is like throwing money down a bottomless pit. They need assurance that the field is finite and that psychiatric treatment is reliable, measurable and provided for people with illnesses that are also objectifiable. DSM–III (APA, 1980) has been the key symbol for objectifiability of psychiatric diagnosis. While not created for that purpose, its impact upon a wide network of fiduciary managers has been important. The APA is also planning to publish a major book on the treatment of psychiatric disorders which will attempt to delineate preferred modes of psychiatric therapies. DSM–III along with a new revised DSM–III-R (APA, 1987) and the book on treatments have stirred lively debates; some of our members fear that these publications will be constrictive and too much like manuals or even cook-books.

Nevertheless, the majority of our members understand the value of the books for their own intrinsic worth and also how they can enhance psychiatry's capacity to cope. The need for objectification is also apparent in our efforts to justify why psychiatric hospital admittance is necessary and how long the patient should be kept in the hospital. Indeed in the United States there is a determined effort by our government (and by insurance carriers) to limit the expensive costs of hospital stays. We are collecting data to see if there are rational principles upon which this system might be anchored.

During the next decade it will be important to strengthen our capacity to increase epidemiological research and to conduct trans-national studies of incidence and prevalence. The stronger our epidemiological base, the more precise we can be in developing or recommending rational policies in services and manpower. Economic research in psychiatry should also receive a higher priority. In the United States we have begun to improve our data base on so called 'offset research'. These studies involve the calculation of cost-savings and increased productivity as a result of psychiatric treatment. For example, to what extent does appropriate treatment for people with manic-depressive illness reduce costs of treatment to these patients' non-psychiatric physicians?

I tend to favour the gradual constriction of the psychiatric boundaries discussed earlier in the paper, so that our role functions become sharper and more delineated from other mental health workers, especially in diagnostic functions. Simultaneously, we need to demonstrate the differences in psychiatric services provided by an internist, a family practitioner, a paediatrician, and other physicians. While constricting many roles in the United States, there is also an effort to re-capture activities which we have under-emphasised such as alcoholism, drug abuse, geriatrics, and mental retardation.

In a previous section of the paper I have commented upon the impact of structural de-medicalisation of psychiatry (Sabshin, 1986). During the last few years we have begun to move towards a structural re-medicalisation of our field. Note that the word 'structural' implies an organised, systematic shift in which the profession as a whole undergoes change. The field is re-emphasising aetiology, diagnosis, treatment, prevention, and epidemiology. We have moved vigorously to develop standards for treatment and for the study of the outcome of treatment. We expect that hypotheses are stated clearly so that they may be tested rigorously and we have become much less likely to accept ideological pronouncements, no matter how brilliantly they may be stated.

Two important caveats should be emphasised at this time. Re-medicalisation does not imply the hegemony of the biological systems over all else in psychiatry. It is important to avoid the pitfalls of biological reductionism which denigrates or trivialises psycho-social variables. Indeed, we expect that psychological and social hypotheses must be tested by rigorous scientific criteria. We recognise the complexities that will be necessary to conduct such research but we are pleased that new technology will assist us through the large array of data necessary to test many psychosocial hypotheses. The dangers of biological reductionism are both subtle and overt. There are many constituencies that have a substantial stake against, for example, the hypothesis that family variables may be significant independent factors involved in the pathogenesis of mental disease. Biological variables are easier to measure and the utilisation of biological treatments may appear, at first glance—and in the short run—to be less expensive. That illusion has great practical impact for cash-poor nations that choose to focus upon psychopharmacology, but fails to provide a system for rehabilitation of chronic patients. Without psychological and social supports, the evidence indicates a much higher rate of relapse, and the psychotherapeutic plus sociotherapeutic skills required to accomplish these therapeutic purposes are often of a high professional order. Technicians at lower levels of mental health workers simply cannot accomplish the task. Furthermore, the psychiatrist who is trained in all of these skills is the key figure to make an accurate diagnosis and to determine the appropriate therapy. The triage role and the mosaic of skills necessary to conduct this triage are the unique professional qualification of the modern psychiatrist. The other mental health professionals and the non-psychiatric physicians do not possess the full range of skills necessary to make a diagnosis and to choose the appropriate course of treatment.

The second important caveat (in addition to biological reductionism) is the need to be aware of some of the limits of empiricism, pragmatism and logical positivism that dominate the new scientific developments in psychiatry and elsewhere. One fundamental concern, of course, relates to the atheoretical proclivities of most current psychiatric researchers.

DSM-III illustrates this process clearly (even if some implicit theoretical biases emerge in a number of instances) in its attempt to deal with limitations in current aetiological knowledge. To many psychiatrists, DSM-III and DSM-III-R appear to be lifeless, dull, and, as some critics say, too much like a printed menu. At one level this variety of criticism may be a subtle form of vitalist philosophy that cannot tolerate what is construed to be a lack of individuality and uniqueness. One more obvious critic of this stripe stated that he would much prefer to diagnose his patient as Raskalnikov or Hamlet rather than use DSM-III terminology. This perspective (or more modest versions of it) often includes a fear that the vitality of clinical interviewing and psychotherapeutic talents will be lost in more standardised procedures of diagnosis and the use of biological medication. On a more fundamental level, the relative paucity of new theoretical constructs in psychiatry, and the domination of what some construe to be more pedestrian research, leads to the fear in some quarters that psychiatry may not attract first-class scientific minds, with brilliance and creativity. This concerns me, too, and it is worth raising our consciousness about these possibilities. One of the reasons I enjoyed Basil James' (1980) 'Psychiatry, Science and the Seduction of Emma Bovary', was his elegant expression of some of these concerns. The very fact of James' paper and other similar essays is a good antidote to stereotyping our thinking as well as our conduct of research. In slight contrast to my good friend, Basil James, I would emphasise that we are in a phase of overcompensating for previous tendencies and perhaps (at least in the United States) this trend may be useful or at least acceptable for a few years. Furthermore, the pragmatic needs in many countries may necessitate the overcompensation in order to reach the decision-makers and the general public.

*Unfortunately*, Hamlet, Emma Bovary, and Raskalnikov stir up images of arts and humanities in ways that perpetuate or reinforce myths and stereotypes about us. I sincerely hope that the current period of proving our scientific credentialling will be effective enough for us to broaden our base in the not too distant future. More importantly, the lack of new theory has a danger of either making us complacent or leading to atrophy that could stifle, and perhaps even impede, our pragmatic objectives.

Despite our legion of critics (including anti-psychiatric psychiatrists) we have moved into a new phase in the history of psychiatry. Nostalgia for our cottage industry days will not suffice. When my colleagues say, ''I don't know if I would go into psychiatry if I were choosing a specialty at this time,'' I answer that they under-estimate the young people coming into our field. The new breeds of psychiatrists will recognise the complexities and live with them in novel ways. Many in my country and yours will become involved in providing the data and the leadership that will develop new strategies. Many will be able to break out of old moulds and chains so we can seize the opportunities. Young people will, I think, understand what I mean by pragmatism and will also recognise that psychiatry must perceive itself confidently as an empirically grounded clinical science of medicine that can also be truly responsive to the needs of our patients. This perspective, of course, is not limited to the new generation. Sir Martin Roth has served as a model for many of us in embodying empiricism and rationality. Hopefully, his approach will become even more dominant in the years to come.

## References

AMERICAN PSYCHIATRIC ASSOCIATION (1980) *Diagnostic and Statistical Manual of Mental Disorders* (3rd edn). Washington, DC: APA.
—— (1987) *Diagnostic and Statistical Manual of Mental Disorder* (3rd edn, revised). Washington, DC: APA.
FREUD, S. (1960) *The Psychopathology of Everyday Life*. London: Hogarth Press and the Institute of Psycho-analysis. (Original work published 1901.)
GRINKER, R. R. (1964) Psychiatry rides madly in all directions. *Archives of General Psychiatry*, **10**, 228–237.
JAMES, B. (1980) Psychiatry, science and the seduction of Emma Bovary. *Australian & New Zealand Journal of Psychiatry*, **14**, 101–107.
KUBIE, L. S. (1949) Medical responsibility for training in clinical psychology. *Journal of Clinical Psychology*, **5**, 94–100.
SABSHIN, M. (1985) Psychoanalysis and psychiatry: Models for potential future relations. *Journal of the American Psychoanalytic Association*, **33**, 473–491.
—— (1986) The future of psychiatry: Coping with ''New Realities''. In *Our Patient's Future in a Changing World* (ed. J. Talbott). Washington, DC: American Psychiatric Press.
SHARFSTEIN, S. S. & BEIGEL, A. (1985) *The New Economics and Psychiatric Care*. Washington, DC: American Psychiatric Press.
SHEPHERD, M. (1965) Psychiatric education in the United States and United Kingdom: Similarities and contrasts. *Comprehensive Psychiatry*, **6**, 246–254.
STRAUSS, A., SCHATZMAN, L., BUCHER, R., EHRLICH, D. & SABSHIN, M. (1981) *Psychiatric Ideologies and Institutions*. London: Transaction Books.

# 2 Martin Roth: Lessons for American psychiatry

**DANIEL X. FREEDMAN**

## A prologue

I have been reflecting on the improbable fact that Martin Roth, who pioneered in studying them, can now call himself a septuagenarian—a fact, as any scan of his recent activities reveals, which he does not appreciate! This is a singular oversight. There are very few facts embracing the span of relevant issues to which he does not attend, but this omission is fortunate for psychiatry. I did try to find the phrase that would epitomise Martin, but found such classification difficult. He is particularly resistant to any kind of categorisation.

Nor, scanning this side of the Atlantic, could I summon the image of a comparable American giant of psychiatry. I could, as if suffering flashbacks, recall phases of dominant emphases in American psychiatry and their leading figures, and have occasionally noted some of these over nearly five decades of scrutiny (e.g., Redlich & Freedman, 1966; Freedman, 1978a, 1978b, 1982, 1987). Thus, after briefly sketching what were, in fact, enthusiastic swings of focus, I will note some current enthusiasms and the potential for a gyroscopic function for these, if in American psychiatry we would but borrow the essential lessons Roth teaches.

## Roth as a subject of description

Even to extract these lessons was not easy. The harder I tried to envisage the investigator, clinician, author, scholarly critic, administrator, innovator in education and in the organisations professionals require—the better I could see how steep the gradient indeed is to grasp the true accomplishment in each of his ventures. Assessing the elusiveness of the desired apt brevity, I realised that his multifaceted life itself exemplifies the themes he fundamentally espouses in his intellectual approach to psychiatry. There he has advocated comprehensiveness and scope but attentiveness to detail. He patiently articulates various complex 'systems' of psychiatry but simultaneously espouses the indefatigable pursuit of leads, of constant but critical search—and, above all, openness.

He is seen by my colleagues as an important teacher of issues of phenomenology and nosology. He is valued for bringing a unique steadfastness of intellect and

12

cheerful ebullience in pursuing the messages the real world of clinical reality generates. He treats these with the use of clinical acuity, of descriptive science's disciplined search for regularities in clinical phenomena, and with a scholarly and critical assessment of methodologies in their analysis.

Where he has found order that might seem to call for reverence and rest, he seems almost mischievously to search for exceptions, *their* meaning, and their consequence upon any of our neater intellectual constructions. In his comprehensiveness and mastery of our field, he has somehow maintained the ability to undertake detailed empirical pursuits of patients and clinical disorders—and to stipulate these with salient case vignettes, an art our research-minded academic leaders and younger educators of the 1960s were accused of neglecting (Freedman, 1971; Kubie, 1971).

Roth sought and assessed 'systems' in the field—whether from Europe or Scandinavia (or Washington, the home of APA and its now life-sustaining series of diagnostic manuals!). But rather than revere 'final solutions' he discovers the problems that systems themselves engender. Touching, as the range of his studies does, the issues of phenomenology and classification I can find some American counterparts. But as Sir Martin reminds us of personality and character problems in diagnostic 'entities' and explores the possibilities of systematising the subjective in diagnostics, as he engages debates centring on typology or dimensions in psychopathology or possible biological markers (Akiskal & Webb, 1978) and keeps the patient alive in so doing, there is a kind of indefatigable seriousness and scope and vibrant communication of it that cannot be matched.

## Our plunge beneath the surface

There is a difference between the kind of sustained openness Roth expounds (it is coupled with and derives from scientific rigour) and the rich and often undisciplined curiosity and explorations into the life of the mind that for two decades characterised (often in caricature) post World War II American psychiatry. I refer, of course, to the excitements attributed to our 'discovery' of psychoanalysis. Its simplest allure was the tenet that things may not be what they seem! The unintelligible surface was to be explained by subterranean configurations with their active historical residues which the gifted could discern; the secret wonders of self could thereby be articulated, if not celebrated. Beneath this there was an unintelligible—or given—set of conflicting operations called the unconscious with its ultimate somatic sources called brain. Its significance, if neurological in consequence, could be attended to, but the job of brain would be ultimately to conform to our subjectivist intuitions and convictions, if not our phenomenologic observations or the inferences of depth psychology.

That the systems of brain might be mindless of what so fills our mind, that various impersonal (though environmentally responsive) signalling processes might operate in their own realm and rules was not in that period of zestful expansion as appreciated as it was by more profound students of human behaviour—Freud, Darwin, Pavlov or, for that matter, Bernard. We, in brief, indulged a widely exploratory and fascinating but, for the most part, unsystematic inquiry into the vicissitudes of self with inevitable consequent solipsism (which, as

I sense it, we have with some relief exported in the 1970s and 1980s as waves of psychoanalytically-derived interests successively capture the imaginations of our friends in different countries abroad). Our reach, I've reflected (Freedman, 1982), at times exceeded our capacity to gasp!

While the *relative* loss of systematics in nosological or clinical investigative pursuit was evident, the intensive probings of mental life of a wide range of the seriously and questionably ill in fact provided us more than an isolated snapshot of disordered behaviour as produced by the rigid mental status examination. As elsewhere noted (Freedman, 1978b, 1982), the intent of many was to know mentally ill individuals as persons—and not solely as psycho-dynamic machines. Accordingly, we can now offer a keener assessment of some of the variation in apparently similar symptomatic presentations and a better understanding of some of the transactions (and stressors) deriving from families and social groups than had been prevalent before 1950. One is not surprised to find panic disorder emerging in the context of a success neurosis—i.e., there are other variables that can be investigated, and perhaps usefully for treatment, than are comprised in the strict nosological frameworks. In fact, as Roth has taught, multi-axial considerations, personality, traits and temperament can be an object of useful scrutiny. Whether or not *specifically* psychoanalytic notions or interventions were requisite for our enlarged scope in that era, there was a lack of focus on consequence and utility of the multiple observations and preoccupations.

In psychiatric education, however, the students' apprehension of transference has enlarged their grasp of otherwise overlooked or distracting elements in transactions with patients. Transference identifies one of man's adaptive techniques in utilising nurturance in phases of dependence and it is essential in growth and development as attachments are constructively utilised. Thus, whether noted (or, as in psychoanalysis, systematically worked with) it is intrinsic to observable patterns of expectations and behaviour in the 'doctor-patient relation-ship'. Further, our enhanced canniness of varied symptomatic presentations derives, in part, from the observations of 'mechanisms of defence'—essentially the tricks the mind can play in its multiple constructive or maladaptive avoidances or in certain dysjunction of self-perceived intent and actual patterns of behaviour. These, in brief, are some abiding residues of that era incorporated by general psychiatry.

But to one of the core lessons I would learn from Roth, the very fact that motivational meaning is attached to all experience does not mean we gain thereby significant leverage effective for behavioural change or the prevention of disorders—and that is the critical question. Rather, in my view, it tells us something about the inevitable functioning of mental life which seems to generate meanings regardless of utility. If so, that striking fact itself requires scrutiny for its consequence.

So it was a struggle in that era to focus as Roth would have us do on differences that make a difference, on observation and testing of those possibly useful notions among the many dynamic psychiatry generated and to investigate simultaneously critical psychosocial and psychobiological determinants of the conditions in which mental life operates. I intend herein no systematic assessment of all this but rather in broad brushstroke to evoke a memory of the swirl of issues and their subsequent transitions.

## *The ascent of the social and biological*

Thus, transitions from the high hopes engendered by the illusion of full comprehension of the interior world shifted in the very early 1960s to equally millenniary expectation of the role of socio-cultural and community factors. As I had noted (Freedman, 1978a), the consequence in terms of the organisation of accountable clinical responsibilities and operations was again a loss of focus. This was evident among the various species of 'mental health workers' engaging in a veritable 'orgy of role transvestism'. At the extremes, the secondary consequences of being ill, 'labelling,' were construed as the real issue and a 'civil right' to be crazy pre-empted concerns for the functional incapacity to *not* be (Freedman, 1987).

At the same time, a quieter development had been shaping as a consequence of effective drugs and their even more consequential 'spin-off'—the discovery of the chemical brain. This was fostered in 1955 and thereafter in this country largely under psychiatric auspices and, in part, by psychiatrists turned into 'psychopharmacologists'. There also grew a mode of proceeding in clinical investigations. This was the ethically accountable engagement of *treated* patients, diagnostically characterised and undergoing assessments of various biological measures made possible by new technologies. This had crystallised as a mode of proceeding by 1966—much faster than anticipated. Thus, in planning for academic departments one had equally to foster access to clinical populations and to adjacent laboratories. This, I believe, became evident in the 1970s and perhaps over-celebrated in this decade as a myriad of new observations have emerged.

All of this has once more resulted in new enthusiasms as psychiatry is claimed to have been re-medicalised and 'biological psychiatry' is hailed as finally having come solidly to the fore. In spite of the new knowledge I have welcomed and fostered in this area I see no cause to close the books and once again replace perspective with the unadulterated joy of enthusiasm. I am reminded of another teacher from Martin's home, Sir Henry Dale, who remarked (as Martin might) that the price of progress had to be assessed in terms of what then is disregarded!

## *Neuroscience as salvation*

I have often noted that 'biological psychiatry' is a redundancy; that our ultimate references are to specific patternings of 'behavings'; that neither modern neuroscience nor clinical investigation has yet unearthed the causes of or predispositions to the postulated initial disequilibria and the cascade of intricate consequences we recognise as symptomatic disease. Rather, for over a century the task of psychiatry—and medicine generally—has been to examine the unity, diversity, and variability of clinical phenomena to see what they reveal about the significance of biological measures and vice versa (Freedman, 1975). That is the uncompleted task that lies ahead.

The availability of useful drugs (some of which are symptomatically specific, but hardly curative) and the precision with which vast unexplored gaps in the physiology of behaviour can now be approached, of course, requires and accounts for our new-found respect for reliable description and classification. But beyond paresis and pellagra, we have little specificity or prevention in hand (as is true for 80% or more of 'medical' diseases). In general, aetiopathology is less developed than various glimpses we have of pathophysiological sequences; our understanding of pharmacotherapeutic mechanisms is far greater than either of the former. It is surely more relevant than it recently was to learn about function from brain lesions or—in our research—to make biological measures. But we tend now to confuse special inquiry and domains of knowledge—drug challenges and neuroendocrine measures, electrophysiologic tests and brain imaging, or psychopharmacology and 'receptorology'—with some kind of new clinical discipline ('neuropsychiatry') rather than recognise the normal adaptation of a clinical specialty to useful tools and relevant new dimensions for scrutiny. Pills have *not* replaced the needed span of inquiry.

We now celebrate 'neuroscience' as a novel and definitive final development. Of course, we have long been accumulating the evidence that the brain is *built* to acquire information, memory and a history; in so doing it constructs an identity and style. We have also known that learned familial rules structure the individual's interpretation of stressors as well as options for coping and that the developing organism needs—seeks—these signals. In brief, we know—or should have known—that the psychosocial is biologically rooted and a part of the regulatory operations with which we function. Simpler operations and their accommodations to signals ('learning') are now receiving molecular definition, excitingly confirming these principles. But, neither pragmatically nor philosophically has 'progress' enabled us to dispense with the various different domains relevant to comprehending or coping with disorders whose presentations are 'behavioural' (a term which conveniently hides the complexity of its multiple components).

So we have not from all our scientific investigation constructed the systematic tools or logical structures to provide us with the convenience of avoiding empirical observations in the clinic. The task of diagnosis and monitoring and rediagnosis of the particular patient remains. I predict that, to some extent, it always will. What we ultimately seek, of course, is to discern the 'logic of nature' to understand the nexus of casual sequences and to find salient points by which we can specifically prevent or repair disorder—whether by understanding the laws of reinforcement or molecular recognition, signalling and regulatory operations. What we seem to forget is that a thorough understanding—if it were attained—would point to the *intrinsic* sources of variability *and* unpredictability in these processes. And it is this contingency (or necessity) that may require us to continue to provide the skilled assessments that clinical interventions provide.

## Sermons to be borrowed from Roth

Now, I can't be blamed for finding in the very breadth of Sir Martin's works the sermons I prefer. I have been describing and wondering about our vulnerability to fad, our rush for premature closure—a kind of intellectual ejaculatio praecox! Why do we rush to be exclusively 'biological,' 'psychosocial,' 'psychodynamic' or 'descriptive'? I believe we do not keep in high focus what Roth essentially practises and teaches to be the overall task of psychiatry.

With Roth, I would believe that psychiatry in all its richness and necessary span of inquiry can grasp that its *defining* business is to be engaged in the study of diseases. This sounds simplistic. It perhaps emphasises the obvious which, however, has a way of eluding us. It even would require that we—no matter how impatient—do first things first (and well!). But our failure to perceive as Roth does this essential task of the study of disease is my diagnosis of our vulnerability to some of the readily caricatured excesses and fads to which we are subject.

I had once been tempted to define psychiatry as a behavioural science. But, whatever it seeks to apprehend in terms of behavioural, neuropsychological, linguistic, affective, psychosocial or physiological processes, it does so with the focus of a *clinical* science. And the job of the clinical sciences in medicine is to comprehend the span of parameters from aetiopathology and precipitating factors and predispositions to the determinants of symptom expression and their secondary and tertiary consequences. The job is to study the course and outcome of disease and to search for mediating mechanisms in pathophysiology and compensatory ones in therapeutics, etc. The clinical sciences of medicine ruthlessly utilise any knowledge source that applies and continually assess the relevance of all findings to those patterned dysregulations that are best studied as disease (Freedman, 1982).

The 'clinical process'—the logic and steps by which we investigate the individual patient—has much in common with the logic of investigative processes. The physician's judgement is informed by the evidence the sciences have adduced and that which investigation of the patient, in fact, reveals. It is not the source of information of the type of intervention or even medicines that make a 'medical model' but rather the *way* all are used in management of a clinical case that is subsumed in the medical model. It is a mode of proceeding—one that is 'open' to relevant data. No single medicine or battery of tests can totally remove us from this mode of practice.

Psychiatry and the rest of medicine (Reich *et al*, 1987) now utilise the same methodologies for identifying vulnerabilities, precipitants, course, outcome and therapeutic efficacy. Prospective, retrospective and clinical trial designs are similar whatever the specialty. In all of medicine, including psychiatry, pathophysiological mechanisms now commonly rest on the identification of molecular and cellular signalling and recognition systems. We all assess their role in the disregulation of metabolic or organ systems—whether these be heart or brain, glucose utilisation or neuroendocrine function.

So fundamentally, in my view, when I am asked what is biological about psychiatry, it is that we and the rest of medicine are a part of the 'life sciences'. Our particular target mediating organ is brain; we have much yet to understand about its multiple ongoing systems and their consequence. And, as does all of medicine, we must also come to understand the range of mechanisms, both endogenous and exogenous to nuclear DNA, by which apparently similar phenotypes are encountered at the level of symptomatic observations.

What we in psychiatry must remember is that the intrinsic genetic design, DNA, 'expects' an environment with which to transact. Its very structure and 'blank' areas provide for order, error, and chance from conception and throughout the life cycle, so, too, for the arrangements of the developing and functioning brain. The instructional and expressive design in nature's logic entails the ceaseless interplay of the 'seeking and the sought' through molecular, cellular and behavioural communications. In embryology we see a nerve seeking the target that signals an 'interest' and in the human we see a search for sources signalling emotional nurturance. The biological response to the milieu that provides for 'directionality' in the simplest of organisms may presage arrangements for 'intentionality' in man. At bottom, then, we are built to behave and in this design the biological requires the behavioural and thus has meaning for psychiatry (Freedman, 1987).

As we achieve a clearer grasp of nature's designs we should gain both in precision and in understanding of the intrinsic sources of variability and unpredictability in regulatory processes relevant to physiology *and* behaviour. But, perhaps some day we may yield the notion that we can rigidly control all outcome in the name of therapeutics or prevention. Nature, as I read it, does not need the illusions of omnipotence that console us.

We can surely anticipate with the current thrust of fundamental clinical and physiological investigations some eventual simplification of the current complexities that perplex us. We can hope for a far better comprehension of workable and more precise alternatives when disease arises. We can anticipate that both medicine and psychiatry will in the future become increasingly unified in what is essentially a dynamic physiology of regulatory functions—and hence the dysregulation we encounter in disease. That, of course, means not only understanding the operations of the varied organ and molecular systems but how they function so as to be coordinated for optimal function in a variable environment. We might then apprehend the intrinsic limitations and 'costs' for any particular 'solution'.

Given this kind of inquiry and willingness to see 'the way things are,' we can grasp what Sir Martin patiently teaches in his view of the comprehensiveness of clinical science. We can understand why it is necessary to have cognisance *both* of regularities and their *inevitable* variations which descriptive psychiatry must record. This focus requires a lively sense of openness but also sustained effort with what concretely is in hand and provides the stabilising 'Rothian' gyroscope we need.

## A postscript

That quality of openness and search is something specially to celebrate for this occasion. I should also add, as a personal note, that I have only *once* known Martin Roth to be all wet! At an early hour that most would eschew (at the 1987 Puerto Rico meeting of the American College of Neuropsychopharmacology) I was obliged to prepare for an early session and was sleepily scanning the deserted beaches. I was startled to see a vigorous lone figure emerging from the ocean and striding in my direction. He greeted me and, while dripping, cheerfully picked up a particular serious conversation we had started several years previously, then sketched his plans for the future edition of his text and other ventures and, in general, left me in desiccated and exhausted admiration. From that kind of vigour and engagement with search we might learn not only the appropriate attitude for our profession but the fact that its pursuit might just be plainly enjoyable!

# *References*

AKISKAL, H . S. & WEBB, W. L. (eds) (1978) *Psychiatric Diagnosis: Exploration of Biological Predictors.* New York: Spectrum Publications

FREEDMAN, D. X. (1971) One to one, or first things first. *Archives of General Psychiatry*, **24**, 97.

—— (ed.) (1975) *The Biology of the Major Psychoses: A Comparative Analysis.* New York: Raven Press.

—— (1978a) Community mental health: Slogan and a history of the mission. In *Controversy in Psychiatry* (eds J. P. Brady & H. K. H. Brodie) Philadelphia: W. B. Saunders.

—— (1978b) From mind to brain: New emphases on psychiatric education. *Yale Journal of Biology and Medicine*, **51**, 117–131.

—— (1982) Presidential address: Science in the service of the ill. *American Journal of Psychiatry*, **139**, 1087–1095.

—— (1987) Strategies for research in biological psychiatry. In *Psychopharmacology, the Third Generation of Progress: The Emergence of Molecular Biology and Biological Psychiatry* (ed. H. Y. Meltzer). New York: Raven Press.

KUBIE, L. S. (1971) The retreat from patients. *Archives of General Psychiatry*, **24**, 98–106.

REDLICH, F. C. & FREEDMAN, D. X. (1966) *The Theory and Practice of Psychiatry.* New York: Basic Books.

REICH, J., BLACK, D. W. & JARJOUA, D. (1987) Architecture of research in psychiatry, 1953 to 1983. *Archives of General Psychiatry*, **44**, 311–313.

# 3 Which therapy is best?
# The role of research design
## GAVIN ANDREWS

The purpose of medicine is to treat disease, which in clinical practice means "cure seldom, relieve often, and comfort always". It is not always straightforward to decide which treatment is most likely to cure or relieve and some treatments, popular with one generation, have not always survived to the next. Treatments which will later be shown to be ineffectual are sometimes accepted because of the charisma associated with the originator, or because the treatment is consistent with current thinking about the disease. It is often presumed that the randomised controlled trial, which implicitly discounts the effect of spontaneous remission, regression to the mean, and placebo response, would allow the true benefits of a treatment to emerge. Sackett, Haynes & Tugwell (1985) recommend relying on randomised controlled trials of practical treatments used on typical patients. If the outcome measures were appropriate, the drop-outs all accounted for, and the result of the trial was clinically and statistically significant, then they consider that one would be on safe ground in accepting the results. While few would quarrel with this formal methodological position, the more important question is whether one can safely accept lesser degrees of evidence and still have a reasonable certainty of not adopting valueless treatments. My early work in Newcastle touched on these issues.

In 1962, in Newcastle-upon-Tyne, I was the recipient of the Metcalf Bequest for research into the aetiology of stuttering (Andrews & Harris, 1964). Early in the life of the project, Professor Roth said that he had heard of a stutterer who had become fluent after two weeks treatment in the Channel Islands. He suggested that we try to emulate that treatment programme. He cautioned that we should make certain that any improvement was due to a specific effect of the treatment and was not evidence of a non-specific placebo response. H. V Hemery, a former Scottish school-teacher, was treating stutterers by teaching them to speak slowly in an even rhythm. After allowing their speech to speed up, he encouraged them to practise their new fluent speech in the local township. The use of rhythmic speech as a fluency-inducing agent was well-known; his contribution was to use a two week, 100 hour, intensive period of treatment. Sydney Brandon, Mary Harris and I then put into practice what we believed to be the Hemery method and discovered that chronic stutterers could indeed stop stuttering.

Was this a genuine treatment effect? In this paper I willl illustrate how a specific treatment effect has been demonstrated in the special case of stuttering without the need for a randomised controlled trial. I will then summarise our experience in reviewing the treatment outcome literature in depression, schizophrenia, and the anxiety disorders for the Australian Quality Assurance Project. It might be helpful if the effects of differences in trial design were made explicit. A placebo controlled trial discounts for placebo response, spontaneous remission and regression to the mean. A comparison trial between two active treatments allows the superiority of one to be established but requires information from a placebo-controlled trial of one of the agents to know how effective the treatment is. A wait-list controlled trial and a base line pre-post controlled trial both discount for remission and regression but not for placebo response. A pre-post trial does not count for any of these factors.

In analysing these sets of data we made use of the meta-analytic technique introduced by Glass (1976). Meta-analysis involves the calculation of a standard measure of improvement called an effect size. In randomised controlled trials it is the difference between the outcomes of the treatment and control groups divided by the standard deviation of the control group on that measure. In comparison trials one follows the same procedure for the new and old treatments, adding the effect size superiority of the new treatment to that already established for the old treatment on the basis of independent placebo controlled trials of the old treatment. In baseline pre-post trials the effect size is calculated from the differences in outcome scores measured before and after therapy divided by the pre-treatment standard deviation and reduced by the effect size due to placebo treatment when that has been established from independent studies. Pre-post studies are handled in the same way, but also need to be corrected for the effects of regression to the mean and spontaneous remission established from independent studies. Clearly, randomised placebo controlled trials are the simplest to process but they are not always available or practical. The meta-analytic technique allows data from different designs to be compared, and the influence of patient differences, different types of measurements, and timing of assessments to be taken into account. The standard measure of improvement is called an effect size (ES). An effect size of 1.0 indicates that after treatment the average patient would have less symptoms than 84% of the untreated control group, a statement that makes some sense clinically.

## *The evaluation of the treatment of stuttering*

Before discussing the results of the treatment of stuttering a brief comment about the nature of the disorder might be in order. Readers who are more interested might care to look at a fuller review (Andrews *et al*, 1983). Idiopathic stuttering afflicts 5% of children, but because of early remission and late onset the incidence never rises above 1%. Thus 80% of afflicted children remit, usually within a year of beginning to stutter. The modal age of onset is five and very few cases begin after puberty. Remission is rare in stutterers whose affliction persists into adulthood. Twin and family studies have repeatedly shown that genetic factors are important and may be a sufficient cause. Studies of the affected twin in monozygotic twins discordant for stuttering, and studies of neurologically damaged children, show that acquired lesions can also be a sufficient cause. In adults, stuttering can follow brain insult, is occasionally seen as a form of malingering, and almost never as a neurotic or hysterical symptom. In fact, stuttering does not co-occur with other emotional symptoms seen in childhood, and stutterers and their mothers are just as, and no more likely to be, emotionally disturbed than normal-speaking children and their mothers. It is not a psychiatric condition. It is a disorder of speech motor control, stutterers being handicapped in the sensory-motor modelling essential for ongoing speech production. Stutterers are frequently late and poor talkers during the time when children are developing speech, have impaired auditory-speech reaction times and become fluent in speech situations that simplify the sensory-motor integration required, e.g., singing, whispering, or speaking very slowly.

We have gradually developed the treatment programme begun in Newcastle and for the last 15 years have been treating 50 new adult stutterers per year. The structure has changed little, and at 12 hours per day for 15 days it remains an intensive and demanding programme even for well-motivated adult stutterers. The original fluency inducing agent, syllable-timed speech, was replaced in 1970 by the more effective prolonged speech, and this in turn has been replaced with a more normal-sounding variant known as smooth speech. In the transfer phase the stutterers still practise their fluency in the town but the third week of treatment is now aimed at rectifying, on an individual basis, any of the three major treatment goals not yet achieved. These goals are reliable fluent stutter-free speech, normalisation of speech attitudes, and internalisation of locus of control. The programme is very effective: most stutterers become stutter-free and, given some modicum of continued care over their speech, are able to function as normal speakers in the long term. Some patients relapse but do better after being retreated. In a recent study, the mean effect size from before treatment to follow-up ten months later was 3.0 ES units, indicating that the average stutterer after treatment was better than 99% of untreated stutterers. The frequency of stuttering, in percentage of syllables stuttered, dropped from 14% to 1%, the S24, a measure of attitudes to speaking, dropped from 19 to the population mean of 9, and 80% of subjects internalised their locus of control (Andrews & Feyer, 1985; Andrews & Craig, 1988). A year later both subjects and employers reported significant improvement in speech related work efficiency and in income.

Now what is the evidence that this is a genuine treatment effect? In a meta-analysis of all reports of stuttering treatment (Andrews *et al*, 1980), we showed that pre-post designs were acceptable because there were data to allow estimation of the effect of a very plausible placebo treatment, and data to show the magnitude of regression to the mean and spontaneous remission in adult stutterers. The cumulative influence of these three factors was estimated at 0.2 ES units whereas the mean improvement of all the studies analysed was more than 1.0 ES unit above this. The fluency training techniques used by ourselves and others (prolonged speech, precision fluency shaping) were found to be significantly better than all other techniques analysed. There are now published data on the use of these techniques with some 600 subjects of both sexes, ranged in age from 10 to 80 years. As these reports come from many centres, and similar results are achieved by therapists who have never met each other, the techniques are reliably effective.

That they are effective can be concluded from the base-line pre-post trials despite the absence of randomised placebo controlled trials. But randomised placebo controlled trials are probably unethical once long-term post-treatment efficacy of a non-drug treatment has been demonstrated. Like wait-list controlled trials, they are probably impractical and unlikely to attract volunteers in any society in which treatment is freely available. Furthermore, they are probably less informative than baseline pre-post trials which use each subject as his own control, a better solution than randomisation. Baseline pre-post trials are particularly satisfactory if placebo response, regression to the mean or likelihood of spontaneous remission have been shown to be minimal, as is the case in stuttering.

Were the measures used reliable and valid? There are published criteria for diagnosing and measuring stuttering. Raters in our unit commonly achieve inter-rater reliabilities of 0.98 using these criteria. But do stutterers speak especially well when they know they are being assessed? This, of course, is a concern in all psychiatry; how can we know that what people do or say in the clinic is representative of their everyday performance? In a series of covert assessments of treated stutterers we have shown that one year after treatment there is no difference between speech in the clinic, speech at home, talking to clinic staff on the telephone, or speech when talking to an opinion poll interviewer who appeared to have no connection with the clinic (Andrews & Craig, 1982). The improvement extends to all aspects of the disorder; there is increased fluency, lessened avoidance of situations and normalised attitudes to speaking. Even the extent to which the new speech sounds normal has been demonstrated.

Thus, on many levels, despite the absence of a randomised controlled trial, there are data to satisfy the claim that the fluency training techniques offer very good hope for stutterers over 10 years of age. But there are two more lines of information to support the specificity of the response to treatment. First, a dose response curve between hours of treatment and outcome has been demonstrated with this technique. Second, we now have evidence from 24 subjects that the prolonged speech technique reduced the abnormality in auditory speech reaction time (Feyer, 1987), putative evidence that this treatment was affecting one manifestation of the aetiological sensory-motor integration deficit. When a treatment is shown to remedy the underlying aetiological defect and a dose response curve is demonstrated then a specific treatment effect exists.

## The evaluation of psychiatric treatment

In 1981 we began a project, supported by the Australian Department of Health and under the aegis of the Royal Australian and New Zealand College of Psychiatrists, to describe treatment outlines for the commoner psychiatric disorders. A principal part of this exercise was to prepare empirical reviews of the literature, using established data bases to search for articles on the outcome of treatment that could be handled by the meta analytic technique. One limitation of this technique is that only studies reporting data from which an effect size can be calculated can be analysed. The virtue is that others repeating the meta-analysis should get precisely the same results, in part because reviewer bias does not intrude into the selection of articles or evaluation of results.

As a preliminary we reanalysed the data of Smith, Glass & Miller on the benefits of psychotherapy (Andrews & Harvey, 1981). Selecting only studies of patients who had been referred or sought treatment for a neurotic condition, we were able to show that there were significant differences in benefit between patients receiving behaviour therapy and patients receiving psychotherapy, and that both treatments seemed more effective than counselling or placebo treatment. The claim that dynamic psychotherapy was more effective than placebo has been disputed because of the paucity of data from randomised placebo controlled trials. Subsequently we conducted a randomised placebo controlled trial of dynamic psychotherapy in general practice attenders and failed to demonstrate that psychotherapy was of more benefit than placebo (Brodaty & Andrews, 1983). The effectiveness of dynamic psychotherapy in patients with anxiety and depression has still not been conclusively demonstrated.

While averaging effect sizes from different studies enabled us to establish a putative case for the psychotherapies, and in particular the behavioural psychotherapies, the review illustrated that while the placebo controlled trial is common in the drug therapies, it is rare in the non-drug therapy field. On reflection, different questions are being asked of drug and non-drug treatments. Drug trials are commonly carried out over a six week period, long enough to demonstrate the pharmacological effect of the drug, but there is almost never any follow-up after the drug is withdrawn to determine whether the patients remain improved. In this context the use of a placebo group is both practical and ethical. Studies of behavioural or dynamic psychotherapy are different. An adequate dose of non-drug treatment is usually spread over many weeks, and follow-up after treatment has ended is expected. Placebo control subjects are difficult to arrange for two reasons: a plausible placebo treatment is difficult to design and it is difficult to persuade patients, provided there are no economic barriers to treatment elsewhere, to comply either with the placebo or remain without treatment over the months of treatment and follow-up required by the study design. Furthermore, it is unlikely that ethics committees would today approve patients being deprived of treatment for such a lengthy period. Hence baseline pre-post designs in which each patient serves as his/her own control may be the best that can be expected in the non-drug therapies, with evidence about placebo response being taken from other published studies.

I turn now to the treatment of specific conditions. In the meta-analysis of the treatment of depressive illness 200 placebo and comparison controlled trials were analysed. The results are displayed in Fig. 1 and are consistent with established knowledge, i.e. ECT and the tricyclic antidepressants are the treatments of choice in endogenous depression, the psychotherapies and the tricyclic antidepressants are most effective for neurotic depression (Quality Assurance Project, 1983). The most disturbing finding was that the median duration of all the drug trials was only four weeks and, while some justification for this might be found in the needs of placebo-treated patients for active treatment for depression, comparison trials of two antidepressant drugs were equally brief. We concluded that a pharmacological rather than a clinical answer may have been of most interest to the researcher or to his source of funding. This finding is particularly disturbing because there is now good evidence that the prognosis for patients admitted to hospital with either endogenous or neurotic depression is surprisingly poor. Only a fifth recover and have no further difficulty, one fifth commit suicide or remain constantly unwell, while the remainder continue to have episodes of depression (Kiloh *et al*, 1988). A four week trial of drug treatment is just not informative about how to manage what will be, for most people, a life-long condition.

While there was research evidence on the benefits of cognitive therapy, that for dynamic psychotherapy in neurotic depression was weak, which is surprising as this condition is a significant indication for long-term intensive psychotherapy (Andrews & Hadzi-Pavlovic, 1988).

The project on the treatment of schizophrenia analysed 216 controlled trials. The results are also presented in Fig. 1 and described in the legend (Quality Assurance Project, 1984). The summary conclusions were that antipsychotic drugs and little else had been shown to inhibit effectively the symptoms of schizophrenia in the short and long term, and that their efficacy could be doubled by the addition of one of the family intervention programmes. We were concerned that, despite the advent of the anti-psychotic drugs, the long-term prognosis for schizophrenia remained poor and that little effort was being made to implement these programmes. It seemed that a costing of the treatment of schizophrenia might provide evidence to support the implementation of the family intervention programmes. The results of our incidence-based costing (Andrews *et al*, 1985) showed that schizophrenia in Australia cost half as much as myocardial infarction, even though it was only one twelfth as common, and that the implementation of family intervention programmes would be very cost effective.

The data on the treatment of anxiety disorders were analysed in three sections: anxiety neurosis, obsessive compulsive disorder and agoraphobia. Different experimental designs predominated in each disorder; randomised controlled designs in the anxiety neuroses, randomised and pre-post designs in OCD, and pre-post designs in agoraphobia. In terms of clinical and statistical significance, the data on agoraphobia are superior to those available for the other disorders, again indicating that the presence of randomised controlled trials do not, by themselves, make a literature informative. We located 81 controlled trials of patients with anxiety neurosis (Quality Assurance Project, 1985), placebo controlled trials for drug treatments and wait-list controlled trials in the case of the behaviour therapies. The benzodiazepines produced a 0.72 standard deviation superiority over placebo, but because of the response of the placebo group, the overall clinical improvement to be expected from a benzodiazepine was quite considerable, 1.43 ES units. The full results are displayed in Fig. 1. The interesting finding was that despite the demonstrated efficacy of the benzodiazepines in reducing anxiety, there was virtually no support for their usage as a critical treatment for anxiety neurosis from either a sample of practising psychiatrists or from psychiatrists nominated as expert in the treatment of anxiety (Andrews *et al*, 1987). This response illustrates that treatments which have shown a statistically significant superiority over placebo are not necessarily of use clinically.

A meta-analysis was also used to integrate the research literature on the treatment of obsessive compulsive disorder (Christensen *et al*, 1987). Three types of trial were analysed: randomised placebo and comparison controlled trials, pre-post trials with interval data, and pre-post trials which reported only ordinal data that had to be transformed by probit. The results from all three sources of data converged and were consistent with antidepressants such as clomipramine and the response prevention behaviour therapies producing a one standard deviation improvement in symptoms over and above that expected from placebo treatment. A consistent finding in this study was that psychiatrists' ratings of improvement generated larger effect sizes than patient self-report measures.

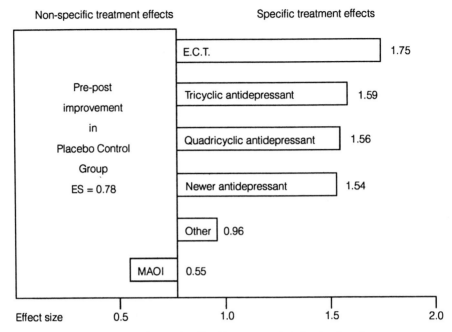

Endogenous depression: Total improvement during treatment

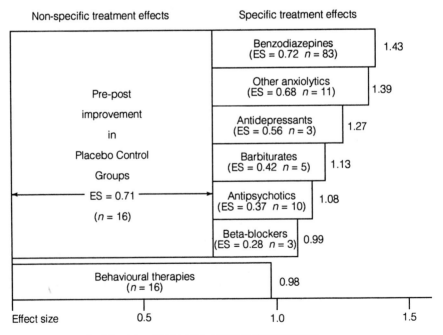

Anxiety states: Total improvement during treatment

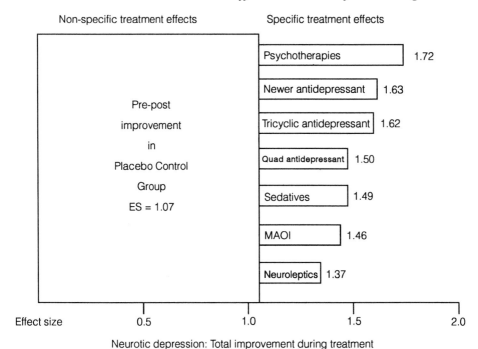

Neurotic depression: Total improvement during treatment

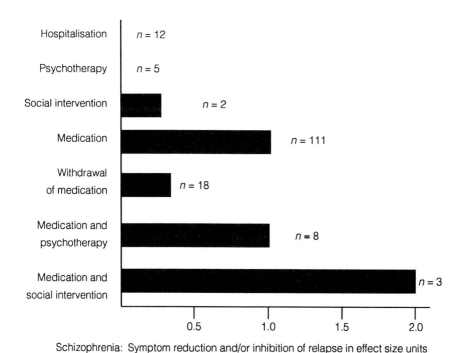

Schizophrenia: Symptom reduction and/or inhibition of relapse in effect size units

This appeared to be a genuine bias and not a scaling artefact. A similar bias was noted in the anxiety neurosis meta-analysis. This raises the issue that psychiatrists habitually over-value their patients' improvement, although it could, of course, be evidence that patients, as they improve, keep raising their expectations as to what constitutes being completely well.

In our most recent enquiry, a meta-analysis of some 80 trials of the treatment of agoraphobia with panic attacks (Andrews & Moran, 1988), we found little support for the view that either imipramine or alprazolam are critical or unique treatments for panic. They produced moderate improvements in panic and smaller changes in phobic behaviour. The best effects on phobia in the short and long term came from treatments that included exposure to feared situations. These behavioural treatments produced a reduction in panic similar to that found with the drugs. The most effective therapies were those which combined either imipramine *or* placebo tablets with a behaviour therapy, a finding that raises the interesting possibility that when patients are learning to control panics, the presumption that a drug is also helping is important to them, even when no active drug is being used.

## Conclusions

Writing this account of treatment evaluation for this tribute has caused me to grapple with some issues that were not previously clear to me. A well-done randomised controlled trial in which the results are unambiguous, and clinically and statistically significant, is clearly better than any other strategy for evaluating a treatment. When trials last only weeks and yet the disorder lasts years, as was the case for the drug trials of depression, then neither randomisation nor any other methodological sophistication will produce data bearing on the long-term care of the patients. The anxiety neurosis literature highlights another way that randomised controlled trials can become irrelevant. There are a large number of controlled trials showing the benefits when benzodiazepine drugs are used with anxious patients. Additional trials will make no difference for, at least in Australia, psychiatrists have decided that benzodiazepine drugs are not

---

Fig. 1. (*previous pages*) *The results of treatment for the endogenous and neurotic depressions, schizophrenia and anxiety. Estimates of the improvement in symptoms that occur during treatment are presented in effect size or standard deviation units. Controlled trials estimate the benefits of the specific treatment being investigated, but patient improvement will often be greater than this because of the non-specific or placebo effect of being in treatment.*

*The upper diagrams refer to depression. In endogenous depression the placebo control groups averaged a 0.78 effect size unit improvement, while the groups treated with ECT averaged an additional 0.97 ES units. Thus the observed clinical improvement would have been 1.75 ES units. In the pooled results for neurotic depression the placebo response was larger (ES = 1.07), and the response to specific treatments smaller.*

*In the lower left figure similar conventions are used to show the anxiolytic power of different drugs in patients with anxiety neurosis. There were no placebo controlled trials of behavioural therapy and the averaged result from the six wait-list controlled trials are shown at the bottom and represents the sum of the specific and non-specific effects (ES = 0.98).*

*The lower right figure concerns schizophrenia. Hospitalisation alone did not produce a change in symptoms, neither did psychotherapy. Anti-psychotic medication produced a one standard deviation improvement (ES = 1.0) and the addition of a social or family intervention package doubled the effectiveness of the drug therapy, the addition of psychotherapy did not (from The Quality Assurance Project 1983, 1984, 1985. Reproduced by kind permission of the* Australian and New Zealand Journal of Psychiatry)

the treatments of choice for the patients they see suffering from anxiety neurosis, presumably because these drugs do not alter the underlying psychopathology and do cause dependence.

In stuttering and agoraphobia, both chronic conditions, there are pre-post trials that are supported by information about regression to the mean and placebo response. Furthermore, they have follow-up periods that provide the necessary clinical information on the long-term outcome to be expected from a particular treatment. In neurotic depression and anxiety neurosis the groups treated with placebo improved considerably. As both conditions tend to be acute-on-chronic in course, the brief randomised trial is not particularly informative. Yet is is with these groups that the pre-post designs can fail, for quite apart from the problems posed by regression and remission, it seems that the belief that 'one is being treated' allows patients to mobilise coping strategies they would not otherwise have used. In these situations the non-specific effects of treatment seem very important.

Data on the outcome of treatments evaluated by different research designs have been presented. Given supporting data appropriate to each of these designs, the information generated by any of them can be sufficient so that one might reasonably accept that the benefits associated with a treatment are due to a specific effect. It would appear that the methodological formalism typified by the single-minded advocacy of the randomised controlled trial ignores that there may be a number of ways of providing data to answer Professor Roth's request to "make certain the improvement is due to a specific effect of the treatment".

# *References*

ANDREWS, G. & CRAIG, A. (1982) Stuttering: Overt and covert measurement of the speech of treated stutterers. *Journal of Speech and Hearing Disorders*, **47**, 96–99.
—— & —— (1988) Prediction of outcome after treatment for stuttering. *British Journal of Psychiatry*, **153**, 236–240.
——, ——, FEYER, A-M., HODDINOTT, S., HOWIE, P. M. & NEILSON, M. (1983) Stuttering: a review of research findings and theories circa 1982. *Journal of Speech and Hearing Disorders*, **48**, 226–246.
—— & FEYER, A-M. (1985) Does behavior therapy still work when the experimenters depart: an analysis of a behavioral treatment program for stuttering. *Behavior Modification*, **9**, 443–457.
——, GUITAR, B. & HOWIE, P. (1980) Meta-analysis of the effects of stuttering treatment. *Journal of Speech and Hearing Disorders*, **45**, 287–307.
—— & HADZI-PAVLOVIC, D. (1988) The work of Australian psychiatrists, circa 1986. *Australian and New Zealand Journal of Psychiatry*, **22**, 153–165.
——, ——, CHRISTENSEN, H. & MATTICK, R. P. (1987) Views of practising psychiatrists on the treatment of anxiety and somatoform disorders. *American Journal of Psychiatry*, **144**, 1331–1334.
——, HALL, W., GOLDSTEIN, G., LAPSLEY, H., BARTELS, R. & SILOVE, D. (1985) The economic costs of schizophrenia: Implications for public policy. *Archives of General Psychiatry*, **42**, 537–543.
—— & HARRIS, M. (1964) The Syndrome of Stuttering. *Clinics in Developmental Medicine*, No. 17. London: Heinemann.
—— & HARVEY, R. (1981) Does psychotherapy benefit neurotic patients? A reanalysis of the Smith, Glass and Miller data. *Archives of General Psychiatry*, **38**, 1203–1208.
ANDREWS, G. & MORAN, C. (1988) Exposure treatment of agoraphobia with panic attacks: Are drugs essential? In *Panic and Phobias 2* (eds. I. Hand and H.-U. Wittchen). Heidelberg: Springer-Verlag.
BRODATY, H. & ANDREWS, G. (1983) Brief psychotherapy in family practice: A controlled prospective intervention trial. *British Journal of Psychiatry*, **143**, 11–19.

CHRISTENSEN, H., HADZI-PAVLOVIC, D., ANDREWS, G. & MATTICK, R. P. (1987) Behaviour therapy and tricyclic medication in the treatment of obsessive compulsive disorder: a quantitative review. *Journal of Consulting and Clinical Psychology*, **55**, 701–711.

FEYER, A-M. (1987) *An Information Processing Analysis of Skill Acquisition in a Treatment Program for Stuttering*. PhD. Thesis, School of Psychiatry, University of New South Wales. Sydney. Australia.

GLASS, G. V. (1976) Primary, secondary and meta-analysis of research. *Primary Researcher*, **10**, 3–8.

KILOH, L. G., ANDREWS, G. & NEILSON, M. D. (1988) The long-term outcome of depression. *British Journal of Psychiatry*, **153**, 752–757.

THE QUALITY ASSURANCE PROJECT (1983) A treatment outline for depressive disorders. *Australian and New Zealand Journal of Psychiatry*, **17**, 129–148.

—— (1984) Treatment outlines for the management of schizophrenia. *Australian and New Zealand Journal of Psychiatry*, **18**, 19–38.

—— (1985) Treatment outlines for the management of anxiety states. *Australian and New Zealand Journal of Psychiatry*, **19**, 138–151.

SACKETT, D. L., HAYNES, R. B. & TUGWELL, P. (1985) *Clinical Epidemiology: A Basic Science for Clinical Medicine*. Boston/Toronto: Little, Brown.

# 4 The uses of psychiatric historiography: the 19th and 20th centuries

## GERMAN E. BERRIOS

Understanding and creativity in psychiatry are enhanced by knowledge of her history. This polymathic approach, uncommon in Great Britain, is, however, well illustrated in the work of Professor Sir Martin Roth. It is, therefore, fitting that this tribute should include a chapter on this aspect of his endeavours. This chapter is about psychiatric historiography in the work of some representative 19th century alienists and of their 20th century counterparts. It is also about methods of history writing available to the clinician.

## *The 19th century*

Researchers are struck by the interest in the history of psychiatry shown by 19th century alienists. Two approaches can be distinguished in their work. Firstly, there is what can be called *dedicated* historical writing illustrated by the work of Calmeil, Morel, Trelat, Semelaigne, Kirshoff, Winslow, Ireland, Mercier, Bucknill and Tuke. These authors carried out primary historical research and regularly published the result of their labours. Secondly, there is what can be described as a *second-hand approach* represented by the historical chapters included in clinical textbooks, such as those by Pinel, Haslam, Heinroth, Guislain, Esquirol, Prichard, Calmeil, Feuchsterleben, Conolly, Griesinger, Bucknill and Tuke, Lucas, Falret, Dagonet, and Giné.

This chapter will explore only the second approach. It will ask: what inspired alienists to write such historical chapters? More technically, was there a recognised historiographic approach and motivation behind their endeavours?

To begin, we must disprove the view that the inclusion of such chapters was customary amongst contemporary *medical* textbook writers. A survey of ten contemporary medical volumes shows that in only one case was there a historical chapter included. So it would seem that an explanation specific to psychiatry is required. In this respect, it would be plausible to suggest that, in contrast to their medical colleagues, 19th century alienists conceived of their subject as 'historical'; i.e. as resulting from a linear developmental process whose operation brought psychiatric knowledge ever nearer the truth. Let us examine seven illustrative cases.

**The illustrative cases**

The first is provided by Haslam's work (1809). The great London apothecary
had a keen eye for the historical etymology of psychiatric terms. He announced
his task thus: "Mad is therefore not a complex idea, as has been supposed, but
a complex term for all the forms and varieties of this disease. Our language has
been enriched with other terms expressive of this affection . . ." (p. 4).

A second illustration is found in Heinroth's *Lehrbuch* (1818). Inspired by the
18th century German 'historicist' tradition (Engel-Janosi, 1944) this alienist
interpreted his own historical work as an effort to rescue lost insights from an
obscure (and probably mythical) psychiatric past. Heinroth subscribed to a
cyclical conception of history. In the modern world, this view had restarted with
Machiavelli and through Vico and Montesquieu had culminated in Gibbon's
*Decline and Fall.* According to this view, history was composed of the periodic
recurrence of a few great themes. Heinroth believed that "the development of
mental forces in humanity is accompanied by an ever advancing, ever more
degraded degeneration of these forces" (p. 40). Psychiatry, however, was set
on a developmental path and real advance could take place: "a study of the
kind and degree of recognition and treatment of mental disturbances observed
in early antiquity shows that these bear a striking imprint of the childhood of
the human spirit" (p. 41).

Prichard's book of 1835 provides the third example. The Bristol scholar utilised
historical material in a very personal way. Influenced by Faculty Psychology
(Berrios, 1988) (and wanting to break away from Associationism), Prichard
attacked the intellectualistic view of insanity: "It has been supposed that the
chief, if not the sole disorder of persons labouring under insanity consists in some
particular false conviction, or in some erroneous notion indelibly impressed upon
belief . . . from Mr Locke's time it has been customary to observe that the insane
reason correctly from wrong premises . . . that this is, by far, too limited
an account of insanity and only comprises one among various forms of mental
derangement, every person must be aware . . ." (p. 3). As counterexamples,
he included in his book many clinical vignettes. The reader might have noticed
how redolent Prichard's statement is of Pinel's early criticism of John Locke
(Pinel, 1809).

The fourth illustration is provided by Pinel's work. It is common knowledge
that the French alienist used in his *Treatise* an unashamedly presentistic approach.
Influenced by the optimistic historiography of the French revolution, he regarded
the past of psychiatry as little more than a museum of failed endeavours. Men,
ideas, and even books were criticised. Typical of this attitude are his pointed
comments on 18th century English books on alienism: "English monographs
on mental alienation during the second half of the 18th century promise a great
deal in view of the avowed intention by their authors to concentrate on specific
topics; but this promise is rarely fulfilled. Vague and repetitious arguments, old
fashioned clinical approach and lack of sufficient clinical facts and doctrine
contribute to this failure" (p. xix).

Few authors of this period made their historiographic tenets as explicit as did
Feuchtersleben (our fifth example) in his magnificent book of 1845. Quoting
Goethe he stated: "All professional men labour under a great disadvantage in
not being allowed to be ignorant of what is useless . . . every one fancies that

he is bound to transmit what is believed to have been known'' (p. 23); then went on to say that only the "empirical sciences" can dispense with their past as a history of errors. In most cases, as indeed in the case of most of medical psychology, "the history of science is properly the science itself''. For him, however, psychiatry "belonged to both spheres": "that part of it which was philosophical contained an abstract of that state of philosophy in every age, while that which is empirical has by no means attained such precision and clearness as to render a knowledge of previous opinions superfluous . . . ''. On account of this need he concludes: "I am therefore obliged to treat the history of our branch of the profession . . ." (p. 24). This he did in a historical chapter 3000 words long.

The sixth example is to be found in Bucknill & Tuke's *Manual* of 1858. It includes various historical chapters: on lay descriptions of insanity, on the 'opinion of medical writers', on the concept of insanity, on historical aspects of treatment, and on historical classifications. The inclusion of abundant material is likely to have resulted from the keen historical interest of both authors. Bucknill was soon after to publish a pathographic book on the *Mad Folk of Shakespeare* (1867) and Tuke his *History of the Insane in the British Isles* (1882).

It is an intriguing point, however, that Bucknill and Tuke, living in a world of Whiggish historiography, managed to care little for historical continuities. Indeed, they emphasised conceptual breaks and remarked upon the relevance of the social context for classifications and descriptions. For example, they rejected (correctly as it transpired) the view that the pre-19th century medical concept of melancholia had any major association with 19th century views (Berrios, 1988).

The seventh and last illustration is provided by the popular Spanish treatise by Giné y Partagás (1876). This author chose to emphasise the possibility that the concept of insanity might reflect social values: "given that the various branches of human knowledge tend to reflect the moral and political development of the nations, there is no better example of this than the branch of medicine that deals with mental illness" (p. 1). Influenced by Comtean and Darwinian ideas, Giné believed that the fact that the concepts of psychiatry seemed to show an independent historical pedigree legitimised its separation from neurology. This was not the first time that historical reasons had been used to argue for the independence of two branches of knowledge.

The seven popular psychiatric textbooks mentioned above sample successive decades of the 19th century and illustrate both the assiduous use of historical material and the varied historiographic motivation of their authors. Anthological, biographical, pathographic, narrative, and conceptual historiographic approaches can be recognised. In general, the authors adhered to a secular view of history according to which progress was linear and accumulative and conceived of psychiatric knowledge as evolving in a stepwise fashion. Later authors such as Maudsley, Ireland, and Mercier made even more explicit their debt to this form of Comtean positivism.

## *The 20th century*

Has this 19th century stylistic fashion of including historical introductions in clinical textbooks lasted into the 20th century? If so, has its historiographic quality been improved? A review of seven randomly chosen textbooks from various parts of the world helps to answer the first question in the positive. Historical introductions are included, for example, in Kaplan & Sadock (1981), Arieti's *American Handbook of Psychiatry* (1974), Henry Ey *et al*'s *Manuel* (1974), Forrest *et al*'s *Companion* (1978), Shepherd *et al*'s *Handbook* (1983), Sluchevski's *Psychiatry* (1960), and Alonso-Fernandez's *Textbook* (1976).

With respect to the second question the answer seems to be that there has been no improvement. Written by clinicians (with the exception of one) these chapters are narrative in style and never contain (as the chapters on clinical issues accompanying them do) adequate reviews of recent *research*.

Neglectful of recent work on the history of psychiatry, their authors can but limit themselves to iterate the conventional. They haltingly rehearse the mythical continuity started in Hippocrates and leading to Areteus, Galen, Platter, Linne, Cullen, Chiarurgi, Pinel, Griesinger, Kraepelin, Freud, Jung and Schneider. Hence, their chapters are repetitious and perpetuate historical errors once upon a time started by Zilboorg, Whitwell and Alexander and Selesnick (their main data sources). Historical information is never organised in terms of hypotheses nor is any conceptual framework provided. Predictably, the same illustrations by Dührer, Hogarth, Arnolds, Floury, Tardieu, and Brouillet are included.

With the exception of Bynum's historical survey (in Shepherd's *Handbook*) the rest have no recognisable historiographic position. So one can conclude that these chapters:

(a)  have not advanced historical knowledge
(b)  have a lesser academic standing than their companion clinical chapters
(c)  have become statutory writings.

## On history writing

### Strategies

The new examination of the Royal College of Psychiatrists is to include (after some prompting) questions on the history of psychiatry. When answering these questions, will the young clinician be helped by the above mentioned textbook chapters? The answer is that he will not. Hence more research and better publications in this area are badly needed. The trainee must gain the impression that the history of psychiatry is also an area of active research rather than a dead chronology.

Research into the history of psychiatry can be justified on a number of grounds but only one will be mentioned here. Psychiatry remains a descriptive discipline, that is, the capture of clinical data is dependent upon the recognition and naming of behavioural forms. The quality of fit between descriptions and behavioural phenomena depends, therefore, upon the quality of the descriptive system and the stability of the phenomena themselves. While the former is a function of semantic organisation (and the rate of change of the psychosocial matrix) the latter is guaranteed by neurobiological mechanisms (Berrios, 1984).

If 'quality of description and fit' are aims to strive for, then strategies to calibrate the language of psychiatry must be developed. At least three spring to mind: clinical, mathematical and historical (Berrios, 1984). Because psychiatry is not a contemplative but a modificatory activity, the clinician is primarily interested in the predictive power of the available descriptions. This predictive power stems from persistent clinical observation unencumbered by semantic confusion. Knowledge of the semantic provenance of all terms is essential. History must study meanings and their interaction with concepts. It must also estimate how much of these meanings can symptom-descriptions retain after they have been transferred from one historical episteme to another. For example, can one assume that the term 'hallucination' means in 1988 the same as it did in 1817 when it was operationalised? If one cannot, what are the crucial differences?

The term 'historical episteme' has been mentioned and deserves to be commented upon. It is used to name (more or less) autonomous ideological domains, contained within recognisable temporal boundaries. These ideological systems feed, so to speak, meaning into all the events and ideas they contain. 'Renaissance' and 'Enlightenment' can be considered as epistemes; from the psychiatric point of view, the period 1820 to the present can be regarded as another.

A common fate befalling the clinical historian is to become locked into a given historical episteme. Once trapped he soon will lose sight of the long-term (trans-epistemic) trends that also characterise the history of medicine. When in this predicament the inexperienced historian is led to adopt a form of relativism which makes him call into question all notions of psychiatric progress.

To escape this danger the clinician must endeavour to seek trans-epistemic invariants. Such can be found in the linguistic, psychological, anatomical, or physiological domains. Clinical historians, understandably, prefer the latter. For example a trans-epistemic history of delirium or dementia is only made possible by assuming the existence of neurobiological invariants (Berrios, 1987). Another solution to the danger of relativism is to concentrate on the history of the present episteme, i.e. of the current psychiatric 'discourse'. As it has been stated elsewhere (Berrios, 1984) the same system of beliefs and concepts has governed psychiatry since the middle of the 19th century.

The psychiatrist may also search for a theoretical solution. An appealing model is provided by Braudel (1980) who depicts history as a harmonic conglomerate of processes of short, medium and long duration. Explanations for the direction and content of psychiatric history can then be sought from these various levels. Some events, like the accident that befell Wernicke (which changed the direction of taxonomy and pathogenesis), make sense as short processes; others, like the impact of Faculty Psychology on psychiatric classification and aetiological theory, are better understood as medium duration processes; yet others, like the changes in the understanding of madness, are better defined as long duration, trans-epistemic processes. The clinician finds in this view escape from the mortal embrace of the episteme.

One of the general objectives of historical research is to break the epistemological code. In this respect, psychiatry seeks to uncover the unsaid rules of the psychiatric discourse or formulate the changing assumptions that have inspired alienists throughout the ages (e.g. concepts of disease and views on the nature of man). By encouraging the clinician-historian to unveil the assumptions underlying the current (and apparently ultimate) psychiatric discourse, history makes sure that psychiatrists lose their conceptual innocence.

There is little doubt that among the various types of psychiatric history, the conceptual history of psychopathology must be considered as its core. If none is available (as has been the case until recently) the psychiatrist must endeavour to write his own. How is he to tackle it? The first thing to remember is that methodological standards in historical research must be as strict as those in neurochemistry. The difficult problem is that these standards must be achieved in a research area that demands tools and canons of proof unfamiliar to the clinician, that contains untamed data and is governed by non-biological forms of thinking. It is no coincidence that good history of psychiatry can only be written by clinicians who have had historical, philosophical or anthropological training.

## Sources and material

In practical terms, historiographic strategies and the definition of what constitutes legitimate historical data are related. For example, the 19th century confronts the clinician with an embarrassment of riches. Lest the clinician-historian ends up writing only superficial chronicles, anthologies or biographies, he must seriously worry about his choice of historiography and about his criteria for data selection. The problem is different from what he is used to in clinical research. In the latter the investigator is comfortably eased into his work by producing an 'integrated review of the relevant'. He rarely (if ever) will question the paradigms and assumptions controlling choice of methods and instruments in his field. Furthermore, he accepts without complaint all dicta from the scientific community he aspires to join (these, in practical terms, come to him via learned journals, funding bodies reports, and the views of his academic boss).

These restrictions, however, are less in some areas of psychiatric historical research. For example, there is yet no clear consensus as to what methodological and presentation formats should be used to make the history of descriptive psychopathology patently clear to the clinician. The clinician-historian yearning for intellectual freedom ought to welcome this refreshing openness. Other forms of history of psychiatry (particularly those dealing with psychiatry as a pure 'social phenomenon') are, however, restrictive. Sociology has also its own mandarins and controlling paradigms. Thus, an anti-scientific attitude accompanied by the mechanical application of devices such as the theory of social control or a self-defeating relativism, mar any results. It is not surprising, therefore, that there is little in the way of fine grain *clinical analysis* in the work of social historians of psychiatry such as Scull, Blassius, Foucault, Dörner or Castel. On inspection,their magnificent historical constructions are strikingly lacking in clinical furniture. What is worse, their theories offer little help to clinicians who want to understand, for example, how and why a shift occurred in the meaning of, say, dementia between 1880 and 1890. To say that dementia is but a social control device, implemented in France in the wake of the Franco Prussian War to get the elderly out of circulation, is instructive but will hardly exhaust the field of explanations.

A useful technique is to 'to-and-fro' between conceptual analysis and reassessment of the historical (clinical) material. This task must be undertaken (as Braudel recommended) against the ideological matrix of a chosen period and always riding on one's clinical skills. For example, it is still possible (both in

Great Britain and in other European countries) to do good research into the evolution of psychiatric descriptions by studying old asylum log-books.

But case-notes are only part of the material available. Books, newspapers, official documents, learned periodicals, personal and institutional archives, epistolary collections and literary remains are also rich sources of information. Clinical colleagues coming across runs of old case-notes often ask what sort of research they can undertake. The answer is that it depends upon the continuity and quality of the material. Document runs may have been broken up by acts of God or wanton destruction by administrators; others may be continuous but of bad quality (for example when not sufficient post-mortem material is included). Continuous and well stratified archives offer invaluable help to study, for example, the evolution of individual symptoms.

Official reports include numeric and diagnostic information on patient movement and can be used to search for trends. A number of mathematical techniques, such as Time Series Analysis, have been adapted to this end; they can help to tease out historical 'harmonics' i.e. combinations of temporal regularities covering different historical periods.

Because of the particular characteristics of the asylum population, the old alienists had the opportunity to observe unspoilt cohorts. Longitudinal analysis is known to magnify the gain of whatever clinical signals may be present in these cohorts. Hence they must be sought for, with the result that disease patterns otherwise invisible to the cross-sectional analysis may appear. Although these configurations may on occasions be artefacts resulting from the operation of social variables, this is not invariable. For example the concept of 'Presbyophrenia' (Berrios, 1986) described as a subtype of dementia by late 19th century alienists (and fallen into desuetude as a result of conceptual, not empirical changes affecting the notion of dementia) has been shown to contain clinical information.

## Conclusion

This chapter, written to celebrate Professor Martin Roth's contribution to psychiatry, has dealt with the uses of historical information by 19th century clinicians and examined seven case-histories. It has also analysed usage by 20th century textbook writers and addressed the practical issues of history writing from the point of view of the clinician. It has shown that the inclusion of historical chapters in 19th century textbooks was due to explicit historiographic needs and suggested that these have been lost in 20th century textbooks. As a consequence historical chapters in these works are stereotyped affairs lacking in objectives and freshness. Of all forms of psychiatric history writing, the history of psychopathology is of greatest interest and usefulness to the clinician and must be tackled with a certain urgency. History writing, however, is not easy and the clinician must be aware of a number of pitfalls. Some of these have also been discussed in this chapter.

## References

ALONSO-FERNÁNDEZ, F. A. (1976) *Fundamentos de la Psiquiatría Actual. Tomo I. Psiquiatría General.* Madrid: Editorial Paz Montalvo.

ARIETI, S. (ed.) (1974) *American Handbook of Psychiatry Vol. 1.* New York: Basic Books.

BERRIOS, G. E. (1984) Descriptive psychopathology: Conceptual and historical aspects. *Psychological Medicine.* **14**, 303–313.

—— (1986) Presbyophrenia: The rise and fall of a concept. *Psychological Medicine*, **16**, 267–275.

—— (1987) Dementia during the seventeenth and eighteenth centuries. A conceptual history. *Psychological Medicine*, **17**, 829–837.

—— (1988) The historical development of abnormal psychology. In *Textbook of Abnormal Psychology* (eds E. Miller and P. J. Cooper). London: Churchill Livingstone, pp. 26–51.

BRAUDEL, F. (1980) *La Historia y las Ciencias.* Madrid: Alianza Editorial.

BUCKNILL, J. C. & TUKE, D. H. (1858) *A Manual of Psychological Medicine.* London: Churchill.

—— (1867) *The Mad Folk of Shakespeare.* London: Macmillan.

ENGEL-JANOSI, F. (1944) *The Growth of German Historicism.* Johns Hopkins University. Studies in History and Political Science, Series 62, No. 2.

EY, H., BERNARD, P. & BRISSET, CH. (1974) *Manuel de Psychiatrie.* Paris: Masson.

FEUCHTERSLEBEN, E, VON (1845) *The Principles of Medical Psychology* (translated by H. E. Lloyd and B. G. Babington) London: Sydenham Society.

FORREST, A. D., AFFLECK, J. W. & ZEALLEY, A. K. (eds) (1978) *Companion to Psychiatric Studies.* Edinburgh: Churchill Livingstone.

GINÉ Y PARTAGÁS, D. (1876) *Tratado Teórico-Práctico de Freno-Patología.* Madrid: Moya y Plaza.

HASLAM, J. (1809) *Observations on Madness.* London: J. Callow.

HEINROTH, J. C. (1818) *Lehrbuch der Störungen des Seelenlebens* (translated by J. Schmorak in 1975), 2 vols. Baltimore: Johns Hopkins Press.

KAPLAN, H. I. & SADOCK, B. J. (1981) *Modern Synopsis of Comprehensive Textbook of Psychiatry/III.* Baltimore: Williams & Wilkins.

PINEL, PH. (1809) *Traité Médico-Philosophique sur l'Alienation Mentale* (second edition) Paris: Brosson.

PRICHARD, J. C. (1835) *A Treatise on Insanity and other Disorders Affecting the Mind.* London: Sherwood, Gilbert and Piper.

TUKE, D. H. (1882) *Chapters in the History of the Insane in the British Isles.* London: Kegan Paul, Trench.

SHEPHERD, M. & ZANGWILL, O. L. (eds) (1983) *Handbook of Psychiatry: Volume 1. General Psychopathology.* Cambridge: Cambridge University Press.

SLUCHEVSKI, I. F. (1960) *Psiquiatria.* Spanish translation by Florencio Villa Landa and Manuel de la Loma. Mexico: Editorial Grijalbo.

# 5 Case history of a spy

## MAX F. PERUTZ, OM

On 10 September 1949 Michael Perrin, one of the directors of the British Atomic Energy Programme, was awakened by an urgent telephone call asking him to come to the communications room in the US London Embassy. There he was asked by the Pentagon to arrange for an RAF plane to check the upper atmosphere for radioactivity, already detected by the US Air Force, that appeared to signal a Soviet atomic explosion.

The public confirmation of this momentous event stunned the scientific community. We had believed that Stalin first heard about the American atomic bomb at the Potsdam Conference in August 1945, and we could not understand how the Russians had been able to overcome the formidable scientific and technical hurdles involved in the construction of the bomb in no more time than the four years, 1941–45, taken by the cream of European and American physicists.

A few weeks before that telephone call, Michael Perrin had received another disturbing piece of news. A coded message sent to Moscow by the Soviet Mission in New York during the war and only recently deciphered by the US Signal Corps indicated that one Klaus Fuchs, a German-born member of the British atom bomb team, had given them information about the atomic bomb project. Fuchs was arrested in London in February 1950, convicted of an offence under the Official Secrets Act, and sentenced to 14 years' imprisonment. What he told the Russians was never revealed and is still classified information in Britain (lest the Russians get to know of it?), but the Americans were told and full details are available in FBI files (Moss, 1987).

Klaus Fuchs was born in 1911, the son of a German pastor with left-wing sympathies, who taught his children the Lutheran precept of acting according to their own consciences rather than obeying established authority. Fuchs became a student at the time when German universities had turned into battlegrounds between the extremes of right and left. At first he sided with the Social Democrats, but when their weak opposition to the Nazis disappointed him he joined the Communist Party. For this he was once beaten up and thrown into a river by Nazi thugs.

When Hitler came to power in March 1933 Fuchs feared for his life and went into hiding until the Communist Party dispatched him to an anti-Fascist meeting in Paris. From Paris he came to England, where he became a research student in Nevill Mott's great school of theoretical physics in Bristol; afterwards he joined the German physicist Max Born, one of the founders of wave mechanics, in Edinburgh. In the spring of 1940 Fuchs was arrested, interned, and later deported to Canada together with hundreds of other German and Austrian refugees, including myself. We were returned to England and released in January 1941.

The atomic bomb project was set in motion in 1940 when two refugee physicists in Birmingham, the German-born Rudolph Peierls and the Austrian-born Otto Robert Frisch, found that the critical mass of the fissile uranium isotope $^{235}U$ needed for an explosion was no more than a few kilograms. In the summer of 1941 Peierls engaged Fuchs to help him with theoretical work on the project. Nine years later Fuchs confessed: "When I learned the purpose of the work, I decided to inform Russia and established contact through another member of the Communist Party." He made this high-handed decision despite having freely signed the Official Secrets Act, which pledged him not to disclose anything he learned in the course of his work to an unauthorised person, and having applied for naturalisation as a British subject. When this was granted he would have to "swear by Almighty God that on becoming a British subject I will be faithful and bear true allegiance to His Majesty King George VI, his heirs and successors according to law."

Fuchs was a brilliant mathematician and physicist with an accurate memory and a remarkable ability to explain difficult concepts lucidly. I experienced the latter attribute when he taught me theoretical physics during our internment at Quebec in the summer of 1940. These talents, and the information accessible to him, enabled him to provide the Russians with extensive instructions for the manufacture of fissile material and the construction of atomic bombs.

On that first occasion, Fuchs told the Russians that the building of an atomic bomb was possible in principle and that Britain was taking the first steps. He also informed them of the critical mass of a uranium bomb and of his own theoretical work on the separation of the rare fissile isotope of uranium-235 from its more abundant non-fissile partner. Later, at Los Alamos, Robert Oppenheimer, the scientific leader of the atomic bomb project, involved Fuchs in scientific discussions on all its aspects, so that Fuchs was better informed than most of the other scientists whose knowledge was restricted to their own special task. Here is an example, in Fuchs' own words, of information handed in one session to a Soviet agent at a town near Los Alamos (Moss, 1987):

Classified data dealing with the whole problem of making an atom bomb from fissionable material as I then knew the problem.

Information as to the principle of the method of detonating an atom bomb.

The possibility of making a plutonium bomb.

The high spontaneous fission rate of plutonium. (It is this which causes fission to occur more quickly than in $^{235}U$.)

Much of what was then known concerning implosion.

The fact that high explosives as a type of compression were considered but had not been entirely decided upon.

The size as to outer dimensions of the high explosive component.

The principle of the lens system which had not at that time been finally adopted.

The difficulties of multi-point detonation, as this was the specific problem on which I was then working.

The comparative critical mass of plutonium as compared with uranium–235.

The approximate amount of plutonium necessary for such a bomb.

Some information as to the type of core.

The current ideas as to the need for an initiator.

On another occasion he handed over 13 papers and a report of 35–40 pages on the separation of the uranium isotopes by diffusion.

How easy it all was! General Groves, the American commander of the project, was notorious among the scientists for his obsession with security, yet Fuchs could load a pile of secret documents, including a scale drawing of the plutonium bomb, into his car and drive out of the Los Alamos compound to hand them to a Soviet agent in a deserted street of the nearest town. Several such meetings took place with Soviet agents in both America and England.

When Fuchs did not have copies of the relevant documents he wrote down the mathematical equations and technical data from memory before meeting the agent. He did all this without ever arousing the suspicion of the young English theoretician with whom he shared an office for two years, nor that of any other of his colleagues. Back in England he was appointed Head of the Theoretical Division of the Atomic Energy Research Establishment at Harwell, in which capacity he told the Russians that Britain was building its own atomic bomb before even the Cabinet knew of it. As a British civil servant he became a stickler for security. At meetings of the Anglo-American Declassification Committee (also attended by Donald Maclean!) he invariably voted for keeping atomic information classified. As a final irony, Fuchs refused to reveal to the Scotland Yard detective who questioned him the technical details he had passed to the Russians on the grounds that the detective was not security-cleared.

When Fuchs was convicted, Parliament and the public wondered how a member of the Communist Party could have been allowed to work on the atomic bomb, but Attlee, who was then Prime Minister, assured the House of Commons:

> "Not long after this man came into this country (in 1933) it was said that he was a Communist. The source of that information was the Gestapo. At that time the Gestapo accused everybody of being a Communist. When the matter was looked into there was no support for this whatever. And from that time on there was no support. A proper watch was kept at intervals."

When I mentioned this to a veteran physicist friend of mine recently, he interjected: "But Fuchs and I were in the same Communist cell when we were students at Bristol." Max Born, Fuchs' former chief at Edinburgh, wrote about him: "He never concealed that he was a convinced Communist. During the Russo-Finnish war everyone's sympathies in our department were with the Finns, while Fuchs was passionately pro-Russian". On the other hand, Peierls had no idea that Fuchs was a Communist.

When Fuchs finally confessed he seems to have had no idea that he had committed a crime, and believed that he could return to Harwell as though nothing had happened. Fuchs had closed his mind to the consequences of his actions, even though he later analysed his behaviour with remarkable insight:

"In the course of this work I began naturally to form bonds of personal friendship and I had concerning them my inner thoughts. I used my Marxist philosophy to establish in my mind two separate compartments. In one compartment I allowed myself to make friendships, to have personal relations, to help people and to be in all personal ways the kind of man I wanted to be and the kind of man which, in personal ways, I had been before with my friends in or near the Communist Party. I could be free and easy and happy with other people without fear of disclosing myself because I knew that the other compartment would step in if I approached the danger point. I could forget the other compartment and still rely on it. It appeared to me at the time that I had become a 'free man' because I had succeeded in the other compartment to establish myself completely independent of the surrounding forces of society. Looking back at it now the best way of expressing it seems to be to call it a controlled schizophrenia."

Fuchs' resolve to decide the fate of the world seems to have been born of an arrogance that bordered on megalomania, as became apparent in prison where he told Peierls that when he had helped the Russians take over everything he would tell their leaders what was wrong with their system. He did not live up to that promise, however, and recently told a Western colleague visiting him in East Germany that Sakharov was a traitor who had deserved harsher punishment than mere exile from Moscow.

When Fuchs and I were interned together in Canada I attended his brilliant lectures, but I had no human contact with that pale, narrow-faced, thin-lipped, austere-looking man. Being more interested in the physics he taught me than in the physicist, I did not mind. People who knew him better thought him a very cold fish. All Fuchs' former colleagues, interviewed by Moss (1987), have stressed his reticence. Edward Teller, the Hungarian-born creator of the hydrogen bomb and *éminence grise* behind Reagan's SDI, found Fuchs "taciturn to a pathological degree". When Teller heard the news of his arrest he is said to have remarked: "So that's what it was!" An aquaintance told Moss that she had never heard Fuchs laugh. He had no close friends, never talked about his German past, and appeared to be sexless.

Moss (1987) attributes Fuchs' reticence to his desire to conceal his Communist past, but Born's autobiography shows that he made no secret of it, at least before he started his double life. I suspect that part of his reticence stemmed from his family background. His grandmother, mother, and one of his sisters all committed suicide in fits of depression; his brother was a tuberculosis sufferer in hospital in Switzerland; and his second sister, who lived in the US, was hospitalised for schizophrenia in the late forties, which suggests that Fuchs knew her to be mentally unbalanced. Fuchs himself may have been abnormal in being able to lock his activities into two watertight compartments and to close his mind to the implications of his spying for the colleagues who trusted him and the country that had given him shelter, but no more abnormal than Anthony Blunt, who made friends with the King while spying for Russia.

It has been said that Fuchs handed atomic secrets to an ally and that he merely put into effect the policy of sharing atomic secrets with the Soviet Union that the great Danish physicist Niels Bohr in vain urged upon Roosevelt and Churchill. There is a world of difference, however, between Bohr's ideal of preventing a nuclear arms race by a policy of mutual trust and Fuchs secretly giving Russia a good start in the race by handing over his colleagues' scientific results.

Before Fuchs was unmasked, the British and the Americans had been discussing ways of continuing their wartime collaboration in peacetime, but afterwards American distrust of British security destroyed all prospects of joint work. According to Dean Acheson, US Secretary of State at the time: "The talks with the British and Canadians returned to square one where there was a deep freeze from which they did not return in my time." Fuchs must have been pleased to have rendered this further gratuitous service to Russia.

That Fuchs put atomic weapons into Stalin's hands sooner than he would otherwise have had them is not in doubt: how much sooner is anyone's guess. Russian physicists were working on the possiblility of making an atomic bomb before they received Fuchs' first report. Moss (1987) cites David Holloway's book *The Soviet Union and the Arms Race* for evidence that it was this report which caused Stalin to give the project the highest priority. The former Head of the Institute of Nuclear Research in East Germany estimates that Fuchs saved the Russians two years; Russian physicists told Peierls that Fuchs saved them between one and two years.

I am sceptical of such estimates. Scientific research is an imaginative activity, dependent on qualities of mind that are beyond our comprehension. There is no linear progression from the appearance of a problem to its solution. During the Second World War the Germans failed even to start a sustained chain reaction in a nuclear pile because they had incorrectly determined one of the vital parameters. It might equally well have taken the Russians many more years to solve the very difficult problems involved, had Fuchs not given them the solutions. What difference that would have made politically is even harder to guess. Moss (1987) cites evidence that Stalin would not have incited North Korea to attack the South if he had not felt secure in the possession of nuclear weapons. Would an American monopoly of nuclear weapons have deterred the Russians from invading Hungary in 1956? We shall never know.

In the late 1940s Fuchs began to have doubts about Russian policy which he expressed in his confession: "It is impossible to give definite incidents because now the control mechanism acted against me, also keeping away from me facts which I could not look in the face, but they did penetrate and eventually I came to a point when I knew I disapproved of a great many actions of the Russian Government and of the Communist Party, but I still believed that they would build a New World and that one day I would take part in it and on that day I would also have to stand up and say to them that there are things which they are doing wrong."

He also began to understand the values that had enabled Britain to prevail against the Nazis: "Before I joined the project most of the English people with whom I had made personal contacts were left-wing, and affected to some degree or other, by the same kind of philosophy. Since coming to Harwell I have met English people of all kinds, and I have come to see in many of them a deep-rooted firmness which enables them to lead a decent way of life. I do not know where this springs from and I don't think they do, but it is there."

On being released from Wakefield Prison in 1959, Fuchs joined his father in East Germany where he married and became an honoured citizen and member of the Politbureau, no longer plagued by doubts about the Communist Party line or by nostalgia for the British way of life, until his death in January 1988. The shutters in his mind seemed to have come down once more and stayed down.

From this case history psychiatrists will, perhaps, be able to decide what diagnostic label, if any, is applicable to this unusual personality who influenced the course of history

## *Reference*

Moss, Norman (1987) *Klaus Fuchs: The Man who Stole the Atom Bomb.* London: Grafton Books.

This article was first published in the *London Review of Books* in June 1987 (vol. 9, no. 12); ©*London Review of Books*.

# II. Issues of classification

# 6 Psychiatric classification simplified

## ERIK ESSEN-MÖLLER

Different syndromes may relate to same aetiologies, and different aetiologies may correspond to identical syndromes. For satisfactory clinical information we are forced to make, as far as possible, a *twofold approach*, one descriptive and the other causative.

The syndromatic diagnosis should never be omitted, not even where aetiology is known. A dissociative picture remains a dissociative picture whatever its cause.

Registration of organic aetiology is mostly restricted to cases that can be attributed to an "independently diagnosable cerebral or systemic disease" (ICD–10 draft). This leaves us with no aetiological diagnosis for the majority of cases. However, to my mind, the diagnoser should be urged also to present his speculations and beliefs. This will stimulate his interest in diagnostics and may occasionally lead to fruitful research. The same view pertains to the group of aetiological or eliciting factors designed as psychogenic or situational.

The vagueness introduced with this freedom on the part of the diagnoser can be conveniently balanced by an index by which the suggested aetiology is graded as 'confident', 'provisional' or 'tentative' (ICD–10 draft). In Lund we used to add the item 'cryptogenic' in order to indicate that the problem of aetiology was left open. In this way the classification became all-covering and obligatory.

The multitude of intercombinations of the two diagnostic systems may appear cumbersome. It may be hard to find the precise fit in both systems simultaneously. Retrieval of records with a specified item will require scanning of the entire field of combinations.

This type of difficulty can be overcome by not using the overall layout of combinations and replacing it by two separate *standard lists*, one of which is descriptive and the other aetiological. The items of each list here have to be coded independently. For every patient, one relevant item (or more) from each list can now be chosen and combined into a joint classification. This simplified procedure will also warrant a freer choice of items, unbiased by the suggestion inherent in preformulated combinations.

There is considerable saving of space and repetitions. While each discovery of a new aetiology or syndrome will generate numerous new entries in the combinatory field, a single entry in the relevant list will do. Correspondingly, the retrieval of all records with a specified item in common is much easier when keeping to the appropriate list.

Transition from the present international systems to the principles here advocated will, of course, require certain condensations and regroupings of the clinical descriptions and the explanatory text. However, a beginning might be made at any time by erecting the two standard lists. Hopefully they will prove as flexible and profitable as did ours in Lund, where the idea was applied for more than 20 years.

## References

ESSEN-MÖLLER, E. & WOHLFAHRT, S. (1944) Preliminärt förslag till ny psykiatrisk nomenklatur. *Svenska psykiatriska föreningens förhandlingar.* p. 28–29.

—— & —— (1947) Ytterligare bearbetning av den psykiatriska diagnostabellan. *Nordisk psykiatrisk medlemsblad,* 1, 48–51.

—— (1947) Suggestions for the amendment of the official Swedish classification of mental disorders. *Eighth Congress of Scandinavian Psychiatrists,* 47, 551–555.

—— (1961) Introduction to problems of taxonomy. Discussion. In *Field Studies in the Mental Disorders.* (J. Zubin) New York: Grune & Stratton, pp. 37–38.

—— (1961) On classification of mental disorders. *Acta Psychiatrica Scandinavica,* 37, 119–126.

—— (1971) Suggestions for further improvement of the international classification of mental disorders. *Psychological Medicine,* 1, 308–311.

—— (1973) Standard lists for three-fold classification of mental disorders. *Acta Psychiatrica Scandinavica,* 49, 198–212.

—— (1982) Gutenberg and the ICD-9 of mental disorders. *British Journal of Psychiatry,* 140, 529–531.

# 7 DSM-III and Europe

## ERIK STRÖMGREN

In most European countries there has been great interest in DSM-III. Many institutions are already using it on a routine basis, others are making more or less systematic trials. Some psychiatrists recommend DSM-III for general official use. The reasons for this positive attitude towards DSM-III can be divided into four main groups:

(a) dissatisfaction with other classifications in use, among them ICD
(b) DSM-III's basic principle with regard to multiaxial classification
(c) the introduction of sharply defined diagnostic criteria
(d) the organisation of the work behind DSM-III and of the tools for its application.

Let us take each of these four groups separately:

(a) Although the great majority of the member states of the United Nations have accepted ICD, satisfaction with this classification is limited. One of the main reasons for dissatisfaction is that about one half of the member states are using ICD-8 and the rest ICD-9. When, in 1975 ICD-9 appeared, most countries were using ICD-8, and in many of them it was felt that it would be too costly and laborious to change horses so soon after the appearance of ICD-9; several countries had been using it for only a few years. Other countries, which in the meantime had become members, would naturally choose the most recent edition, ICD-9. Unfortunately, the differences between the two editions are in some points so substantial, especially with regard to classification of depressive states, that they are practically incompatible. On the other hand, the section on mental disorders has one great advantage, as compared with other sections of the ICD, namely the inclusion of a glossary with definitions and descriptions of terms contained in the section. This glossary is, however, not complete, a number of important terms not being defined. During the preparatory work for ICD-10 it has been one of the main tasks to create a glossary which will be really comprehensive. It is, however, obvious that as ICD-8 and 9 stand now they cannot compete with DSM-III in this respect.

(b) DSM-III's fundamental principle of a multiaxial classification is in accordance with an universally increasing interest in this type of classification. Some 40 years ago Essen-Möller & Wohlfart (1947) advocated multiaxial classification, and further publications by Essen-Möller (1961, 1971) and by Ottosson & Perris (1973) have provided more refined examples. From 1952 to 1965 the official Danish classification (1952) was biaxial, a system which worked

49

well and was only given up because ICD-8 had appeared and for reasons of international understanding was chosen to substitute the Danish classification. Finally, a modification of ICD specifically for child psychiatry is multiaxial and seems to be well accepted by those using it.

(c) The diagnostic criteria applied in DSM-III are felt by many psychiatrists to be clearer than those applied in other classifications. The different 'decision trees' are appealing and do not seem to leave anybody in doubt. Most psychiatrists are busy people, and sometimes they may feel attracted to directions for use which are easy to apply, even if they do not feel sure that they provide an adequate description of realities.

(d) Everybody must be impressed by the extensive amount of work which lies behind the construction of the DSM-III. Many competent experts have been in collaboration, and the coordination of the different trials has obviously been on a high level. In many respects the organisers of the DSM-III have been in a more favourable position than those of the ICD. The World Health Organization has been in a strained financial position for many years, which has hampered the preparatory work with regard to arrangement of meetings, trials, etc. In addition, WHO has naturally more international obligations to take into consideration than could ever be relevant for the American Psychiatric Association. DSM-III is a national classification, tailored for the needs of American psychiatrists and institutions, whereas WHO has to consider the needs of some hundred countries. APA seems to have been able to finance the work with DSM-III generously, thus enabling rapid publication and distribution of documents, whereas publication of WHO material is necessarily a complicated and time-consuming process. Finally, the section on 'Mental Disorders' of the ICD is just one section of the total ICD, which implies that the basic structure has been elaborated by other forces than those concerned with the construction of the psychiatric part.

It is thus obvious that the constructors of the ICD will always be in a much more difficult position than those responsible for the creation of DSM-III and its modifications. It is no wonder that DSM-III has been able to aquire some very favourable qualities as compared with ICD. On the other hand, nobody will claim that DSM-III is the ideal solution. Many, some severe, criticisms have been expressed. They can be divided into three groups:

(a) Although the general attitude to the principle of multiaxial classification is definitely favourable, this attitude does not apply to all the axes within DSM-III. Axes I and II are regarded as useful or even necessary. The placement of different items within these two axes can, however, be discussed. There will be many objections to the placement of mental retardation within axis I which seems less appropriate than within axis II. This criticism has been accepted in DSM-III-R. The description of the schizotypal personality disorder, on the other hand, gives many readers the impression of a variant of a schizophrenic process which would then rather belong to axis I. Axis III is generally felt to be useful and necessary as it stands. The most widespread criticism concerns axes IV and V, respectively. They are regarded as inapplicable for international use and even for the use in many countries with a social structure similar to that of the United States. The quantifications are felt to be quite ambiguous.

The whole discussion on the DSM-III axes makes it clear that there is no agreement on what the term 'axis' really implies. Is it just synonymous with the older term 'dimension' which has been in wide use especially in the German-speaking psychiatry? Many fundamental publications by Ernst Kretschmer and his pupils apply a multidimensional description of cases. A similar but more systematic approach was applied by Karl Birnbaum in his classic monograph *The Making of a Psychosis* in which he performed a 'structural analysis', distinguishing between predisposing, preforming, pathogenetic, pathoplastic, and precipitating factors. Are such dimensions or factors also instances of axes?

The five axes of DSM-III do not constitute a logical system; they were obviously chosen solely for practical purposes. Many other criteria could as well have been selected as 'axes'—for instance age, course, duration, etc. Some of these criteria (e.g., course, duration) occasionally play important roles among DSM-III's diagnostic criteria. They are, however, used only in certain chapters, which is probably why they were not promoted to the rank of axes.

But even when several axes are applied, it may be difficult to visualise the patient behind the description. Even a very short narrative account, or a 'vignette', will obviously be much more informative, although unfortunately not easily quantifiable for statistical purposes.

(b) The basic principle in DSM-III is not aetiological. This principle is, however, discarded on several occasions. In other instances, such as the dementias, it is felt unnatural that aetiology is kept so far in the background.

Although the terms psychosis and neurosis are not parts of this classification, these terms are used on several occasions. It is, of course, true that it may be difficult to define them, especially neurosis; a classification which does not use the psychosis criterion will, however, be inadequate for those working in forensic psychiatry, which in many countries places psychotics as quite distinct from other mentally deviant persons, in accordance with existing legislation.

(c) The elaboration of diagnostic criteria in DSM-III has a great appeal to many psychiatrists. Most of them are so clear that their probably high reliability will make it possible for different psychiatrists to delimit similar groups of these disorders, regardless of whether the groups correspond to any kinds of nosological entities. They can, at any rate, be regarded as representing international diagnostic conventions.

There are, however, some of DSM-III's diagnostic criteria which to many psychiatrists represent minor or major catastrophes, particularly the frequently used type of criterion that consists in ascertainment of a certain minimum number of symptoms (or other subcriteria) among a larger number of possible symptoms. For instance, one of the main criteria for "major depressive episode" is "at least four of the following symptoms", following which eight different symptoms are mentioned. What seems quite unsatisfactory in this procedure is that the eight symptoms mentioned are obviously regarded as equivalent, in spite of the fact that some of them are far more specific for major depressive episodes than the rest. For example, "poor appetite or significant weight loss . . . or increased appetite or significant weight gain, insomnia or hypersomnia, and loss of energy, fatigue" are not nearly as specific for the diagnosis of a major depressive episode as "feelings of worthlessness, self reproach, or excessive or inappropriate guilt". It is thus possible to select four of the eight symptoms mentioned also in cases that definitely do not belong to the group "major depressive episode", whereas just one or two of the more specific symptoms will be sufficient to make the diagnosis of this particular disorder certain. It seems most unsatisfactory that no quantification of the very different degrees of importance of the symptoms is attempted. It is to be hoped that further practical trials will provide materials that will allow calculation of coefficients ('weights') for each of these symptoms. Until such coefficients have been calculated on the basis of research, it will probably be much better to apply estimated coefficients, based on clinical experience, than to regard all symptoms as equivalent which must necessarily be unrealistic.

The criticism expressed here can, of course, be applied with equal right to most existing rating scales, including some of the most popular and widely used 'research diagnostic criteria', some of which have attained an importance that, in the opinion of many psychiatrists, they certainly do not deserve. They are tools, just tools, and often very crude tools, the handiness and pseudo-exactness of which has obviously given them an influence for which there is no scientific foundation.

The most controversial of all the criteria specified in DSM–III is probably that of duration of episodes, which plays a crucial role in several sections of the classification, especially in the section on 'Psychotic Disorders Not Elsewhere Classified', in which the decisive criterion for distinction between "schizophreniform disorder", "brief reactive psychosis", and "atypical psychosis" is just the duration of the episode. Here the classification depends primarily on whether duration is less than two weeks, between two weeks and six months, or more than six months. Such limits do not seem acceptable. First, it is, of course, quite arbitrary whether one uses these time limits or others that deviate more or less from them; it is just a question of convention. Second, and more important, even if such conventions were permissible, and in some cases might be necessary, their application would be dubious, in the sense that determination of duration can be difficult or impossible; in so many cases it is retrospectively impossible to say exactly when an episode began. And third: as time passes, several cases will automatically have to change diagnosis.

Concerning "brief reactive psychosis" the confusion increases when no "psycho-social stressor" can be ascertained; in this case the psychosis is degraded to "atypical psychosis" which brings it into a waste bag, which also contains all schizophrenic disorders arising after the age of 45.

With regard to the criteria for the diagnosis of schizophrenic disorder, it should be mentioned that to most European psychiatrists it will be incomprehensible that in the discussion of schizophrenic symptoms the term autism does not occur at all. Eugen Bleuler regarded autism as one of the central symptoms of schizophrenia, and Manfred Bleuler, the psychiatrist who probably has the most intimate knowledge of a great number of schizophrenics, tends to stress autism as perhaps the only really pathognomonic symptom in schizophrenia. In DSM–III the term autism only occurs in connection with infantile autism, Kanner's syndrome, a disease which has nothing to do with schizophrenia and in which 'autism' is fundamentally different from the autism described by Eugen Bleuler who originally invented and defined the term.

With regard to DSM–III's concept of schizoid personality disorder and schizotypal personality disorder, respectively, there will be much uncertainty. As mentioned before, schizotypal personality disorder as described in DSM–III will be felt to be a psychotic disorder by many psychiatrists. The term "schizoid" is used in a sense which differs from that used by its originator Eugen Bleuler, especially since it excludes the positive personality features which, according to Bleuler, are also characteristic of schizoid persons.

The criticisms mentioned in the preceding pages are expressed widely by European psychiatrists. In addition, some more specific comments are heard from continental psychiatrists, coloured by the traditions and schools prevailing in the respective countries.

German-speaking psychiatrists have expressed their great satisfaction with the multiaxial principle of DSM–III but stress the main weakness to be DSM–III's compromise character which counterbalances not only the efforts of standardisation but also the multiaxial design itself. And the general comment is made that, although for the purpose of health statistics a world-wide common diagnostic system is desirable, this should not be accomplished at the expense of clarity and an openness to new developments. Useful as DSM–III might be for purposes of health statistics, it is not regarded as a diagnostic classification system to be recommended for research.

In Belgium, reactions have been different in the Dutch-speaking and the French-speaking part, respectively. In the first named area DSM–III has been well accepted, it is already in use in many institutions, and several more intend to use it in the future. French-speaking psychiatrists in Belgium are much more close to French psychiatry. They feel that ICD–9 is more compatible with the French way of conceptualising mental disorders than DSM–III. It is regretted that DSM–III is inadequate in its description of reactional psychosis and depressive psychosis. It is stressed that DSM–III should not replace existing psychiatric knowledge. There will be a real danger that new generations of physicians or psychiatrists will think only in terms of DSM–III diagnosis: "mere knowledge of DSM–III's diagnostic criteria can give the illusion of a thorough knowledge of psychopathology. The same applies to other professional groups, such as lawyers, who are also interested in DSM–III as it relates to criminology: lawyers and others involved in legal proceedings may now, through knowledge of DSM–III criteria, think they have aquired an understanding of psychopathology" (Cosyns *et al*, 1983). One more problem is that it can be difficult to have to choose between the presence or absence of a criterion when, as is often the case, an intermediary level is met in clinical reality.

In the Netherlands, the attitudes towards DSM–III have in general been very favourable, and there seems to be a possibility that the Dutch government and the Dutch Psychiatric Association will decide to adopt DSM–III officially. On the other hand, a number of general and specific criticisms have been expressed. For instance it is regretted that DSM–III does not contain clear counterparts to psychogenic psychosis, hysterical psychosis and a number of other concepts which are used widely in the Netherlands. It has been suggested that a three dimensional approach to classifying depressions should rate symptoms, aetiology and course independently.

Among Italian psychiatrists the attitude to DSM–III seems to be negative. The omission of some of the most widely used categories such as neurosis, neurotic depression, endogenous depression etc. will not be accepted easily because they are deeply embedded in the cultural background of Italian psychiatrists who will also be very resistant to the introduction of completely new diagnostic categories such as schizotypal personality disorder, cyclothymic and dysthymic disorders and somatoform disorders. On the whole, the radical changes made in DSM–III are felt as revolutionary and as an imposition of, or intrusion by, North American Thought and Culture (Cassano & Maggini, 1983).

In Spain the interest in DSM–III has been great and the attitude on the whole positive. Juan López-Ibor & José López-Ibor (1983) state that "Spanish psychiatrists do not believe that the American Psychiatric Association is going to rest on its laurels and the admiration of the rest of the countries of the world"; it is suggested that the APA might consider adopting a wider interactive or phenomenological concept of symptoms, one that includes the context in which they develop; increasing the validity of the diagnostic criteria in a way that will facilitate international communication and improve every day clinical care.

Reactions of French psychiatrists to DSM–III have been described by Professor Pichot and co-workers (1983) who stress that the conceptual world of French psychiatry is far from that which lies behind DSM–III, and that it will become very difficult to induce the majority of French psychiatrists to adopt DSM–III. These authors, however, draw attention to some practical circumstances which may induce some French psychiatrists to use DSM–III in their publications, probably parallel with the existing French classifications. First, many French researchers intend to publish their work in the journals that appear in the United States and they feel that the use of DSM–III will further understanding of their results by American readers; next, many pharmaceutical companies request physicians to conduct clinical trials using the DSM–III, hoping eventually to obtain authorisation to enter the American market by performing clinical trials in Europe, and that the use of the DSM–III will be a factor in acceptance by the FDA.

In the five North European countries the interest in DSM–III has been great. Many trials are going on. It is quite understandable that one of the main objections towards DSM–III is that it is very difficult to place in it the large group of psychoses which in Scandinavian countries traditionally are labelled reactive or psychogenic psychoses.

In summary, it can be stated that there seems to be general agreement that DSM–III in many ways is superior to other existing classifications and that it will have a lasting impact on classifications to come. Its basic principle of multiaxial classification is sound, but the choice of axes certainly cannot be definitive. DSM–III's refined and comprehensive use of diagnostic criteria is in principle to be recommended highly. In many cases, however, the diagnostic distinctions are felt to be artificial and to make unnatural dividing lines between groups which, from a clinical viewpoint, belong together while, conversely, they combine in some groups a heterogeneous selection of cases. It can, on the other hand, be claimed that exact clinical diagnostic criteria will allow clinicians to use the same language and to understand each other, thus improving scientific communication. It is, of course, very nice if scientists from many countries can use the same language. But sometimes one does not feel certain that it is clinical reality they are talking about.

There is no doubt that systems of diagnostic research criteria can be useful and even necessary for some purposes. But they can never contribute to the natural evolution of clinical psychiatry. On the contrary, they may even counteract it, especially if they are applied as substitutions for clinical, empathic diagnostication.

When contemplating these dangers I am sometimes reminded of an old anecdote about a Scandinavian who had emigrated to the United States. On one of his visits to the old country he, like other Scandinavian Americans, talked much about technical progress in the United States. He claimed, for instance, that a practical invention had been made which made it unnecessary for people to shave themselves. In a number of public places there were certain automatic machines and, if you put your head into them, in ten seconds you got shaved. When a sceptic among his listeners objected that all heads do not have the same shape the answer was: "No, not from the beginning—but they acquire it".

Time will show whether in psychiatric diagnostication the machines or the heads will prove to be the most solid part.

## References

AMERICAN PSYCHIATRIC ASSOCIATION (1980) *Diagnostic and Statistical Manual of Mental Disorders* (3rd edn.) Washington, DC: APA.

CASSANO, G. B. & MAGGINI, C. (1983) DSM-III and Italian psychiatry. In *International Perspectives on DSM-III*. (eds R. L. Spitzer, J. B. W. Williams & A. E. Skodol) Washington, DC: American Psychiatric Press. pp. 75–183.

COSYNS, P., ANSSEAU, M. & BOBON, D. P. (1983) The use of DSM-III in Belgium. In *International Perspectives on DSM-III*. (eds R. L. Spitzer, J. B. W. Williams & A. E. Skodol) Washington, DC: American Psychiatric Press. pp. 127–134.

DANSK PSYKIATRISK SELSKAB (1952) Diagnoseliste med kommentarer. *Nordisk psykiatrisk medlemsblad*, **6**, 272–295.

ESSEN-MÖLLER, E. (1961) On classification of mental disorders. *Acta Psychiatica Scandinavica*, **37**, 119–126.

—— (1971) Suggestions for further improvement of the international classification of mental disorders. *Psychological Medicine*, **1**, 308–311.

—— & WOHLFART, S. (1947) Suggestions for the amendment of the official Swedish classification of mental disorders. *Acta Psychiatica Scandinavica*, suppl. **47**, 551–555.

LÓPEZ-IBOR, J. & LÓPEZ-IBOR, J. M. (1983) Spanish psychiatry and DSM-III. In *International Perspectives on DSM-III*. (eds R. L. Spitzer, J. B. W. Williams & A. E. Skodol) Washington, DC: American Psychiatric Press. pp. 251–256.

OTTOSSON, J.-O. & PERRIS, C. (1973) Multidimensional classification of mental disorders. *Psychological Medicine*, **3**, 238–243.

PICHOT, P., GUELFI, J. D. & KROLL, J. (1983) French perspectives on DSM-III. In *International Perspectives on DSM-III*. (eds R. L. Spitzer, J. B. W. Williams & A. E. Skodol) Washington, DC: American Psychiatric Press. pp. 155–176.

SPITZER, R. L., WILLIAMS, J. B. W. & SKODOL, A. E. (1983) *International Perspectives on DSM-III*. Washington, DC: American Psychiatric Press.

WHO (1967) *International Classification of Diseases*. 1965 Revision. Geneva: World Health Organization.

—— (1977) *International Classification of Diseases*. 1975 Revision. Geneva: World Health Organization.

# III.  Depression and anxiety

# 8 Single genes productive of affective disorder

## ELLIOT S. GERSHON

Single-locus inheritance in the affective disorders was not demonstrable in segregation analysis of diagnosis, but has been discovered through linkage to chromosomal markers in pedigrees. The finding of linkage to chromosome 11 markers in a bipolar pedigree from a population isolate (the Amish), and the controversial finding of linkage to X-chromosome markers in several but not all studies, imply that a single causative gene for at least a proportion of bipolar and related illnesses may soon be discovered.

In the affective disorders, the fact that multifactorial models are consistent with some studies and that single locus models are usually rejected does not necessarily rule out single locus inheritance. The power of these methods to detect major loci in complex diseases may be low. Goldin *et al* (1984) found by simulation that a single locus for a disease could not be identified for certain modes of inheritance, especially 'quasi-recessive' inheritance where the heterozygote individuals have low, but not zero penetrance. In addition, if affective disorders are genetically heterogeneous, the detection of single locus genetic mechanisms may require a valid linkage marker or single-gene vulnerability factor.

The importance of finding a genetic marker, whether as an inherited vulnerability factor or as a chromosomal linkage marker, is self-evident. It would provide important information on the inherited pathophysiological event, and have immediate application to prevention and treatment.

Gene mapping provides a general approach to locating single locus markers. One can systematically study all genes active in the central nervous system, or specific to the central nervous system, or active in specific chromosomal regions about which one has a hypothesis. With the advent of molecular genetic methods, mapping of the entire human genome with respect to an illness is now close to a practical possibility. The gene mapping approach using restriction fragment length polymorphisms (RFLPs) of genomic DNA has proved valuable in several recent studies in neurologic and psychiatric disorders, including the affective disorders.

The power of a linkage demonstration is that it unequivocally ties the transmission of illness to a particular gene region, although it does not actually

Paper presented at the International Congress on New Directions in Affective Disorders, Jerusalem, Israel, 7 April, 1987. A preliminary version of this paper is to be published as 'Single locus markers in affective disorder', in *New Directions in Affective Disorders*, (eds. B. Lerer and S. Gershon). Springer Verlag, New York.

specify which gene within that region is responsible for the illness. Linkage also aids greatly in resolving genetic heterogeneity once it is established, although it should be noted that the presence of heterogeneity makes linkage more difficult to detect.

## Restriction fragment length polymorphisms on chromosome 11

The use of very large pedigrees in linkage studies is based on the assumption that, even in an illness that is genetically heterogeneous, there will be genetic homogeneity within pedigrees. This is questionable for a common disease in a large population, where persons marrying into the pedigree may bring in different forms of illness, but in a population isolate homogeneity may be considered more likely, at least within a pedigree. The Amish population studied by Egeland is an isolate in which several large pedigrees segregating for affective illness have been identified. In one pedigree, Egeland *et al* (1987) found autosomal dominant transmission and linkage of bipolar and unipolar illness to the Insulin-ras oncogene region of the short arm of chromosome 11. In Bethesda, MD, we (Detera-Wadleigh *et al*, 1987) have found this linkage not to be present in three smaller pedigrees, and Hodgkinson *et al*, (1987) in three Icelandic pedigrees, also do not find this linkage. It is difficult to find methodologic fault with the Amish finding, since the pedigrees were cultured, with the diagnoses and cells available to interested scientists, before the chromosome 11 markers were applied to it. The non-replication seems to be due to genetic heterogeneity in this case, with the implication that the Amish form of manic-depressive illness is genetically uncommon in the other populations studied.

## Colourblindness region of X-chromosome

Between 1969 and 1974, Winokur and his colleagues, and shortly afterwards Mendlewicz and co-workers, reported that bipolar illness is linked to the X-chromosome markers Xg blood group and Protan/Deutan colourblindness. At the time of the initial reports, it was not known that these results were inconsistent with each other, because linkage of bipolar illness to both Xg and to protan and deutan colourblindness is not compatible with the known large chromosomal map distance between the Xg locus (on the short arm) and the protan-deutan region (at the tip of the long arm).

We were unable to replicate either of these linkages in our own data. For both Xg and protan-deutan colourblindness, close linkage to affective illness was ruled out (Leckman *et al*, 1979; Gershon *et al*, 1979). Our pedigrees were not heterogeneous with respect to each other and there were no single pedigrees strongly suggesting linkage to either marker. Mendlewicz and associates (1979), on the other hand, reported eight new families in Belgium and suggested linkage to colourblindness in at least one.

It has been argued (Risch & Baron, 1982) that there is linkage to colourblindness but not Xg blood group, and that heterogeneity accounts for differences between investigators. This is difficult to accept when the initial series was so strikingly positive and the replication series so negative, and also in view of the inconsistency of the initial finding that both Xg and colourblindness were linked to bipolar illness. If methodological errors in diagnostic or ascertainment procedures produced the unique homogeneity of the 1972–1974 pedigree series of Mendlewicz and colleagues, that would explain why the strikingly positive results are not replicated either in our series or in the later series of Mendlewicz *et al* (1979).

Strongly positive, multigenerational, pedigrees for the red-green colourblindness linkage have since been reported by Baron *et al* (1987), and Mendlewicz and co-workers have reported linkage to the glucose-6-phosphate dehydrogenase (G6PD) locus (a marker on the X-chromosome very close to the red-green colourblindness loci) (Mendlewicz *et al*, 1980) and to the blood clotting Factor IX, which is within 15–30 centimorgans of the red-green colourblindness region (Mendlewicz *et al*, 1987.)

Since DNA probes for this region of the X-chromosome now exist, their use may make virtually all pedigrees informative for linkage and lead to a resolution of the controversy of whether or not there is a generally reproducible finding of linkage to the colourblindness region in a portion of manic-depressive patients. My colleagues Berrettini, Gelernter and Detera-Wadleigh, and I, have recently applied the St14 probe of Oberle *et al* (1985), which marks the colourblindness of the X-chromosome, to new manic-depressive pedigrees, and continue to find linkage to be excluded; further pedigrees will be studied before these results are published.

## HLA complex

Although claims of linkage between bipolar and unipolar illness have appeared, the analytic methods employed have been criticised (Goldin *et al*, 1982, Suarez *et al*, 1982), and the reports are not generally accepted.

## References

BARON, M., RISCH, N., HAMBURGER, R. *et al* (1987) Genetic linkage between X-chromosome markers and bipolar affective illness. *Nature*, **326**, 289–292.
DETERA-WADLEIGH, S. D., BERRETTINI, W. H., GOLDIN, L. R., BOORMAN, D., ANDERSON, S. & GERSHON, E. S. (1987) Close linkage of c-Harvey-ras-1 and the insulin gene to affective disorder is ruled out in three North American pedigrees. *Nature*, **325**, 806–808.
EGELAND, J. A., GERHARD, D. S., PAULS, D. L., SUSSEX, J. N., KIDD, K. K., ALLEN, C. R., HOSTETTER, A. M. & HOUSMAN, D. E. (1987) Bipolar affective disorders linked to DNA markers on chromosome 11. *Nature*, **325**, 783–787.
GERSHON, E. S., TARGUM, S. D., MATTHYSSE, S. & BUNNEY, W. E. Jr. (1979) Color blindness not closely linked to bipolar illness. *Archives of General Psychiatry*, **36**, 1423–1430.
GOLDIN, L. R., CLERGET-DARPOUX, F. & GERSHON, E. S. (1982) Relationship of HLA to major affective disorders not supported. *Psychiatry Research*, **7**, 19–25.
——, COX, N. J., PAULS, D. L., GERSHON, E. S. & KIDD, K. K. (1984) The detection of major loci by segregation and linkage analysis: a simulation study. *Genetic Epidemiology*, **1**, 285–296.
HODGKINSON, S., SHERRINGTON, R., GURLING, H., MARCHBANKS, R., REEDERS, S., MALLET, J., McINNIS, M., PETURSSON, H. & BRYNJOLFSSON, J. (1987) Molecular genetic evidence for heterogeneity in manic depression. *Nature*, **325**, 804–806.
LECKMAN, J. F., GERSHON, E. S., McGINNISS, M. H. *et al* (1979) New data do not suggest linkage between the Xg blood group and bipolar illness. *Archives of General Psychiatry*, **36**, 1435–1441.

MENDLEWICZ, J., LINKOWSKI, P., GUROFF, J. J. *et al* (1979) Color blindness linkage to bipolar manic-depressive illness: New evidence. *Archives of General Psychiatry*, **36**, 1442–1447.

——, —— & WILMOTTE, J. (1980) Linkage between glucose-6-phosphate dehydrogenase deficiency and manic-depressive psychosis. *British Journal of Psychiatry*, **137**, 337–342.

——, SEVY, S., BROCAS, H. *et al* (1987) Polymorphic DNA marker on X chromosome and manic depression. *Lancet*, **i** 1230–1232.

OBERLE, I., DRAYNA, D., CAMERINO, G., WHITE, R. & MANDEL, J. L. (1985) The telomeric region of the human X chromosome long arm: Presence of a highly polymorphic DNA marker and analysis of recombination frequency. *Proceedings of the National Academy of Sciences of the USA*, **82**, 2824–2828.

RISCH, N. & BARON, M. (1982) X-Linkage and genetic heterogeneity in bipolar-related major affective illness: reanalysis of linkage data. *Annals of Human Genetics*, **46**, 153–166.

SUAREZ, B. K. & CROUGHAN, J. (1982) Is the major histocompatibility complex linked to genes that increase susceptibility to affective disorder? A critical appraisal. *Psychiatry Research*, **7**, 29–45.

# 9 The clinical separation of anxiety and depression: Old issues, new disputes

## GERALD L. KLERMAN

For almost a century, psychiatrists, psychologists, and biologists have debated the nature of anxiety and depression. A recurrent theme in these debates has been the controversies between those who see these conditions as a single clinical condition (unitary point of view), and those who see them as two or more separate conditions (dualistic or pluralistic points of view). These debates are related to larger issues in psychiatric classification where there has always been a tension between the 'lumpers' and the 'splitters'. 'Lumpers', such as Adolf Meyer and others, employ broad categories to pull together diverse phenomena, particularly if they can discern an underlying or common causal mechanism. In contrast, the 'splitters' seek to identify multiple discrete syndromes and disorders, with the goal of distinguishing separate diagnostic and disease entities, each with its own unique aetiology, symptom pattern, and clinical course. This point of view is often identified with Emil Kraepelin and the continental school of psychiatry (1921).

In the decades since World War II, this controversy intensified when applied to neurotic conditions, conditions without psychotic manifestations. In particular, disputes arose as to the separation of anxiety disorders and depressive disorders from each other and from the larger category of neurotic conditions. Within the group of depressive disorders, numerous distinctions had been proposed: unipolar, bipolar, agitated/retarded, psychotic/neurotic, endogenous/reactive, biological/environmental. Within the group of anxiety disorders, it had been proposed that the previously widely accepted category of anxiety neurosis be separated into panic anxiety and generalised anxiety; and further, that panic disorder be linked with agoraphobia. Research previously had demonstrated the validity of separating phobias into agoraphobia, simple phobia, and social phobia. Even finer distinctions within the phobia group have been proposed, such as blood/injury phobias and performance phobias, such as public speaking and musical performance (Marks, 1987).

Sir Martin Roth and his associates, particularly during the period when he was a Professor at Newcastle, played a significant and enduring role in these developments. Three aspects of the contributions made by Roth and his associates are worthy of special consideration. These are:

(a) the application of multivariate statistical techniques to symptom and psychopathological data sets

(b) investigation of the response to treatments, particularly tricyclic anti-depressants and ECT, as validators of diagnostic distinctions

(c) reaffirmation and modification of the classic Kraepelinian point of view into a neo-Kraepelinian paradigm.

In this chapter, each of these three aspects will be explored in some detail and related to current disputes, particularly those arising since the promulgation in 1980 of the *Diagnostic and Statistical Manual III* (DSM–III) by the American Psychiatric Association (APA) (1980).

## Contributions of Roth and the Newcastle school

During the period when Roth was the Professor of Psychiatry at Newcastle, he gathered around him a group of talented clinical investigators. The Newcastle school pursued a series of studies which have created new standards for clinical research in the post-World War II period.

They made use of new technologies, particularly multivariate statistical techniques, high speed electronic calculators (computers) and new psycho-pharmacologic agents. They applied these new technologies within a larger theoretical and conceptual framework, initiating the formation of what we have termed the ''neo-Kraepelinian'' paradigm, using Kuhn's term ''paradigm'' derived from the writings of Kraepelin (1921).

### Application of multivariate statistical techniques to problems in psychopathology

Roth and his associates (Kiloh, Garside, 1963) (Schapira *et al*, 1972) undertook a series of investigations of the clinical presentation, symptomatology and clinical course of patients with neurotic, non-psychotic, conditions, particularly depressive and anxiety states.

For many decades, British and North American psychiatry had been involved in controversies concerning the unity of neurosis and the value of various separations within the depressive states. Sir Aubrey Lewis (1930), the most influential British psychiatrist in the period immediately after World War II and an acknowledged student of Adolf Meyer at Johns Hopkins University in Baltimore, Maryland, USA (Klerman, 1979), had challenged the popular distinction between endogenous-reactive depression (Gillespie, 1929) and had contributed to the development of the concept of depressive neuroses. He extended his unitary view and proposed that anxiety and depressive states should be considered a single clinical entity. He proposed that the concept of affective disorder include both anxious and depressive states, although in his own work he devoted most attention to countering dualistic approaches to depression, particularly the psychotic/neurotic distinction, closely related to the endogenous/reactive distinction.

Lewis' papers in the early 1930s, based in part upon his MD thesis at Adelaide, Australia, were a challenge to the earlier paper by Gillespie, which emphasised the distinction between endogenous and reactive depressions (Gillespie, 1929) (Lewis, 1930, 1934a, 1934b).

Given the many historic contributions of English statisticians, notably Galton, Pearson, and Fisher, it is appropriate that the application of multivariate methods to psychiatric data should also have been undertaken by English investigators.

Multivariate methods, such as factor analysis and discriminant function, had been developed before World War II, but their application had been hindered by the tedious and time-consuming hand computations required. The availability of newly developed high speed electronic calculators (computers) in the 1960s changed that situation and allowed the increasingly wide application of multivariate statistics to clinical data.

Roth was among the earliest to apply these methods to demonstrate the validity of the distinction between endogenous and neurotic depression; an endogenous/depressive factor was often to be found as one of the solutions of factor analysis. Furthermore, when the items identified by factor analysis were arranged into a psychometric scale (the well-known Newcastle Scale) it formed a useful diagnostic test, which, when applied to various populations, produced what was interpreted as a bimodal distribution, further supporting the separation of endogenous from neurotic depression.

Within a few years, a large number of factor analytic studies of many clinical conditions were reported; schizophrenia and depression were the most widely studied conditions. The research on psychotic states, particularly by Lorr (1962), led to the development of standardised rating scales, the IMPS, from which Overall & Gorham (1962) developed the BPRS, which is the standard clinical assessment technique for psychotic patients, particularly those psychotic patients who are admitted to hospital.

Controversy was greatest in the area of depression. Disagreement followed, particularly from the London group. Robert Kendell, one of Lewis' most gifted students, undertook a series of comprehensive studies of psychopathology, including an important monograph on the nature of classification of depressive states (1968). Kendell and others challenged the extent to which multivariate statistical techniques generated objective and independent tests of psychopathologic hypotheses (1986). In particular, Kendell pointed to the opportunities for attitudes and theoretical biases of the investigators to enter into clinical judgements, selection of samples and interpretation of data (1988).

### Differential response to treatments

In parallel with these psychopathological investigations, studies were undertaken of the differential responses to somatic treatment, particularly to tricyclic antidepressants and to electroconvulsive therapy (ECT). Attempts were made to identify clinical features of depressed patients predictive of response to these biological treatments and to interpret these response patterns as validators of the clinical syndromes previously identified by clinical observation and by statistical investigations.

The most widely accepted result of this approach has been the association of positive response to tricyclic antidepressants with the symptom pattern of endogenous depression. Roland Kuhn (to be distinguished from Thomas Kuhn, the historian and philosopher of science), the Swiss psychiatrist, in reporting the first observations of the therapeutic effectiveness of imipramine, noted that patients with endogenous types of depression responded to tricyclics. Imipramine had been developed by Geigy Pharmaceutical Company in Switzerland as a potential neuroleptic because of its similarity in chemical structure to the phenothiazines. However, it was observed in early clinical trials that schizophrenic and other psychotic patients admitted to hospital were not benefited; in fact, some patients seemed to have intensification of their hallucinations, delusions and other psychotic symptoms, while patients with depressive features, described by Kuhn as "endogenous", seemed to respond. This observation led to investigation of the therapeutic uses of imipramine, which has become established as the standard antidepressant, and a subsequent large number of related tricyclic compounds have been developed.

Kiloh & Garside (1963), working with Roth at Newcastle, applied multivariate statistical techniques to symptom sets of patients being treated with tricyclics and reported that those patients who responded well to the tricyclic imipramine had clinical features usually interpreted as endogenous depression with emphasis on retardation, weight loss, sleep difficulty, and diurnal variation. This study contributed to the acceptance of the endogenous syndrome as the subtype of depression responsive to tricyclic and other biologic treatments and most likely to have a biological basis. The majority of studies undertaken to investigate the psychophysiology of depression, such as neuroendocrine studies and studies of the transmitter system, selected patients considered endogenous based on the assumption that within the heterogeneous group of depressive subjects, the endogenous subtype would be the form of depression most likely to exhibit biological correlation.

Similar approaches were also undertaken to predict response to ECT. The controversy about the effectiveness of ECT in the United Kingdom led to the development of randomised trials including the use of 'sham' ECT as a placebo control. Most notable is the Leicester ECT study undertaken by Brandon (1985), an associate of Roth at Newcastle, who had become professor of psychiatry at the new medical school in Leicester. The Leicester studies demonstrated the feasibility of placebo control, using 'sham ECT', and demonstrated that the efficacy of ECT was related to its electrophysiologic activity and not to placebo effects. They also identified delusional depressive features as predictive of possible response to ECT, which was cited as another source of evidence for the validity of subtyping depressive disorders, in this case the psychotic or delusional subtype.

Another set of observations concerning differential response to drug treatment was reported by clinicians in London at St Thomas's Hospital (Sargant, 1960) (West & Dally, 1959), who described the characteristics of patients responding to iproniazid, the first of the MAO inhibitor antidepressants. They observed that patients responding to MAO inhibitors had 'atypical' depression. Their clinical picture was different from endogenous depression, with the presence of anxiety and phobic symptoms and the absence of diurnal variation. This has led to an extensive clinical search for characteristics predictive of response to MAO inhibitors in depression (Nies *et al*, 1977). MAO inhibitors were also reported to be of value in phobic anxiety and agoraphobia (Sheehan *et al*, 1980; Tyrer, 1986).

The differential response to medication as a validator of diagnostic types has become a major theme in the work of Donald Klein in the United States. Klein has called this approach "pharmacologic dissection". He has elaborated the use of this approach to delineate different clinical syndromes responsive to medication, not only providing valuable guides in clinical decision making but also as providing possible clues for pathophysiology and aetiology mechanisms (Klein, 1981).

**Reaffirmation of Kraepelinian and 'medical' psychiatry**

These specific clinical and research activities were not isolated empiricism but rather the expression of a distinct point of view about the nature of psychopathology and psychiatry. British psychiatry through the 1940s and 1950s, like North American psychiatry, had been dominated by the ideas of Adolf Meyer and the psychobiological school (1957): the most influential British textbook had been that of Henderson & Gillespie (1927). Sir Aubrey Lewis became the leading British psychiatrist after World War II and organised the development of the Institute of Psychiatry at the University of London. He had studied with Meyer and adopted many of Meyer's ideas, particularly those in opposition to the Kraepelinian system. Whereas Adolf Meyer had written an intensive critique of Kraepelin's concept of dementia praecox, Lewis extended Meyer's approach to a critique of the concept of manic-depressive insanity and the Kraepelinian approach to depressions, particularly as represented in the concept of endogenous depression. Arguing against sharp splits between biological and environmental, he affirmed the importance of studying the individual case. He was one of the leaders of social psychiatry and the honorary director of the social psychiatry unit at the Maudsley, out of which came the pioneering work of John Wing (1980) and the other British social epidemiologists.

An alternative point of view was first articulated by Mayer-Gross, Slater & Roth (1954) in the first edition of their influential textbook. The introduction to this textbook was strongly critical of psychoanalysis, psychotherapy and social psychiatry and provided an aggressive reaffirmation of the Kraepelinian tradition, with emphasis on discrete nosologic categories, the importance of proper diagnosis and the role of genetic and constitutional factors in the aetiology of psychiatric disorders. Although subsequent editions edited by Roth were to soften the tone of criticism, the basic approach remained, with great emphasis on descriptive psychopathology, the careful assessment of patients' history and symptoms and the delineation of psychiatric disorders and, particularly within the group of depressions, the separation of endogenous from neurotic depression.

This work provided the intellectual background for the group led by Robins and Guze at Washington University at St Louis, whose activities in the US were to formulate the neo-Kraepelinian paradigm, culminating in the APA DSM–III (Akiskal *et al*, 1977) (Klerman, 1986).

## *The neo-Kraepelinian paradigm and DSM–III*

Although the Mayer-Gross, Slater and Roth textbook appeared in 1954, it had relatively little immediate impact upon North American psychiatry. In the decades immediately after World War II, descriptive psychopathology, diagnosis and classification were in disrepute. The concept of mental illness itself was challenged by antipsychiatry and by other critics, including the labelling theorists in social psychology and by the cultural relativists from anthropology and their allies in the developing countries.

Confronted by these challenges, groups within the US research community responded vigorously. By the late 1960s, there was a growing awareness among clinicians and researchers that the absence of an objective and reliable system for description of psychopathology and for diagnosis was limiting progress. In 1965, the NIMH Psychopharmacology Research Branch sponsored a conference on classification in psychiatry, noting the problems created by inadequate knowledge of diagnosis and classification (Cole *et al*, 1978).

Lehmann (1970), commenting on the long period of neglect of diagnosis, nosology and classification in North American psychiatry, predicted a renaissance of interest. His words were prophetic: within a few years the Washington University criteria for operational diagnosis were published, and, soon afterward, the Schedule for Affective Disorders and Schizophrenia (SADS) and Research Diagnostic Criteria (RDC) were developed by the NIMH Collaborative Program on Psychobiology of Depression (Katz & Klerman, 1979). A number of other developments occurred: the advance of new therapeutic modalities, especially the new psychopharmacologic agents, but also new behavioural and brief psychotherapeutic methods; the availability of high-speed electronic computers allowing management of large-scale data sets and the application of multivariate statistics; and the use of rating scales and other psychometric techniques for quantitative assessment of symptoms, behaviour and personality.

Biological treatments, notably psychopharmacologic drugs, were shown to be useful, not only in psychotic states (mania, paranoia, schizophrenia) but also in many neurotic conditions (obsessive/compulsive states, phobias, anxiety disorders). Findings from these therapeutic studies were related to family aggregation studies and pathophysiology research to suggest biological bases for many neurotic conditions and for some personality disorders. By themselves, however, these developments could not have constituted a paradigm shift. They created the climate for change, but did not define the nature of the change. That was to be the role of the 'neo-Kraepelinians'.

At this point, it is useful to apply Kuhn's theory of scientific progress. Kuhn proposes that scientific progress occurs when a new paradigm emerges to resolve an impasse or to solve a crisis. A crisis had occurred in psychopathology after World War II. The new paradigm that emerged in the early 1970s involved the reaffirmation of the concept of multiple discrete disorders and the use of operational criteria for making diagnostic judgments of a categorical (nosological) nature.

A large number of reliable and valid scales were developed in the late 1950s and 1960s, first for psychotic patients and then for depressed and anxious patients. Lorr, Klett, McNair & Lasky (1963), Hamilton (1960), Zung (1965), Beck (1969) and Overall & Gorham (1962) were the leaders in these efforts. There was active interchange among psychiatrists, clinical psychologists, pathophysiologists and psychopharmacologists. They were able to draw upon the extensive knowledge in psychometrics initially developed in the assessment of intelligence and other areas of educational and social performance, but gradually applied to psychopathology and abnormal behaviour from the late 1930s until 1950.

By the late 1960s, however, considerable difficulty was encountered because of the lack of reliable, valid and standardised techniques for individual patient diagnosis and for the selection of samples for research and treatment studies. Psychiatrists and other clinicians had been relying heavily on a categorical (nosological) approach, in contrast to the dimensional methods employed in rating scales and personality inventories. There was considerable dissatisfaction with existing diagnostic practices, both in clinical practice and in research, because of the evidence of the unreliability of existing psychiatric diagnoses.

The development of the new paradigm helped to resolve the 'crisis' of psychotic diagnoses. The operational criteria formulated by the Washington University-St Louis group and codified in the 1972 paper by Feighner and associates (Feighner *et al*, 1972) led the way for improved reliability and empirical tests of validity. Fleiss and associates (1972) developed the Kappa technique for quantifying diagnostic reliability and categorical judgements, and this technique was applied by Spitzer and associates to a wide range of data on psychopathology.

Considerable earlier progress in this area had been made by Wing and his associates in developing the Present State Examination (PSE) (Wing *et al*, 1974) which was adopted by the World Health Organization (WHO) in the International Pilot Study of Schizophrenia (IPSS) which demonstrated the feasibility of structured interviews for current mental status and the availability to train psychiatrists from many countries to achieve reliability in data gathering. The development of operational criteria constituted the main technical innovation of the new paradigm; operational criteria reduced the problems of reliability that paralysed research on psychopathology and diagnosis and classification through the 1950s and 1960s.

Although the neo-Kraepelinians tend to be most interested in biological, especially genetic, explanations for mental illnesses, a focus on a categorical (nosological) approach is not necessarily unique to the biological school of psychiatry. For example, Freud and many of his early followers, such as Abraham and Glover, proposed a classification of mental illness based on psychosexual stages of development. In current research and clinical practice, however, most neo-Kraepelinians emphasise the biological bases of mental disorders. As a group they are neutral, ambivalent (at times hostile) toward psychodynamic, interpersonal or social approaches.

## The impact of DSM–III

The DSM–III may be regarded as the culmination of the ' paradigm shift' that had taken place during the 1970s. Although Spitzer, the Chair of the APA Task Force that generated the DSM–III, has denied his personal inclination to be considered a neo-Kraepelinian, the approach to the DSM–III, particularly the emphasis on operational criteria, the elimination of the category of neurosis and the development of the multiaxial system represent ideas, concepts and methods from the neo-Kraepelinian paradigm.

The DSM–III has been criticised from many sources. The psychoanalysts were critical of the elimination of neurosis as a diagnostic category and abandonment of psychodynamic conflict as causative of anxiety neuroses and other states. Psychologists, social workers and other mental health professionals were cautious and sceptical lest the DSM–III represent an attempt on the part of psychiatrists to assert professional dominance. One of the controversial issues was whether the conditions in the DSM–III should be regarded as 'medical disorders', as distinct from mental disorders. The DSM–III has proven a major challenge to the World Health Organization's Official ICD classification. Many European psychiatrists have been critical that the US APA did not accept the WHO-ICD-9 (1977), but chose to proceed independently. Nevertheless, the DSM–III has been translated into many languages and many of the features novel to the DSM–III are to be incorporated in the proposed draft of the World Health Organization International Classification of Disorders 10th ed. (ICD-10).

After the promulgation of the DSM–III, the new paradigm became the standard and a period followed which Kuhn called "normal science". There was expansion of structured interviews and application to epidemiology, family/genetics, follow-up studies and a marked increase in research on personality disorders as conceptualised in axis II.

## Current disputes

Viewed from the vantage point of the late 1980s, the issues with which Roth and his colleagues in the Newcastle school grappled in the 1960s are still current, although they have taken on new forms. In large part, the current disputes have been prompted by the DSM–III and the reactions to those proposals. Four areas of dispute are:

  (a) 'neuroses' as a diagnostic category
  (b) separations within the category of anxiety disorders
  (c) separations within the category of mood disorders
  (d) the concept of mixed anxiety and depression.

### The value of neuroses

Nineteenth century neuropsychiatry had defined a group of organic conditions; the remaining conditions were called 'non-organic,' or, more often, 'functional'. There was ambiguity in the term 'functional'. Originally, it referred to conditions due to presumed biological changes in the central nervous system, but which were not apparent by the usual histopathologic means. Hence, the impairment was in the functioning, rather than in the structure of the nervous system. Later, the term became synonymous with conditions presumed to be due to environmental or non-biological causes.

Further, the functional disorders have usually been subdivided according to the psychotic-neurotic distinction. The criteria for the distinction between psychotic and neurotic states were formulated at the turn of the century in the writings of Freud and Kraepelin. Freud, in particular, wrote a series of influential papers correlating the differences between neurotic and psychotic states with symptoms, type of psychological impairment, and, from the psychodynamic point of view, level of regression and extent of loss of secondary process and manifestation of primary process thinking.

The psychotic/neurotic distinction had considerable appeal: it simultaneously combined five aspects of psychopathology: descriptive symptoms, causation, psycho-dynamics, justification for hospital admission, and treatment recommendation.

The psychotic disorders had in common impairment of higher mental faculties, as manifested by hallucinations, delusions, disorientation and impairment of perception, memory and thought. It was presumed they were due to constitutional (biological) causes—either hereditary, biochemical or physiological—and provided justification of hospital admission, and, if necessary, involuntary hospital admission and commitment. Where treatments were available, these would usually be somatic (biological) treatments, such as lobotomy, electric convulsive treatment and the psychopharmacologic agents which became available in the 1950s.

In contrast, the neurotic conditions were characterised by the absence of impairment of higher mental faculties and by the patient's subjective experience of distress, which often provided the impetus for the patient to seek medical care.

It was generally agreed that the neurotic conditions were due to learning and experience, the two dominant aetiologic theories being conditioning and psychodynamics. Moreover, treatment seldom required prolonged stays in hospital but, rather, some form of out-patient psychotherapy—individual, group, family—based either on behavioural, psychodynamic or interpersonal principles.

In the US, the major opposition to the elimination of the concept of neurotic disorders has come from within the psychoanalytic community (Klerman *et al*, 1984). Whereas DSM–II had incorporated strong features of the psychodynamic concept that neurotic symptoms were more the manifestation of unconscious mental conflict than defences against anxiety, the DSM–III, in the attempt to be atheoretical with regard to the causation of specific disorders, explicitly eliminated the concept of neurosis because it was, in the opinion of the formulators of DSM–III, too tied to the psychodynamic theory symptom formation.

In contrast, many leading British psychopathologists have argued for the validity and utility of the category of neurosis. While not accepting the psychodynamic theory of symptom formation, nevertheless they feel there is a strong unity to the neurotic symptom process caused by a neurotic hereditary constitution and the learning of maladaptive patterns of social and personality functioning. Thus, Tyrer (1984), Sims (1986) and Roth (1984) have argued against the elimination of the category of neurotic disorders and the draft of the ICD-10 does continue its category of neurotic disorders, although not as prominently as in the ICD-8 and ICD-9.

### Divisions within the group of anxiety disorders

In addition to abolishing the general concept of neurotic disorders, the DSM–III established a separate category of anxiety disorders, and included within this category the separation of panic anxiety from generalised anxiety. This has also been one of the controversial features of the DSM–III and an issue which has divided American and British psychiatrists. This US-UK split was based upon British studies of psychopathology and the efficacy of MAO inhibitors in the treatment of atypical depression and phobic anxiety disorders. A major point at issue is the continuity and discontinuity between panic anxiety and other forms of anxiety and the potential unique nature of panic anxiety.

Related to the dispute over the status of generalised anxiety has been the controversy regarding the relationship between panic disorder and agoraphobia. According to Klein's theory (Klein, 1981), agoraphobia is a conditioned, learned reaction to spontaneous panic attacks; a view that has been adopted by many clinicians and researchers who hold that agoraphobia does not occur without history of current or past panic disorder.

The most intense disputes regarding this relationship have come from proponents of behaviour therapy (Marks, 1987). Opinions on the psycho-pathologic and diagnostic issues are confounded by opinions as to the relative value of pharmacologic and behavioural treatments for these conditions. Biologically oriented psychiatrists, such as Klein and Sheehan, emphasise the primacy of the panic attack and its discontinuity from normal anxiety and attribute the predisposition to panic attacks to a genetically determined endogenous/ biochemical abnormality and, consequently, justify the use of medications. In contrast, behaviourally oriented psychiatrists and psychologists, such as Marks and Foa, interpret the panic attack as a continuum of severity along with 'normal' and 'generalised' anxiety and do not regard the panic attack as the driving force in the pathogenesis of phobic avoidance, particularly in agoraphobia. They emphasise the therapeutic value of behavioural and cognitive-behavioural techniques, not only for the treatment of agoraphobic avoidance (Marks, 1983), but also for the treatment of panic attacks (Schear & Barlow, 1988).

## Divisions within the group of 'mood disorders'

In the 1960s and 1970s, the most intense controversies were in regard to the best methods for subdividing depressive disorders, particularly the dualistic theories around the endogenous-neurotic depression. In the 1980s, the source of controversy seemed most intense around the anxiety disorders. The DSM–III was the first diagnostic system to designate the affective disorders as a separate category. This has been accepted in the draft of the ICD-10, although the title of the group of disorders has been modified from Affective Disorders to Mood Disorders. The separation between psychotic and neurotic forms of depression, which appears in ICD-8 and ICD-9, does not appear in ICD-10. The ICD-10 section on mood disorders is very close to that of the DSM–III and the DSM–III-R.

There is wide agreement on the heterogeneity of the mood disorders and the likelihood that there are multiple aetiologies. Individual conditions have varying mixtures of genetic, environmental, and medical causes. The best accepted distinction is the bipolar distinction, but the validity of psychotic/delusional types of depression has been widely accepted, particularly as it predicts response to ECT as well as the continued reliability of the endogenous concept.

In the DSM–III-R, the concept of endogenous depression was modified into that of melancholic depression. The controversies around the validity of endogenous/melancholic depression persists, not only with regard to predictive value for differential response to treatment, but with regard to biological marker, particularly the extensive amount of research devoted to the dexamethasone depression test (DST).

## Mixed anxiety and depression

A number of investigators have undertaken studies of psychiatric morbidity among patients seen in general medical settings, particularly in general practice (UK) and primary care (US). The pioneering work in this endeavour was by Shepherd and his associates in their studies of London (Shepherd *et al*, 1966), out of which came the work of Goldberg in his studies of psychiatric problems in general practice patients in Manchester. These studies demonstrated a high prevalence of psychiatric symptoms and morbidity in patients seeking medical assistance from general practitioners. As part of the methodologic advances in these investigations, Goldberg developed the General Health Questionnaire (GHQ) (Goldberg, 1978; 1979).

Previous work in the military mainly during World War II, had made use of similar instruments, such as the Cornell Medical Index and the Health Opinion

Survey (HOS). These were extensively studied for reliability and discriminant validity using psychometric techniques; however, the Goldberg GHQ has become the most widely used mode of assessing psychiatric morbidity in general medical settings. Investigations using the GHQ and similar techniques have documented high rates of psychiatric morbidity, often manifested in anxiety and depression symptoms. These symptoms were usually unrecognised and untreated by the general physician, who tends to interpret patients' complaints in terms of traditional medical diagnoses. These studies, showing high degrees of association between anxiety and depression, questioned the clinical value as well as the epidemiologic validity of psychiatric diagnostic systems which attempted to identify discrete syndromes.

Goldberg has extended his use of new multivariate statistics and recently reported the application of latent trait analyses to the problem of anxiety and depression (Grayson *et al*, 1987) (Goldberg *et al*, 1987). Goldberg continues the application of multivariate techniques originated by the Newcastle group, but now applies more advanced techniques, particularly those derived from Rausch, concluding that the use of latent trait analysis shows high degrees of correlation between anxiety and depression (in the range of 0.7) and substantiates the criteria strongly advocated by Kendell.

## Conclusions

The relationship of anxiety and depression has preoccupied psychiatry for almost one hundred years. As new technologies and new treatments have become available, they have been applied to the unity or separation of these two conditions.

The work of Roth and his associates in the use of multivariate statistical techniques, in the investigation of response to treatments as validators or diagnostic distinctions, and in the reaffirmation, through modification, of the Kraepelinian point of view set the standards after World War II for the research and treatment of these mental illnesses. Current efforts are refining the solutions he and his associates fashioned.

## Acknowledgements

This contribution is supported in part by grants RO1 MH 43044 and UO1 MH 43077 from the Anxiety and Affective Disorders Research Branch, Division of Clinical Research, National Institute of Mental Health, Alcohol, Drug Abuse, Mental Health Administration, Public Health Service, Department of Health and Human Services, Washington, DC. Gratitude is expressed for the contribution of Lorraine Lubin in the development of this manuscript.

## References

AKISKAL, H. S., DJENDEREDJIAN, A. H., ROSENTHAL, R. H. & KHANI, M. K. (1977) Cyclothymic disorder: validating criteria for inclusion in the bipolar affective group. *American Journal of Psychiatry*, **134**, 1227–1233.

AMERICAN PSYCHIATRIC ASSOCIATION (1980) *Diagnostic and Statistical Manual of Mental Disorders*, 3rd edn. *(DSM-III)*, Washington, DC: APA.

BRANDON, S., COWLEY, P., MCDONALD, C., NEVILLE, P., PALMER R. & WELLSTOOD-EASON, S. (1984) Electro-convulsive therapy: results in depressive illness from the Leicester trial. *British Medical Journal*, **288**, 22-25.

——, ——, ——, ——, —— & —— (1985) Leicester ECT trial: results in schizophrenia. *British Journal of Psychiatry*, **146**, 177-183.

BECK, A. T. (1969) *Depression: Clinical, Experimental and Theoretical Aspects*. New York: Harper & Row.

COLE, J. O., SCHATZBERG, A. F. & FRAZIER, S. H. (1978) *Depression: Biology, Psychodynamics and Treatment*. New York: Plenum Press.

FEIGHNER, J., ROBINS, E., GUZE, S. B., WOODRUFF, R. J., WINOKUR, G. & MUNOZ, R. (1972) Diagnostic criteria for use in psychiatric research. *Archives of General Psychiatry*, **26**, 57-63.

FLEISS, J. L., SPITZER, R. L., ENDICOTT, J., et al (1972) Quantification of agreement in multiple psychiatric diagnoses. *Ibid.* **26**, 168-171.

GILLESPIE, R. D. (1929) The clinical differentiation of types of depression. *Guy's Hospital Reports*, **79**, 306-344.

GOLDBERG, D. P. (1978) *Manual of the General Health Questionnaire*. London: NFER Publishing.

—— (1979) Training family physicians in mental health skills: implications of recent findings. Paper presented at the Institute of Medicine Conference on Primary Care, Washington, DC.

——, BRIDGES, K., DUNCAN-JONES, P. & GRAYSON, D. A. (1987) Dimensions of neuroses seen in primary-care settings. *Psychological Medicine*, **17**, 461-470.

GRAYSON, D. A., BRIDGES, K., DUNCAN-JONES, P. & GOLDBERG, D. P. (1987) The relationship between symptoms and diagnosis of minor psychiatric disorder in general practice. *Ibid.*, **17**, 933-942.

HAMILTON, M. A. (1960) A rating scale for depression. *Journal of Neurology, Neurosurgery & Psychiatry*. **23**, 56-62.

HAND, I. & WITTCHEN, H. U. (eds) (1986) *Panic and Phobias*. New York: Springer.

HENDERSON, D. K. & GILLESPIE, R. D. (1927) *A Textbook for Students and Practitioners*. London: Oxford University Press.

KATZ, M. & KLERMAN, G. L. (1979) Introduction: Overview of the clinical studies program. *American Journal of Psychiatry*, **136**, 49-51.

KENDELL, R. E. (1968) *The Classification of Depressive Illnesses*. Maudsley Monograph No 18, New York: Oxford University Press.

—— (1986) What are mental disorders? In *Issues in Psychiatric Classification* (eds A. M. Freedman, R. Brotman, I. Silverson & D. Hutson) New York: Human Sciences Press.

—— (1988) What is a case? Food for thought for epidemiologists. *Archives of General Psychiatry*, **45**, 374-376.

KILOH, L. G. & GARSIDE, R. F. (1963) The independence of neurotic depression and endogenous depression. *British Journal of Psychiatry*, **109**, 451-463.

KLEIN, D. F. & DAVIES, J. M. (1980) *Diagnosis and Drug Treatment of Psychiatric Disorders: Adults and Children*. 2nd edition. Baltimore: Williams & Wilkins.

—— (1981) Anxiety reconceptualized. In *Anxiety: New Research and Changing Concepts* (eds D. F. Klein & J. G. Rabkin) pp. 235-263. New York: Raven Press.

—— (1988) Letter to the Editor. *Archives of General Psychiatry*, **45**, 387-388.

KLERMAN, G. L. (1979) The psychobiology of affective states: the legacy of Adolf Meyer. In *Research in the Psychobiology of Human Behavior*. (eds E. Meyer & J. Bradley) pp. 115-131. Baltimore: Johns Hopkins University Press.

—— (1983) The significance of DSM-III in American psychiatry. In *International Perspectives on DSM-III* (eds R. L. Spitzer, J. B. W. Williams & A. E. Skodal) pp. 3-25. Washington, DC: American Psychiatric Press.

——, SPITZER, R. L., VAILLANT, G. & MICHELS, R. (1984) A debate on DSM-III. *American Journal of Psychiatry*, **141**, 539-553.

—— (1986) Historical perspective on contemporary schools of psychopathology. In *Contemporary Directions in Psychopathology* (eds T. Millon & G. L. Klerman) pp. 3-28, New York: Guildford Press.

KRAEPELIN, E. (1921) *Manic-Depressive Insanity and Paranoia*. Translated M. Barclay, Edinburgh: Livingstone.

KUHN, T. (1970) *The Structure of Scientific Revolutions*. (2nd ed.) Vol 2, No 2. Chicago: University of Chicago Press.

LEHMANN, H. (1970) Epidemiology of depressive disorders. In *Depression in the 1970s* (ed. R. R. Fieve) New York: Excerpta Medica.

LEWIS, A. (1930) *Investigation into the Clinical Features of Melancholia*. MD Thesis: University of Adelaide.

—— (1934a) Melancholia: a historical review. *Journal of Mental Science*, **80**, 1–142.

—— (1934b) Melancholia: a clinical survey of depressive states. *Ibid.*, **80**, 277–378.

LORR, M., KLETT, C. J., MCNAIR, D. M., & LASKEY, J. J. (1963) *Manual: In-Patient Multi-Dimensional Psychiatric Scale (IMPS)*. Palo Alto, CA: Consulting Psychologists Press.

——, MCNAIR, D. M., KLETT, C. J. & LASKEY, J. J. (1962) Evidence of ten psychiatric syndromes. *Journal of Consulting Psychology*, **26**, 185–189.

MARKS, I. M. (1983) Panic attacks in phobia treatment studies. *Archives of General Psychiatry*, **40**, 1150–1152.

—— (1987) *Fears, Phobias and Rituals*. Oxford: Oxford University Press.

MAYER-GROSS, W., SLATER, E. & ROTH, M. (1954) *Clinical Psychiatry*. Baltimore: Williams & Wilkins.

MEYER, A. (1957) *Psychobiology: a Science of Man*. Springfield, Ill: Charles C. Thomas.

NIES, A., ROBINSON, D. S., BARTLETT, D. & LAMBORN, K. R. (1977) MAO inhibitors in clinical practice: principles based on recent research. *Psychopharmacology Bulletin*. **13**, 54.

OVERALL, J. E. & GORHAM, D. P. (1962) The brief psychiatric rating scale. *Psychological Reports*. **10**, 799–812.

ROTH, M. (1960) The phobic anxiety-depersonalisation syndrome and some general aetiological problems in psychiatry. *Journal of Neuropsychiatry*, **1**, 293–306.

—— & MYERS, D. H. (1969) Anxiety neuroses and phobic states. II. Diagnosis and management. *British Medical Journal*, **1**, 559.

—— (1984) Agoraphobia, panic disorder and generalized anxiety disorder: some implications of recent advances. *Psychiatric Developments*, **2**, 31–52.

—— & KROLL, J. (1987) *The Reality of Mental Illness*. Cambridge: Cambridge University Press.

SARGANT, W. (1960) Some newer drugs in the treatment of depression and their relation to other somatic treatments. *Psychosomatics*, **1**, 14–17.

SCHAPIRA, K., ROTH, M., KERR, T. A. & GURNEY, C. (1972) The prognosis of affective disorders: the differentiation of anxiety states from depressive states. *British Journal of Psychiatry*, **121**, 175–181.

SCHEAR, M. K. & BARLOW, D. (eds) (1988) Panic Disorder Section: *Annual Review of Psychiatry*, Vol 8. Washington, DC: American Psychiatric Press.

SHEEHAN, D. V., BALLENGER, J. C. & JACOBSON, G. (1980) Treatment of endogenous anxiety with phobic, hysterical and hypochondriacal symptoms. *Archives of General Psychiatry*, **37**, 51–57.

—— (1982) Current concepts in psychiatry: panic attacks and phobias. *New England Journal of Medicine*, **307**, 156–158.

SHEPHERD, M., COOPER, B. & BROWN, A. C. (1966) *Psychiatric Illness in General Practice*. London: Oxford University Press.

SIMS, A. (1986) Perspectives in the study of neuroses in contemporary psychiatric practice. *Psychiatric Developments*, **4**, 273–288.

SPITZER, R. L., ENDICOTT, J. & ROBINS, E. (1978) Research diagnostic criteria: rationale and reliability. *Archives of General Psychiatry*, **35**, 773–782.

TYRER, P. (1984) Neurosis divisible. *Lancet*, *i*, 685–688.

—— (1986) Classification of anxiety disorders. *Journal of Anxiety Disorders*, **11**, 99–104.

WEST, E. D. & DALLY, P. J. (1959) Effects of iproniazid in depressive syndromes. *British Medical Journal*, **1**, 1491–1494.

WING, J., COOPER, J. & SARTORIUS, N. (1974) *The Measurement and Classification of Psychiatric Symptoms*. Cambridge: Cambridge University Press.

—— (1980) Social psychiatry in the United Kingdom: the approach to schizophrenia. *Schizophrenia Bulletin*, **6**, 556–565.

WORLD HEALTH ORGANIZATION (1973) *The International Pilot Study of Schizophrenia*. Geneva: WHO.

—— (1977) *International Classification of Diseases*, 9th ed. (ICD-9) Geneva: WHO.

ZUNG, W. W. (1965) A self-rating depression scale. *Archives of General Psychiatry*, **12**, 63–76.

# 10 Subcategories of depression

## GIOVANNI B. CASSANO, assisted by Laura Musetti and Giulio Perugi

The identification of new drugs that are effective in treating mood disorders has led to clearer conceptualisation and more accurate diagnosis. The usefulness of previous dichotomous classifications of depression was linked to a temporal dimension, the obsolescence of the endogeneous-reactive dichotomy was followed by that of the psychotic-neurotic (Klerman *et al*, 1979; Akiskal *et al*, 1978), since then, even the bipolar-unipolar distinction has been challenged by several investigators (Gershon *et al*, 1982; Taylor & Abrahms, 1980; Akiskal, 1983).

In a cross-sectional evaluation of major depressive episode (MDE), DSM–III criteria provide distinctions between melancholia and non-melancholia, between psychotic and non-psychotic features, and between congruous and incongruous prevailing mood. Psychotic features and incongruous mood (Leckman *et al*, 1984), and atypical depression (Quitkin *et al*, 1979) in particular, may be relevant to a definition of the effectiveness of new drugs. Moreover, the DSM–III criteria tell us little about the longitudinal characteristics of depressive disorders, except the unipolar-bipolar distinction.

Coupling lithium salts with the bipolar disorder had a greater reinforcing effect upon the original unipolar-bipolar distinction proposed by Leonhard (1957), Angst (1966), and Perris (1966) than the present array of contradictory, clinical, psychopathological, and biological findings (Depue & Monroe, 1978; Angst *et al*, 1979; Angst, 1981; Gershon *et al*, 1982; Goodwin & Jamison, 1984; Nurnberger & Gershon, 1984).

Growing knowledge about the limitations of long-term tricyclic antidepressant (TCA) treatments and the availability of new compounds such as carbamazepine, valproic acid, and calcium antagonists for long-term prevention has led to a reconsideration of the spectrum of mood disorders. A current, unitarian view is based on the course of illness characteristics; it stresses the roles of both polarity and periodicity as unifying diagnostic dimensions for the affective disorders (Akiskal, 1983). As a result, the boundaries of mood disorders are undergoing a redefinition which necessarily entails a significant change in our concept of other disorders.

The clinical domain of the mood disorders has expanded in most directions, especially into the traditional rubrics of the schizoaffective and schizophrenic disorders (Clayton, 1986) and the personality disorders (Akiskal, 1986, 1987). Besides this, 'mixed states', which were sometimes misdiagnosed, are now usually recognised as affective disorders.

The exceptions have been the anxiety, somatoform and adjustment disorders. DSM–III (1980) defined these more accurately, and sharpened the distinctions between them and the genuine mood disorders. In this field, a very important contribution has been made by the studies of Sir Martin Roth and the Newcastle group; these authors showed that there is a clear distinction between clinical groups of anxious and depressed patients in terms of clinical symptoms, personality, treatment response, course and prognosis (Roth *et al*, 1972; Schapira *et al*, 1972). Though several overlapping areas have still to be thoroughly explored, anxiety and mood disorders may now be considered independent nosographic entities.

The current diagnostic definition of MDE made by DSM–III, however, remains overly broad, since it probably includes several subcategories of mood disorder. The major empirical justification for such over-inclusive classification is that most MDE respond favourably and predictably to TCA or electro-convulsive treatment (ECT).

Because the criteria for a diagnosis of MDE may separate genuine from nongenuine primary mood disorders, they can be regarded as a tool for identifying a population for further research. Subsequent studies can then aim to isolate discrete clinical subtypes within a diagnosis of MDE. Such attempts may include pharmacological dissection, identification of biological markers, or clinical and psychopathological descriptive classification. This last approach has been utilised in the studies carried out at the Institute of Psychiatry, Pisa University (Italy). These studies had three major aims: to define MDE more clearly; to identify homogeneous subcategories within MDE; to assess both preepisodic and postepisodic temperamental profiles and to evaluate symptom patterns and social adjustment during the interepisode intervals. The methodology involved an examination of depression that considered the affective disorder in its longitudinal perspective, including abnormalities of temperament, full-blown manifest symptomatology, residual symptoms, and social adjustment.

Several previous studies (Prien, 1978; Angst, 1981; Dunner, 1983; Squillace *et al*, 1984; Coryell & Winokur, 1984; Winokur, 1986) used both cross-sectional and longitudinal approaches in attempts to classify affective disorders and to distinguish between depressive states. Variability in the symptomatology and the course of these disorders and differences between clinical settings, and the methodologies applied in them, were all factors leading to differences between the various patient samples and, therefore, to discrepancies between results.

In planning the study reported here, it was assumed that the presence of MDE would identify the most common and most easily assessable index episode. By taking MDE as the index episode we were enabled:

(a) to explore most of the range of mood disorders
(b) to ascertain the genuine nature of the mood disorder
(c) to identify the most common population of patients
(d) to identify groups most often selected for clinical trials.

## The study

The sample comprised 405 depressive patients (364 out-patients and 41 in-patients) who met the DSM–III-R Draft (1985) criteria for MDE. In order to

TABLE I
*Diagnosis distribution of 405 patients with major depressive episode*

|  | Number | % |
|---|---|---|
| Bipolar I | 25 | 6.2 |
| Bipolar II | 107 | 26.4 |
| Bipolar III | 5 | 1.2 |
| Recurrent | 174 | 43.0 |
| Single episode | 94 | 23.2 |

obtain a homogeneous sample of primary affective disorders, patients were excluded if they suffered from organic mental disorder, psychoactive substance use disorder, chronic and incapacitating physical illness, or mood disorder concomitant with panic, obsessive-compulsive, phobic, somatoform, and eating disorders.

The sample included 128 (31.6%) males and 277 (68.4%) females. Their mean age was 50.6 (s.d. = 13.8). Table I shows the diagnostic subcategories in our sample.

The Semistructured Interview for Depression, SID, (Cassano *et al*, 1988) was developed to diagnose MDE (DSM–III-R Draft) and to collect anamnestic data concerning the course of illness, the family history, temperament characteristics, the residual and interval phenomena, and the response to previous treatments. The SID also incorporates a decision tree paradigm to identify five subtypes of MDE:

    (a) typical bipolar I
    (b) bipolar II, defined according to whether MDE preceded, or was followed by, hyperthymia or hypomania
    (c) bipolar III, comprising patients not meeting bipolar I or II criteria but who have first-degree relatives with bipolar disorders
    (d) recurrent unipolar depression—cases with neither hyperthymia nor hypomania
    (e) single episode depression.

The last diagnosis is, to some degree, a residual category.

Our criteria differed somewhat from prior studies. Dunner *et al* (1976a) and Gershon *et al* (1982) categorised depressed patients as bipolar I only if they required prior admission to hospital for mania. The SID definition of bipolar II includes not only hypomanic episodes but also the presence of hyperthymic temperament. We classified either spontaneously or pharmacologically induced hypomania as bipolar II because of the difficulty in determining exact relationships between hypomanic switches and treatment events. Others have regarded only spontaneous hypomania as bipolar II (Akiskal, 1983). We also considered temperamental hyperthymia alternating with short swings of subclinical magnitude in the depressive direction (cyclothymia) as a bipolar II condition.

The terminology 'temperament' was adopted following Kraepelin (1921) to emphasise the weighting of the premorbid subclinical features. In fact, evidence of increased activity and elevated mood in an expansive direction is not always paralleled by forms of behaviour commonly recognised as pathological. Other researchers too have stressed the importance of premorbid hyperthymic temperamental traits in reaching decisions about the pharmacological treatment of depression (Kukopulos *et al*, 1983; Akiskal, 1986, 1987).

In addition to the SID, we used a separate form to collect additional anamnestic and demographic data. For the assessment of symptomatology, psychiatrists completed the Hamilton Psychiatric Rating Scale for Depression (HAM-D) and the Retardation Rating Scale (RRS) of Widlocher (1983), and patients completed the Hopkins Symptoms Checklist (HSCL-90).

The statistical methods included ANOVA followed by Neuman-Keuls comparisons of pairs of means for the continuous dimensional variables, and Chi-square for the categorical data.

## The findings

*Bipolar I* The bipolar I group was a clearly distinguishable 6.2% of the total sample; the selection of patients on the basis of MDE as the index episode probably reduced the percentage of bipolar I and increased that of bipolar II and of recurrent unipolar. Consistent with previous reports (Beigel & Murphy, 1971; Depue & Monroe, 1978; Angst, 1981; Gershon *et al*, 1982; Akiskal, 1983; Coryell *et al*, 1985), they had an earlier age at onset, more prior depressive episodes, more hospital stays and the youngest age at their first admission to hospital. (Table II). Bipolar I depression is clearly identified by these findings as the most severe form. It also has the highest rate of suicidal attempts (Table III); this finding appears to be consistent with some previous reports (Perris, 1966; Johnson & Hunt, 1979). On the other hand, Dunner *et al* (1976b) and Dunner (1987) found the highest suicidal rate in bipolar II depression, but Dunner's requirement of hospital admittance for mania for a bipolar I diagnosis may have resulted in classifying cases that were really bipolar I as bipolar II.

The bipolar I chronicity rate (current duration of present episode over two years), was quite close to that for bipolar II and recurrent unipolar depression (Table III). Bipolar I had a higher rate of complete remission between episodes than recurrent unipolar, the lowest presence of reported stressors during the six months preceding the episode, and the most frequent onset of pharmacologic hypomania. The prevalence of the melancholic features was no greater than that observed in bipolar II or in recurrent unipolar (Table IV).

TABLE II

| *Age, age at onset, prior treatment, and characteristics of affective disorder by diagnostic group* | | | | | | |
|---|---|---|---|---|---|---|
| *Diagnostic group* | *B1* | *B2* | *R* | *SE* | | |
| | *M* | *M* | *M* | *M* | *F* | |
| Age | 44.0 | 49.4 | 52.3 | 50.4 | 3.12* | B1 < R |
| Age at onset | 28.4 | 35.7 | 36.6 | 48.7 | 24.13*** | B1 < B2, R < SE |
| Length of the illness | 15.6 | 13.7 | 15.7 | 1.7 | 40.9*** | SE < B2, B1, R |
| Number of depressive episodes | 7.8 | 4.8 | 5.4 | — | 3.08* | B2, R < B1 |
| Number of manic episodes | 2.5 | — | — | — | | |
| Number of hospital stays | 4.2 | 1.3 | 1.5 | 0.2 | 15.5*** | SE < B2, R < B1 |
| (Number) | (25) | (107) | (174) | (94) | | |
| Age 1st hospital stay | 29.1 | 36.8 | 38.1 | 47.3 | 5.19** | B1 < B2, R < SE |
| (Number) | (16) | (45) | (80) | (16) | | |

B1 = Bipolar I, B2 = Bipolar II, R = Recurrent, SE = Single episode
*P < 0.05
**P < 0.01
***P < 0.001

TABLE III
*Chronic course, hypomania, temperament, interepisodic characteristics, and stressors by diagnostic group*

| Diagnostic group | B1 | B2 | R | SE | | |
|---|---|---|---|---|---|---|
| | % | % | % | % | $X^2$ | df |
| Chronic course (>24 months) | 12.0 | 13.1 | 12.1 | 25.5 | 9.49* | 3 |
| Hypomania | 64.0 | 65.4 | — | — | 0.01 | 1 |
| Pharmacologic hypomania | 36.0 | 21.5 | — | — | 1.60 | 1 |
| Hyperthymic temperament | 20.0 | 46.7 | — | — | 4.90* | 1 |
| Depressive temperament | 36.0 | 15.0 | 51.7 | 39.4 | 38.15*** | 3 |
| Suicide attempts | 32.0 | 12.1 | 13.2 | 4.3 | 15.05** | 3 |
| 'Stressors' | 44.0 | 55.7 | 49.4 | 66.0 | 7.95* | 3 |
| (Number) | (25) | (107) | (174) | (94) | | |
| Complete remission between episodes | 62.5 | 62.2 | 48.9 | — | 5.00 | 2 |
| (Number) | (25) | (90) | (174) | | | |

B1 = Bipolar I, B2 = Bipolar II, R = Recurrent, SE = Single episode
*$P<0.05$; **$P<0.01$; ***$P<0.001$

TABLE IV
*Melancholia and psychotic features*

| Diagnostic group | B1 | B2 | R | SE | | |
|---|---|---|---|---|---|---|
| | % | % | % | % | $X^2$ | df |
| Melancholia | 64.0 | 82.2 | 81.0 | 42.6 | 52.87*** | 3 |
| Psychotic features | | | | | | |
| Congruent | 8.0 | 7.5 | 7.5 | 5.3 | 0.54 | 3 |
| Incongruent | 0.0 | 2.8 | 1.1 | 0.0 | 3.61 | 3 |
| (Number) | (25) | (107) | (174) | (94) | | |

B = Bipolar I, B2 = Bipolar II, R = Recurrent, SE = Single Episode
***$P<0.001$

*Bipolar II* This group made up 26.4% of the total sample; it has acquired special clinical importance because of the accumulating evidence in favour of positive lithium or carbamazepine response, and because of reports that long-term high dosages of TCA drugs may trigger continuous cyclicity (Wehr & Goodwin, 1979; Lerer *et al*, 1980; Oppenheim, 1982; Kukopulos *et al*, 1983, 1985). Diagnostically bipolar II occupies an intermediate position between bipolar I and recurrent unipolar, but it appears to be a quite stable category (Coryell *et al*, 1984; Endicott *et al*, 1985) and not a transitional stage.

In our sample, age at onset for bipolar II was significantly above that for bipolar I (Table II), suggesting an attenuated, late onset type of bipolar illness. They had a younger age at onset, however, than recurrent unipolar. The sex distribution in bipolar II was closer to bipolar I than to recurrent unipolar (Table V). The bipolar II group, in fact, had the highest percentage of males of all groups, and, in this respect, differed most from recurrent unipolar.

The bipolar II group was also consistently intermediate between bipolar I and recurrent unipolar depression in the number of depressive episodes, suicidal attempts, and complete interepisode remissions (Table III). They shared temperamental hypomanic features and pharmacologic response patterns with bipolar I.

These findings, which apparently confirm the bipolar-unipolar dichotomy, can explain why other studies have assimilated bipolar II either to bipolar I (Angst *et al*, 1980) or to recurrent unipolar (Dunner *et al*, 1976a). Considered in detail,

TABLE V
*Sex distribution*

| Diagnostic group | B1 | B2 | R | SE | Total |
|---|---|---|---|---|---|
| | % | % | % | % | % |
| Male | 40.0 | 43.9 | 22.4 | 33.0 | 31.8 |
| Female | 60.0 | 56.1 | 77.6 | 67.0 | 68.3 |

$\chi^2 = 15.17$ ($P < 0.01$)
B1 = Bipolar I, B2 = Bipolar II, R = Recurrent, SE = Single episode

the data support an intermediate or bridge position for bipolar II between typical bipolar I and typical recurrent unipolar (Akiskal, 1983).

*Bipolar III* Only five patients (1.2%) met the bipolar III criteria—too few for meaningful analysis. An unknown number may have been unrecognised due to the difficulty of obtaining valid family histories for the full range of manic states. Any such unrecognised bipolar III disorders would have been misclassified by our methods as unipolar recurrent or single episode. On the other hand, it is quite possible that there may be a very low percentage of patients who fail to show either hypomanic episodes or hyperthymic temperament but who have a positive family history for bipolar disorders. In other words, bipolar III may be very rare.

*Recurrent unipolar* Nearly half (43%) of the sample had recurrent unipolar depression. This percentage was perhaps increased by the selection of a MDE as the index episode. They had the highest proportion of women (Table V), and they were the oldest (Table II). Age at onset, however, was about the same as bipolar II. They were also like bipolar II, and unlike bipolar I, with respect to age at first hospital admittance and number of hospital stays. Recurrent unipolar had the smallest proportion of complete remission between episodes, and they had the highest prevalence of lifelong depressive temperament (Table III). Thus, recurrent depression and depressive temperament are mostly associated with females, while mania, hypomania, and hyperthymic temperament are mostly associated with males. It is possible that in some patients depressive temperaments actually represented a chronic dysthymic disorder, such patients who display a superimposed MDE are sometimes described as having double depression (Keller & Shapiro, 1982; Keller *et al*, 1983).

*Single episode* Subjects with single episodes represented 23.2% of the total sample. It is not possible, of course, to know which of these patients may have subsequent episodes of either depression or mania. These depressed patients had a later onset (Table II), a higher rate of chronicity, a higher prevalence of reported stressors during the six months preceding the index episode (Table III), and the lowest prevalence of melancholia (Table IV). They may comprise different kinds of depression. Attempts should be made to differentiate single episode patients who are potentially bipolars or recurrent unipolars from patients who may have a single lifetime episode. Since more than half this group were over 45 years old at the onset of the index episode, it seems plausible that the first episode of depression experienced so late in life may represent a final common pathway for the expression of many kinds of psychological and organic stress that may have a more or less chronic course.

TABLE VI
Ham-D factor and total scores

| Diagnostic group | B1 | | B2 | | R | | SE | |
|---|---|---|---|---|---|---|---|---|
| | M | s | M | s | M | s | M | s |
| Anxiety/somatisation | 0.92 | 0.4 | 0.97 | 0.4 | 1.07 | 0.4 | 1.02 | 0.4 |
| Weight | 0.32 | 0.6 | 0.47 | 0.7 | 0.40 | 0.6 | 0.52 | 0.7 |
| Cognitive disorders | 0.50 | 0.3 | 0.60 | 0.3 | 0.59 | 0.4 | 0.50 | 0.3 |
| Diurnal variation | 0.60 | 0.7 | 0.96 | 0.8 | 0.98 | 0.7 | 0.89 | 0.7 |
| Motor retardation | 1.64 | 0.6 | 1.74 | 0.6 | 1.77 | 0.6 | 1.72 | 0.6 |
| Sleep disorders | 0.85 | 0.5 | 0.79 | 0.6 | 0.89 | 0.5 | 0.80 | 0.6 |
| Total Ham-D | 18.60 | 5.1 | 20.23 | 5.3 | 21.31 | 5.9 | 19.97 | 5.4 |
| Number | (25) | | (107) | | (174) | | (94) | |

B1 = Bipolar I, B2 = Bipolar II, R = Recurrent, SE = Single episode

TABLE VII
RRS items and total score

| Diagnostic group | B1 | | B2 | | R | | SE | |
|---|---|---|---|---|---|---|---|---|
| | M | s | M | s | M | s | M | s |
| Gait | 1.00 | 1.0 | 1.13 | 1.0 | 1.03 | 0.9 | 1.05 | 0.9 |
| Movement | 1.32 | 0.9 | 1.05 | 1.0 | 1.06 | 0.9 | 1.02 | 0.9 |
| Mimetic | 1.48 | 1.1 | 1.27 | 0.9 | 1.29 | 0.9 | 1.24 | 0.9 |
| Language | 1.08 | 1.0 | 0.83 | 0.9 | 0.85 | 0.9 | 0.91 | 0.9 |
| Voice | 0.76 | 0.7 | 0.76 | 0.7 | 0.71 | 0.7 | 0.77 | 0.7 |
| Brevity | 0.92 | 1.0 | 0.84 | 0.9 | 0.75 | 0.9 | 0.93 | 0.9 |
| Variety | 1.08 | 1.2 | 1.07 | 1.0 | 1.14 | 1.0 | 1.18 | 0.9 |
| Richness | 1.20 | 1.2 | 1.15 | 1.1 | 1.12 | 1.0 | 1.17 | 1.0 |
| Ruminations | 1.72 | 1.2 | 1.99 | 1.1 | 1.85 | 1.1 | 1.82 | 0.9 |
| Fatigability | 2.08 | 1.2 | 2.07 | 1.1 | 2.06 | 1.0 | 1.82 | 0.9 |
| Interest | 2.28 | 1.0 | 2.10 | 1.0 | 2.12 | 0.8 | 2.12 | 1.0 |
| Time perception | 1.44 | 1.3 | 1.50 | 1.3 | 1.42 | 1.3 | 1.50 | 1.3 |
| Memory | 0.88 | 0.9 | 1.17 | 1.0 | 1.07 | 0.9 | 0.89 | 0.9 |
| Concentration | 2.08 | 0.9 | 1.97 | 0.9 | 1.92 | 0.8 | 1.89 | 0.9 |
| Total | 19.32 | 10.2 | 18.90 | 9.7 | 18.39 | 8.7 | 18.32 | 8.9 |
| (Number) | (25) | | (107) | | (174) | | (94) | |

B1 = Bipolar I, B2 = Bipolar II, R = Recurrent, SE = Single episode

TABLE VIII
HSCL-90 factor scores

| Diagnostic group | B1 | | B2 | | R | | SE | |
|---|---|---|---|---|---|---|---|---|
| | M | s | M | s | M | s | M | s |
| Somatisation | 1.23 | 0.8 | 1.18 | 0.6 | 1.38 | 0.8 | 1.40 | 0.8 |
| Obsession-compulsion | 1.99 | 0.8 | 1.87 | 0.7 | 2.05 | 0.8 | 1.86 | 0.8 |
| Sensitivity | 1.60 | 0.9 | 1.29 | 0.8 | 1.27 | 0.8 | 1.18 | 0.9 |
| Depression | 2.14 | 0.9 | 2.14 | 0.7 | 2.21 | 0.7 | 2.18 | 0.7 |
| Anxiety | 1.71 | 1.0 | 1.58 | 0.8 | 1.61 | 0.8 | 1.64 | 0.8 |
| Hostility-anger | 0.99 | 0.8 | 0.84 | 0.8 | 0.86 | 0.7 | 1.04 | 0.7 |
| Phobic anxiety | 1.32 | 1.0 | 0.97 | 0.9 | 1.02 | 0.8 | 0.99 | 0.9 |
| Paranoidism | 1.27 | 0.7 | 1.12 | 0.8 | 1.11 | 0.8 | 1.13 | 0.9 |
| Psychoticism | 1.12 | 0.6 | 1.09 | 0.7 | 1.03 | 0.6 | 1.05 | 0.6 |
| (Number) | (25) | | (107) | | (174) | | (94) | |

B1 = Bipolar I, B2 = Bipolar II, R = Recurrent, SE = Single episode

*Symptomatological features* No significant differences were found among the four subtypes in the symptomatologic profiles assessed by the HAM-D (Table VI), RRS (Table VII), and HSCL-90 (Table VIII) scales. These widely used standardised measures were selected with the aim of identifying differences between the manifest symptom patterns presented by the four types, especially those generally referred to as criteria which allow differentiation between typical bipolar and unipolar disorders (motor retardation vegetative symptoms etc.). The mean total HAM-D scores for the four groups ranged narrowly from 18.6 to 21.3; the Widlocher RRS suggested a trend for more severe retardation in bipolar I (19.3) than in single episode (18.3), with an intermediate position taken by the bipolar II and recurrent groups. The absence of significant differences on these measures and the high percentage of melancholic features in the sample suggest that MDE diagnosis identified affective mood disorders widely representative of the entire spectrum, with rather uniform and homogeneous manifest symptomatology. It also tends to justify the focus on the course of illness and evolution of the disorder in subclassification efforts.

## Discussion

This study sample was selected by requiring the presence of a full-blown index depressive episode and by excluding secondary affective disorders as well as co-morbid panic, obsessive-compulsive, phobic, somatoform, and eating disorders. The selection method identified a large sample of genuine mood disorders. This may explain why some symptomatological differences between unipolar and bipolar patients reported in the literature (Depue & Monroe, 1978) were not confirmed here. It is likely that past studies compared affective bipolars with mixed groups of affective and nonaffective disorders. For the same reasons, prior reports of successful differentiations between unipolars and bipolars on the basis of biological markers must be considered as of uncertain validity due to the many inconsistencies between the classification methods used.

The finding that the manifest symptomatology of MDE did not differ substantially among the four groups is consistent with the view that such episodes are features of several types of genuine mood disorder that differ markedly along other dimensions.

Clinical guidelines and criteria for distinguishing subtypes were derived here not only from the assessment of the symptomatology of the acute episodes of mania and depression, but also from the course of the illness during the patient's lifetime. Correct assessment of the presence and frequency of recurrence of episodes, characteristics of the intervals between episodes, and the fundamental personality temperament are of basic importance. Diagnostic subgroups of mood disorders were examined for their therapeutic relevance.

Bipolar I, as identified by the SID, appears to be a very homogeneous group characterised by a high frequency of manic and hypomanic episodes, a high prevalence of depressive and hyperthymic temperaments, and the highest rate of complete interepisodic remission. Comparison with the bipolar II or recurrent unipolar disorders show it to be the most severe of the mood disorders, since it displays an earlier onset, longer duration, a greater number of episodes, and earlier and more frequent hospital admissions. It requires different preventive and long-term treatment management, as there is a higher risk of suicide attempts. Moreover, the high prevalence of pharmacologically induced hypomania requires caution in treating these patients with antidepressants (Lerer *et al*, 1980; Akiskal, 1983, 1986, 1987; Kukopulos *et al*, 1985). It is suggested that lithium or carbamazepine be added to TCAs, which should begin at lower than customary dosages. Follow-up studies should be undertaken to determine whether TCA treatments will differentially influence the future course of the disorder. Considering recent claims by several investigators, we believe that the scientific community of psychiatrists should plan and undertake a multi-centre long-term study to determine whether TCA treatments induce chronic mixed states, shorter and more frequent cycles, and slow or rapid continuous cyclicity.

The validity of the bipolar II category is still questioned by various researchers. Some combine this group with bipolar I (Angst *et al*, 1980), some regard it as a variant of recurrent unipolar depression, and still others consider it to be a bipolar condition with a premorbid personality disorder (Coryell *et al*, 1984). In our study, as far as the course of illness is concerned, the bipolar II category overlaps with pure recurrent unipolar and other aspects of the illness show similarities with those in bipolar I. Thus bipolar II occupies an intermediate position between bipolar I and pure recurrent unipolar (Akiskal, 1983).

The features noted which make this disorder close to bipolar I should stimulate further comparative research on the way that each responds to lithium and carbamazepine treatments, and the probability that each will lead to TCA-induced chronicity. Previous studies (Coppen *et al*, 1971; Quitkin *et al*, 1978) which failed to find significant differences between the long-term maintenance effects of lithium and TCA in recurrent unipolars may be due to the fact that in these samples the type of bipolar II identified here was not distinguished from recurrent unipolars.

On the other hand, Prien *et al* (1973) found that recurrent unipolars responded better to TCA than to lithium in long-term treatment; however, no diagnostic distinction was made between bipolar II and recurrent unipolar. Comparative studies should now be performed on bipolar II and on recurrent unipolars after excluding cases with hyperthymia and hypomania.

We found a high percentage of depressive as well as hyperthymic temperaments in our sample. These temperamental patterns are relatively easily detectable and assessable for research and clinical purposes. Following Akiskal (1986, 1987) and Kukopulos *et al* (1985), the evaluation and diagnosis of bipolarity should include the assessment of cycles which may be constituted by full blown episodes, intervals of remission, and mild temperamental, subaffective, and long lasting attenuated states of mood elevation or depression.

## Conclusion

The nosographic systematisation of mood disorders is a direct expression of the continuous evolution of knowledge of therapeutics and aetiology. The present classifications and the new definitions in terms of categories are to be considered essential tools for communication and research models, and they are fundamental to improving treatment choices.

The rigidity of the unipolar-bipolar dichotomy limits its clinical usefulness. The categories of mood disorders, especially at the depressive pole, must be considered along the bipolar spectrum according to a multidimensional evaluation of such clinical aspects as family history, temperamental pathology, age at onset, number and type of previous episodes, prior treatment response, interphase recovery and adjustment, and cycle frequency. In short, much more is required than the standard evaluation of present symptomatology and its accompanying features and complications.

## Acknowledgement

This study was supported by a grant from the Ministero della Pubblica Istruzione, Italy.

## References

AKISKAL, H. S., BITAR, A. H. & PUZANTIAN, V. R. (1978) The nosological status of neurotic depression: a prospective 3–4 year follow-up examination in the light of the primary-secondary and the unipolar-bipolar dichotomies. *Archives of General Psychiatry*, **35**, 756–766.

—— (1983) The bipolar spectrum: new concepts in classification and diagnosis. In *Psychiatry Update* (ed. C. Grinspoon) Vol. II pp. 271–292 Washington, DC: American Psychiatric Press.

—— (1986) The clinical significance of the ''soft'' bipolar spectrum. *Psychiatric Annals*, **16**, 667–671.

—— (1987) The milder spectrum of Bipolar Disorders: diagnostic, characterologic and pharmacologic aspects. *Psychiatric Annals*, **17**, 33–37.

AMERICAN PSYCHIATRIC ASSOCIATION: DSM–III (1980) *Diagnostic and Statistical Manual of Mental Disorders*, 3rd edn. Washington, DC: APA.

—— WORK GROUP TO REVISE DSM–III (1985) *Draft DSM–III-R in development*, Washington, DC: American Psychiatric Association.

ANGST, J. (1966) *Zur Ätiologie und Nosologie endogener depressiver Psychosen. Monographien aus dem Gesamtgebiete der Neurologie und Psychiatrie.* Berlin: Springer-Verlag.

——, FELDER, W. & FREY R. (1979) The course of unipolar and bipolar affective disorders. In *Origin, Prevention and Treatment of Affective Disorders* (eds M. Schou & E. Strömgren), pp. 215–226. London: Academic Press.

—— FREY, R., LOHMEYER, B. & ZERBIN-RUDIN, E. (1980) Bipolar manic-depressive psychoses: results of a genetic investigation. *Human Genetics*, **55**, 237–254.

—— (1981) Course of affective disorders. In *Handbook of Biological Psychiatry* (eds Van Praag *et al*), pp. 225–242. New York: Marcel Dekker.

BEIGEL, A. & MURPHY, D. L. (1971) Unipolar and bipolar affective illness: differences in clinical characteristics accompanying depression. *Archives of General Psychiatry*, **24**, 215–229.

CASSANO, G. B., MUSETTI, L., PERUGI, G., MIGNANI, V., SORIANI, A., MCNAIR, D. M. & AKISKAL, H. S. (1988) Major depression subcategories: their potentiality for clinical research. Proceeding of Symposium: *Diagnosis and treatment of depression: ''Quo vadis?''*, SANOFI Group, May 11–12, 1987, Montpelier.

CLAYTON, P. J. (1986) Bipolar Illness. In *The Medical Basis of Psychiatry* (eds G. Winokur & P. Clayton), pp. 39–59. Philadelphia: W. B. Saunders.

COPPEN, A., NOGUERA, R., BAILEY, J., BURNS, B., SWAMI, M., HARE, E. & GARDNER, R. (1971) Prophylactic lithium in affective disorders. *Lancet*, *ii*, 275–283.

CORYELL, W. & WINOKUR, G. (1984) Depression spectrum disorders: clinical diagnosis and biological implications. In: *Neurobiology of Mood Disorders* (eds R. M. Post & J. C. Ballenger), pp. 102–112. Baltimore/London: Williams & Wilkins.

——, ENDICOTT, J. & REICH, T. (1984) A family study of bipolar II disorder. *British Journal of Psychiatry*, **145**, 49–54.

——, ——, ANDREASEN, N. & KELLER, M. (1985) Bipolar I, bipolar II, and nonbipolar major depression among the relatives of affectively ill probands. *American Journal of Psychiatry*, **142**, 817–823.

DEPUE, R. A. & MONROE, S. M. (1978) The unipolar-bipolar distinction in the depressive disorders. *Psychological Bulletin*, **85**, 1001–1029.

DUNNER, D. L., FLEISS, J. L. & FIEVE, R. R. (1976a) The course of development of mania in patients with recurrent depression. *American Journal of Psychiatry*, **133**, 905–908.

——, GERSHON, E. S. & GOODWIN, F. K. (1976b) Heritable factors in the severity of affective illness. *Biological Psychiatry*, **11**, 31–42.

—— (1983) Sub-types of bipolar affective disorder with particular regard to bipolar II. *Psychiatric Developments*, **I**, 75–86.

—— (1987) Stability of bipolar II affective disorder as a diagnostic entity. *Psychiatric Annals*, **17**, 18–20.

ENDICOTT, J., NEE, J., ANDREASEN, N., CLAYTON, P., KELLER, M. & CORYELL, W. (1985) Bipolar II: Combine or keep separate? *Journal of Affective Disorders*, **8**, 17–28.

GERSHON, E. S., HAMOVIT, J., GUROFF, J. J., DIBBLE, E., LECKMAN, J. F., SCEERY, W., TARGUM, S. D., NURNBERGER, J. I. Jr., GOLDIN, L. R. & BUNNEY, W. E. Jr. (1982) A family study of schizoaffective, bipolar I, bipolar II, unipolar, and normal control probands. *Archives of General Psychiatry*, **39**, 1157–1167.

GOODWIN, F. K. & JAMISON, K.-R. (1984) The natural course of manic-depressive illness. In *Neurobiology of Mood Disorders* (eds R. M. Post & J. C. Ballenger), pp. 20–37. Baltimore/London: Williams & Wilkins.

JOHNSON, G. F. & HUNT, G. (1979). Suicidal behavior in bipolar manic-depressive patients and their families. *Comprehensive Psychiatry*, **20**, 159–167.

KELLER, M. B. & SHAPIRO, R. W. (1982) Double depression: superimposition of acute depressive episodes on chronic depressive disorders. *American Journal of Psychiatry*, **139**, 438–442.

——, LAVORI, P. W., ENDICOTT, J., CORYELL, W. & KLERMAN, G. L. (1983) Double depression: two year follow-up. *American Journal of Psychiatry*, **140**, 689–694.

KLERMAN, G. L., ENDICOTT, J., SPITZER, R. & HIRSCHFELD, R. (1979) Neurotic depression: a systematic analysis of multiple criteria and meanings. *American Journal of Psychiatry*, **136**, 57–61.

KRAEPELIN, E. (1921) *Manic-Depressive Insanity and Paranoia*. Edinburgh: E. & S. Livingstone.

KUKOPULOS, A., CALIARI, B., TUNDO, A., MINNAI, G., FLORIS, G., REGINALDI, D. & TONDO, L. (1983) Rapid cyclers temperament and antidepressants. *Comprehensive Psychiatry*, **24**, 249–258.

——, REGINALDI, D. & CALIARI, B. (1985) New approaches to the treatment of lithium non-responders. In *Psychiatry: The State of the Art*, (eds P. Pichot *et al*), pp. 425–429. New York: Plenum.

LECKMAN, J. F., WEISSMAN, M. M., PRUSOFF, B. A., CARUSO, K. A., MERIKANGAS, K. R., PAULS, D. L. & KIDD, K. K. (1984) Subtypes of depression: a family study perspective. *Archives of General Psychiatry*, **41**, 833–888.

LEONHARD, K. (1957) *Aufteilung der endogenen Psychosen*. Berlin: Akademic Verlag.

LERER, B., BIRMACHER, B. & EBSTEIN, R. P. (1980) 48-hours depressive cycling induced by antidepressants. *British Journal Psychiatry*, **137**, 183–185.

NURNBERGER, J. I. & GERSHON, E. S. (1984) Genetics of affective disorders. In *Neurobiology of Mood Disorders*, (eds R. M. Post & J. C. Ballenger), pp. 76–101. Baltimore/London: Williams & Wilkins.

OPPENHEIM, G. (1982) Drug-induced rapid cycling: possible outcomes and management. *American Journal of Psychiatry*, **137**, 939–943.

PERRIS, C. (1966) A study of bipolar (manic-depressive) and unipolar recurrent depressive psychoses. *Acta Psychiatrica Scandinavica*, **42**, (suppl. 194): 1–188.

PRIEN, R. F., KLETT, C. J. & CAFFEY, E. M. (1973) Lithium carbonate and imipramine in prevention of affective episodes. *Archives of General Psychiatry*, **29**, 420–433.

—— (1978) Lithium in the treatment of affective disorders. In *Clinical Neuropharmacology* (ed. H. L. Klawans), pp. 113–119. New York: Raven Press.

QUITKIN, F. M., RIFKIN, A., KANE, J., RAMOS, L. Jr., & KLEIN, D. F. (1978) Prophylactic effect of lithium and imipramine in unipolar and bipolar II patients: A preliminary report. *American Journal of Psychiatry*, **135**, 570–575.

——, —— & KLEIN, D. F. (1979) Monoamine oxidase inhibitors: a review of antidepressant effectiveness. *Archives of General Psychiatry*, **36**, 749–760.

ROTH, M., GURNEY, G., GARSIDE, R. F. & KERR, T. A. (1972) The relationship between anxiety states and depressive illnesses. Part I. *British Journal of Psychiatry*, **121**, 147–161.

SCHAPIRA, K., ROTH, M. & KERR, T. A. (1972) The prognosis of affective disorder: the differentiation of anxiety states from depressive illness. *British Journal of Psychiatry*, **122**, 175–181.

SQUILLACE, K., POST, R. M., SAVARD, R. & ERWIN-GORMAN, M. (1984) Life charting of the longitudinal course of recurrent affective illness. In *Neurobiology of Mood Disorders*, (eds R. M. Post & J. C. Ballenger) pp. 38–57. Baltimore/London: Williams & Wilkins.

TAYLOR, M. A. & ABRAMS, R. (1980) Reassessing the bipolar-unipolar dichotomy. *Journal of Affective Disorders*, **2**, 197–205.

WEHR, T. A. & GOODWIN, F. K. (1979) Rapid cycling in manic depressive induced by tricyclic antidepressants. *Archives of General Psychiatry*, **36**, 555–559.

WIDLOCHER, D. (1983) A basic emotional response? In *The Affective Disorders*, (eds J. M. Davis & J. W. Maas). Washington, DC: American Psychiatric Press.

WINOKUR, G. Unipolar depression (1986) In *The Medical Basis of Psychiatry*, (eds G. Winokur & P. Clayton), pp. 60–79. Philadelphia: W. B. Saunders.

# 11   Delineating chronic affective subtypes: towards a science of out-patient psychiatry

**HAGOP S. AKISKAL**

Martin Roth pioneered the extension of the Kraepelinian approach to the neuroses and affective morbidity in the out-patient setting, areas long dominated by metapsychology. Kraepelin (1921), in his historic delineation of the psychopathology and the course of the major psychoses, had paid little attention to individual biography. Kurt Schneider (1923), in declaring that there were no neuroses—only neurotics—was expressing his reservation toward the application of the rigour of medical science to the large universe of ambulatory mental disorders. Martin Roth's writings (1959, 1960, 1963, 1984) challenge this viewpoint. His phenomenologic precision in depicting the inner world of neurotic suffering remains unsurpassed. What is unique to his endeavour is the elegant synthesis of nosologic rigour and phenomenologic subtlety. Martin Roth is thus natural heir to the two giants of German psychiatry—Emil Kraepelin and Karl Jaspers. Jaspers (1963) had delineated the conceptual framework for a science of subjective psychopathologic experiences, but the clinical application of his ideas to the neuroses proved difficult. Martin Roth's descriptions of the various forms of neurotic and ambulatory affective suffering provide psychiatry with naturalistic tableaux of lasting value. Indeed, it can be said that the science in his writings is more compelling because of its aesthetic qualities.

Martin Roth's classification (1978) of the affective disorders into endogenous and the affective neuroses represents a challenge to the unitarian viewpoint that saw a pathogenetic continuum underlying the apparent clinical overlap of the various affective conditions in the clinic. Subdivisions within these two general categories represent clinical entities validated with painstaking detail in personality functioning, signs and symptoms and course. This work has further led to the demarcations of the anxiety from the depressive states (Roth et al, 1972; Schapira et al, 1972; Kerr et al, 1974; Roth & Mountjoy, 1982). Distinctions within the anxiety states (e.g., social phobia, anxiety neurosis, agoraphobia) are more tentative, but the emphasis on delineating their individual clinical phenomenology embodies the hypothesis that diverse aetiologic factors modify the clinical expression of special subtypes of anxiety disorders.

The clinical overlap between anxiety and depressive disorders is particularly confusing at the milder symptomatic level of suffering that often pursues a course of intermittent chronicity. Sufferers of such chronic dysphoric conditions, variously termed 'atypical', 'anxious', and 'characterologic' depressive subjects, represent major diagnostic and therapeutic challenges to clinicians working in out-patient settings in both psychiatry and general medical practice. More recently, the American Psychiatric Association (1980) created the 'dysthymic' rubric for these patients. This term, which literally means 'ill-humoured', refers to a temperamental inclination to negative affective arousal; it has been applied to all unpleasant affective states with depressive, anxious, and obsessional qualities.

Although the inclusion of this rubric into the official American classification has brought attention to a large universe of chronic affective morbidity, 'dysthymia' is an over-inclusive concept which tends to obliterate important phenomenologic distinctions in anxiety and depressive disorders. This paper reviews research conducted at the University of Tennessee (Akiskal, 1983), which supports Martin Roth's broad outline on the clinical utility of delineating phenomenologically distinct subtypes within this heterogeneous realm. The review is limited to three subtypes that have received the greatest support from external validating strategies: patients where low-grade dysphoric manifestations represent the residual phase of a partially remitted depressive episode; lifelong dysthymias originating in childhood; and chronic admixtures of anxiety and depressive symptomatology with reverse vegetative signs.

## Residual depressive states

The course of late onset depressive illness can be quite protracted (Akiskal, *et al*, 1981); residual symptoms are common, and chronicity may develop after one or several episodes that fail to remit fully. During this residual phase, which may last two to five years or even longer, 'characterologic' manifestations—a sense of resignation, generalised fear of inability to cope, emotional lability, and/or inhibited communication—often dominate the clinical picture, with depressive symptoms pushed to the background (Cassano *et al*, 1983). The lives of these individuals are often characterised by overdedication to work and inability to enjoy leisure activities (DeLisio *et al*, 1986). Marital conflict takes the form of chronic deadlock, where patients neither reconcile with, nor divorce their spouses. In other patients, the residual state is dominated by somatic manifestations involving vegetative or autonomic nervous system irregularities that mimic anxiety symptoms.

Sleep EEG evaluation at our Centre has shown that rapid eye movement (REM) latency is shortened not only during the acute episode but also during the chronic phase (Akiskal, 1982). This neurophysiologic similarity suggests the value of conceptualising the chronic phase as an affective process. Gender, developmental loss of parent(s), and personality failed to distinguish chronic depressive subjects from a control group of episodic depressive subjects who recovered fully. However, positive family history for mood disorders was significantly more common in the chronic group. Furthermore, chronic depressive subjects were significantly more likely to have disabled spouses, multiple losses of immediate family members through death, concurrent disabling medical illness, use of catecholamine-depleting antihypertensive agents and excessive use of alcohol and sedative-hypnotic agents. It would therefore appear that multiple factors are involved in the incomplete recovery from depressive episodes. A recent study from Newcastle (Scott *et al*, 1988), which employed a different strategy, supports many of these clinical findings.

Patients suffering from residual depression require long-term treatment with tricyclic antidepressants (TCAs); ECT may also benefit some. In patients refractory to these measures, the possibility of occult malignancies, endocrine abnormalities, or neurologic disease should always be kept in mind (Akiskal, 1985).

Residual depressions, then, represent either inadequately treated depressive patients or those rendered refractory because of concurrent systemic or cerebral disease. It has also been recently suggested that in some premorbidly hyperthymic or cyclothymic individuals, continued TCA treatment of depressive episodes in middle or late life may lead not only to rapid-cycling (Kukopulos *et al*, 1980), but also to chronicisation (Akiskal & Mallya, 1987). These highly unpleasant residual states are characterised by unrelenting dysphoria which manifests by irascibility, severe agitation and refractory anxiety; unendurable sexual excitement, intractable insomnia, and suicidal obsessions or impulses; and 'histrionic' demeanour—yet genuine expressions of intense suffering. Thus, the residual chronicity in some recurrent depressions in reality represents a protracted mixed state. These residual mixed states respond best to substitution of lithium, carbamazepine, or short-term neuroleptics for TCAs.

## Early onset dysthymias

In these patients, low-grade depressive symptomatology is not the residuum of a major depressive episode. The onset of the illness is insidious—typically before age 25, and often going as far back as childhood—and the course is intermittent (Akiskal, 1983). Brooding about negative events, the gloomy outlook, self-hatred, and self-denigration are so deeply ingrained in these dysthymic individuals that they appear to be part of the character structure. The clinical dilemmas faced by physicians in their clinical encounters with such patients may be related to their demanding natures which, in the extreme, can manifest by an almost exhibitionistic flaunting of suffering. Dysthymic patients studied at Tennessee (Akiskal, 1983), have made statements such as "I feel depressed all the time," and "I am the most miserable creature on earth". These hyperbolic descriptions of suffering contrast so strongly with the relative absence of objectively ascertainable illness that the diagnosis of "characterologic depression" is often invoked during clinical disquisitions. This clinical colloquialism is apt inasmuch as it connotes the difficulty of clinically separating the depressive attributes from the character structure. This is a heterogeneous group of patients conventionally considered resistant to most treatment modalities.

In our approach (Akiskal *et al*, 1980) to this therapeutic challenge, we hypothesised that the generally disappointing results with pharmacotherapy could be explained by failure to address these patients' lack of social adroitness; by contrast, psychotherapies seem impotent in reversing the temperamentally based inertia characteristic of many such patients. To address these issues, in our study we combined 'practical' psychotherapeutic modalities like social skills training with a vigorous trial of several TCAs and/or lithium carbonate. Patients who responded to such combined treatment were considered to constitute an attenuated or a *subaffective* dysthymic group in view of family history, superimposed major depressive episodes, and hypomanic responses to antidepressant drugs.

Furthermore, even when examined in their habitual condition—i.e., when not in a definable depressive episode—these patients had the abnormally shortened REM latency characteristic of primary depressive states. By contrast, the nonresponsive group conformed to a primary characterologic disorder with unstable features, normal REM latency, familial alcoholism, familial assortative mating, and high rates of developmental object loss and, therefore, was classified as having a *character-spectrum* disorder. Recent work at the Dartmouth Sleep Clinic (Hauri & Sateia, 1984), which defined two subtypes of chronic dysthymia based on the subaffective and character-spectrum categories delineated by us, has replicated the differentiating sleep EEG findings reported above.

The results overall support the notion that some personalities with introverted-obsessoid features, who are habitually brooding, guilt-ridden, gloomy, pessimistic, self-denigrating, anhedonic, and tend to oversleep—features reminiscent of Schneider's (1923) description of the depressive psychopath—are suffering from a genetically attenuated but lifelong form of recurrent mood disorder. Careful evaluation of their lethargy will often reveal psychomotor inertia, which is worse in the morning. Furthermore, although habitually introverted, these patients sometimes appear extroverted and driven for short periods of time. These hypomanic tendencies can be accentuated by TCAs, thereby suggesting the potential benefits of a lithium trial. As suggested elsewhere (Akiskal, 1983), and in keeping with tradition, it is best to limit the operational territory of the term 'dysthymia' to this subaffective group of chronic depressives.

## Anxious depressions

Some middle-aged and elderly depressive patients present with severe anxiety, or such symptoms may dominate the residual phase of their illness as described earlier. Insomnia, anxiety and related neurotic symptoms—including panic attacks during the early part of the night and daytime fatigue—occurring for the first time after the age of 40 are usually manifestations of depressive illness. This conclusion, based in part on sleep EEG findings that have revealed that late-onset neurotic syndromes share the REM abnormalities observed in depressive disorders (Akiskal & Lemmi, 1987), supports earlier suggestions by Roth & Mountjoy (1982).

The more common presentation of mixed anxiety and depressive symptoms has a different chronology. These patients are younger and, before developing depressive symptoms, seek help from general practitioners for such 'alarming' autonomic nervous system manifestations as palpitations, chest pain, and light-headedness. Clinical attention and treatment are directed toward these anxiety symptoms, and psychiatric referral is often delayed until depressive or phobic symptoms become incapacitating. When first evaluated by psychiatrists, these patients appear discouraged and helpless; they are at least moderately disabled in their personal and vocational lives, and lack self-confidence; that is, a high level of demoralisation is superimposed on the dysphoric anxious mood. When seen in Sleep Disorder Centres, anxious depressive patients present a clinical picture characterised by excessive daytime irritability, weariness, fatigue and daytime napping. Patients may or may not complain of initial insomnia; however, careful questioning will reveal intermittent initial insomnia.

To clarify the nosologic status of the younger group of anxious depressive patients, we compared the sleep EEG of anxious depressive patients with that of dysthymic patients and a control group of subjects without sleep and psychiatric disorders and who were undergoing various polysomnographic montages (Akiskal *et al*, 1984). Despite major clinical overlap, sleep measures distinguished the anxious and dysthymic groups. Significant findings included greater disturbances in sleep continuity—especially in the first half of the night—in the anxious and short REM latency in the dysthymic groups. These data suggest that the majority of anxious depressions are more like anxiety disorders than primary depressive illness. Similar data have been reported by Duke *et al* (1985).

Our analyses (Akiskal & Lemmi, 1987) in the dysthymic subjects have further shown little night to night variability in sleep measures; by contrast, the anxious depressive subjects exhibited significant variability of sleep measures from night to night and, most importantly, sleep continuity measures did not return to normal after the night of 'adaptation'. That these results in the anxious group represented an inherent psychophysiologic characteristic—and not merely a stress response—can be seen in the fact that essentially all deviant sleep measures in control subjects returned to normal after the first night of adaptation. It would appear that anxious depressive patients, like all patients with anxiety neuroses, are overwhelmed by new environmental conditions—especially those that involve being monitored and scrutinised and where the opportunity of escape is low, as is the case with the sleep laboratory which recreates the typically dreaded phobic stimuli for many of these patients. This would explain why in real life they experience psychophysiologic arousal and insomnia on an intermittent basis—depending on the perceived novelty of challenges that they face in day-to-day living. The intial insomnia in the first part of the night in many anxious patients gives rise to a tendency to oversleep toward the morning; if unable to sleep late in the morning in view of educational, vocational, or domestic pursuits, they experience extreme fatigue and irritability during the day—with a tendency to hypersomnolence. Daytime napping would further predispose to sleep-wake schedule disturbances, thereby creating a vicious cycle of more initial insomnia and daytime somnolence. This is then our hypothesised mechanism for the genesis of many of the reverse vegetative signs considered characteristic of "atypical depressions".

From the perspective of our sleep studies, the majority of anxious depressions emerge as forms of chronic neuroses rather than of primary mood disorders. This conclusion is concordant with the original British reports (West & Dally, 1959) delineating the atypical depressions of neurasthenic patients who had previously attended medical clinics because of symptoms referable to the autonomic nervous system. The concept of atypical depression currently occupies an unresolved territory in psychiatric nosology. Suffice it to state here that hypersomnic depressive conditions are heterogeneous and embrace anxiety neuroses on the one hand and mild bipolar variants—fluctuating depressions with infrequent hypomania—on the other. Feeling worse in the evening and initial insomnia, with the tendency to feel sleepy and fatigued during the day, further characterise the anxious depressions; feeling worse in the morning and tendency to oversleep are more characteristic of the bipolar variants, including the subaffective dysthymias described earlier. MAOIs are generally considered superior to TCAs for many of these 'atypical' patients. The higher level of the enzyme MAO in the brains of women may in part account for the higher prevalence of atypical depressive conditions in women and their preferential response to MAOIs (Davidson & Pelton, 1986).

## Comment

In this tribute to Martin Roth, I have reviewed recent research findings which exemplify the heuristic and clinical utility of nosologic subtyping within the large universe of chronic dysphoric states seen in ambulatory clinic settings. Such patients have been traditionally lumped under vague rubrics such as 'character neurosis', 'atypical depression', or 'borderline states'. The delineation of specific affective subtypes has been accomplished by combining developmental, familial, phenomenologic, and sleep EEG data. The differential therapeutic response of the affective subtypes so delineated offers new hope for chronic sufferers of affective illness who are among the most common utilisers of out-patient services in both psychiatry and general medical practice. The findings summarised here are presented as examples of the progress towards a science of out-patient psychiatry which rests on the seminal contribution of Martin Roth.

## References

AKISKAL, H. S., KING, D., ROSENTHAL, T. L., ROBINSON, D. & SCOTT-STRAUSS, A. (1981) Chronic depressions: Part I. Clinical and familial characteristics in 137 probands. *Journal of Affective Disorders*, **3**, 297–315.
—— (1982) Factors associated with incomplete recovery in primary depressive illness. *Journal of Clinical Psychiatry*, **43**, 266–271.
—— (1983) Dysthymic disorder: Psychopathology of proposed chronic depressive subtypes. *American Journal of Psychiatry*, **140**, 11–20.
—— (1985) A proposed clinical approach to clinical and "resistant" depressions: Evaluation and treatment. *Journal of Clinical Psychiatry*, **43**, 31–36.
—— & LEMMI, H. (1987) Sleep EEG findings bearing on the relationship of anxiety and depressive disorders. In *Anxious Depressions: Assessment and Treatment*. (eds G. Racagni & E. Smeraldi). New York: Raven Press.
——, ——, DICKSON, H., KING, D., YEREVANIAN, B. I. & VAN VALKENBURG, C. (1984) Chronic depressions: Part 1. Sleep EEG differentiation of primary dysthymic disorders from anxious depressions. *Journal of Affective Disorders*, **6**, 287–295.
—— & MALLYA, G. (1987) Criteria for the "soft" bipolar spectrum—Treatment implications. *Psychopharmacology Bulletin*, **23**, 68–73.
——, ROSENTHAL, T. L., HAYKAL, R. F., LEMMI, H., ROSENTHAL, R. H. & SCOTT-STRAUSS, A. (1980) Characterological depressions: Clinical and sleep EEG findings separating "subaffective dysthymias" from "character-spectrum" disorders. *Archives of General Psychiatry*, **37**, 777–783.
AMERICAN PSYCHIATRIC ASSOCIATION (1980) *DSM-III: Diagnostic and Statistical Manual of Mental Disorders*, (3rd edn.) Washington, DC: APA.
CASSANO, G. B., MAGGINI, C. & AKISKAL, H. S. (1983) Short-term, subchronic, and chronic sequelae of affective disorders. *Psychiatric Clinics of North America*, **6**, 55–67.
DAVIDSON, J. & PELTON, S. (1986) Forms of atypical depression and their response to antidepressant drugs. *Psychiatry Research*, **17**, 87–95.
DELISIO, G., MAREMMANI, I., PERUGI, G., CASSANO, G. B., DELTITO, J. & AKISKAL, H. S. (1986) Impairment of work and leisure in depressed outpatients: A preliminary communication. *Journal of Affective Disorders*, **10**, 79–84.
DUKE, S., KUMAR, N., ETTEDGUI, E., POHL, R., JONES, D. & SITARAM, N. (1985) Cholinergic REM induction responses: separation of anxiety and depression. *Biological Psychiatry*, **20**, 408–418.
HAURI, P. & SATEIA, M. J. (1984) REM sleep in dysthymic disorders. *Sleep Research*, **13**, 119.

JASPERS, K. (1963) *General Psychopathology* (trans. by J. Hoenig & M. W. Hamilton). Manchester: Manchester University Press.

KERR, T. A., ROTH, M. & SCHAPIRA, K. (1974) Prediction of outcome in anxiety states and depressive illnesses. *British Journal of Psychiatry*, **124**, 125–133.

KRAEPELIN, E. (1921) *Manic-depressive Insanity and Paranoia*. Edinburgh: E. & S. Livingstone.

KUKOPULOS, A., REGINALDI, R., FLORIS, G., SERRA, G. & TONDO, L. (1980) Course of the manic-depressive cycle in changes caused by treatment. *Pharmakosychiatrie Neuro-psykopharmakologie*, **13**, 156–167.

ROTH, M. (1959) The phobic anxiety-depersonalization syndrome. *Proceedings of Royal Society of Medicine*, **52**, 587–595.

—— (1960) The phobic anxiety-depersonalization syndrome and some general aetiological problems in psychiatry. *Journal of Neuropsychiatry*, **1**, 293–306.

—— (1963) Neurosis, psychosis and the concept of disease in psychiatry. *Acta Psychiatria Scandinavica*, **39**, 128–145.

——, GURNEY, C., GARSIDE, R. F., KERR, T. A. & SCHAPIRA, K. (1972) Studies in the classification of affective disorders. The relationship between anxiety states and depressive illnesses. I. *British Journal of Psychiatry*, **121**, 147–161.

—— (1978) The classification of affective disorders. *Pharmakopsykie*, **11**, 27–42.

—— & MOUNTJOY, C. Q. (1982). The distinction between anxiety states and depressive disorders. In *Handbook of Affective Disorders* (ed. E. Paykel). London: Churchill Livingstone.

—— (1984) Agoraphobia, panic disorder and generalized anxiety disorder: Some implications of recent advances. *Psychiatric Developments*, **2**, 31–52.

SARGANT, W. (1962) The treatment of anxiety states and atypical depressions by the monoamine oxidase inhibitor drugs. *Journal of Neuropsychiatry*, **3**, 96–103.

SCHAPIRA, K., ROTH, M., KERR, T. A. & GURNEY, C. (1972) The prognosis of affective disorders: The differentiation of anxiety states from depressive illnesses. *British Journal of Psychiatry*, **121**, 175–181.

SCHNEIDER, K. (1923) *Psychopathic Personalities*. Translated by M. W. Hamilton. London: Cassell (1958).

SCOTT, J., BARKER, W. A. & ECCLESTON, D. (1988) The Newcastle chronic depression study: Patient characteristics and factors associated with chronicity. *British Journal of Psychiatry*, **152**, 28–33.

WEST, E. D. & DALLY, P. J. (1959) Effects of iproniazid in depressive syndromes. *British Medical Journal*, **1**, 1491–1494.

# 12  Some reflections on the concept of endogenous depression

## NANCY C. ANDREASEN

One of the most fundamental questions concerning the concept of depression is whether it is homogeneous or heterogeneous. While Martin Roth has made many contributions to psychiatry, one of his most important was to this issue. One of the purposes of Festschrift is to honour such contributions and to reflect upon their influence throughout time and space.

While many members of the psychiatric establishment in Great Britain, especially Aubrey Lewis and his co-workers at the Maudsley, were arguing that all depressions represented the same basic phenomenon, Lewis (1938, 1971; Kendell, 1968, 1976), Martin Roth's group at Newcastle took a dissenting position (Carney et al, 1965). They completed a series of empirical studies designed to identify subtypes of depression, especially subtypes that would be useful in predicting response to treatment. On the opposite of the Atlantic, in a department also isolated from its own national psychiatric establishment, investigators in Iowa City led by Paul Huston were pursuing similar goals and reaching similar conclusions (Huston & Locher, 1948).

As a young clinician receiving my training in Iowa City during the late 1960s and early 1970s, I was taught to search carefully in order to identify characteristic features of 'real' depression that would be likely to respond to somatic therapies such as tricyclics or ECT. At that time, the distinction between endogenous and reactive depression was one of the few things that I was taught that seemed supported both by common sense and by clinical observation. Patients suffering from hysteria were not very common and did not respond well to efforts to relieve their repressed memories through psychodynamic psychotherapy or hypnosis. Schizophrenic patients did not always have thought disorder, while many manic patients did. Patients suffering from anxiety and panic usually could not recall any early life precipitants or triggers. Vigorous therapy with neuroleptics and careful surveillance did not prevent schizophrenic patients from relapsing or deteriorating. These teachings were usually buttressed by appeal to authority and tradition rather than to data.

In this environment, the work being done in Great Britain struck a chord that resonated with a frequency that seemed intuitively correct. Whatever individual differences they might have, investigators like Martin Roth, Robert Kendell, Eugene Paykel and John Wing were pursuing the proper strategy: defining methods and measurements carefully, exploring their fundamental assumptions, and subjecting them to quantitative scrutiny. I read their work with admiration and respect. They set high standards that provided important teachings to me and to others of my (only slightly younger) generation of investigators in America. Later, it became one of the great pleasures of my life that I was eventually able to meet and know as colleagues and even friends many of these psychiatrists whose work I read as a young person.

However much I admired the conceptual rigour of the Maudsley group as they discussed the continuum concept of depression, my own training and intuition tended toward subtyping and favoured a distinction between endogenous and reactive depression. Joined by a talented younger colleague, William Grove, and supported by access to a large data set collected through the NIMH Collaborative Study of the Psychobiology of Depression, I pursued a series of studies that pay homage to Martin Roth in particular, and to the tradition of British empiricism in general. Truth is to be found wherever our data lead us.

## Conceptual issues

The original concept of endogenous depression as developed in the Newcastle Scale attempted to operationalise features that would predict a good response to treatment (Carney *et al*, 1965). Their basic strategy was to collect a broad base of empirical data that characterised the group of patients suffering from depression and then to identify and weight those characteristics associated with a good outcome. They suggested that the following items were strongly and positively associated with good outcome and should therefore be given a weighting of + 2: no adequate psychogenesis, weight loss, depressive psychomotor activity, and nihilistic delusions. Normal personality, a distinct quality to the depressive mood, the existence of previous episodes and the presence of guilt were also associated with good outcome, although less strongly, and were therefore given a positive weighting of + 1. A tendency to blame others and the presence of anxiety were negatively weighted and therefore given a score of − 1. When these items were added, a score of 6 was considered to represent a criterion for endogenous depression.

While the Newcastle Scale became an important measure for predicting treatment response, its mixture of cross-sectional and longitudinal features posed psychometric problems for subsequent nosological research. It could be argued that, if purely cross-sectional features could be identified, then longitudinal features could be treated as dependent or outcome measures and used as potential validators. Using this approach, one would attempt to define core or characteristic cross-sectional symptoms, and then determine whether these were associated with differences in onset, outcome, or personality traits. In addition to allowing for additional nosological validators, this approach also has the strength that it limits defining features to those currently present in the patient and therefore enhances the likelihood of establishing a reliable definition.

Consequently, several alternatives to the Newcastle Scale were subsequently developed in the United States. Two that gained wide currency were the Research Diagnostic Criteria (RDC) (Spitzer *et al*, 1975) and DSM–III (1980). These definitions drew on the work of Roth and others and attempted to identify a clustering of symptoms that would isolate a subtype of depression that was probably biologically based as opposed to purely situational. Because clinicians

TABLE I
*Newcastle scale (endogenous depression)*

| Symptom | Criterion for diagnosis |
|---|---|
| No adequate psychogenesis (weight, +2) | Score >6 |
| Weight loss (+2) | |
| Depressive psychomotor activity (+2) | |
| Nihilistic delusions (+2) | |
| Adequate personality (+1) | |
| Distinct quality (+1) | |
| Previous episode (+1) | |
| Guilt (+1) | |
| Blame others (-1) | |
| Anxiety (-1) | |

*Research diagnostic criteria (endogenous depression)*

| Symptom | Criterion for diagnosis |
|---|---|
| Group A | Exhibiting 6 symptoms |
| Distinct quality | including >1 from Group A |
| Autonomy of mood | |
| Mood worse in a.m. | |
| Pervasive loss of interest or pleasure | |
| Group B | |
| Self-reproach or excessive guilt | |
| Terminal or middle insomnia | |
| Psychomotor agitation or retardation | |
| Poor appetite | |
| Weight loss | |
| Decreased sex drive, loss of interest or pleasure | |

*DSM–III (melancholia)*

| Symptom | Criterion for diagnosis |
|---|---|
| A. Pervasive loss of interest or pleasure (anhedonia) | Must exhibit A, B and C |
| B. Nonreactivity of mood (autonomy) | |
| C. At least 3 of the following: | |
|     Distinct quality | |
|     Mood worse in a.m. | |
|     Terminal insomnia | |
|     Anorexia or weight loss | |
|     Psychomotor agitation or retardation | |
|     Excessive or inappropriate guilt | |

increasingly recognised that environmental stresses could precipitate biological events such as reactions in the neuroendocrine system that could trigger depression, the DSM–III definition dropped the term ''endogenous'' altogether and substituted ''melancholic'' instead.

The defining features of these three widely used definitions are summarised in Table I.

## Exploring the validity of the endogenous concept

We used two strategies to examine the validity of the endogenous concept. One involves internal validators such as cluster analysis, and the other involves external validators such as familial aggregation. In these studies, completed at the University of Iowa during the past ten years, we were able to draw on the growing data set generated through the NIMH Collaborative Study of the

Psychobiology of Depression. The complete data set is now quite extensive and consists of a total of 942 probands with major depression, 612 of whom were included in a family study. Direct interview data are available for 2,226 of their first degree relatives, and family history data are available for an additional 1,197 relatives included in the family study and another 1,703 relatives not included in the family study (Andreasen *et al*, 1986).

Cluster analysis is a mathematical technique that is used to scan groups of individuals and to chunk them together in clusters which share a number of common features. Cluster analysis can be used to develop new nosological systems, but it can also be used to determine whether clusters generated represent those produced through some other existing classification system such as the RDC. If the clusters generated through this empirical mathematical technique resemble an existing nosology, then the existing nosology can be considered to be at least partially validated (Andreasen *et al*, 1980).

A variety of techniques has been proposed in order to conduct cluster analysis. The major methodological problems include the choice of variables to generate the clusters, the type of clustering procedures (i.e., hierarchical v. overlapping, agglomerative v. divisive), the mathematical criterion used to determine group membership, and the appropriate number of clusters to generate. We found that an hierarchical agglomerative method, sometimes referred to as Ward's method (Ward, 1963) is most useful, confirming observations made previously by Paykel (1971). In this method, the mathematical criterion to determine group membership is to minimise the error sum of squares so that patients are assigned to groups in such a way that the within-group sum of squares is as small as possible. This method tends to find tight clusters of approximately equal size and of relatively homogeneous individuals.

Applying cluster analysis to the Collaborative Depression data set, we have completed three different cluster analytic studies. The results of the studies have been similar and lend some credence to the existence of an endogenous depressive subtype.

In our first cluster study, we evaluated 86 patients with an RDC diagnosis of major depression (Andreasen *et al*, 1980). In this study, three clusters were generated. Cluster I consisted of a group of patients who had relatively characteristic endogenous depression with vegetative features. Cluster II consisted of patients with milder depression who frequently had precipitating events and prominent anxiety, while Cluster III was a group of patients with relatively chronic depression. Fifty nine per cent of the patients in Cluster I met RDC criteria for endogenous depression, while none of the patients in Cluster II were classified as endogenous by RDC criteria. The endogenous group differed significantly from the other two in having greater diurnal variation, psychomotor retardation, nonreactivity of mood, decreased interest, loss of appetite, and terminal insomnia.

In a second cluster analysis study, we evaluated a larger sample of 228 patients with RDC major depression (Andreasen & Grove, 1982). In this somewhat larger sample we found four clusters. Again, Cluster I consisted of patients with endogenous depression with prominent vegetative features. Cluster II consisted of patients with milder depression. Because this sample was larger and broader, we also identified two additional clusters not previously seen in Cluster Study I. Cluster III consisted of patients with bipolar depression who tended to cycle within the episode, while Cluster IV consisted of patients with depression accompanied by psychotic features. In this study, 71% of the patients in Cluster I met RDC criteria for endogenous depression.

As intake in the Collaborative Depression Study reached completion and a much larger sample of patients was available for investigation, we conducted a third cluster study (Grove *et al*, 1987). In this study, we decided to focus on a somewhat narrower group of patients and to exclude those who had features of bipolar illness or schizoaffective disorder. This yielded a sample of 569 patients who met RDC criteria for major depression who were neither bipolar nor schizoaffective. When these patients were excluded, we identified two large clusters. Cluster I again consisted of a group of patients with endogenous depression, while the second consisted of patients who were non-endogenous. In this study, the clinical characteristics that were most prominent in Cluster I included anorexia, weight loss, insomnia, psychomotor agitation, loss of interest or pleasure, feelings of worthlessness, suicidal thoughts and extremely severe dysphoric mood.

While the defining features consistently generated by these three cluster studies are not identical to those identified in the Newcastle Scale, they are relatively similar. An endogenous cluster was consistently identified, and this cluster tended to be marked by vegetative features similar to those identified by the Newcastle Scale. In our third cluster study, we had sufficient data to look at a variety of longitudinal features in addition to cross-sectional ones. The results of this study were somewhat disappointing, in that the endogenous subgroup did not have the expected absence of precipitants, good outcome, or normal personality.

If endogenous depression is in some sense biologically mediated, then one might expect it to be more familial because it would be based on a genetic diathesis. The weaknesses of this assumption are, of course, obvious, in that learned behaviour can also be familial, and therefore family studies must always be subjected to careful scrutiny and independently validated through other more purely genetic methods such as twin studies, adoption studies, and molecular genetic studies. Nevertheless, family studies provide an important initial beginning for exploring possible genetic factors.

We therefore used the Collaborative Depression Family Study sample in order to evaluate familial transmission as an external validator for endogenous depression. Table II compares familial prevalence using three different definitions of endogenous depression: the Newcastle Scale, the RDC, and DSM–III. Table II summarises results using the family history method. Somewhat surprisingly,

TABLE II

*Familial rates of illness in probands suffering from endogenous v. non-endogenous depression*

| Diagnosis in relatives (N = 2492) | Proband diagnosis using three different definitions | | | | | |
| | Newcastle | | RDC | | DSM–III | |
| | Endogenous | Non-endogenous | Endogenous | Non-endogenous | Endogenous | Non-endogenous |
|---|---|---|---|---|---|---|
| Mania | 0.7% | 0.7% | 0.8% | 0.5% | 1.6% | 0.4%* |
| Depression | 19.9% | 19.1% | 19.4% | 19.2% | 22.0% | 18.3%* |
| Recurrent unipolar | 6.0% | 3.8%** | 4.8% | 4.1% | 4.9% | 4.4%* |
| Other | 15.8% | 19.7%** | 17.1% | 20.8%** | 16.4% | 19.2%* |

*$P < 0.05$
**$P < 0.01$

the family history method yielded more prominent patterns of familial transmission than did the family study approach based on direct interview. The DSM–III definition of endogenous depression appears to be the most powerful in detecting familial correlates of endogenous depression. When the DSM–III definition is used, the relatives of endogenous patients have higher rates of mania, depression, and recurrent unipolar disorder, as well as lower rates of other psychiatric disorder. An interesting finding emerges from the use of the Newcastle Scale, however. Using this scale, a higher rate of recurrent unipolar disorder is observed in the families of the patients with endogenous depression. This is a rather interesting finding, since the Newcastle Scale uses recurrence as one of its definitional elements. These results tend to suggest that recurrence may tend to 'breed true' within families, a finding that suggests that longitudinal components to a definition may have a major clinical significance.

Overall, we found our family studies somewhat disappointing. We had anticipated that patients with endogenous depression would have higher rates of depression than did the non-endogenous patients. This was not, however, the case. Thus, the results of this study must be considered inconclusive. The familiality of recurrence identified by the Newcastle Scale and of mania, depression and recurrence using DSM–III, provide positive statistical evidence, but it is not overwhelming.

## Conclusion

Another of my British friends, John Donne, once wrote.

> On a huge hill,
> Cragged and steep, Truth stands, and hee that will
> Reach her, about must, and about must goe;
> And what the hills suddennes resists, winne so;
> Yet strive so, that before age, deaths twilight,
> Thy Soule rest, for none can worke in that night.

That summarises my own thinking about the nature of endogenous depression and our attempts to validate it. I still suspect depression constitutes a heterogeneous group of subtypes. The Platonic idea of a subtype that is biologically mediated and can be biologically relieved through somatic therapy remains very real to me. My pursuit of it, and that of many other investigators, has been a hard climb up a purgatorial mountain, and we still have not got very far. I personally believe that the pursuit is still worthwhile and likely to lead to some long-term scientific rewards that will eventually increase our understanding of both diagnosis and treatment of serious depressions. In that pursuit, we must simply rework our strategies and perhaps return again to ideas developed by the Newcastle group. Perhaps we need to include longitudinal features in order to identify a homogeneous subtype of biological or nuclear depression. Perhaps identifying a subgroup of patients with a good response to somatic therapy is still the best initial step.

# Acknowledgement

This research was supported in part by NIMH grants MH31593 and MH40856; a Scottish Rite Schizophrenia Research Grant; The Nellie Ball Trust Research Fund, Iowa State Bank & Trust Company, Trustee; a Research Scientist Award, MH00625; and Grant Rr59 from the General Clinical Research Centers Program, Division of Research Resources, NIH.

# References

AMERICAN PSYCHIATRIC ASSOCIATION (1980) *DSM–III: Diagnostic and Statistical Manual of Mental Disorders*, (3rd edn.) Washington, DC: APA.

ANDREASEN, N. C. & GROVE, W. M. (1982) The classification of depression: traditional versus mathematical approaches. *American Journal of Psychiatry*, **139**, 45–52.

——, —— & MAURER, R. (1980) Cluster analysis and the classification of depression. *British Journal of Psychiatry*, **137**, 256–265.

——, SCHEFTNER, W., REICH, T., HIRSCHFELD, R. M., ENDICOTT, J. & KELLER, M. B. (1986) The validation of the concept of endogenous depression. *Archives of General Psychiatry*, **43**, 246–251.

CARNEY, M. W. P., ROTH, M. & GARSIDE, R. F. (1965) The diagnosis of depressive syndromes and the prediction of ECT response. *British Journal of Psychiatry*, **111**, 659–674.

DONNE, J. (1912) Satyre III. In *The Poems of John Donne*, vol. 1 (ed. H. J. C. Grierson). London: Oxford University Press.

GROVE, W. M., ANDREASEN, N. C., YOUNG, M., ENDICOTT, J., KELLER, M. B., HIRSCHFELD, R. M. A. & REICH, T. (1987) Isolation and characterization of a nuclear depressive syndrome. *Psychological Medicine*, **11**, 471–484.

HUSTON, P. E. & LOCHER, L. M. (1948) Involutional psychosis: course when treated and untreated with electric shock. *Archives of Neurology & Psychiatry*, **59**, 385–394.

KENDELL, R. E. (1968) *The Classification of Depressive Illness*. London: Oxford University Press.

—— (1976) The classification of depression: a review of contemporary confusion. *British Journal of Psychiatry*, **109**, 261–266.

LEWIS, A. (1938) States of depression: their clinical and aetiological differentiation. *Journal of Mental Science*, **84**, 875–878.

—— (1971) 'Endogenous' and 'exogenous': a useful dichotomy? *Psychological Medicine*, **1**, 191–196.

PAYKEL, E. S. (1971) Classification of depressed patients: a cluster analysis derived grouping. *British Journal of Psychiatry*, **118**, 257–288.

SPITZER, R., ENDICOTT, J. & ROBINS, E. (1975) *Research Diagnostic Criteria*. New York: New York State Psychiatric Institute.

WARD, J. JR. (1963) Hierarchical grouping to optimize an objective function. *Journal of the American Statistical Association*, **58**, 236–244.

# 13 Biological markers and the diagnostic status of schizo-affective depression

**CORNELIUS L. E. KATONA**

This paper describes, and sets in the context of past and subsequent research, a study (Katona & Roth, 1985) that I carried out in collaboration with Sir Martin Roth while I was a registrar at Fulbourn Hospital in 1982. The study was suggested to me by Sir Martin, who encouraged me to apply to the Wellcome Trust for funding and supported my successful application to them.

## Background

The development and validation of a classificatory system of psychiatric diagnosis has been one of the most important connecting threads in Sir Martin Roth's varied and distinguished contribution to psychiatric research. Reviewing the classification of affective disorders (Roth & Barnes, 1981), he clarifies the contrasting requirements of classificatory schemes for research and clinical use. Diagnostic criteria for use by psychiatric researchers must primarily serve the "severely pragmatic purpose of securing uniformity in their findings". To achieve such high inter-rater reliability, a classification that relies primarily on current mental state phenomena may be satisfactory. Clinical diagnosis, however, must be multi-dimensional and take full account of such factors as past and family history, personality, treatment response and prognosis.

The status of schizo-affective psychosis has posed particular problems in psychiatric classifications. The term was originally coined by Kasanin (1933) who referred to psychoses that "occur in young men and women and tend to repeat themselves". Since Kasanin's original postulate, there has been a wide variety of proposed definitions for schizo-affective illness, most of which (Brockington & Meltzer, 1983) would not accommodate the cases Kasanin described. These definitions have been succinctly reviewed by Brockington & Leff (1979), who applied eight possible definitions to a sample of 119 psychotic first admission patients. Although 10% of the sample fulfilled three or more of the diagnostic criteria, the mutual concordance between definitions was very low, with a mean of 0.19. Roth & Barnes (1981) stressed the possible kinship between schizo-affective disorders and both affective illness and schizophrenia, suggesting that "if some clarity and order could be imported into the area (of schizo-affective illness) a number of problems of classification of schizophrenia, affective psychosis and the neuroses would be closer to resolution". It is particularly unfortunate that there should be such marked contrast between the definitions of schizo-affective illness adopted by the most widely used research classificatory systems. This is highlighted by Hirschowitz *et al* (1986) who compare diagnostic categories allocated to a group of patients using Research Diagnostic Criteria: RDC (Spitzer & Endicott, 1978), ICD-9 (World Health Organization, 1977), and DSM–III (American Psychiatric Association, 1980) criteria. Of 18 patients fulfilling RDC criteria for schizo-affective illness the majority are similarly diagnosed using ICD-9, but most of those fulfilling the criteria for the RDC schizophrenic subtype are diagnosed in DSM–III as schizophreniform psychosis, leaving a variety of diagnoses for the RDC affective subtype. It is clear that such a lack of diagnostic clarity has clinical as well as research relevance; as Bouman *et al* (1986) point out "as long as a generally accepted definition of schizo-affective illness is lacking it will remain difficult to ascertain the effectiveness of lithium prophylaxis in this group".

Several strategies have been adopted to resolve these difficulties. These have included studies of inheritance, treatment response, course and outcome (Brockington & Meltzer, 1983), and involve the search for clinically distinct schizo-affective subgroups, as well as comparisons with pure affective or schizophrenic illnesses. Pope & Lipinski (1978) review a number of early phenomenological studies to show that the presence of schizophrenic symptoms contributes little to diagnosis, prognosis, or treatment response in psychotic patients. Brockington & Leff (1979) carried out a discriminant function analysis on a group of patients with relatively clear diagnoses of affective disorder or schizophrenia. The resultant function, which consisted mainly of outcome rather than baseline clinical variables, separated the schizophrenic and affective subjects in this sample with reasonable success, but failed to generate any clear delineation of subgroups when applied to a separate sample diagnosed clinically as schizo-affective.

Several studies of outcome in schizo-affective patients were reviewed by Harrow & Grossman (1984) who concluded that, in general, outcome was intermediate between that in affective disorder and in schizophrenia, and that mood-incongruent psychotic features were themselves predictive of poor outcome. More recently, McGlashan & Williams (1987); Williams & McGlashan (1987) examined long-term outcome in unipolar depressed, manic, bipolar, and schizo-affective depressed subjects. In general, schizo-affective subjects had better short-term but worse long-term outcome than purely depressive subjects, and the depressive subtype of schizo-affective illness had better long-term outcome than the other schizo-affective subtypes, the latter difference not reaching statistical significance.

Studies of treatment response (Goodnick & Meltzer, 1984) suggest that acute schizo-affective illness responds somewhat better to neuroleptics than to antidepressants, and better to the combination than to either drug alone. Response to antidepressants is clearly poorer than in pure depressive illness, but the differences are small in those studies that specifically use psychotically depressed comparison subjects. Lithium prophylaxis was found to be effective in schizo-affective illness in the review by Goodnick & Meltzer (1984); more recently this has been investigated by Maj (1984) and by Bouman *et al* (1986). Both reported favourable responses to lithium prophylaxis, and Maj (1984) found that a past or family history of pure affective illness was a specific predictor of good response to lithium.

Genetic evidence also suggests that schizo-affective depression is a hetero-geneous grouping. Mendlewicz *et al* (1980) reviewed a number of early studies, as well as presenting their own findings on the genetics of schizo-affective illness. Using the Feighner *et al* (1972) criteria for diagnosing their schizo-affective subjects, they reported excess family history of both affective and, less markedly, schizophrenic psychoses in first-degree relatives of schizo-affective subjects, and a strikingly rarity of family history of schizo-affective illness. They suggested that the majority of their subjects therefore had an affective genotype, but a minority had atypical expressions of schizophrenic illness. Unfortunately their findings are not expressed in terms of subtypes of schizo-affective illness. Baron *et al* (1982), however, compared psychiatric illness in the first degree relatives of RDC schizo-affective subjects with that in unipolar and bipolar depressive subjects and schizophrenic subjects, and also separated the mainly affective and mainly schizophrenic subtypes of RDC schizo-affective illness. Morbidity risk for unipolar depression was high in the relatives of the mainly affective schizo-affective subjects; and that for both unipolar depression and schizophrenia increased in the relatives of the mainly schizophrenic schizo-affective subjects. Morbid risk for bipolar depressive illness, as well as for schizo-affective illness itself, was hardly raised in relatives of the schizo-affective subjects. Several other studies reviewed by Brockington & Meltzer (1983) concur broadly with these findings, although there are several reports of a minority of families in which schizo-affective illness breeds true.

The findings discussed above have provided some evidence for the existence of distinct subtypes of schizo-affective illness. The clinical criteria used have, however, clearly proved insufficient to resolve the rightful position of schizo-affective psychosis in the hierarchy of psychiatric diagnosis. It is not, therefore, surprising that in the specific context of schizo-affective illness, as elsewhere in psychiatry, "numerous attempts have been made in recent decades to relate psychiatric classification to biochemical incidences that might place them on a sound and objective biological basis" (Roth & Barnes, 1981).

A variety of physiological responses, biochemical measures in plasma and CSF and peripheral markers of CNS neurotransmitter receptors have been studied (Meltzer *et al*, 1984). Neuroendocrine markers are perhaps the most promising 'windows' to examine CNS function in schizo-affective illness. Growth hormone (GH) responses to apomorphine (measuring dopaminergic function) is reported as increased in schizo-affective illness compared with schizophrenia and mania (Hirschowitz *et al*, 1986). GH response to clonidine (a measure of post-synaptic alpha-2 adrenoceptor function) was, however, decreased to the same extent as in depression when compared with control subjects; in contrast to this, the responses in schizophrenic subjects were enhanced (Matussek *et al*, 1980), though the latter study used only ICD-8 diagnoses. Sternberg *et al* (1982) reported that the clonidine induced decrease in plasma MHPG (reflecting pre-synaptic alpha-2 adrenoceptor function) was blunted in a combined sample of RDC schizophrenic and schizo-affective subjects but not in depressive subjects; only four schizo-affective subjects were included.

Thyroid-stimulating hormone (TSH) responses to thyrotropin (TRH) have been the subject of many studies in depressive illness. These are reviewed by

Loosen (1985), who concludes that blunted responses are present in about a quarter of endogenously depressed subjects and that such abnormality is no commoner in schizophrenic than in control subjects. Few studies have specifically examined responses to TRH in schizo-affective illness. Targum (1983) studied 21 patients with DSM–III schizophreniform disorder, most of whom had high Hamilton depression rating (HDRS; Hamilton 1960) scores and were therefore likely to fulfil RDC criteria for schizo-affective depression. Six subjects had blunted TRH responses, and there was a tendency for this to be associated with good prognosis. Sauer *et al* (1984) compared TSH responses to TRH in a highly selected group of RDC schizo-affective patients, 18 depressive patients and 12 manic subtype patients, all of whom simultaneously fulfilled criteria for both schizophrenic and affective syndromes at the time of testing. Schizo-affective patients, unlike depressed control subjects, did not show any blunting of TSH response.

The dexamethasone suppression test (DST), initially reported as being a highly specific diagnostic test for melancholia (Carroll, 1982), has recently been widely investigated both in schizophrenia and in schizo-affective disorder. Myers (1984) reports serial DSTs in five chronic schizophrenic patients selected specifically for variability in behaviour. Each subject was tested weekly for 12 weeks, and three of the five showed an abnormal response on at least one occasion. Unfortunately no concurrent mood ratings are reported and one of the five patients was being treated with an antidepressant. Sauer *et al* (1984) found similar rates of abnormal DST result in schizophrenia (7 out of 28) as in depression (6 out of 22). Siris *et al* (1984) reported on a group of 16 patients with post-schizophrenic depressions, an unspecified majority of whom fulfilled RDC criteria for schizo-affective illness at the time of testing. None of these showed abnormal DST result.

## *The dexamethasone suppression test in schizo-affective depression (Katona & Roth 1985)*

In this study, the DST was administered to a group of schizo-affective depressed subjects in order to test the hypothesis that the DST non-suppressors would be clinically distinct from the suppressors and have a presentation and outcome more like that of endogenous depression.

**Methods**

*(a) Subject selection*

Case notes of all acute admission patients to a psychiatric hospital and the attenders at its depot neuroleptic clinic during a six month period were reviewed. Patients were considered for inclusion subject to fulfilling the criteria for schizo-affective depression either of the RDC or of a modification of those proposed by Kendell (Brockington & Leff, 1979), requiring two rather than one nuclear symptoms in the diagnosis of a schizophrenic syndrome. Inclusion was also subject to written informed consent.

(b) *DST procedure*

The DST exclusion criteria of Carroll (1982) were used. Dexamethasone 1 mg was administered at 11 pm and blood taken for cortisol assay at 4 pm and 11 pm the following day. Plasma was stored at 4°C for a maximum of 24 hours prior to cortisol assay, which was performed using the Amerlex radioimmunoassay kit (Amersham International). Non-suppression was defined as either of the post-dexamethasone cortisols being $> 138$ nmol/l.

(c) *Clinical ratings*

Patients were rated using the Schedule for Affective Disorders and Schizophrenia (SADS; Spitzer & Endicott, 1979), the HDRS, and the Comprehensive Psychopathological Rating Scale (CPRS; Åsberg *et al*, 1978) within 48 hours of the administration of the DST. Where possible, HDRS and CPRS ratings were repeated two months later.

**Results**

(a) *Diagnosis*. Of 387 patients reviewed, 37 fulfilled one or other of the inclusion criteria, and 30 agreed to participate. Of these, 20 fulfilled both RDC and Kendell criteria for schizo-affective depression; 23 fulfilling RDC criteria and 27 Kendell criteria.

(b) *DST results*. Of the 30 subjects, 10 were non-suppressors. This may be compared with non-suppression in 1/10 healthy volunteers and 15/26 *RDC* major depressives having ECT (Katona *et al*, 1987). There was a non-significant tendency for non-suppressors to be older (8/10 non-suppressors and only 8/20 suppressors aged $> 40$), but their demographic profile was otherwise similar to that of suppressors. Suppressors and non-suppressors did not differ significantly in severity of psychosis (CPRS total) or depression (HDRS total) and of 17 items extracted from the SADS, characteristic either of depression or schizophrenia, no statistically significant differences between suppressors and non-suppressors were found after allowing for multiple comparisons. There were also no significant differences in outcome (in terms of hospital bed occupancy or change in CPRS or HDRS ratings) between suppressors and non-suppressors.

*Conclusions*

These results confirm that schizo-affective depression is a relatively frequent diagnosis within acute adult psychiatry. They are broadly in line with other studies of the DST in RDC schizo-affective depression summarised in Table I.

DST methodology is broadly similar between the studies, although that by Aguilar *et al* (1984) is unusual in routinely administering a barbiturate along with the dexamethasone. Despite the methodological problems involved, relatively clear conclusions emerge from pooling the results of these studies. Several resctricted themselves to schizophrenic or affective subtype, or expressed their results separately for the two. DST non-suppression is, overall, commoner in those with affective subtype (overall 45 out of 85 non-suppressors; 53%)

TABLE I
*Dexamethasone suppression test in RDC schizo-affective depression*

| Study | n | Subtype | Non-suppressors | Suppressors | Major depression (non-suppressor/suppressor) |
|---|---|---|---|---|---|
| Aguilar *et al* (1984) | 13 | — | 9 | 4 | 40/37 |
| Coccaro *et al* (1985) | 9 | Mainly schizophrenic | 2 | 7 | 9/1 |
| Greden *et al* (1981) | 25 | — | 6 | 19 | 25/21 |
| Katona & Roth | 17 | Mainly affective | 6 | 11 | |
| (1985) | 6 | Mainly schizophrenic | 1 | 5 | |
| | 12 | Acute | 4 | 8 | 15/11 |
| | 11 | Chronic | 3 | 8 | |
| Maj (1986) | 8 | Mainly affective | 2 | 6 | |
| | 4 | Intermediate | 1 | 3 | 21/31 |
| | 8 | Mainly schizophrenic | 2 | 6 | |
| Meltzer *et al* (1984) | 14 | Mainly affective | 4 | 10 | 26/27 |
| | 12 | Mainly schizophrenic | 4 | 8 | |
| Sauer *et al* (1984) | 18 | Acute | 16 | 2 | 17/13 |
| Schlesser M. A. | 46 | Mainly affective | 33 | 13 | |
| (pers. comm.) | 25 | Intermediate | 16 | 9 | 120/50 |
| | 6 | Mainly schizophrenic | 0 | 6 | |

than with schizophrenic subtype (8 non-suppressors out of 37; 22%). Only Katona & Roth (1985) and Sauer *et al* (1984) classified their subjects as acute or chronic; the pooled results again suggest that the DST discriminates, 20/30 of the acute subtype, but only 3/11 of the chronic being non-suppressors.

It therefore appears that the dexamethasone suppression test has produced relatively consistent results in schizo-affective depression. The affective and acute subtypes show non-suppression to a degree roughly similar to that in endogenous depression, whereas the schizophrenic and chronic subtypes do not differ from schizophrenic or control patients. This mirrors the subdivisions suggested by genetic studies and validates the RDC subtyping system.

It is interesting that these RDC subtypes, which were lost in DSM–III (American Psychiatric Association, 1980) with virtually all RDC schizo-affective illness being subsumed within affective illness, have to some extent reappeared in the recent revision of DSM–III, DSM–III-R (American Psychiatric Association, 1987) in which the RDC 'mainly affective' subtype has an approximate equivalent in major depressive episode with mood-incongruent psychotic features, and the mainly schizophrenic subtype appears as a distinct subdivision of schizophrenia.

The DST alone does not resolve the issue of whether the affective subtype of RDC schizo-affective depression is biologically distinct from endogenous depression. The data of Sauer *et al* (1984) as well as the work of Banki *et al* (1985, 1986) suggest that the combined use of DST and TRH tests may discriminate better than either test alone. Specifically Sauer *et al* report that TSH response to TRH is blunted in endogenous but not schizo-affective depression, whereas the DST is abnormal in both. The finding that single biological tests are less satisfactory than combinations of such tests in delineating biologically distinct subtypes is echoed in the recent finding by Katona *et al* (1986) that, although neither the DST nor the growth hormone response to clonidine distinguished clinically identifiable subtypes of depression, abnormalities in the two were significantly associated. Siever & Davies (1985) have suggested that in depressive illness several neurotransmitter systems may simultaneously be dysregulated and that this may be reflected in a variety of abnormal neuroendocrine and peripheral neurotransmitter marker responses.

Dexamethasone suppression test results have provided considerable evidence for the hypothesis that there are identifiable subgroupings within schizo-affective depression. This adds support both to the suggested placement of schizo-affective illness in the diagnostic hierarchy of Roth & Barnes (1981) and also to the value they place on using biological markers in refining psychiatric diagnosis. It is likely that future biological research will further resolve the diagnostic status of schizo-affective illness through similar strategies, though the likely focus of such studies will be on patterns of dysregulation between multiple biological markers rather than on isolated biochemical abnormalities.

# References

AGUILAR, TOSCAŅO, M., LEMAIRE, M., CASTRO, P., LIBOTTE, M., REYNDERS, J. & HERCHUELZ, A. (1984) Study of the diagnostic value of the dexamethasone suppression test in endogenous depression. *Journal of Affective Disorders*, **6**, 33–42.

AMERICAN PSYCHIATRIC ASSOCIATION (1980) *Diagnostic and Statistical Manual of Mental Disorders* (3rd edn.) Washington, DC: APA.

—— (1987) *Diagnostic and Statistical Manual of Mental Disorders* (3rd edn.–revised) Washington, DC: APA.

ÅSBERG, M., MONTGOMERY, S. A., PERRIS, C., SCHALLING, C. & SEDVALL, G. (1978) The CPRS—development and application of a psychiatric rating scale. *Acta Psychiatrica Scandinavica*, Suppl. 271, 5–27.

BANKI, M. C., VOJNIK, M., ARATO, M., PAPP, Z. & KOVACS, Z. (1985) Dexamethasone suppression and multiple hormonal responses (TSH, prolactin and growth hormone) to TRH in some psychiatric disorders. *European Archives of Psychiatry and Neurological Sciences*, **235**, 32–37.

——, ARATO, M., PAPP, Z., RIHMER, Z. & KOVACS, Z. (1986) Associations among dexamethasone non-suppression and TRH-induced hormonal responses: increased specificity for melancholia? *Psychoneuroendocrinology*, **11**, 205–211.

BARON, M., GRUEN, R., ASNIS, L. & KANE, J. (1982) Schizoaffective illness, schizophrenia and affective disorders: morbidity risk and genetic transmission. *Acta Psychiatrica Scandinavica*, **65**, 253–262.

BOUMAN, T. K., NIEMANTSVERDRIET-VAN KAMPEN, B. B. G., ORMEL, J. & SLOOFF, S. J. (1986) The effectiveness of lithium prophylaxis in bipolar and unipolar depressions and schizo-affective disorders. *Journal of Affective Disorders*, **11**, 275–280.

BROCKINGTON, I. F. & LEFF, J. P. (1979) Schizo-affective psychosis: definitions and incidence. *Psychological Medicine*, **9**, 91–99.

—— & MELTZER, H. Y. (1983) The nosology of schizoaffective psychosis. *Psychiatric Developments*, **4**, 317–338.

CARROLL, B. J. (1982) The dexamethasone suppression test for melancholia. *British Journal of Psychiatry*, **140**, 292–304.

COCCARO, E. F., PRUDIC, J., ROTHPEARL, A. & NURNBERG, H. G. (1985) The dexamethasone suppression test in depressive, non-depressive and schizoaffective psychosis. *Journal of Affective Disorders*, **9**, 107–113.

FEIGHNER, J. P., ROBINS, E., GUZE, S. B., WOODRUFF, R. A., WINOKUR, G. & MUNOZ, R. (1972) Diagnostic criteria for use in psychiatric research. *Archives of General Psychiatry*, **26**, 57–63.

GOODNICK, P. J. & MELTZER, H. Y. (1984) Treatment of schizoaffective disorders. *Schizophrenia Bulletin*, **10**, 30–48.

GREDEN, J. F., KRONFOL, Z., GARDNER, R., FEINBERG, M. & CARROLL, B. J. (1981) Neuroendocrine evaluation of schizoaffectives with the dexamethasone suppression test. In *Biological Psychiatry 1981* (eds C. Perris, G. Struwe & B. Janssen). Amsterdam: Elsevier/North Holland Biomedical Press.

HAMILTON, M. (1960) A rating scale for depression. *Journal of Neurology, Neurosurgery and Psychiatry*, **23**, 56–62.

HARROW, M. & GROSSMAN, L. S. (1984) Outcome in schizoaffective disorders: A critical review and re-evaluation of the literature. *Schizophrenia Bulletin*, **10**, 87–108.
HIRSCHOWITZ, J., ZEMAN, F. P., HITZEMANN, R. J., FLEISCHMANN, R. L. & GARVER, D. L. (1986) Growth hormone response to apomorphine and diagnosis: a comparison of three diagnostic systems. *Biological Psychiatry*, **21**, 445–454.
KASANIN, J. (1933) The acute schizoaffective psychoses. *American Journal of Psychiatry*, **13**, 97–126.
KATONA, C. L. E., ALDRIDGE, C. R., ROTH, M. & HYDE, J. (1987) The dexamethasone suppression test and prediction of outcome in patients receiving ECT. *British Journal of Psychiatry*, **150**, 315–318.
—— & ROTH, M. (1985) The dexamethasone suppression test in schizoaffective depression. *Journal of Affective Disorders*, **8**, 107–112.
——, THEODOROU, A. E., DAVIES, S. L., YAMAGUCHI, Y., TUNNICLIFFE, C. A., HALE, A. S., HORTON, R. W., KELLY, J. S. & PAYKEL, E. S. (1986) Platelet binding and neuroendocrine responses in depression. *The Biology of Depression* (ed. J. F. W. Deakin). London: Gaskell (Royal College of Psychiatrists).
LOOSEN, P. T. (1985) The TRH-induced TSH response in psychiatric patients: a possible neuroendocrine marker. *Psychoneuroendocrinology*, **10**, 237–260.
McGLASHAN, T. H. & WILLIAMS, P. V. (1987) Schizoaffective psychosis: II. Manic, bipolar, and depressive subtypes. *Archives of General Psychiatry*, **44**, 138–139.
MAJ, M. (1984) Effectiveness of lithium prophylaxis in schizoaffective psychoses: application of a polydiagnostic approach. *Acta Psychiatrica Scandinavica*, **70**, 228–234.
—— (1986) Response to the dexamethasone suppression test in schizoaffective disorder, depressed type. *Journal of Affective Disorders*, **11**, 63–67.
MATUSSEK, N., ACHENHEIL, M., HIPPIUS, H., MULLER, F., SCHRODER, H-TH., SCHULTES, H. & WASILEWSKI, B. (1980) Effect of clonidine on growth hormone reliance in psychiatric patients and controls. *Psychiatry Research* **2**, 25–36.
MELTZER, H. Y., ARORA, R. C. & METZ, J. (1984) Biological studies of schizoaffective disorders. *Schizophrenia Bulletin*, **10**, 49–70.
MENDLEWICZ, J., LINKOWSKI, P. & WILMOTTE, J. (1980) Relationship between schizoaffective illness and affective disorders or schizophrenia. *Journal of Affective Disorders*, **2**, 289–302.
MYERS, E. D. (1984) Serial dexamethasone suppression tests in male chronic schizophrenic patients. *American Journal of Psychiatry*, **141**, 904–905.
POPE, H. G. & LIPINSKI, J. F. (1978) Diagnosis in schizophrenia and manic-depressive illness: a reassessment of the specificity of "schizophrenic" symptoms in the light of current research. *Archives of General Psychiatry*, **35**, 811–828.
ROTH, M. & BARNES, T. R. E. (1981) The classification of affective disorders: a synthesis of old and new concepts. *Comprehensive Psychiatry*, **22**, 54–77.
SAUER, H., KOEHLER, K. G., SASS, H., HORNSTEIN, C. & MINNE, H. W. (1984) The dexamethasone suppression test and thyroid stimulating hormone response to TRH in RDC schizoaffective patients. *European Archives of Psychiatry and Neurological Science*, **234**, 264–267.
SIEVER, L. J. & DAVIES, K. L. (1985) Overview: toward a dysregulation hypothesis of depression. *American Journal of Psychiatry*, **142**, 1017–1031.
SIRIS, S. G., RIFKIN, A., REARDON, G. T., DODDI, S. R., FOSTER, P., STRAHAN, A. & MORGAN, V. (1984) The dexamethasone suppression test in patients with postpsychotic depressions. *Biological Psychiatry*, **19**, 1351–1356.
SPITZER, R. L. & ENDICOTT, J. (1978) *Research Diagnostic Criteria for a Selected Group of Functional Disorders* (3rd edn). New York: New York State Psychiatric Institute.
—— & —— (1979) *Schedule for Affective Disorders and Schizophrenia* (3rd edn). New York: New York State Psychiatric Institute.
STERNBERG, D. E., CHARNEY, D. S., HENINGER, G. R., LECKMAN, J. F., HAFSTAD, K. M. & LANDIS, H. (1982) Impaired presynaptic regulation of norepinephrine in schizophrenia. *Archives of General Psychiatry*, **39**, 285–289.
TARGUM, S. D. (1983) Neuroendocrine dysfunction in schizophreniform disorder: correlation with six month clinical outcome. *American Journal of Psychiatry*, **140**, 309–313.
WILLIAMS, P. V. & McGLASHAN, T. H. (1987) Schizoaffective Psychosis: I. Comparative long term outcome. *Archives of General Psychiatry*, **44**, 130–137.
WORLD HEALTH ORGANIZATION (1977) *Manual of the International Statistical Classification of Diseases, Injuries, and Causes of Death*, 9th revision. Geneva: WHO.

# 14 The differential diagnosis of depression and the prediction of response to ECT: a continuing odyssey

**MICHAEL W. P. CARNEY**

When I started work with Sir Martin in Newcastle upon Tyne in 1960 we were both impressed with the work of Crooks *et al* (1959) on diagnostic indices for separating thyrotoxic from euthyroid patients. Contemporaneously, Professor Kiloh and his co-workers were applying the methods of multivariate analysis to the problem of predicting response to the (then) new antidepressant drug, imipramine (Kiloh *et al*, 1962). At the suggestion of Sir Martin, I compiled a list of clinical features culled from the literature and credited with value in making the distinction between endogenous and neurotic depression, and weighted them in proportion to their apparent importance in making this discrimination. I then used these weighted features to analyse retrospectively the records of in-patients at the Newcastle General Hospital, admitted and treated with ECT, over the preceding three years. I found a good separation between the endogenous depressive patients, who mostly had responded well, and the neurotic patients who had not.

Encouraged by this finding, I carried out a prospective investigation of depressed patients admitted for that reason to the psychiatric facilities of Newcastle upon Tyne. From statistical analyses of these data, Garside computed two sets of weighted features, one for differential diagnosis and the other for predicting response to ECT (Carney *et al*, 1965). Subsequently, Gurney and her co-workers (1972) produced a set of weighted features to distinguish between depression and anxiety. All three sets of features have been called 'Newcastle Index' but in this paper, I shall reserve the term for the two sets of weighted

TABLE I
*Diagnosis Scale*

| Feature | Weights |
|---|---|
| Adequate personality | + 1 |
| No adequate psychogenesis | + 2 |
| Distinct quality | + 1 |
| Weight loss | + 2 |
| Previous episode | + 1 |
| Depressive psychomotor activity | + 2 |
| Anxiety | − 1 |
| Nihilistic delusions | + 2 |
| Blame others | − 1 |
| Guilt | + 1 |

Score > 6 = endogenous depression

110

TABLE II
*ECT prediction scale*

| Feature | Weights |
| --- | --- |
| Weight loss | + 3 |
| Pyknic | + 3 |
| Early wakening | + 2 |
| Anxiety | − 2 |
| Somatic delusions | + 2 |
| Paranoid delusions | + 1 |
| Worse p.m. | − 3 |
| Self pity | − 1 |
| Hypochondriacal | − 3 |
| Hysterical | − 3 |

Score >1 = good response

features produced by Carney *et al*, (1965)—the Newcastle Diagnosis Scale and the Newcastle ECT Prediction Scale. (Tables I and II.)

## Validity of the scale

The Newcastle Scales are valid. This is supported by statistical, biochemical, therapeutic, other physiological, clinical and tomographical evidence. A rating scale is also validated if the original results are replicated in different years, regions, populations and cultures. Kendell & Post (1973), hardly likely to favour the dualist view, confirmed the presence of an endogenous-neurotic continuum, i.e. that not all variation in depression was due to severity, and thus supported the validity of the endogenous-neurotic dichotomy.

Roth & Garside (1973) maintained that bimodality, no matter how derived, always favoured two distinct populations whereas unimodality can be taken to indicate a homogeneous population or a bimodal distribution obscured by other factors. Moreover, further analysis of Kendell's group B revealed a distribution significantly deviant from normality (Garside, 1973). Hope (1969), on replicating Kendell's discriminant function analysis, concluded that Kendell's own findings supported a bimodal distribution of his patients' scores.

Carney & Sheffield (1972) applied the index to a group of Lancashire in-patient depressive subjects, all treated with ECT. They were able to replicate the Newcastle bimodal distribution, one 'hump' comprising endogenous patients, and the other, neurotic depressive subjects. The former were responsive, and the latter poorly responsive, to ECT. It is noteworthy that these patients were drawn from a different population from the original Newcastle depressive subjects.

An inventory of items taken largely from the 'Newcastle Scales' of Carney *et al* (1965) and Gurney *et al* (1972) was devised by Bech *et al* (1980) for comparison with WHO's schedule for the Standardised Assessment of Depressive Disorders (SADD). The authors applied this to in-patients classified as endogenous by these scales and found significant relationships between plasma levels of imipramine and clomipramine and antidepressant effectiveness. On the other hand, non-endogenous patients showed no similar correlation. Montgomery *et al* (1978) have reported a similar finding with mianserin. Like Carney *et al* (1965), they also found that the initial severity of depression in patients diagnosed as endogenous, non-endogenous and doubtful diagnosis did not differ on mean Hamilton score, i.e. severity of depression. Feinberg & Carroll (1982) also separated two depressive types, using discriminant function analysis and criterion diagnoses derived from two certainly diagnosed groups of depressive patients. They validated the scale thus obtained by applying it to a second group of depressed patients and achieved a similar separation. They commented on the similarity of their items to the Newcastle items. Of their patients, 80% were correctly classified by their index which achieved an agreement with the original clinical diagnosis of 90%. The authors also validated their index by means of the Dexamethasone Suppression Test (DST). Carney & Sheffield (1972) conducted a blind assessment of 165 patients one month after courses of ECT. These patients had participated in various research projects and had been rated on the Newcastle Scale. One hundred and one had a 'good outcome' and 64 a 'poor outcome'. The mean Newcastle Score of the good outcome patients was found to be significantly higher, i.e. more endogenous ($P<0.001$), than the poor outcome patients. The same authors also found a significant rank order correlation between mean fall in Hamilton Score (i.e. extent of improvement) and magnitude of original Newcastle ECT prediction score.

## Biochemical evidence of validity

Naylor *et al* (1971) measured erythrocyte sodium and potassium concentrations in 11 neurotic and 14 psychotic depressive patients, the diagnostic type being determined by the Newcastle and Kendell Scales. There was complete agreement between these scales in allocating patients to one category or the other. Though there was no change in plasma sodium on recovery and no change at any time in potassium, the mean erythrocyte sodium in the neurotic patients was lower than that of the psychotic depressive subjects and remained so after recovery. Naylor and his colleagues elsewhere (1974) reported good concordance between Newcastle and Kendell Scales and between both these devices and cyclic AMP in recovering endogenous depressives (ICD 296.2).

Montgomery *et al* (1978) measured plasma levels of mianserin in patients treated with the drug divided into Newcastle Scale endogenous and neurotic depression. A significant relationship between plasma level and response was found in endogenous depression but not in non-endogenous depression. In 98 patients allocated to endogenous and neurotic groups by the Scale, a significant relationship between plasma level and response to imipramine and clomipramine was found in the endogenous depressive subjects but not in the neurotic depressive subjects (Bech *et al*, 1980).

The relationships of growth hormone responses to clonidine and apo-morphine in a group of eight drug-free patients with Newcastle endogenous depression were explored by Corn *et al* (1984). Growth hormone responses were significantly smaller than responses to apo-morphine and similar to responses found with normal subjects. The authors felt their findings supported a defect in the adenergic but not in the dopaminergic regulation of growth hormone in endogenous depression.

An investigation of CSF vasopressin, adrenaline and nor-adrenaline and in plasma vasopressin and osmolarity in 37 depressed patients and 10 normal controls (Gjerris *et al*, 1985) failed to reveal differences between Newcastle endogenous and non-endogenous patients, but CSF vasopressin was significantly lower in depressive subjects than in normal control subjects.

The Newcastle Index was used in an investigation of melatonin and cortisol values during treatment with desipramine (Thompson *et al*, 1985). However, no differences between endogenous and non-endogenous patients were recorded. On the other hand, in a study of platelet alpha 2 and lymphocyte beta 2 adrenoceptors, plasma nor-adrenaline and serum cortisol in nine Newcastle endogenous depressive patients one week after a course of ECT (Cooper *et al*, 1985), the mean plasma nor-adrenaline was found to be initially high but fell as the ECT course proceeded, matching the degree of clinical recovery.

### Dexamethasone Suppression Test (DST)

Holden (1982) reported DST results in 41 depressive patients allocated to endogenous or neurotic depression by Newcastle Score. The results correlated with the Newcastle diagnosis of endogenous depression with a specificity of 89%, a sensitivity of 82% and a diagnostic confidence of 94%. Coppen *et al* (1983) showed that 89% of patients with a Newcastle Score for endogenous depression had an abnormal DST response compared to only 49% of those with non-endogenous depression.

A number of recent studies of the DST employed the Newcastle Diagnosis Index with conflicting results. Thus Ames *et al* (1984) described 90 patients with primary depressive illness, all of whom were given the DST before treatment. With respect to the first treatment response, the non-suppressors did better than the suppressors but there was no correlation between overall response and diagnosis score or response and DST suppression. On the other hand, Klein *et al* (1984) found the DST to discriminate to a significant degree between Newcastle endogenous depression and neurotic depression and noted that baseline and post-dexamethasone control levels were reduced by minor tranquillisers but not by major tranquillisers or antidepressants. However, they did not find that the DST results could be used as a reliable indicator of prognosis. MacKeith (1984), using the Newcastle Scale, found that the DST was a valid diagnostic test for endogenous depression thus defined, but of no value in distinguishing dementia from depressive illness. Another study (Berger *et al*, 1984) found the DST to be of limited value in separating endogenous from non-endogenous depression as defined by the Newcastle Diagnostic Index. Nevertheless, a review of 20 studies dealing with DST non-suppression in endogenous and non-endogenous depression diagnosed by a variety of methods (Braddock, 1986) indicated that there is a higher non-suppression rate in Newcastle Diagnosis Scale endogenous depressives than in non-endogenous depressives. Moreover, Coppen *et al* (1985) found post-dexamethasone cortisol to be significantly correlated with Newcastle Scores after Hamilton Scores (severity of depression) were partialled out. Using a DST cut-off point of 100 ng/ml with respect to plasma cortisol, patients with intermediate Newcastle Scores (i.e. 4–8) did better after ECT or antidepressant drugs than those with higher or lower scores.

The DST was applied to 143 patients with major depression (Coppen *et al*, 1983) classified into those scoring positively for the Newcastle Diagnosis item 'weight loss' and those not scoring on this item; 73% of patients with the item and 61% of the rest showed abnormal DST. Moreover, 13 patients on prophylactic lithium carbonate were found to have changed their DST status over a period of 14 months, but did not change their weight.

The associations of life events, the pituitary-adrenal axis and the DST were explored in 72 depressed patients (Dolan *et al*, 1985). Though associations were found between antecedent life events on the one hand and first episodes and greater severity of depression on the other, this feature did not associate with endogenous or non-endogenous depression as diagnosed by the Newcastle Diagnosis Scale or with DST status, though urinary cortisol levels were found to be higher in those patients who had experienced stressful life events.

Coppen and his colleagues (1983, 1985) carried out major studies of the value of the DST in predicting treatment response in depression. They showed that patients with intermediate Newcastle Diagnosis Scores (4–8) showed a superior response to antidepressant drugs than those with higher or lower scores. They also found post-dexamethasone cortisol to be significantly correlated with the Newcastle Score after the Hamilton Score (severity of depression) was partialled out.

Sireling (1986) applied the DST to 12 mentally-handicapped depressive patients classified by several scales including the Newcastle Diagnosis Index. There was no correlation between Newcastle Diagnosis and DST results and the authors suggested that the Newcastle Diagnosis Index was unreliable in this group. However, Braddock (1986), reviewing 20 studies of DST suppression and non-suppression rates in endogenous and non-endogenous depression, thought that the Newcastle Diagnostic Index gave the best differentiation between the two kinds of depression in terms of DST results. In general, there was a higher non-suppression rate in endogenous as identified by the Newcastle and Carroll Scales than in non-endogenous depression. Zimmerman *et al* (1986) also found a significantly higher rate of DST non-suppression in Newcastle endogenous depressive patients than in non-endogenous depressive patients. The authors cited this as evidence of discontinuity between endogenous and non-endogenous depressive patients. In a later study (Zimmerman *et al*, 1987) they showed that the morbid risk for alcoholism was lower in Newcastle endogenous depressive patients than in non-endogenous depressive patients and that the relationship between Newcastle Score and these variables was non-linear, indicating that endogenous and non-endogenous depressive subjects did not come from the same population.

Discontinuity between Newcastle endogenous and non-endogenous depressive patients was also found in the investigations of Davidson *et al* (1984) and Carney *et al* (1987). The former team studied the Newcastle Index in 36 depressed patients: endogenous and non-endogenous depressive subjects thus defined responded differently to isocarboxazid.

## Physiological

Mirkin & Coppen (1980) measured electrodermal activity in 18 depressed patients to whom the Newcastle Scale had been applied and compared their response with that of 15 controls. The endogenous depressives had significantly lower skin conductance and lower 5-HT uptake than the non-endogenous depressives. In two studies of depressed patients, negative (depressing) thoughts were reduced by the presentation of external information at a high rate. This reduction negatively correlated with Newcastle Score, being greater for neurotic and less for endogenous patients (Teasdale & Rezin, 1978).

## Cerebral tomography

Jacoby & Levy (1980) investigated 41 elderly depressed patients with computed cerebral tomography. They identified a sub-group of patients, older than the rest, with higher mean Newcastle Scores, later onset of depression and enlarged cerebral ventricles, possibly due to organic cerebral factors. Followed up one year later, this sub-group was found to be persistently depressed as judged by the Hamilton Rating Scale and had a higher mortality than the other patients.

## Treatment

Carney & Sheffield (1972) in a study of depressed patients treated with ECT showed that those scoring 6 or more on the diagnosis scale (endogenous) did significantly better in terms of social and clinical recovery, both immediately and at three months after treatment, than the remaining patients. The same authors (1973) subsequently carried out a blind assessment, one month after ECT, of 165 depressives who had been rated on the Newcastle Scale in the course of several projects; 101 patients had made a full social recovery and 64 patients had not done so. There was a highly significant difference between them in terms of mean results with ECT, Newcastle endogenous patients doing better than Newcastle neurotic patients. The predictive value of the Newcastle Diagnosis Scale in depressed patients treated with ECT was also confirmed by Vlissades & Jenner (1982).

Rao & Coppen (1979) rated 54 depressed patients on the Scale before giving amitriptyline. When reassessed six weeks later, patients scoring 4–8 on the Newcastle Scale did significantly better than those with higher or lower scores, a difference not accounted for by differences in pre-treatment severity of depression as measured by the Hamilton Scale. On the other hand, Lambourn & Gill (1978), using the diagnosis scale in a controlled comparison of simulated and real pulse ECT, found no difference between the two groups but more recently doubt has been cast on this conclusion by the finding that the low energy pulse ECT used in this investigation is relatively ineffective (Robin & De Tissera, 1982).

Carney and his colleagues (1987) used the Newcastle Diagnosis Scale to classify patients as endogenous and non-endogenous in several trials of S-adenosyl methionine (SAM). The endogenous patients consistently did well with SAM whereas the neurotic patients showed a negligible response.

The Newcastle Scale has also been used to classify patients as endogenous or non-endogenous in studies of ECT and pituitary response (Slade & Checkley, 1980), desipramine and central adenergic function (Glass *et al*, 1982); as well as with methylamphetamine and clonidine and central alpha adrenoceptors

(Checkley *et al*, 1981). Differences with respect to endogenous and neurotic depression emerged in these studies.

Robin & De Tissera (1982) employed both diagnosis and ECT scales in an investigation comparing the efficacy of low-energy ECT, high-energy pulses and pulsed current ECT. Most endogenous depressive patients did well whereas those given low-energy pulse current did not. In a double-blind placebo-controlled trial of phenelzine and amitriptyline in patients with Newcastle Scores greater than 8 (Robinson *et al*, 1973) there was no clear evidence of clinical sub-groups responding preferentially to one drug or the other. Johnstone *et al* (1980) used the scale to define more exactly patients admitted to the Northwick Park trial of real and simulated ECT. Coppen *et al* (1983) defined his depressive patients with the scale. In a placebo-controlled trial of lithium carbonate in a group of 38 depressive patients following ECT, both treatment groups had similar (endogenous) mean Newcastle Scores and lithium was found to be more effective than placebo in preventing relapse.

Montgomery (1981) examined the validity of several scales used in research. He believed the Medical Research Council criteria (1965) to be inadequate and unreliable while the Present State Examination failed to distinguish between primary depression and that associated with alcohol, drugs, etc. The Research Diagnostic Criteria (Spitzer & Endicott, 1978) used a definition too heavily weighted towards endogenous depression; and he doubted whether the DSM–III (1980) was adequate. However, he regarded the Newcastle Diagnosis Scale (1965) and that of Gurney *et al* (1972) as being adequate. Nevertheless, it must be admitted that the Newcastle Diagnosis Scale has been much more used than the Newcastle ECT Scale (see below).

The results of clinical investigations and treatment with S-adenosyl methionine (SAM) have been clarified by the use of the Scale (Reynolds *et al*, 1984; Carney *et al*, 1987). SAM metabolism is intimately connected with folate and monoamine metabolism and may have other actions in the nervous system with respect to cell membranes and neurotransmission (Reynolds & Stramentinoli, 1983). SAM is synthesised in the body and a major source of methyl groups. Preliminary results in the United Kingdom (Carney *et al*, 1983) indicated that the substance had an antidepressant action in endogenous depression and was associated with switches into elated mood. In a later paper on the prediction of outcome by the Newcastle Scale, Carney *et al* (1987) described a series of depressed patients admitted to three trials of SAM: a placebo-controlled trial, a pilot trial and a controlled comparison of SAM and amitriptyline. It was found that the Newcastle Diagnosis Scores were not normally distributed but bimodally distributed. Evidence for discontinuity in these distributions was adduced from the contrast in outcome between Newcastle endogenous and Newcastle neurotic depressive patients, the former faring consistently better than the latter. On the other hand, the unipolar/bipolar classification failed to predict differing results for these categories and the DSM–III criteria also failed to identify sub-groups of differing prognoses.

## Cognitive therapy

Teasdale & Rezin (1978) examined the extent to which distracting patients from preoccupying negative thoughts reduced their frequency and thus alleviated depression. They found that patients with "more neurotic symptoms" as judged on the Newcastle Diagnosis Index achieved greater negative thought reduction than more "endogenous" patients. This was confirmed by Davies (1982), using a different population and a different distraction task. The subject of cognitive therapy and major depression is reviewed by Williams (1984).

## Clinical

An American study which throws doubt on the concept of endogenous depression but which employed, among others, the Newcastle Diagnosis Index is that of Young *et al* (1986). These workers studied symptom ratings from 788 major depressive patients participating in the NIMH Collaborative Depression Study. Though the results did not show that the symptoms specified a dichotomous classification (melancholic and non-melancholic, or endogenous and non-endogenous) the results did support two typings, 'anhedonia' and 'vegetative'. Some support to a hierarchical classification based on these symptoms was suggested by the fact that the vegetative features rarely occurred in non-anhedonic patients.

The Newcastle Index was used in the study of clinical features in a comparison of general practice (GP) and out-patient depressives, treated with antidepressants (Sireling *et al*, 1985). The GP depressives were less severely ill than the out-patients and had fewer depressive symptoms and a shorter duration of illness. There were also fewer primary depressives and fewer endogenous depressives (as defined by Newcastle Index) among the GP patients.

## ECT Prediction Scale

There have been few investigations on the other scale proposed by Carney *et al* (1965)—the ECT Prediction Scale. Carney & Sheffield (1972) applied it to a small group of severely depressed patients treated with ECT and reported it to be both valid and reliable. In the Northwick Park ECT Trial (1984), no significant correlation between Newcastle ECT Score and improvement was found after real or simulated ECT. Katona *et al* (1987), however, applied the Newcastle ECT Scale to a group of major depressive patients given ECT. The Scale successfully predicted both intermediate outcome and outcome at six months following ECT, whereas the Newcastle Diagnosis Scale (Carney *et al*, 1965), the Newcastle Scale of Gurney *et al* (1972) and the DST failed to do so.

## Reliability

Carney & Sheffield (1972) found the Newcastle Diagnosis Scale to be reliable in a small number of patients. In a small pilot investigation of SAM-treated patients, Martin & Nissenbaum (unpublished) found the Newcastle Diagnosis Scale to be reliable, as did the WHO collaborative study involving 13 research centres in 12 countries (Coppen & Metcalfe, 1987). However, it must be admitted that this topic has not been adequately investigated.

## Conclusions

Few psychiatric topics of this century have generated more controversy than the question of the classification of depression—by severity alone or by the additional source of variation contributed by the endogenous and neurotic sub-types. Some years ago the argument raged about the question of the bimodal or unimodal distributions of Newcastle Diagnosis Scores. As Roth & Garside (1973) pointed out, only a bimodal distribution of scores could provide an unequivocal verdict— in favour of two distinct sub-populations. Finding a unimodal distribution is equivocal, either favouring bimodality obscured by other factors, or pointing to a single homogeneous population. A new slant to the question has been given, however, by recent discussions concerning the implications of continuity or discontinuity as evidenced by some independent criterion, like response to treatment or a biochemical measure. Preliminary appraisal of the results of such studies supports the validity of the distinction, even when the Newcastle Diagnosis Scores have been unimodally distributed. There can be little doubt of the validity of the Newcastle Diagnosis Index in distinguishing between endogenous and non-endogenous depressions and this is reflected in the increasing number of studies employing the device.

Should then traditional methods of diagnosis be replaced by this kind of device? It is arguable that diagnosis should be more than a system of numerical taxonomy. For the practising clinician, a diagnosis is a simple guide to treatment in the medical sense, other forms of management and prognosis. Moreover, trying to remember a number of weighted features is onerous for many people whereas a clinical diagnosis is a stable, simple entity which medically-trained clinicians can readily grasp.

Similar arguments are relevant to the question of predicting response to a given treatment by means of a number of weighted indices. Moreover, treatment fashions come and go. Are we to have a different set of items for each new treatment? Diagnosis on the other hand is a more enduring entity and carries with it implications for the kind of management appropriate to it. There can be little argument though that in the areas of research, communication of data and standardisation of classification, sets of indices are more precise and relevant.

The reliability of the Newcastle Diagnosis Index, however, is much less investigated than the question of validity, and much remains to be done. Likewise, the Newcastle ECT Prediction Index has received comparatively little attention but the recent pioneering study of Katona *et al* (1987) should provide a useful impetus to this avenue of enquiry.

Growing acceptance of the pragmatic value of the Newcastle Diagnosis Index and the ECT Prediction Index is reflected in the increasing interest in these fields. Though much remains to be done in different cultures and in different regions, these devices are increasingly judged to be of universal relevance. Recent contributions have come from France and the World Health Organization. Ansseau *et al* (1987) have shown that the distribution of Newcastle scores from 41 depressed patients tended to be bimodal. The Newcastle endogenous patients were more often severely depressed and were more often of the primary, endogenous, agitated and simple RDC sub-types as compared with those judged to be neurotic by the Scale. The diagnosis scale has also been adopted by the World Health Organization (Bech *et al*, 1984). In a collaborative study involving

13 research centres in 12 countries, the Scale was used to define endogenous and neurotic depression in 543 depressed patients and 246 healthy controls. In four of five countries contributing sufficient endogenous patients to be statistically meaningful, the Newcastle endogenous depressives had higher mean post-dexamethasone plasma control concentrations than the Newcastle neurotic depressives (Coppen & Metcalfe, 1987).

From my own point of view, I feel a sense of quiet satisfaction that these scales, born of the interest of Sir Martin, Roger Garside and myself in these topics so many years ago, after so much controversy, have given rise to so many productive enquiries, useful results and now an increasing measure of agreement. The odyssey, however, continues.

## References and further reading

AMERICAN PSYCHIATRIC ASSOCIATION (1980) *Diagnostic and Statistical Manual of Mental Disorders* (3rd edn). Washington, DC: APA.

AMES, D., BURROWS, G., DAVIES, B., MAGUIRE, K. & NORMAN, T. (1984) A study of the Dexamethasone Suppression Test in hospitalised depressed patients. *British Journal of Psychiatry*, **144**, 311–313.

ANSSEAU, M., CERFINTAIRE, J. L., VON FRENCKELL, R., CHERBS, G., DAPART, P. & FRANCK, G. (1987) L'index pour le diagnostic de depression endogene. *L'Encephale*, **13**, 67–72.

ANDREASEN, N. C., GROVE, W. M. & MAURER, R. (1980) Cluster analysis and classification of depression. *British Journal of Psychiatry*, **137**, 256–265.

BECH, P., GRAM, L. F., REISBY, N. & RAFAELSEN, O. J. (1980) The WHO Depression Scale: relationship to the Newcastle Scales. *Acta Psychiatrica Scandinavica*, **62**, 140–153.

——, GASTPAR, M. & MOROZOV, P. V. (1984) Clinical Assessment Scales for biological psychiatry to be used in WHO studies. *Progress in Neuropsychopharmacology & Biological Psychiatry*, **8**, 190–196.

BERGER, M., PIRKE, K-M., DOERR, P., KRIEG, J-C. & ZERSSEN, D. VON (1984) The limited utility of the Dexamethasone Suppression Test for the diagnostic process in psychiatry. *British Journal of Psychiatry*, **145**, 372–382.

BRADDOCK, L. M. (1986) The Dexamethasone Suppression Test: fact and artefact. *British Journal of Psychiatry*, **148**, 363–374.

CARNEY, M. W. P. & SHEFFIELD, B. F. (1972) Depression and the Newcastle Scale. The relationship to Hamilton Scale. *British Journal of Psychiatry*, **121**, 35–40.

—— & —— (1973) The depressive illnesses of late life. *British Journal of Psychiatry*, **123**, 723–725.

——, ROTH, M. & GARSIDE, R. F. (1965) The diagnosis of depressive syndromes and the prediction of ECT response. *British Journal of Psychiatry*, **111**, 651–674.

——, MARTIN, R., BOTTIGLIERI, T., TOONE, B. K., NISSENBAUM, H., REYNOLDS, E. H. & SHEFFIELD, B. F. (1983) The switch mechanism in affective illness and SAM. *Lancet*, **i**, 820–821.

——, EDEH, J., REYNOLDS, E. H., TOONE, B. K., THOMAS, C. & SHEFFIELD, B. F. (1987) Prediction of outcome in depressive illness by the Newcastle Scale. Its relationship with the Unipolar/Bipolar and DSM III systems. *British Journal of Psychiatry*, **150**, 43–48.

CHECKLEY, S. A., SLADE, A. P. & SHUR, E. (1981) Growth hormone and other responses to clonidine in patients with endogenous depression. *British Journal of Psychiatry*, **138**, 531–551.

COOPER, S. J., KELLY, J. G. & KING, D. J. (1985) Adrenergic receptors in depression. Effects of electro-convulsive therapy. *British Journal of Psychiatry*, **147**, 23–29.

COPPEN, A., ABOU-SALEH, M., MILLN, P., METCALFE, M., HARWOOD, J. & BAILEY, J. (1983) Dexamethasone suppression test in depression and other psychiatric illness. *British Journal of Psychiatry*, **142**, 498–504.

——, MILLN, P., HARWOOD, J. & WOOD, K. (1985) Does the Dexamethasone Suppression Test predict antidepressant treatment success? *British Journal of Psychiatry*, **146**, 294–296.

—— & METCALFE, M. (1987) The Dexamethasone Suppression Test in depression. A World Health Organization collaborative study. *British Journal of Psychiatry*, **150**, 459–462.

CORN, T. H., HALE, A. S., THOMPSON, C., BRIDGES, P. K. & CHECKLEY, S. A. (1984) A comparison of the growth hormone responses to clonidine and apomorphine in the same patients with endogenous depression. *British Journal of Psychiatry*, **144**, 636–639.

CROOKS, J., MURRAY, I. P. & WAYNE, E. J. (1959) Statistical methods applied to the clinical diagnosis of thyrotoxicosis. *Quarterly Journal of Medicine*, **28**, 211.

CURRAN, D., MALLINSON, W. P. (1941) Depressive states in war. *British Medical Journal*, **i**, 305.

DAVIDSON, J., STRICKLAND, R., TURNBULL, C., MELYEA, M. & MILLER, R. D. (1984) The Newcastle Endogenous Depression Index: validity and reliability. *Acta Psychiatrica Scandinavica*, **69**, 220–230.

DAVIES, E. (1982) An investigation into the effects of internally and externally focused tasks on depressed mood (Unpublished MSc thesis, Department of Psychiatry, University of Newcastle upon Tyne).

DOLAN, R. J., CALLOWAY, S. P., FONAGY, P., DE SOUZA, F. V. A. & WAKELING, A. (1985) Life events, depression and hypothalamic-pituitary-adrenal axis function. *British Journal of Psychiatry*, **147**, 429–433.

EYSENCK, H. J. (1970) The classification of depressive illness. *British Journal of Psychiatry*, **117**, 241–250.

FEINBERG, M. & CARROLL, E. J. (1982) Separation of the sub-types of depression using discriminant function analysis. *British Journal of Psychiatry*, **140**, 384–390.

GARMANY, G. (1958) Depressive states: their aetiology and treatment. *British Medical Journal*, ii, 341.

GARSIDE, R. F., KAY, D. W., WILSON, I., DENTON, I. B. & ROTH, M. (1971) Depressive syndromes and classification of patients. *Psychological Medicine*, **1**, 333–338.

—— (1973) Depressive illness in late life. *British Journal of Psychiatry*, **122**, 118–119.

GJERRIS, A., HAMMER, M., VENDSBORG, P., CHRISTENSEN, N. J. & RAFAELSEN, O. J. (1985) Cerebro-spinal fluid vasopressin—changes in depression. *British Journal of Psychiatry*, **147**, 696–701.

GLASS, I. R., CHECKLEY, S. A., SHUR, E. & DARLING, S. (1982) Effect of desipramine upon central adenergic function in depressed patients. *British Journal of Psychiatry*, **141**, 372–376.

GURNEY, C., ROTH, M., GARSIDE, R. F., KERR, T. A. & SCHAPIRA, K. (1972) Studies in the classification of affective disorders. *British Journal of Psychiatry*, **121**, 162–166.

HOLDEN, N. L. (1982) Depression and the Newcastle Scale: their relationship to the Dexamethasone Suppression Test. *British Journal of Psychiatry*, **142**, 505–507.

HOPE, K. (1969) Review of the classification of depressive illnesses by R. E. Kendell. *British Journal of Psychiatry*, **115**, 731–734.

JACOBY, R. J. & LEVY, R. (1980) Computed tomography in the elderly. 3: affective disorders. *British Journal of Psychiatry*, **136**, 270–275.

JOHNSTONE, E. C., DEAKIN, J. F. W., LAWLER, P., FRITH, F. D., STEVENS, N., McPHERSON, K. & CROW, T. J. (1980) The Northwick Park electro-convulsive therapy trial. *Lancet*, ii, 1317–1320.

KALINOWSKY, L. B., (1959) Organic non-drug therapy of depression. *Canadian Psychiatric Association Journal* (Special Supplement), **4**, 138.

KATONA, C. L. E., ALDRIDGE, C. R., ROTH, M. & HYDE, J. (1987) The Dexamethasone Suppression Test and prediction of outcome in patients receiving ECT. *British Journal of Psychiatry*, **150**, 315–318.

KAY, D. W., GARSIDE, R. F., ROY, J. R., BEAMISH, P. B. (1969) Endogenous and neurotic syndromes of depression. *British Journal of Psychiatry*, **115**, 389–399.

KENDELL, R. E. & POST, F. (1973) Depressive illnesses in late life. *British Journal of Psychiatry*, **112**, 657–677.

—— (1982) The choice of diagnostic criteria for biological research. *Archives of General Psychiatry*, **39**, 1334–1339.

KILOH, L. G., BALL, J. R. B. & GARSIDE, R. F. (1962) Prognostic factors in the treatment of depressive states with imipramine. *British Medical Journal*, i, 12–25.

—— & GARSIDE, R. F. (1963) The independence of neurotic depression and endogenous depression. *British Journal of Psychiatry*, **109**, 451.

——, ANDREWS, G., NEILSON, M. & BIANCHI, G. N. (1972) The relationship of the syndromes called endogenous and neurotic depression. *British Journal of Psychiatry*, **121**, 183–196.

KLEIN, M. E., BENDER, W., MAYR, H., NEIDERSCHWEIBERER, A. & SCHMAUSS, M. (1984) The DST and its relationship to psychiatric diagnosis and treatment outcome. *British Journal of Psychiatry*, **145**, 591–599.

KRAEPELIN, E. (1927) *Physique and Character*. Berlin, Heidelburg, New York: Springer.

LAMBOURN, J. & GILL, D. (1978) A controlled comparison of simulated and real ECT. *British Journal of Psychiatry*, **133**, 514–519.

LEWIS, A. J. (1934) Melancholia: a clinical survey of depressive states. *Journal of Mental Science*, **80**, 277.

—— (1936) Melancholia: prognostic study in case material. *Journal of Mental Science*, **82**, 488.

MACKEITH, I. G. (1984) Clinical use of DST in a psychogeriatric population. *British Journal of Psychiatry*, **145**, 389–393.

MATUSSEK, P., SOLDNER, M. & NADEL, D. (1981) Identification of the endogenous depressive syndrome based on symptoms and characteristics of the course. *British Journal of Psychiatry*, **138**, 361–372.

MEDICAL RESEARCH COUNCIL (1965) Clinical trial of the treatment of depressive illness. *British Medical Journal*, i, 881–886.

MENDELS, J. & COCHRANE, C. (1968) The nosology of depression. The endogenous-reactive concept. *American Journal of Psychiatry*, **124**, 1–11.

MIRKIN, A. M. & COPPEN, A. (1980) Electro-dermal activity in depression: clinical and biochemical correlates. *British Journal of Psychiatry*, **137**, 93–97.

MONTGOMERY, S. A. (1981) Measurement of Serum Blood Levels in the Assessment of Anti-depressants. In *Central Nervous System* (eds M. Lader & A. Richens), pp. 61–68. London: MacMillan.

——, MONTGOMERY, D. B., McAULEY, R. & RANI, S. J. (1978) Mianserin plasma levels and differential clinical response in endogenous and neurotic depression. *Acta Psychiatrica Belgica*, **78**, 798–812.

MOWBRAY, R. M. (1969) Classification of depressive illness. *British Journal of Psychiatry*, **115**, 1344–1345.

NAYLOR, J. G., McNAMEE, H. B. & MOODY, G. P. (1971) Changes in erythrocyte sodium and potassium on recovery from a depressive illness. *British Journal of Psychiatry*, **118**, 219–223.

——, STANFIELD, D. A., WHITE, S. F. & HUTCHINSON, F. (1974) Urinary excretion of adenosine—3 : 5-cyclic monophosphate in depressive illness. *British Journal of Psychiatry*, **125**, 268–274.

PILOWSKY, I., LEVINE, S. & BOULTON, B. M. (1969) The classification of depression by numerical taxonomy. *British Journal of Psychiatry*, **115**, 937–945.

PAYKEL, B. S., PRUSOFF, B. A. & TANNER, J. (1976) Temporal stability of symptom patterns in depression. *British Journal of Psychiatry*, **128**, 369–374.

RAO, R. & COPPEN, A. (1979) Classification of depression and response to amitriptyline therapy. *Psychological Medicine*, **9**, 321–325.

REYNOLDS, E. H., CARNEY, M. W. P. & TOONE, B. K. (1984) Methylation and mood. *Lancet*, ii, 196–197.

REYNOLDS, E. H. & STRAMENTINOLI, G. (1983) Folic acid, S-adenosylmethionine and affective disorder. *Psychological Medicine*, **13**, 705–710.

ROBIN, A. & DE TISSERA, S. (1982) Double-blind controlled comparison of the therapeutic effects of low and high energy electro-convulsive therapies. *British Journal of Psychiatry*, **141**, 357–366.

ROBINSON, A., NIES, A. & RAVARIS, L. (1973) The monoamine oxidase inhibitor phenelzine in the treatment of depressive anxiety states: a controlled clinical trial. *Archives of General Psychiatry*, **129**, 407–413.

ROTH, M. (1959) The phenomenology of depressive states *Canadian Psychiatric Association Journal* (Special Supplement). **4**, 532.

—— & GARSIDE, R. F. (1973) Depressive illness in late life. *British Journal of Psychiatry*, **123**, 373–375.

—— & BARNES, T. R. E. (1981) The classification of affective disorders: the synthesis of old and new concepts. *Comprehensive Psychiatry*, **22**, 54–77.

SANDIFER, M., WILSON, I. C. & GREEN, L. (1966) The 2-type thesis of depressive disorders. *American Journal of Psychiatry*, **123**, 93–97.

SIRELING, L. I., FREELING, P., PAYKEL, E. S. & RAO, D. M. (1985) Depression in general practice: clinical features and comparison with out-patients. *British Journal of Psychiatry*, **147**, 119–126.

——, L. (1986) Depression in mentally handicapped patients: diagnostic and neuroendocrine evaluation. *British Journal of Psychiatry*, **149**, 274–278.

SLADE, A. P. & CHECKLEY, S. A. (1980) A neuroendocrine study of the mechanism of the action of ECT. *British Journal of Psychiatry*, **137**, 217–221.

SPITZER, R. L. & ENDICOTT, J. (1978) *Schedule for Affective Disorders and Schizophrenia*. Biometric Research. New York State Psychiatric Institute.

TEASDALE, J. D. & REZIN, V. (1978) The effects of reducing frequency of negative thoughts in the mood of depressed patients—tests of a cognitive model of depression. *British Journal of Clinical Psychology*, **17**, 65–74.

TEJA, J. S., NARANG, R. I. & AGGARWAL, A. K. (1971) Depression across cultures. *British Journal of Psychiatry*, **119**, 253–263.

THOMPSON, C., MEZEY, G., CORN, T., FRANEY, C., ENGLISH, J., ARENDT, J. & CHECKLEY, S. A. (1985) The effects of desipramine upon melatonin and cortisol secretion in depressed and normal subjects. *British Journal of Psychiatry*, **147**, 389–393.

TREDGOLD, R. F. (1941) Depressive states in the soldier. *British Journal of Psychiatry*, **2**, 709.

VENKOBA RAO, A. (1966) Depression—a psychiatric analysis of 30 cases. *Indian Journal of Psychiatry*, **8**, 143–154.

VLISSADES, B. N. & JENNER, F. A. (1982) The response of endogenously & reactively depressed patients to electro-convulsive therapy. *British Journal of Psychiatry*, **141**, 239–242.

WILLIAMS, J. M. G. (1984) Cognitive behaviour therapy for depression: problems and perspectives. *British Journal of Psychiatry*, **145**, 254–262.

WING, J. K., COOPER, J. E. & SARTORIUS, N. (1974) *The Measurement and Classification of Psychiatric Symptoms: An Instruction Manual for the PSE and Catego Program*. Cambridge University Press.

YOUNG, M. A., SCHEFTNER, W. A., KLERMAN, G. L., ANDREASEN, N. C. & HIRSCHFELD, R. M. A. (1986) The endogenous sub-type of depression: a study of its internal construct validity. *British Journal of Psychiatry*, **148**, 257–267.

ZIMMERMAN, M., PFOHL, B., STANGL, D. & CORYELL, W. (1986) An American study of the Newcastle Diagnostic Scale I. Its relationship with the Dexamethasone Suppression Test. *British Journal of Psychiatry*, **149**, 627–630.

——, CORYELL, W., PFOHL, B. & STANGL, D. (1987) An American validation study of the Newcastle Diagnostic Scale II. Relationship with clinical, demographic, familial and psychosocial features. *British Journal of Psychiatry*, **150**, 526–532.

# 15 The measurement and classification of the affective disorders

## JAMES A. MULLANEY

The work inspired by Professor Sir Martin Roth has been in the fore-front of clinical psychiatric classification for over a quarter of a century. He has merited many honours and tributes, not least the affection in which he is held by those who have been privileged to be guided and to learn from him. As one so privileged, this chapter reviews the last of a number of studies on classification in the affective disorders begun under Sir Martin in Newcastle. The approach in this investigation was to bring the confluence of two streams, that of multivariate statistics and of psychometric instrumental design, to bear on the issue of classification within the affective disorders.

A number of issues which had not satisfactorily been resolved were to preoccupy me, and the late Dr Roger Garside, to whom I am eternally indebted. The first was the growing recognition as earlier data were perused, that there had been a consistent failure to search diligently enough for comparative results in classifying syndromes, before proceeding to classify persons. No less was the tendency to reify disease entities, such as neurotic or endogenous depression, and to accept their existence as disorders on *a priori* grounds. Defining a syndrome presents more difficulties than we may suppose. Labelling a cluster of clinical features a syndrome is one thing but defining it in a scientific or mathematical sense is another. These latter objectives imply some form of measurement and purification of syndromes. Hence we must first identify the important replicable syndromes, and then develop pure measures of these. Lastly we must relate these to the classification of persons, a *sine qua non* of clinically derived classification. Unfortunately this is an approach that has been singularly rare in classification studies of depression.

The term affective disorder used here implies a group of conditions in which a primary mood change of anxiety or depression constitutes the cardinal features from which all other symptoms are directly or indirectly derived. Anxiety and depression in various forms have been found to be the most prominent of psychiatric disorders in epidemiological studies.

As Lewis (1934a) observed, the history of melancholia is the history of psychiatry, and the literature on the classification of depression is too voluminous therefore to encompass here. However, beyond the mid part of this century the problem, according to Becker (1974), crystallised among Western psychiatrists into those who held opposing views as to whether depression was a unitary entity

123

(represented by the Maudsley school) or better represented by two (Newcastle), or more entities (mainland Europe and North America).

While many from the Meyerian school regard phenomenological classification as a somewhat dubious exercise, those from Kraepelian backgrounds tend to emphasise the isolation of endogenous or other subgroups. For such reasons anxiety has been largely ignored in depression studies. This is because it has been considered an inferior dimension or construct and also it has generally been assumed that in selecting depressive populations anxiety syndromes have been excluded. For reasons discussed below many researchers are in error on this account.

Kendell (1976), in relation to the classification of depressive illness, concluded that "we now have more not fewer competing classifications than we had a generation ago and in those areas where a consensus has emerged multivariate analysis has not played a crucial role" (p. 26). This pessimistic conclusion has had the effect of influencing researchers so that in recent times only cursory attention has been paid to the areas of research detailed here, in comparison to neurochemical and pharmacological studies.

## The First Study: syndromes of anxiety and depression

In our first study, plots were drawn from the first two unrotated components reported in 40 principal component analysis reports in the literature 1934–1977 (Mullaney, 1984; 1986). Two clusters of features were found in each plot and the composition of each was consistent from one analysis to the next. Close inspection indicated one cluster comprised items consistent with general notions of fear, apprehension, physiological arousal and anxiety, the other, to consist of sadness, loss of vitality and depression. The clusters correspond to clinical anxiety and depression respectively. Lines projected from the centres of these clusters to the points of origin give dimensions of anxiety and depression which tend to vary around the orthogonal. The geometric distance and separation of clusters in the plots is equivalent to a diminishing statistical correlation between them. Reviews of these studies in the past have concentrated on comparing the relative factor loadings in one or more of the major components and have ignored the geometric configuration. Indeed general opinion in recent times has veered between regarding the studies under scrutiny as of little or no value or as providing limited descriptive validity for neurotic and psychotic depression (Mendels, 1968; Mendels & Cochrane, 1968; Lorr, 1969; Costello, 1970; Frank, 1976; Kendell, 1976; MacFadyen, 1977; Garside, 1976; Blashfield, 1984).

In these studies the authors themselves, and later reviewers, failed to recognise the occurrence of these dimensions or their true nature. This resulted from a preoccupation with subgrouping depression, a lack of attention to comparative aspects, and perhaps over-valuing the display of data in algebraic as opposed to geometric form.

These two clusters occur in all relevant studies irrespective of the sub-type designation of the affective group under scrutiny. They occur in
(a) consecutive in-patient, out-patient, and day patient depressions
(b) general practice and research group depressives and
(c) anxious neurotic out-patients and even some 'normal' populations.

Further, the clusters are not simply an artefact of any particular rating system as they occur where the domains sampled have varied, and also occur both in self rating and observer rated studies.

The most novel and salient finding is that the two clusters do not represent neurotic (reactive) and psychotic (endogenous) depression. This mislabelling has complicated interpretation of much of the general affective literature. The two clusters are unequivocally those of anxiety and depression. Appending these new labels induces a radical revision in interpretations placed on clinical, psychometric, physiological, sociological and classificatory studies in depression particularly, but also in anxiety. The number of analyses examined, their wide geographical distribution, the variation in theoretical outlook and in the instruments included, all underline the remarkable comparability in the results. This is all the more surprising considering the heterogeneity of the material and the care taken to exclude specifically anxiety neurosis in some of the reviewed analyses (Carney *et al*, 1965; Raskin *et al*, 1974) or, in others, to exclude depression (Williams *et al*, 1968; Lipman *et al*, 1969).

The lack of clear orthogonality between the axes of these syndromes suggests two independent conditions which are not mutually exclusive. Such a state of affairs is likely to complicate the interpretation of distributions of persons along any single axis. Leaving aside considerations referable to the distributions of persons, there would seem to be some general agreement that if replicable factors or dimensions are established, one could use patient scores on these factors for purposes of description of patterns of illness (Rosenthal & Gudeman, 1967).

It follows that the design and validation of psychometric instruments reflecting clinical anxiety and depression can thereby be improved. Descriptive measures of each condition should lie within the clusters and along the descriptive dimensions. The greater the distance they lie from the origin, the more will they reflect severity. It has always been difficult to design validating criteria for descriptive scales, but this framework applied appropriately offers considerable promise.

## The Second Study: descriptive and severity scales of anxiety and depression

For practical purposes, clinical scales in psychiatry have been divided by Garside (1976) into four main types, each with distinct characteristics. The first type is the assessment or descriptive scale that can be used to assess the degree of illness such as depression, for example the Hamilton Depression Scale (HDS) (Hamilton, 1967). The second is discriminatory rather than descriptive, and may be useful in arriving at a psychiatric diagnosis, for example the Newcastle Diagnostic Index (Carney *et al*, 1965). The essential feature of a descriptive scale is that individual items should correlate more highly among themselves and give rise to a general factor indicating that it is meaningful to describe patients along such a dimension, i.e. convergent validity. In diagnostic scales it is essential that the items produce separate correlational groups, i.e. discriminant validity. While there is general agreement on empirical findings with the use of descriptive scales (Pichot, 1974), there has been little agreement on findings on diagnostic

TABLE I
*Descriptive scales of anxiety and depression*

*Anxiety*
    Zung Anxiety Scale (ZAS)
    Hamilton Anxiety Scale (HAS)
*Depression*
    Zung Depression Scale (ZDS)
    Hamilton Depression Scale (HDS)
    Beck Depression Inventory (BDI)
    Wakefield
*Separate measure of both*
    Hopkins Symptom Check List (HSCL)
    SCL-90-R
    McNair Scales
    Middlesex Hospital Questionnaire (MHQ)
    Leeds Anxiety and Depression Scales
    Snaith Hospital Anxiety and Depression Scales

scales in depression. Descriptive scales have also been referred to as quantitative scales to distinguish them from qualitative ones, e.g. discriminatory or diagnostic scales (Bech, 1983). The other type of scales are predictive, in the sense of predicting the course and outcome of particular psychiatric conditions, as in Kerr *et al* (1972), or the results of specific treatments, as with Kiloh *et al* (1962), Paykel (1972) and Carney *et al* (1965).

There are a number of commonly used and established descriptive scales for measuring anxiety and depression (Table I). The main uncertainty in their use centres on the question of validity. There are uncomfortably high correlations between any of the scales listed measuring depression and those designed to measure anxiety (Mullaney, 1986). For instance, the Hamilton Depression and Hamilton Anxiety Scales show intercorrelations of around 0.5 to 0.6. This could suggest that clinical anxiety and depression are highly correlated. However, impure scales could magnify this relationship, and most of our present scales fail to distinguish anxiety from depression adequately enough. What if, for instance, the HDS was not a sufficiently pure measure of the illness termed depression? After all, it was designed on a logical-empirical basis by Max Hamilton, although he did go on to examine its psychometric properties. What if the margin of error in accuracy was say 10% or even 30%, where would that leave interpretations of amine levels or pharmacological treatment indices, when the HDS is the critical variable?

Since most descriptive clinical scales lay claim to reflect a dimension of individual difference then estimation of construct validity is appropriate if not obligatory (Fiske, 1971; Cronback & Meehl, 1955). The establishment of construct validity is contingent on the functioning of a scale or dimension as a high level concept or as a hypothetical construct within a theory from which it derives its definition. The validity of the scale as a measure of the construct is bound up with the extent to which predictions derived from the theory but using the scale are refuted or confirmed. An important criterion of validity has been elucidated above, in that a valid descriptive scale of anxiety and depression should correlate highly with their respective syndromes derived from an appropriate principal components analysis. If they fail to do so then their validity is seriously in doubt. This is a direct useful progression of the formal model or hypothesis above that clinical syndromes of anxiety and depression are distinct.

The second part of this work involved a specific study of consecutive affective patients ($n = 180$) selected by exclusion criteria alone (Mullaney, 1986). Primary aims were to examine the relative claims for validity of commonly used descriptive scales of anxiety and depression, e.g. Hamilton Depression and Anxiety Scales, Zung Depression and Anxiety Scales, SCL-90-R and Beck Depression Index. It was anticipated that, because of the high correlations alluded to above, some of these scales would be found to be impure. As part of the purification of the syndromes above, it was proposed to design and validate superior scales of anxiety and depression. Eventually two pure dimensions crystallised and a 12 item anxiety and a 14 item depression scale were derived (Mullaney, 1986, 1987). These were composed of clinical items in the factor space formed by the two first components. Inspection ensured that only those that achieved the widest separation across the factor plot of components I and II and which also showed highest continguity within the separate clusters of anxiety and depressive features were chosen.

Striking similarities were found for the scales for mean scores, ranges, profile item scores and factorial structures between this study with a broad affective designation, and those studies quoting selected depression or anxiety groups. This underlined the difficulty in separating groups of patients. Nonetheless, separation of the syndromes was distinct and showed that the Beck when administered as a self-rated instrument and the Zung Depression Scales poorly reflected depression in a descriptive sense. Although they might be of value for rating mood change over time (Kendell, 1975), they would appear to function as 'extensive' measures of mood (Wittenborn, 1975) but not 'intensive' measures of depression. The Hamilton Anxiety scale was a less than impressive measure of anxiety and the Hamilton Depression scale an imperfect measure of depression. The depression scale of the SCL-90-R showed serious descriptive deficiencies. Table II shows the relative magnitudes of the correlations of the new dimensions or scales compared with the HDS and HAS. This measure of extensive severity is simply the extensive measure of mood referred to earlier, i.e. scores on the general factor. The new anxiety scale and the new depression scale have reasonably good correlations with this general dimension of mood disorder. The new depression scale correlation is as good as the HDS. The correlation between the two Hamilton scales is 0.55, a consistent finding in the literature. The new anxiety scale has a high correlation with the HAS and likewise the new depression

TABLE II
*Some scales correlations from this study* (n = 180)

| | |
|---|---|
| New Anxiety/Depression Scales | – 0.19 |
| Global Severity/New Depression Scale | 0.63 |
| Global Severity/New Anxiety Scale | 0.57 |
| Global Severity/HAS | 0.36 |
| Global Severity/HDS | 0.65 |
| HAS/HDS | 0.55 |
| HAS/New Depression Scale | 0.14 |
| HAS/New Anxiety Scale | 0.66 |
| HDS/New Depression Scale | 0.71 |
| HDS/New Anxiety Scale | 0.19 |

scale has a high correlation with the HDS, yet their correlations are of a magnitude of − 0.19. They are therefore more or less independent, far more so than the existing Hamilton scales.

The general factor derived from items of the new depression scale has a variance of over 40%. This compares favourably with the HDS in which it has been consistently found to be around 20% both in his study and the literature. The anxiety general factor has a variance of 28% which is still impressive when compared with general factor 'g' in intelligence testing (Vernon, 1961). Although not ideal, these two scales contain a higher proportion of variance than other scales such as HDS and HAS.

Some indication of the purification achieved along these lines can be gauged from analysis of the data collected by Lewis (1934b) and re-analysed by Kiloh & Garside (1973). They were unable to demonstrate a general factor when using Lewis' neurotic items. The point has already been made that the diagnosis of 'neurotic' depression is in this context inappropriate. In a more recent study by Roth *et al* (1972) of anxiety and depressive patients, separate analysis of anxiety and depressive items yielded general factors of 16.7% and 19% respectively. The present findings compare favourably with these figures.

Little has been said of the relationship of these new scales and the established descriptive scales to independent criteria, such as type of treatment allocation, outcome at discharge or follow-up. Suffice to say that the new scales of anxiety and depression were superior at predicting independent treatment allocation in the index episode. Further, they were better at predicting outcome at both discharge and over the following year.

## Empirical studies on the relationship of anxiety and depression

Both the ICD-9, 10 and DSM–III and its later revisions (Spitzer & Williams, 1983) inexplicably exclude anxiety from consideration within the affective disorders. It is not surprising therefore that most clinical studies on classification of depression have tended to ignore the valid inclusion of anxiety mood state. As Lewis (1971) put it, "it (anxiety) has had a short life as far as psychiatry in the English speaking countries goes, and has not endeared itself to French and German authorities on psychiatric terminology". Similarly, the category of neurotic-depressive reaction has only had a brief history in terms of main-stream psychiatric practice, being introduced into the American Psychiatric Association *Diagnostic and Statistical Manual* as late as 1963. For these reasons mainly, systematic clinical studies bearing on the relationship of anxiety and depression are of recent origin.

The relationships pertaining to anxiety and depression can be summarised from the literature into the following models:
   (a) Anxiety and depression are closely interwoven affects. (Psychoanalytic and behaviourist theorists).
   (b) Anxiety state and depression (whether neurotic or endogenous) are separate disorders (Roth *et al*, 1972; Gurney *et al*, 1972; Kerr, 1974; Roth & Mountjoy, 1982).

(c) Anxiety is part of a depressive disorder and possibly comprises an anxious–depressive subgroup (Paykel, 1971).

(d) Anxiety and depression are symptomatically distinct but are not mutually exclusive disorders (Finlay-Jones & Brown, 1981).

(e) Depression and anxiety generally occur together but depression can occur as a distinct entity (Zung, 1971).

(f) There is a hierarchical arrangement in terms of specific symptoms with specific depressive symptoms further up the hierarchy (Foulds & Bedford, 1976).

(g) It is not possible to distinguish anxiety neurotics from depressive neurotics and any distinction between them is of little value for purposes of drug treatment (Johnstone *et al*, 1980).

(h) There are qualitative as well as quantitative differences between anxiety and depression but it is not possible to specify them clearly (Derogatis *et al*, 1972a; Derogatis & Cleary, 1977).

With the exception of the general viewpoint expressed in the first model all other authors have quoted empirical data supporting their theoretical viewpoints. However, consideration of the inter-relationship of anxiety and depression is far from complete when confined to studies focusing solely on patients designated as suffering from depression or mixed anxiety-depression. Clinical data derived from almost all previous affective classifications are relevant.

It might be helpful at this point to summarise the important distinctions from the various schools of psychiatry along the lines proposed by Eysenck (1970). An adaptation of his framework to encompass the broader definition of affective disturbance rather than just 'depression' is required in order to do justice to empirical findings (Study 1). This list of possible classifications is useful in that it is particularly applicable to multivariate data. He drew attention to the general agreement that there were two important descriptive factors or syndromes apparent in most studies of depression but little agreement on methods of classifying persons. Nonetheless his theoretical scheme is relevant in that it lays down the general outlines of how syndromes might influence the classification of persons. To some extent the issue revolves on whether categorical or dimensional models best fit the data. The models include:

(a) a unitary and categorical one (favoured by Mapother, Lewis)

(b) a unitary and dimensional one (favoured by Kendell, Freud)

(c) a binary and categorical one (early Newcastle studies)

(d) a binary and dimensional one (Eysenck)

(e) binary, both categorical and dimensional (Kiloh, Fahy, Everitt, Wing).

## The Third Study: classifications of anxiety and depression

Much of the earlier controversies using factor analysis focused on the distribution of factor scores and whether it was possible to demonstrate bimodality (Garside & Roth, 1978) or points of rarity (Kendell, 1982). This issue has also been reviewed by Mullaney (1985) in regard to discriminant function. There is in fact a further application of factor analysis particularly applicable to descriptive dimensions and this refers to the issue of factor invariance. Most developers of descriptive scales have presumed that their scales possess this important characteristic and have failed to recognise the need for empirical demonstrations.

If significant differences occur in the structuring of what are thought to be similar or identical descriptive dimensions, i.e. in groups characterised by differences in gender or age, it limits greatly any broad application of such dimensions in different clinical groups. A dimension in this sense is simply an aggregate of symptoms with defined mathematical inter-relationships e.g. the new descriptive scales here. Examination of this issue contributes to assessing the limits in the application of any particular scale to different clinical populations (Derogatis & Cleary, 1977). The invariance characteristics of the Hopkins Symptom Scale (Derogatis *et al*, 1971; 1972b), and its later development the SCL-90 (Derogatis, 1977), have been detailed, but doubts expressed in Study 1 above concerning the validity of the subscales, particularly those of anxiety and depression, render the results ambiguous. In spite of technical accomplishments in recent years in the measurement of invariance, a definite measure has yet to be developed. All methods have been found to have limitations (Gorsuch, 1974).

The aim of this part of the work was to apply these new scales to an affective population to see whether, and in what manner, the patient groups could be discriminated from each other; in other words, to challenge the null hypothesis that the two main identifiable clinical syndromes derived earlier merge imperceptibly into one another. Invariance presents a method of elucidating evidence for discontinuity and demonstrating whether there are qualitative differences in clinical syndromes between designated sub-groups. In the first instance, one must have reasonable grounds for deciding that mathematically derived descriptive syndromes can be derived. The new descriptive scales for the dimensions of anxiety and depression form a useful starting point. General factors for the new scales were derived for sub-populations of the main body of 180 consecutive affectives above. These compressed sub-divisions by age, gender, social class, and hospital status (in-patient versus day, and out-patient combined). The general factors were then compared with each other and the results shown in Table III. The method is crude but nonetheless robust, and indicates that subgrouping in this manner does not invalidate the invariance of anxiety and depression as defined in these publications.

TABLE III
*Invariance of scales of anxiety and depression*

|  | Anxiety scale items (12) Rank correlation | Depression scale items (14) Rank correlation |
|---|---|---|
| Age: <40 n = 104 | 0.73* | 0.58* |
| >40 n = 76 | | |
| Sex: Male = 67 | 0.55* | 0.43* |
| Female = 113 | | |
| Hospital status | | |
| In-patient = 136 | 0.41 | 0.74* |
| OP & DP = 44 | | |
| Social class | | |
| 1 + 2    = 36 | 0.55* | 0.63* |
| 3 + 4 + 5 = 129 | | |

For 12 pairs of scores, when $r > 0.43$ $P < 0.05$
For 14 pairs of scores, when $r > 0.39$ $P < 0.05$   (Kendall's tau)

However, it is instructive to compare these results with those found when even this simplified procedure is applied to samples where a putative diagnostic division can be imposed. If factor invariance fails to occur across diagnostic boundaries but yet can be demonstrated for other indices, it favours a valid distinction of a qualitative kind. The random hospital population of affectives ($n = 180$) described earlier was dichotomised on the basis of individual scores, above or below zero, attained on the bipolar component in the initial analysis. This component resulted from an analysis of 82 variables and included symptoms, personality and biographical data, descriptive scale scores, and scores on two personality questionnaires. The populations were designated as 'anxious' ($n = 100$) and 'depressed ($n = 73$), reflecting the distribution of clinical features on this component (shown in Mullaney, 1987).

The distributions of the total, and the two sub-populations above, were examined for:
  (a)  the general and bipolar components derived in Study 2
  (b)  the descriptive dimensions of anxiety and depression also derived in Study 2
  (c)  the general factors derived from the new descriptive scales' items.
Little evidence favouring bimodality was adduced. However, for the descriptive dimensions there were clear differences in distribution for the two populations, on the anxiety dimension ($P<0.05$) and for the depressive dimension ($P<0.001$).

Principal component analyses of the items of each scale were separately analysed in both sub-populations, and in each case a general factor was extracted. This resulted in two general factors for population BPO, for anxiety and depression; similarly extracted were general factors of anxiety and depression for population BPI. As retardation did not attain any score in the anxious BPO population, in order to compare the general factor of depression across the two populations, it was necessary to reduce analysis of the depression scale to 13 from 14 items. In addition the hierarchy of items from each general factor was compared with the hierarchical correlations of items of each factor with the 'diagnostic' boundary, i.e. the correlations of items separately with the allocation into BPO or BPI groups.

The questions at issue are whether anxiety and depression are the same for the two sub-populations, and whether anxiety or depression as defined by these descriptive dimensions or scales was independent or significantly correlated with this dichotomy. The correlations of the general factors of anxiety and depression with the 'diagnostic' column allow us to examine the latter. If the construct anxiety proved similar in both sub-populations BPO and BPI, then a diagnostic division on this basis would have little to commend it. Should the converse result ensue, clear qualitative differences could be said to exist between the sub-populations.

The anxiety scale was found to be invariant across the 'diagnostic' boundary ($P<0.05$) (Table IV). It was not correlated with the diagnostic boundary, the correlations were non-significant and both were close to 0. This suggests that anxiety, as defined by the anxiety scale, was co-extensive across the 'diagnostic' boundary i.e. all the patients, whether depressed or not, were anxious. There was no similarity between depression as defined by the depression factors in the BPO and BPI populations. The depression scale was highly significantly

TABLE IV
*Invariance of scales of anxiety and depression*

(a) *Anxiety scale general factor (12 item)*
Rank correlation
   Populations BPO, 'anxiety' with BPI, 'depression' = 0.55 $P<0.05$
   Population BPO, 'anxiety' with Dichotomy Column = 0.08 N.S.
   Population BPI, 'depression' with Dichotomy Column = 0.07 N.S.
(b) *Depression scale general factor (13 item)*
Rank correlation
   Populations BPO, 'anxiety' with BPI, 'depression' = 0.000 N.S.
   Population BPO, 'anxiety' with Dichotomy Column = 0.38*
   Population BPI, 'depression' with Dichotomy Column = 0.73 $P<0.01$

*$P$ just fails to meet 5% level of significance (Kendall's tau)

correlated with the 'diagnostic' dichotomy. Unlike anxiety, depression was not co-extensive in these two sub-populations. Such a result is in agreement with the bivariate plots and not only argues for a qualitative distinction between population BPO and BPI but specifies the nature of this distinction.

There is one caveat to these results. The 26 items forming the descriptive dimensions were included in the 82 items determining the bipolar component. Hence, having shared items the descriptive dimensions and the bipolar component were not clearly independent of each other. Therefore claims as to the utility of this classification require further validation or confirmation in a replication study.

## Qualitative distinctions

The null hypothesis also holds that there are no qualitative distinctions in syndromes of anxiety and depression in designated sub-groups of the affective population. Sub-groups here are BPO 'anxious' and BPI 'depressed' populations. Few studies have previously addressed this question. Here the structure of depression and anxiety in the two populations was examined using the items of the two dimensions. Retardation was found to be absent in the anxious group, and this represents one qualitative difference between the two groups.

### The hierarchical relationship between anxiety and depression

Most clinical as opposed to research classifications of mental illness implicitly accept a hierarchy of disorders whereby each tier is allowed to exhibit the characteristic features of lower tiers. The international classification (ICD-9) starts with the organic psychoses (categories 290–294). Next comes schizophrenia (295), followed by affective and other functional psychoses (296–299), neurotic disorders (300), and personality disorders (301). Schneider's (1957) dictum that his 'symptoms of first rank' are pathognomonic of schizophrenia 'except in the presence of coarse brain disease' is an implicit recognition of schizophrenia's status in the hierarchy. Neurotic illness, the fourth tier, can only be diagnosed in the absence of all psychotic symptoms although there is no objection to the presence of characteristic features of a lower tier, e.g. personality disorder. This scheme has evolved largely by accident rather than design. From a research point of view, studies examining the validity of hierarchical systems have only recently been forthcoming.

Overall, the results here indicate that the anxiety scale is invariant across the diagnostic boundary, i.e. all the patients, whether depressed or not, are anxious. The depression scale is not invariant and, unlike anxiety, the quality of depression is not co-extensive in anxious and depressed patients. A patient either has, or has not got depression. A patient with depression is likely to have anxiety in addition. The patient who suffers from an 'anxiety' illness does not necessarily have depression. The findings here are substantially in agreement with Zung's (1971) and Fould's hypothesis concerning the hierarchical nature of depressive illness (Foulds & Bedford, 1976). However, here it would seem that clinical mood disturbance can be resolved into a hierarchical arrangement whereby all patients with depression have anxiety in addition, but not all patients with clinical anxiety have depression.

This interpretation is not so far removed from Torgerson's (1968) suggestion that a set of classes representing specific disorders with one or more quantitative dimensions superimposed might eventually prove to be the best solution to psychiatric classification. Kiloh *et al* (1972), and Costello *et al* (1974), arrived at the same general conclusion in relation to depression but were unable to specify more precisely what constituted the general dimension involved.

The results suggest that the null hypothesis be rejected. All the affective patients have anxiety but not all have depression. Maxwell (1972) suggested that the majority of patients tend to have a basic core of symptoms, neurotic in type, which lend themselves to a dimensional description. Here that neurotic core has been shown to be that of anxiety. Recent empirical studies have tended with some variations to support this hierarchical position. These include Foulds & Bedford (1975); Bagshaw (1977); Surtees & Kendell (1979); Sturt (1981) and Morey (1985).

Tyrer (1985) argued against the use of hierarchical symptoms for neurotic syndromes but implicitly accepted that for schizophrenia and psychotic depression such systems probably did operate. However, he was at a loss to suggest where the dividing line should be drawn in relation to depressions of various kinds and the general neurotic syndromes which he felt were underpinned by anxiety (Tyrer, 1984).

It will be appreciated that the binary, both categorical and dimensional, model discussed in the literature review (Fahy, 1969; Wing *et al*, 1978; Kiloh *et al*, 1972; Everitt *et al*, 1971) appears to fit the data. Yet such a model fails to do justice to the relationship between the two main mood syndromes. For here the categorical entity depression is dimensional within the group to which it applies, i.e. true depression. Further, the relationship between the two is hierarchical. Neither of these conditions would appear to have been considered by earlier proponents of this binary model.

## The descriptive dimension of depression

It is an appropriate question as to where the scale or concept of depression developed here fits into the classical descriptions of depression. Terms such as melancholia, endogenous, endogenomorphic, vital and autonomous depression have frequently been applied to what Kendell referred to as Type A depression. Other depressions in contrast have included such designations as neurotic, reactive, situational, atypical and anxious depressions. Klerman (1977) has counselled against the use of terms which carry aetiological implications, and this would seem sensible in view of our continuing ignorance concerning aetiology.

Although Carney *et al* (1965), employed principal component analysis in the early part of their study, its function was simply to show that two clusters were a meaningful partialling of the data. However, when these workers came to derive item weights, these were obtained by discriminant function using clinical diagnosis as the critical variable. So the principal component analysis and the discriminant function were quite independent. Hence, though the Carney scale is discriminant, its discrimination does not reflect directly in a mathematical sense the bipolar component here, or in the original study of Carney *et al* (1965).

This consideration also applies to the Anxiety Depression and Depression Scales of Gurney (Gurney *et al*, 1972). It has been found that the unipolar and bipolar groups here ($n = 28$) account for the high scorers on the Carney scale (Mullaney, 1985). Such a result implies that the Carney definition is more restrictive than that attained for depression using the bipolar component. Of course, unlike the above scales, the new scale is descriptive, i.e. all mood disordered patients will likely attain some positive scores on it. However, if not suffering from a structural depression, scores will be low. If 'anxiety' syndrome patients did not also experience some depressive symptoms there would be no need to engage in such an intricate analysis as the present one.

There is strong similarity between the descriptive items selected here and the results derived from other multivariate studies (Kiloh & Garside, 1963; Kiloh *et al*, 1972; Mendels & Cochrane, 1968). Nelson & Charney (1981) sought to isolate 'the common characteristics of the various descriptions of major depressive illness' applied in the literature. They employed the term 'autonomous depression' as inclusive of a constellation of symptoms present in over 20 studies which had used discriminant function, counts of symptom frequency, instrumental measures and symptoms correlated with treatment response. With the exclusion of agitation this depression mirrors the items of the depression scale here. Matussek *et al* (1981) highlighted the chief features of the endogenous depressive syndrome derived empirically from two separate cluster methods of analysis, plus an examination of clinical diagnostic practice in Germany. Again, the items selected were similar to this study.

It is not possible here to deal with the issue of neurotic depression except to state that when scrutinised fairly closely neurotic/reactive depression falls into a number of ill defined syndromes; it is only very recently that attention has been paid to this commonly labelled disorder. Endogenous features have always been the main focus of interest in classification and multivariate studies. Little attention has been paid to where neurotic depression might fit within the spectrum of affective disorder. More pertinent is the question as to whether this syndrome which has been commonly defined as a 'depression' might be more logically labelled otherwise. Anxiety forms a prominent and recurrent feature of these entities, yet in many instances it has either been ignored, or its importance minimised. The results here not only cast serious doubt on the existence of such an entity but also provide a more consistent descriptive framework for patients previously diagnosed as suffering from neurotic depression.

Descriptively the second dimension here is clearly consistent with general notions and appellations of anxiety. It behaves in a unitary manner and is superior in this regard to any other available clinical measures of this concept. There is no attempt to suggest that it is the only other aspect of descriptive clinical importance (along with depression) yet it is one of the two more important descriptive aspects. All these patients share this dimension in varying quantities and in the majority it would appear to be the primary syndrome of mood disturbance. This interpretation is a radical departure from orthodox psychiatric opinion, though at least, there are indications that this position may alter (Tyrer, 1984; 1985).

The extent to which this dimension applies to non-hospitalised affective cases is unknown. The extent to which this syndrome as a general unitary dimension underlines the majority of cases with milder dysthymic conditions in the community and in general practice is unknown. There is currently an active and inconclusive debate as to the proper identification and description of these conditions. This debate lacks an appreciation of the simplification afforded by the resolution of the classification of anxiety and depression here. It will be appreciated that Mapother's (1926) conclusions and Lewis's (1966) further elaborations are strongly refuted by these results. Anxiety does not merge by a series of gradations into melancholia; there is a categorical shift into depression.

In these studies the null hypothesis was adjudged rejected, in that while all affective patients were alike in respect of sharing an identical syndrome of anxiety, only some suffered from depression. The variation in the anxiety syndrome was of a purely quantitative nature. This implies that the relationship between anxiety and depression is a hierarchical one. It is suggested that these new Newcastle Scales of anxiety and depression offer considerable promise in relation to research and clinical practice.

## References

BAGSHAW, V. E. (1977) A replication study of Foulds and Bedfords hierarchical model of depression. *British Journal of Psychiatry*, **131**, 53–55.

BECH, P. (1983) Assessment scales for depression: The next 20 years. *Acta Psychiatrica Scandinavica*, Supplement, **310**, 117–130.

BECKER, J. (1974) *Depression, Theory and Research*. Washington, DC: Winston V. H. & Sons.

BLASHFIELD, R. K. (1984) *The Classification of Psychopathology*. New York: Plenum Press.

CARNEY, M. W. P., ROTH, M. & GARSIDE, R. F. (1965) The diagnosis of depressive syndromes and prediction of ECT response. *British Journal of Psychiatry*, **111**, 659–674.

COSTELLO, C. G. (1970) Classification and psychopathology. In *Symptoms of Psychopathology*, pp. 1–26 (ed. C. G. Costello). New York: John Wiley.

——, CHRISTENSEN, S. J. & ROGERS, T. B. (1974) The relationships between measures of general depression and the endogenous versus reactive classification. *Canadian Association Psychiatric Journal*, **19**, 259–256.

CRONBACK, L. & MEEHL, P. (1955) Construct validity in psychological tests. *Psychological Bulletin*, **52**, 281–302.

DEROGATIS, R., LIPMAN, R., COVI, L. & RICKELS, K. (1971) Neurotic symptom dimensions as perceived by psychiatrists and patients of various social classes. *Archives of General Psychiatry*, **24**, 454–464.

DEROGATIS, L. R. (1977) The SCL-90 Manual 1; Scoring, administration, and procedures for the SCL-90. Baltimore: Johns Hopkins University School of Medicine. Clinical Psychometrics Unit.

——, KLERMAN, G. L. & LIPMAN, R. S. (1972a) Anxiety states and depressive neuroses. *Journal of Nervous and Mental Disease*, **155**, 392–403.

——, LIPMAN, R. S., COVI, L. & RICKELS, K. (1972b) Factorial invariance of symptom dimensions in anxious and depressive neuroses. *Archives of General Psychiatry*, **27**, 659–665.

—— & CLEARY, P. A. (1977) Confirmation of the dimensional structure of the SCL-90: A study in Construct Validation. *Journal of Clinical Psychology*, **33**, 981–989.

EVERITT, B. S., GOURLAY, A. J. & KENDELL, R. E. (1971) An attempt at validation of traditional psychiatric syndromes by cluster analysis. *British Journal of Psychiatry*, **119**, 399–412.

EYSENCK, H. J. (1970) The classification of depressive illness. *British Journal of Psychiatry*, **117**, 241–250.

FAHY, T. J. (1969) The Phenomenology of Depression in Hospital and in the Community. MD Thesis. University College of Dublin.

FINLAY-JONES, R. & BROWN, G. W. (1981) Types of stressful life events and the onset of anxiety and depressive disorders. *Psychological Medicine*, **11**, 803–815.

FISKE, D. W. (1971) *Measuring for the Concepts of Personality*. Chicago: Adline.

FOULDS, G. A. & BEDFORD, A. (1975) Hierarchy of classes of personal illness. *Psychological Medicine*, **5**, 181–192.

—— & —— (1976) Classification of depressive illness: a re-evaluation. *Psychological Medicine*, **6**, 15–19.

FRANK, G. (1976) *Psychiatric Diagnosis: A Review of Research*. Oxford: Pergamon Press.

GARSIDE, R. F. (1976) The comparative value of types of rating scales. *British Journal of Clinical Pharmacology*, Supplement, 61–67.

—— & ROTH, M. (1978) Multivariate statistical methods and problems of classification in psychiatry. *British Journal of Psychiatry*, **133**, 53–67.

GORSUCH, R. L. (1974) *Factor Analysis*. Philadelphia: Saunders.

GURNEY, C., ROTH, M., GARSIDE, R. F., KERR, T. A. & SCHAPIRA, K. (1972) Studies in the classification of affective disorders: the relationship between anxiety states and depressive illnesses II. *British Journal of Psychiatry*, **121**, 162–166.

HAMILTON, M. W. (1967) Development of a rating scale for primary depressive illness. *Journal of Clinical and Social Psychology*, **6**, 278–296.

JOHNSTONE, E. C., CUNNINGHAM-OWENS, D. G., FRITH, C. D., MCPHERSON, K., DOWIE, C., RILEY, G. & GOLD, A. (1980) Neurotic illness and its response to anxiolytic and antidepressant treatment. *Psychological Medicine*, **20**, 321–328.

KENDELL, R. E. (1975) *The Role of Diagnosis in Psychiatry*. Oxford: Blackwell.

—— (1976) The classification of depressions: A review of contemporary confusion. *British Journal of Psychiatry*, **129**, 15–28.

—— (1982) The choice of diagnostic criteria for biological research. *Archives of General Psychiatry*, **39**, 1134–1139.

KERR, T. A., ROTH, M., SCHAPIRA, K. & GURNEY, C. (1972) The assessment and prediction of outcome in affective disorders. *British Journal of Psychiatry*, **121**, 167–174.

—— (1974) The Prognosis of Affective Disorders with Special Reference to Problems of Classification. MD Thesis. University of Leeds, UK.

KILOH, L. G., BALL, J. R. B. & GARSIDE, R. F. (1962) Prognostic factors in treatment of depressive states with imipramine. *British Medical Journal*, i, 1225–1227.

—— & GARSIDE, R. F. (1963) The independence of neurotic depression and endogenous depression. *British Journal of Psychiatry*, **109**, 451–463.

——, ANDREWS, G., NEILSON, M., BIANCHI, G. N. (1972) The relationship of the syndromes called endogenous and neurotic depression. *British Journal of Psychiatry*, **121**, 183–186.

—— & GARSIDE, R. F. (1973) Depression: A multivariate study of Sir Aubrey Lewis's data on melancholia. *Australian & New Zealand Journal of Psychiatry*, **11**, 149–56.

KLERMAN, G. L. (1977) Anxiety and depression. In *Handbook of Studies on Depression* (ed. G. Burrows). Amsterdam: Excerpta Medica.

LEWIS, A. J. (1934a) Melancholia: a historical review. *Journal of Mental Science*, **80**, 1–42.

—— (1934b) Melancholia: A clinical survey of depressive states. *Journal of Mental Science*, **80**, 227–378.

—— (1938) States of depression: their clinical aetiological differentiation. *British Medical Journal*, ii, 875–878.

—— (1966) In *Price's Textbook of the Practice of Medicine* (ed. R. B. Scott). Oxford University Press.

—— (1971) The ambiguous word "anxiety". *International Journal of Psychiatry*, **9**, 62–79.

LIPMAN, R. S., RICKELS, K., COVI, L., DEROGATIS, L. R. & UHLENHUTH, E. H. (1969) Factors of symptoms distress. Doctor ratings of anxious, neurotic outpatients. *Archives of General Psychiatry*, **21**, 328–338.

LORR, M. (1969) The depressive syndromes and the endogenous versus reactive dichotomy: on integration. Paper delivered at the American Psychological Association Meeting. Available from author at Catholic University of America.

McFADYEN, H. W. (1977) The classification of depressive disorders. Archives of the Behavioural Sciences Monograph Series. Clinical Psychology Publishing Co. Inc., 4 Conant Square, Brandon, VT 05733, Canada. Also in McFADYEN, H. W. (1975) *The Journal of Clinical Psychology*, **31**, 380–394.

MAPOTHER, E. (1926) Discussion on manic depressive psychosis. *British Medical Journal*, *ii*, 872.

MATUSSEK, P., SOLDNER, M. & NAGEL, D. (1981) Identification of the endogenous depressive syndrome based on the symptoms and the characteristics of the course. *British Journal of Psychiatry*, **138**, 361–372.

MAXWELL, A. E. (1972) Difficulties in a dimensional description of symptomatology. *British Journal of Psychiatry*, **121**, 19–26.

MENDELS, J. (1968) Depression: The distinction between syndrome and symptom. *British Journal of Psychiatry*, **114**, 1549–1554.

—— & COCHRANE, C. (1968) The nosology of depression; the endogenous reactive concept. *American Journal of Psychiatry*, **124**, (supplement) 1–11.

MOREY, L. C. (1985) A comparative validation of the Foulds and Bedford hierarchy of psychiatric symptomatology. *British Journal of Psychiatry*, **146**, 424–428.

MULLANEY, J. A. (1984) The relationship between anxiety and depression: A review of some principal component analytic studies. *Journal of Affective Disorders*, **7**, 139–148.

—— (1985) The validity of two Newcastle Diagnostic Scales in the affective disorders: Bimodality and other correlates. *Journal of Affective Disorders*, **9**, 239–274.

—— (1986) The Development of Severity and Descriptive Scales in the Affective Disorders. MD Thesis, University College, Dublin.

—— (1987) Measurement of anxiety and depression. In *Anxious Depression, Assessment and Treatment* p. 7–19 (eds G. Ragagni & E. Smeraldi). New York: Raven Press.

NELSON, J. C. & CHARNEY, D. S. (1981) The symptoms of major depressive illness. *American Journal of Psychiatry*, **138**, 161–163.

PAYKEL, E. S. (1971) Classification of depressed patients: A cluster analysis derived grouping. *British Journal of Psychiatry*, **118**, 275–288.

—— (1972) Depressive typologies and response to amitryptiline. *British Journal of Psychiatry*, **120**, 147–156.

PICHOT, P. (1974) Psychological measurement in psychopharmacology. Introduction in *Modern Problems in Pharmaco Psychiatry*. Basle: S. Karger. 7(0), 1–7.

RASKIN, A., SCHULTERBRANT, J. C., REATIG, N., CROOK, T. H. & OLDE, D. (1974) Depression subtypes and response to phenelzine, diazepam and placebo. *Archives of General Psychiatry*, **30**, 66–95.

ROSENTHAL, S. H. & GUDEMAN, J. E. (1967) The endogenous depressive pattern. *Archives of General Psychiatry*, **16**, 241–249.

ROTH, M., GURNEY, C., GARSIDE, R. F., KERR, T. A. (1972) Studies in the classification of affective disorders: The relationship between anxiety states and depressive illness I. *British Journal of Psychiatry*, **121**, 147–161.

—— & MOUNTJOY, C. Q. (1982) The distinction between anxiety and depressive disorders. In *Handbook of Affective Disorders* (ed. E. S. Paykel), pp. 70–92. Edinburgh: Churchill Livingstone.

SCHNEIDER, K. (1957) Primäre und secondäre Symptome bei der Schizophrenie. *Forschritte der Neurologie Und Psychiatrie*, **25**, 487–490.

SPITZER, R. L. & WILLIAMS, J. B. (1983) The DSM–III Classification of Affective Disorders. *Acta Psychiatrica Scandinavica*, **310**, 106–116.

STURT, E. (1981) Hierarchical patterns in the distribution of psychiatric symptoms. *Psychological Medicine*, **11**, 783–794.

SURTEES, P. G. & KENDELL, R. E. (1979) The hierarchy model of psychiatric symptomatology: An investigation based on present state examination ratings. *British Journal of Psychiatry*, **135**, 438–443.

TORGERSON, W. S. (1968) Multidimensional representation of similarity structures. In *Classification in Psychiatry and Psychopathology* (eds M. Katz, J. O. Cole & W. Barton). Washington, DC: U.S. Department of Health Education and Welfare. P.H. Publication No. 1584.

TYRER, P. (1984) Classification of anxiety. *British Journal of Psychiatry*, **144**, 78–83.

—— (1985) Neurosis divisible. *Lancet*, *i*, 685–688.

VERNON, P. E. (1961) The structure of human abilities (2nd edn). London: Methuen.

WILLIAMS, H. V., LIPMAN, R. S., RICKELS, K., COVI, L., UHLENHUTH, E. H. & MATTSON NILS, B. (1968) Replication of symptom distress factors in anxious neurotic outpatients. *Multivariate Behavioural Research*, **3**, 199–212.

WING, J. K., MANN, S. A., LEFF, J. P. & NIXON, J. M. (1978) The concept of a "case" in psychiatric population surveys. *Psychological Medicine*, **7**, 505–516.

WITTENBORN, J. R. (1975) Different types and concepts of rating scales (eds J. R. Bossier, H. Hippius & P. Pichot) *Excerpta Medica*. Amsterdam, New York: American Elsevier Publishing. pp. 27–31. International Congress Series No. 359.

ZUNG, W. W. K. (1971) The differentiation of anxiety and depressive disorders. A biometric approach. *Psychosomatics*, **12**, 380–384.

# 16 The neurology of affective disorder and suicide

## F. ANTHONY WHITLOCK

The importance of organic brain disease and dysfunction as causes of psychological disorder scarcely needs re-emphasis today. In this respect the value of a proper understanding of neurology can hardly be over-estimated. Feighner *et al* (1972) used the term "secondary affective disorder" to denote such disturbances in the presence of other psychiatric conditions, organic brain disease and serious medical illnesses. I prefer "symptomatic affective disorder" when depressive and manic syndromes develop in these circumstances. Such a mood of depression is to be differentiated from discrete symptoms of this disorder which might be understandable reactions to adversity, pain, illness and handicap—grief reactions in short.

## Infections

The list of conditions giving rise to symptomatic depression and mania is extensive and includes a number of infectious diseases affecting the CNS, among which should be mentioned influenza (Tuke, 1892; Menninger, 1919; Editorial, *British Medical Journal*, 1976) which can cause an encephalitis with evidence of perivascular demyelination. Mania is less common but does occur (Steinberg *et al*, 1972). Another disorder, infectious mononucleosis (IM) may involve the CNS in 0.7–26.5% of cases (Silverstein, 1978). In my experience, severe and protracted depression following an attack of infectious mononucleosis appears commoner among younger patients, particularly students who may have to give up their studies for a time on account of this complication. A recent account of two young patients with delusional depression after attacks of IM recorded signs of encephalopathy in one who was extensively investigated (White & Lewis, 1987). One might conjecture that less severe cases of depression following attacks of IM could also have similar cerebral involvement. The status of benign epidemic myalgic encephalomyelitis, Royal Free disease, continues to be a matter of debate. Whereas some writers (McEvedy & Beard, 1970, 1973; Easton, 1978) have classed the condition as one of epidemic hysteria, others (Kendell, 1967; Wookey, 1978; Ramsay, 1978; Church, 1980) have reported patients who manifested severe, recurrent depression. On at least one occasion such depression ended with suicide (Kendell, 1967). The most recent contribution to this controversy under the title of post-viral fatigue syndrome centres on the possibility that it is caused by Coxsackie B infection (for review see Dawson, 1987).

General paralysis of the insane (GPI), a relative rarity today, can cause depression, euphoria and hypomania. Traditionally, the hypomanic features have been emphasised but more recent reports (Steel, 1960; Dewhurst, 1969; Storm-Mathieson, 1969) have shown that major depressive symptoms are by no means unusual.

## Head injuries

There is an increasing number of head injuries in civilian life, mainly following car crashes. In 1974 the rate of hospital attendance for such damage was 1700 per 100 000 of the population (Jennett & MacMillan, 1981). Lishman (1978), in a study of 144 head injured patients with severe psychiatric disability following war injuries, found that 58% were episodically or continuously depressed. The severity of these affective disorders often bore little relationship to the degree of damage sustained. In another investigation 37% of patients with simple concussion became depressed (Kay *et al*, 1971) and, in a detailed examination of 27 patients following minor head injuries, seven showed typical features of endogenous depression and another 19 had depression as a symptom (Merskey & Woodforde, 1972). Simple concussion can cause more brain damage than is sometimes supposed, damage which includes slowing of cerebral blood flow (Taylor & Bell, 1966), changes in permeability of the blood-brain barrier and disturbances of vestibular function (Taylor, 1967). At post-mortem examination diffuse capillary haemorrhages as well as actual severance of nerve fibres in many parts of the brain can be seen (Oppenheimer, 1968). The relevance of these findings to compensation cases with persistent psychiatric impairment following concussion is sometimes overlooked. The cases described by Merskey & Woodforde (1972) had no past history of psychiatric illness. It follows that cerebral pathology following head injury can on occasion cause long-standing, refractory affective disorder.

## Cerebrovascular disease

In some 9-12% of elderly depressives, cerebrovascular disease was present before affective symptoms developed (Kay, 1962). In Post's series (1962) the majority of his patients became depressed after cerebrovascular accident, and Roth (1971) observed that in 17-18% of cases of cerebrovascular disease an associated affective disorder could be the harbinger of dementia from progressive brain damage.

In fact, severe depression is a not uncommon sequel to strokes and other cerebrovascular accidents (Adams & Hurwitz, 1963; Folstein *et al*, 1977; Wade *et al*, 1987). With respect to subarachnoid haemorrhages, depressive complications are more likely to follow rupture of aneurysms of the posterior communicating artery, possibly because of hypothalamic damage (Storey, 1967, 1970, 1972). Patients who became depressed in the absence of brain damage were more likely to have suffered from affective disorder in the past. By contrast, those who sustained brain damage and then became depressed more often had robust and energetic premorbid personalities and may have been reacting adversely to the limitations imposed by their disabilities.

## Cerebral tumours

Many authors have recorded the frequency of affective symptoms preceding or accompanying cerebral tumours. Keschner *et al* (1938), for example, in a study of 530 patients, found that 46% suffered from such symptoms, approximately the same number being associated with temporal lobe as with frontal lobe tumours, although by no means all patients were severely depressed. Selecki *et al* (1965) surveyed the frequency of cerebral tumours found in mental hospital autopsies and commented on how often these had not been diagnosed during the patients' lifetime. In this context Pool & Carroll (1958) described 25 patients who had received psychotherapy for 1–13 years before the tumours, the true causes of their psychiatric symptoms, were diagnosed.

Among the different kinds of tumours, meningiomas figure prominently, possibly because of their slow growth and an absence of overt neurological symptoms until comparatively late in their development. The classic signs and symptoms of a space-occupying lesion in the brain are often absent or overlooked, although raised intra-cranial pressure—more liable to occur in posterior fossa tumours—is not a likely cause of psychiatric symptoms. Depression is commoner than mania, although some of Avery's (1971) patients with meningiomas had episodes of mania or hypomania. In some cases epilepsy could contribute to the pathogenesis of recurrent depression (Malamud, 1967).

## Basal ganglia syndromes

Lishman (1978) writes that there is a well established association between parkinsonism and depression and that, of the psychiatric disorders observed in this condition, affective symptoms are the commonest. A recent review (Whitlock, 1986a) found that depression, both reactive and endogenous, occurred in as many as 90% of patients with Parkinson's disease. The pathological changes in the striatum, substantia nigra and locus coeruleus yield clues to the pathogenesis of some examples of depression as the loss of noradrenergic neurones from the locus coeruleus and its connections with the nucleus accumbens and limbic forebrain structures (Horneykiewicz, 1977; Farley *et al*, 1977) would be compatible with the biogenic amine theory of affective disorder.

When compared with patients suffering from equivalent handicaps, depression is often more severe in cases of paralysis agitans (Warburton, 1967; Robins, 1976). On occasion depression has preceded the onset of major neurological symptoms by a considerable period of time (Jackson *et al*, 1923; Kearney, 1964; Celesia & Wanamaker, 1972). To some extent the psychological and physical symptoms are independent of one another, as treatment of depression can be successful in spite of lack of improvement in the patient's physical condition (Mindham, 1970) while conversely, amelioration of the physical symptoms does not invariably produce a corresponding benefit to the patient's psychological state.

It is well known that Huntington's disease can be heralded by depression and suicidal attempts well before the onset of the typical neurological signs and symptoms. Relatives of patients, although not affected themselves, may also have a high incidence of psychotic depression and suicidal behaviour. Whether there is a separate genetic loading for affective disorder in Huntington's disease cannot at present be decided (Oliver, 1970) but Folstein and colleagues (1983) consider that the association between major affective disorder and neurological symptoms may be an indication of genetic heterogeneity in Huntington's disease.

## Multiple sclerosis

Barbellion, in his *Diary of a Disappointed Man* (1919), recorded severe depression and suicidal thoughts well before his neurological symptoms developed, and depression as a prodrome of MS has been described by a number of writers (Bignami *et al*, 1961; Pommé *et al*, 1963; Mür *et al*, 1966; Young *et al*, 1976; Whitlock & Siskind, 1980). This sequence of events has received comparatively little attention as, in one survey of 200 reports, a common pathogenesis for both phenomena was mentioned only in five (Goodstein & Ferrel, 1977).

The inappropriate euphoria described by Cottrell & Wilson (1926), long believed to be the most typical affective change in MS, is now regarded as a sign of organic deterioration. Typical mania (Targowla *et al*, 1928; Cremieux *et al*, 1957) is far rarer than depression but a patient known to me developed bipolar manic-depressive psychosis *after* the onset of neurological symptoms and finally committed suicide during an episode of depression. In an investigation in Brisbane (Whitlock & Siskind, 1980) more evidence of depression among MS patients was recorded than in a matched control sample of patients with other types of incapacitating neurological illnesses. Of the 30 MS patients, eight had experienced depression before the onset of diagnosable neurological symptoms.

Post-mortem examinations of MS patients with severe depression or mania have revealed lesions in the hypothalamus, cerebral peduncles and pons in one case (Bigmani *et al*, 1961) and brain stem lesions in others (Cremieux *et al*, 1957; O'Malley, 1966). Involvement of parts of the limbic brain in some cases could be the basis for major affective disturbances in MS patients.

## Epilepsy

Ictal emotions were described in great detail by Williams in his Bradshaw lecture (1956). Twenty-one of his 100 patients suffered from depression, with or without suicidal feelings, lasting from one hour to three days. Maudsley, writing in 1895, gave an excellent account of an epileptic aura when he described episodes of melancholia associated with changes in consciousness and "a strange and riotous sensation toward the head from the region of the heart or of the epigastrium". He referred to these phenomena as "mental epilepsy". Their true nature was recognised by Reynolds (1861) when he mentioned sudden depression of spirits as part of an epileptic aura. Wells (1975) carried out EEG recordings on two patients with prolonged ictal depression and noted features of epileptic status which ceased with appropriate anticonvulsant treatment. The clinical features of affective disturbances in epilepsy have not been examined so thoroughly as in the case of the schizophrenia-like psychoses. The relatives of epileptic patients have a higher frequency of major psychiatric disorders (Jensen & Larsen, 1979) so possibly genetic and constitutional factors could contribute to the occurrence of affective disorders in epileptics, some of whom will have past personal and family histories of such illnesses. On balance, the evidence supports the belief that severe endogenous depression and mania can develop as ictal and interictal disturbances, disorders which are more likely to occur in patients with temporal lobe epilepsy.

## Cancer

It is known that neurological symptoms can be the precursors of cancer well before the tumours themselves are diagnosed. Until recently less attention has been given to the possibility that major affective symptoms can also be the harbingers of malignancy. The important study by Schmale & Iker (1971) detected signs of depression and hopelessness in a number of women who subsequently developed carcinoma of the cervix. Follow-up investigations of patients in middle life or older who had been treated for depression revealed a higher than expected number of male deaths from cancer during the next four years (Kerr *et al*, 1969; Whitlock & Siskind, 1979). When a cohort of suicide victims was compared with individuals killed in car crashes, the suicides had significantly more malignant tumours revealed at post-mortem investigation (Whitlock, 1978).

The precise reason for this relationship between depression and later carcinoma is not known. Possibly the affective disorder impairs the immunological defences which might then allow malignant cells to gain a foothold and proliferate into diagnosable tumours. It is also known that certain paraneoplastic syndromes such as Cushing's syndrome (Armatruda & Upton, 1974) and hyperparathyroidism (Gordon, 1974) can cause major symptoms of depression which would appear before malignant tumours have declared themselves clinically.

## Systemic lupus erythematosus (SLE) and giant-cell arteritis

Many systemic conditions can cause secondary involvement of the CNS with ensuing psychiatric disturbances. It is not possible to consider all these conditions but two should be mentioned: SLE and giant-cell arteritis.

SLE has a prevalence rate of 2 to 3 per 100 000 (Harrison, 1977) and there are signs of CNS involvement in 60% of patients (Granville-Grossman, 1971). In 15 studies the incidence of psychiatric symptoms varied from 17% to 80%, of which 18.5% to 86% were affective in nature (Whitlock, 1982). Most of these patients suffered from depressive psychoses but in some instances the predominant mood was one of euphoria and even mania (Johnson & Richardson, 1968). Although many of these patients would have been receiving steroids which could influence mood it seems generally to be accepted that neurological damage rather than treatment is responsible for psychiatric disturbances. In fact, increasing steroid therapy often reduces both neurological and psychiatric symptoms. A study of 15 patients with a variety of associated psychiatric disorders demonstrated abnormalities of cerebral blood flow, most marked in the frontal areas of the brain. Raised levels of brain-reactive lymphocytotoxic antibodies were detected which, through leakage due to cerebral vasculitis, could cause brain damage and neuropsychiatric symptoms (Bresnihan *et al*, 1979).

Giant-cell arteritis, which principally affects women, is a condition by no means confined to the temporal arteries, the commonest site for the production of symptoms. The intra-cranial vasculature and blood vessels in other parts of the body may also be affected. Depression can be a prominent complication (Robertson, 1947; Vererker, 1952; Ross Russell, 1959; Von Knorring *et al*, 1966). A patient with severe depression and markedly raised ESR may well be suffering from giant-cell arteritis. One such case with an ESR of 100 recovered from her depression when treated with steroids. There was no previous history of affective disorder (Hughes, 1977).

## Suicide

Depression is one of the commonest causes of suicide and one might, therefore, expect that some patients with cerebral disorder and depression would take their own lives. The far higher rates of suicide and attempted suicide by epileptic patients are testimony to this fact. It has been calculated that death by suicide is five times more frequent in epileptics compared with the general population (Prudhomme, 1941). Suicide attempts are also commoner and from five investigations (Sclare & Hamilton, 1964; Taylor *et al*, 1964; Lawson & Mitchell, 1972; Whitlock & Schapira, 1967; Edwards & Whitlock, 1968) it can be shown that such behaviour is 1.7 to 6.5 times greater in comparison with the non-epileptic population.

On the other hand, suicide is relatively rare in patients afflicted with the other cerebral disorders mentioned in this paper. One exception is Huntington's disease in which suicide accounts for up to 7% of deaths (McHugh & Folstein, 1975), a fact recognised by Huntington (1872) when he mentioned "a tendency to insanity and suicide" as cardinal features of the condition.

An investigation, based on coroners' reports of 1000 suicides in England and Wales, found that at least 89 cases showed evidence of present or past cerebral disease (Whitlock, 1986). The commonest conditions recorded were cerebrovascular disease, epilepsy, dementia and head injury. There were six cases of MS, although most authorities comment on the rarity of suicide by MS sufferers (McAlpine *et al*, 1965; Kurzke, 1970). In one small series of patients there was one suicide attempt, 13 patients admitted to suicidal thoughts and there was one suicide by a patient with manic-depressive psychosis (Whitlock & Siskind, 1980). Epilepsy can affect about 2% of MS patients, and in one report on 27 such patients there were six suicide attempts and one completed suicide (Elian & Dean, 1977). In contrast, in spite of the frequency of depression, few patients with Parkinson's disease take their own lives, although suicidal ideation is not unusual (Warburton, 1967; Robins, 1976; Celesia & Wanamaker, 1972; Asnis, 1977). Parant (1892) commented on the frequency of melancholia in paralysis agitans and considered that this entailed a severe risk of suicide.

# Summary

This survey points to a number of important conclusions. Firstly, many neurological diseases may present as major affective illnesses well before objective physical signs appear. Secondly, a careful investigation of the neuropathology of neurological and co-existing affective syndromes may tell us something about the likely pathogenesis and neurological basis of some varieties of depression and mania. In addition some support for the biogenic amine theory of affective disorders might be obtained from our better understanding of the biochemical disturbances detected in some basal ganglia syndromes. Thirdly, although many of the conditions mentioned cannot always be completely cured, depression, if it develops, can often be successfully treated. Fourthly, in such illnesses the risk of suicide seems greater when depression is a complication of epilepsy or when epilepsy and depression occur in the course of other neurological syndromes.

Finally, a plea should be made to our colleagues in general medicine and neurology that they should be better acquainted with the phenomena of psychiatric disorder and record any observed emotional disturbances in more precise language. We in psychiatry are required to keep abreast with the major developments in general medicine but for a physician to be ignorant of psychiatric terminology is by no means unusual and not regarded with any overt degree of discredit. The evidence collected in this paper makes it clear that a sound working knowledge of general medicine, neurology and psychiatry is essential if we are to diagnose and treat our patients efficiently. Perhaps I might end by repeating Richard Hunter's rather provocative words (1973): "Progress in psychiatry is inevitably and irrevocably from the psychological to the physical—never the other way round". Never? Well hardly ever.

# Acknowledgement

I am indebted to Professor Gordon Parker, editor of the *Australian and New Zealand Journal of Psychiatry*, for permission to reproduce this modified version of my 1981 Beattie Smith Lecture, published in that journal in 1982. *Australian and New Zealand Journal of Psychiatry*, 1982, **16**, 1–12.

# References

ADAMS, G. F. & HURWITZ, L. J. (1963) Mental barriers to recovery from strokes. *Lancet*, ii, 533–537.

ARMATRUDA, T. A. & UPTON, J. V. (1974) Hyperadrenocorticism and ACTH-releasing factor. *Annals of the New York Academy of Science*, **230**, 168–169.

ASNIS, G. (1977) Parkinson's disease, depression and ECT: A review of a case study. *American Journal of Psychiatry*, **134**, 191–195.

AVERY, T. L. (1971) Seven cases of frontal tumour with psychiatric presentation. *British Journal of Psychiatry*, **119**, 19–23.

BARBELLION, W. N. P. (1919) *Diary of a Disappointed Man*. London: Chatto & Windus.

BIGNAMI, A., GERHARDI, D. & GALLO, G. (1961) Sclerosi a placche acuta a localizzazione i potolamica con sintomologia psychica di tipo malinconico. *Revista Neurologica*, **31**, 240–268.

BRESNIHAN, B., HOHMEISTER, R., CUTTING, J., et al (1979) The neuropsychiatric disorder in SLE: Evidence for both vascular and immune mechanisms. *Annals of the Rheumatic Diseases*, **38**, 301–306.

CELESIA, G. G. & WANAMAKER, W. M. (1972) Psychiatric disturbances in Parkinson's disease. *Diseases of the Nervous System*, **33**, 577–583.

CHURCH, A. G. (1980) Myalgic encephalomyelitis, 'an obscene cosmic joke'. *Medical Journal of Australia*, **1**, 307–308.

COTTRELL, S. S. & WILSON, S. A. K. (1926) The affective symptomatology of disseminated sclerosis. *Journal of Neurology and Psychopathology*, **7**, 1–30.

CRÉMIEUX, A., ALLIEZ, J., TONGA, M. & PACHE, R. (1957) Sclerose en plaques a debut par troubles mentaux: étude anatomo-clinique. *Revue Neurologique (Paris)*, **101**, 45–51.

DAWSON, J. (1987) Royal Free disease: perplexity continues. *British Medical Journal*, *i*, 327–328.

DEWHURST, K. (1969) The neurosyphilitic psychoses today. *British Journal of Psychiatry*, **115**, 31–38.

EASTON, H. G. (1978) Epidemic myalgic encephalomyelitis. *British Medical Journal*, *i*, 1969.

EDITORIAL, BRITISH MEDICAL JOURNAL (1976) Low spirits after virus infections. *British Medical Journal*, *ii*, 440.

EDWARDS, J. E. & WHITLOCK, F. A. (1968) Suicide and attempted suicide in Brisbane. *Medical Journal of Australia*, **1**, 932 and 989.

ELIAN, M. & DEAN, G. (1977) Multiple sclerosis and seizures. In *Epilepsy, 8th International Symposium* (ed. J. K. Penry), pp. 341–344.

FARLEY, I. J., PRICE, K. S. & HORNYKIEWICZ, O. (1977) Dopamine in the limbic regions of the human brain: normal and abnormal. *Advances in Biochemical Psychopharmacology*, **16**, 57–64.

FEIGHNER, J. P., ROBINS, E., GUZE, S. B., *et al* (1972) Diagnostic criteria for use in psychiatric research. *Archives of General Psychiatry*, **6**, 57–64.

FOLSTEIN, M. F., MAIBERGER, R., MCHUGH, P. R. (1977) Mood disorder as a specific complication of stroke. *Journal of Neurology, Neurosurgery and Psychiatry*, **40**, 1018–1020.

FOLSTEIN, S. E., ABBOTT, M. H., CHASE, G. A., JENSEN, B. A. & FOLSTEIN, M. F. (1983) The association of affective disorders with Huntington's disease in a case series and in families. *Psychological Medicine*, **13**, 537–542.

GOODSTEIN, R. K. & FERRELL, R. B. (1977) Multiple sclerosis presenting as a depressive illness. *Diseases of the Nervous System*, **38**, 127–131.

GORDON, G. S. (1974) Hyper and hypocalcaemia: Pathogenesis and treatment. *Annals of the New York Academy of Science*, **230**, 181–186.

GRANVILLE-GROSSMAN, K. (1971) *Recent Advances in Clinical Psychiatry*, pp. 231–234. London: Churchill.

HARRISON'S *Principles of Medicine* 8th edn (1977) (eds G. W. Thorn, R. D. Adams, E. Brounwald *et al*). New York: McGraw Hill.

HORNYKIEWICZ, O. (1977) Biogenic amines in the central nervous system. In *Handbook of Clinical Neurology*, **29**, 459–483. (eds P. J. Vinken & G. W. Bruyn). Amsterdam: North Holland Publishing.

HUGHES, G. R. F. (1977) *Connective Tissue Diseases*. Oxford: Blackwell Scientific, p. 221.

HUNTER, R. (1973) Psychosyndrome or brain disease. *Proceedings of the Royal Society of Medicine*, **66**, 359–364.

HUNTINGTON, G. (1872) On chorea. *Medical-Surgical Reports of Philadelphia*, **26**, 317–321.

JACKSON, J. A., FREE, G. B. M. & PIKE, H. V. (1923) The psychic manifestations in paralysis agitans. *Archives of Neurology and Psychiatry*, **10**, 680–684.

JENNETT, B. & MACMILLAN, R. (1981) Epidemiology of head injury. *British Medical Journal*, *i*, 101–104.

JENSEN, I. & LARSEN, J. K. (1979) Mental aspects of temporal lobe epilepsy. *Journal of Neurology, Neurosurgery and Psychiatry*, **42**, 256–265.

JOHNSON, R. T. & RICHARDSON, E. P. (1968) The neurological complications of systemic lupus erythematosus. *Medicine*, **47**, 337–369.

KAY, D. W. K. (1962) Outcome and cause of death in mental disorders of old age: A long-term follow-up of functional and organic psychosis. *Acta Psychiatrica Scandinavica*, **38**, 249–276.

——, KERR, T. A. & LASSMAN, L. P. (1971) Brain trauma and the post-concussion caused by minor head injuries. *Lancet*, *ii*, 1052–1055.

KEARNEY, T. R. (1964) Parkinson's disease presenting as a depressive illness. *Journal of the Irish Medical Association*, **54**, 117–119.

KENDELL, R. E. (1967) The psychiatric sequelae of benign myalgic encephalitis. *British Journal of Psychiatry*, **113**, 833–840.

KERR, T. A., SCHAPIRA, K. & ROTH, M. (1969) The relationship between premature death and affective disorders. *British Journal of Psychiatry*, **115**, 1277–1282.

KESCHNER, M., BENDER, M. V. & STRAUSS, I. (1938) Mental symptoms associated with brain tumours. *Journal of the American Medical Association*, **110**, 714–718.

KURZKE, J. G. (1970) Clinical manifestations of multiple sclerosis. In *Handbook of Clinical Neurology*, **9**, 161–216, (eds P. J. Vinken & G. W. Bruyn). Amsterdam: North Holland Publishing.

LAWSON, A. H. H. & MITCHELL, I. (1972) Patients with acute poisoning seen in a general medical unit 1960–1971. *British Medical Journal*, **4**, 153–156.

LISHMAN, W. A. (1978) *Organic Psychiatry*. Oxford: Blackwell.

McALPINE, D., LUMSDEN, C. E. & ACHESON, E. D. (1965) *Multiple Sclerosis: A Reappraisal*, p. 154. Edinburgh: E. & S. Livingston.

McEVEDY, C. P. & BEARD, A. W. (1970) Royal Free epidemic of 1955: a reconsideration. *British Medical Journal*, i, 7–11.

—— & —— (1973) A controlled follow-up of cases involved in an epidemic of benign myalgic encephalomyelitis. *British Journal of Psychiatry*, 122, 141–150.

McHUGH, P. R. & FOLSTEIN, M. F. (1975) Psychiatric syndromes of Huntington's chorea. In *Psychiatric Aspects of Neurologic Disease* (eds F. Benson & D. Blumer), pp. 267–285. New York: Grune & Stratton.

MALAMUD, N. (1967) Psychiatric disorder with intracranial tumours of the limbic system. *Archives of Neurology*, 17, 113–123.

MAUDSLEY, H. (1895) *The Pathology of Mind*. Facsimile edition (1979) p. 116. London: Julian Friedmann.

MENNINGER, K. A. (1919) Psychoses associated with influenza. *Journal of the American Medical Association*, 72, 235–241.

MERSKEY, H. M. & WOODFORDE, J. M. (1972) Psychiatric sequelae of minor head injury, *Brain*, 95, 521–528.

MINDHAM, R. H. S. (1970) Psychiatric symptoms in Parkinsonism. *Journal of Neurology, Neurosurgery and Psychiatry*, 33, 188–191.

MÜR, J., KÜMPEL, G. & DOSTÁL, S. (1966) An anergic phase of disseminated sclerosis with psychiatric course. *Confinia Neurologica*, 28, 37–49.

OLIVER, J. E. (1970) Huntington's chorea in Northamptonshire. *British Journal of Psychiatry*, 116, 241–255.

O'MALLEY, P. P. (1966) Severe mental symptoms in disseminated sclerosis: A neuropathological study. *Journal of the Irish Medical Association*, 55, 115–127.

OPPENHEIMER, D. R. (1968) Microscopic lesions in the brain following head injury. *Journal of Neurology, Neurosurgery and Psychiatry*, 31, 299–306.

PARANT, V. (1892) Paralysis agitans, insanity associated with. In *Dictionary of Psychological Medicine* p. 884–886 (ed. D. H. Tuke). London: Churchill)

POMMÉ, B., GIRARD, J. & PLANCHE, R. (1963) Forme depressive de debut d'une sclerose en plaques. *Annales Medico-Psychologique* (Paris), 121, 133.

POOL, J. L. & CARROLL, J. W. (1958) Psychiatric symptoms masking brain tumours. *Journal of the Medical Society of New Jersey*, 55, 4–9.

POST, F. (1962) *The Significance of Affective Symptoms in Old Age*. London: Oxford University Press.

PRUDHOMME, C. (1941) Epilepsy and suicide. *Journal of Nervous and Mental Diseases*, 94, 722–731.

RAMSAY, A. M. (1978) Epidemic neuromyasthenia. *Postgraduate Medical Journal*, 57, 718–721.

REYNOLDS, J. R. (1861) *Epilepsy: Its Symptoms, Treatment and Relation to the Chronic Convulsive Disease*. London: Churchill.

ROBERTSON, K. (1947) Temporal or giant-cell arteritis. *British Medical Journal*, ii, 168–170.

ROBINS, A. H. (1976) Depression in patients with Parkinsonism. *British Journal of Psychiatry*, 128, 141–145.

ROSS RUSSELL, R. W. (1959) Giant-cell arteritis. *Quarterly Journal of Medicine*, 28, 471–489.

ROTH, M. (1971) Classification and aetiology in mental disorders in old age: some recent developments. In *Recent Developments in Psychogeriatrics* (eds D. W. K. Kay & A. Walk). Ashford: Headley Brothers p. 1–18.

SCHMALE, A. H. & IKER, H. (1971) Hopelessness as a predictor of cervical cancer. *Social Science and Medicine*, 5, 95–100.

SCLARE, A. B. & HAMILTON, C. M. (1964) Attempted suicide in Glasgow. *British Journal of Psychiatry*, 109, 609–615.

SELECKI, B. R. (1965) Intracranial space-occupying lesions. *Medical Journal of Australia*, 1, 383–390.

SILVERSTEIN, A. (1978) E B Virus infection of the nervous system. In *Handbook of Clinical Neurology* Volume 34 (eds P. J. Vinken & G. W. Bruyn). Amsterdam, North Holland Publishing, p. 185.

STEEL, R. (1960) G.P.I. in an observation ward. *Lancet*, i, 121–123.

STEINBERG, D., HIRSCH, S. R., MARSDEN, S. D. *et al* (1972) Influenza infection causing manic psychosis. *British Journal of Psychiatry*, 120, 531–538.

STOREY, P. B. (1967) Psychiatric sequelae of subarachnoid haemorrhage. *British Medical Journal*, iii, 261–266.

—— (1970) Brain damage and personality change after subarachnoid haemorrhage. *British Journal of Psychiatry*, 117, 129–142.

—— (1972) Emotional disturbances before and after subarachnoid haemorrhage. In *Physiology, Emotion and Psychosomatic Illness*, p. 333–347. Amsterdam: Elsevier.

STORM-MATHIESON, A. (1969) General paresis: A follow-up study of 203 patients. *Acta Psychiatrica Scandinavica*, **45**, 118–132.

TARGOWLA, SEVIN & OBREDANE (1928) *Encéphale* 614. Quoted Surridge, D. (1969) An investigation into some psychiatric aspects of multiple sclerosis. *British Journal of Psychiatry*, **115**, 749–764.

TAYLOR, A. R. (1967) Post-concussional sequelae. *British Medical Journal*, *iii*, 67–71.

—— & BELL, T. K. (1966) Slowing of cerebral circulation after concussional head injury. *Lancet*, *ii*, 178–180.

TAYLOR, D. J. E., DUDLEY HART, F. & BURLEY, D. (1964) Suicide in South London. *Practitioner*, **192**, 251–256.

TUKE, D. H. (1892) Influenza and mental disorders following. In *Dictionary of Psychological Medicine*, 688–691 (ed. D. H. Tuke). London: Churchill.

VERERKER, R. (1952) The psychiatric aspects of temporal arteritis. *Journal of Mental Science*, **98**, 280–286.

VON KNORRING, J., ERMA, B. & LINDSTRÖM, B. (1966) The clinical manifestations of temporal arteritis. *Acta Medica Scandinavica*, **179**, 691–702.

WADE, D. T., LEGH-SMITH, J. & HEWER, R. A. (1987) Depressed mood after stroke: a community study of its frequency. *British Journal of Psychiatry*, **151**, 200–205.

WARBURTON, J. W. (1967) Depressive symptoms in Parkinson patients referred for thalamotomy. *Journal of Neurology, Neurosurgery and Psychiatry*, **30**, 368–370.

WELLS, C. E. (1975) Transient ictal psychosis. *Archives of General Psychiatry*, **32**, 1201–1203.

WHITE, P. B. & LEWIS, S. W. (1987) Delusional depression after infectious mononucleosis. *British Medical Journal*, *ii*, 97–98.

WHITLOCK, F. A. (1986) Suicide and Physical Illness. In *Suicide* p. 151–170 (ed. A. Roy). Baltimore: Williams and Wilkins.

—— (1986a) The psychiatric complications of Parkinson's disease. *Australia and New Zealand Journal of Psychiatry*, **20**, 114–121.

—— (1982) *Symptomatic Affective Disorders*. Sydney: Academic Press, p. 138–143.

—— (1978) Suicide, cancer and depression. *British Journal of Psychiatry*, **132**, 269–274.

—— & SCHAPIRA, K. (1967) Attempted suicide in Newcastle upon Tyne. *British Journal of Psychiatry* **113**, 423–434.

—— & SISKIND, M. M. (1979) Depression and cancer: a follow-up study. *Psychological Medicine*, **9**, 747–752.

—— & —— (1980) Depression as a major symptom of multiple sclerosis. *Journal of Neurology, Neurosurgery and Psychiatry*, **43**, 861–865.

WILLIAMS, D. (1956) The structure of emotions reflected in epileptic experiences. *Brain*, **79**, 28–57.

WOOKEY, C. (1978) Epidemic myalgic encephalomyelitis. *British Medical Journal*, *ii*, 202.

YOUNG, A. C., SAUNDERS, J. & PONSFORD, J. R. (1976) Mental change as an early feature of multiple sclerosis. *Journal of Neurology, Neurosurgery and Psychiatry*, **39**, 1008–1013.

# 17 The Newcastle child depression project: Studies in the diagnosis and classification of childhood depression

**ISRAEL KOLVIN**

in collaboration with L. Barrett, T. P. Berney, S. R. Bhate,
O. O. Famuyiwa, T. Fundudis and S. Tyrer

The last decade has seen a surge of interest in childhood depression, with the main thrust originating in the United States. There has been a slower build up of research in the United Kingdom. Two fundamental issues in the current debate about depression in childhood concern the *validity of screen and diagnostic criteria*, and how best the *classification of depression* in children should proceed. Some, like Puig-Antich (1980), consider it possible to diagnose major depression in childhood using criteria identical to those in adults. However, others emphasise that in younger children depressive experience is less well defined. These differences are reflected in the various combinations of symptoms in diagnostic schemata, such as, Weinberg *et al* (1973), in the USA, and Kolvin *et al* (1984) in Newcastle. How valid are each of these in the diagnosis of depression? As yet this is an unresolved matter, despite its fundamental relevance to the whole topic.

The other issue of importance is how depression should be classified. This is a notoriously complex area in the adult field, and even if childhood depression were exactly similar to adult depression, classificatory problems would be compounded by child development issues. In this paper we address some of these issues using multivariate statistical approaches. In the United Kingdom, the inspiration for multivariate exploration of depression data was the original work of the Newcastle School of Psychiatry, as exemplified by Martin Roth and Roger Garside (Kiloh & Garside, 1963; Carney, Roth & Garside, 1965).

The Newcastle Child Depression Project is a collaborative exercise undertaken by a large team. The aims of this part of the study were two-fold:
(a) to study the validity of screen and diagnostic schemata
(b) to examine classification issues. This includes the value of the parental and child interview data in diagnosis and classification; and the factorial validity of the depressive syndrome.

## Diagnostic issues

A number of instruments have emerged for rating depression in childhood; they are of two kinds, self-rating measures and interview techniques. There are two self-rating instruments, the Child Depression Inventory (CDI) (27 items) which has been developed by Kovacs (1978) in the United States, and the Birleson Inventory (1981) (18 items) in the United Kingdom. The CDI has been widely used in research but because of the relatively high mis-classification rate, it is considered to be only moderately useful as a screen instrument; the same has been shown to be true for the Birleson (Fundudis *et al*, 1989). On the other hand, a number of new diagnostic schemata have been developed based on interview questionnaires.

*The Kiddie-SADS*: the Kiddie-SADS is essentially a modification by Puig-Antich and colleagues (Orvaschel *et al*, 1982; Chambers *et al*, 1985) of the Schedule for Affective Disorders and Schizophrenia (Spitzer & Endicott, 1978) for use with children between 6 and 17 years of age. It has been shown to be a reliable instrument for symptoms of depression and conduct disorder, although the measure of anxiety disorder has not been so consistent. In the original procedure the parents are usually interviewed first, then the child; the interviewer of the child is guided by information provided by the parents' account of each symptom; the examiner is required to make a clinical judgement of the presence or absence of the symptom and, if present, its severity; that is, the onset and duration of symptoms is used to rate severity of each symptom. The rating is a synthesis of all the information available on the child and provides the basis for the diagnosis. Although the Kiddie-SADS was felt to be the best instrument for assessing childhood depression, one essential modification in the procedure was effected in the Newcastle Study. Independent interviewing of parent and child by different interviewers was carried out, thus avoiding contamination effects for the rating of symptoms. Independent ratings of the severity of each symptom were made by each examiner, based on his or her interview with the child or parent *alone*, followed by an independent summary rating. Composite ratings and diagnosis were then established based on a synthesis of all the information.

*The Weinberg Schema of Criteria for Diagnosis*: Weinberg *et al* (1973) have offered a list of primary and secondary symptoms based on the criteria for diagnosis of depression in adulthood (Feighner *et al*, 1972). In order to be diagnosed as depressed, children need to have the primary symptom of dysphoric mood and self-depreciation plus an additional two out of a further eight symptoms which include: aggressive behaviour, sleep disturbance, changes in school performance, social withdrawal, somatic complaints, loss of usual energy, appetite changes and change in attitude to school. There are no guidelines as to the duration and severity of disturbance. Subsequently, Puig-Antich (1980) advanced the hypothesis that depressive disorder in childhood could be diagnosed using unmodified Research Diagnostic Criteria (Spitzer *et al*, 1978). For diagnosis, the child had to have depressed mood or pervasive anhedonia, energy changes, appetite changes, sleep problems, poor concentration, psychomotor retardation, and suicidal thoughts.

*The Newcastle Instrument*: Our research group has also developed a brief set of key diagnostic criteria (Kolvin *et al*, 1984) which are listed in Table I. They differ from the criteria advanced by the North American Research Groups (Weinberg, 1973; Puig-Antich, 1980), but there are more similarities than differences in relation to the Puig-Antich schema than the Weinberg variation. Further work needs to be undertaken to establish whether the Newcastle Schema, specifically developed for separating school phobics into those with and without depression, will have a wider application in the diagnosis before and after puberty. In the current project we have been able to validate the Newcastle Schema as an effective instrument for diagnosing depression in a child psychiatric

TABLE I
*Newcastle diagnostic schema*

1. Dysphoric mood
2. Weeping
3. Sense of emptiness/isolation
4. Sense of being unloved
5. Exaggerated illness behaviour
6. Loss of interest
7. Loss of energy
8. Initial insomnia
9. Nocturnal restlessness
10. Feeling life is not worth living
11. Depersonalisation

| | |
|---|---|
| Scored as ordinal scale | (1, 2, 3, 4) |
| Recorded as binary scale | (0, 0, 1, 1) |
| Best cut: 6 plus on binary scale | |

clinic population. This was achieved by experienced psychiatrists interviewing the child using the Goldberg *et al* (1970) standardised interview to diagnose depression and checking the schemata against this diagnosis. Little differences in validity are found between the different instruments provided severity and duration are taken into consideration (Kolvin *et al*, 1989). We, therefore, concluded that the use of such schemata depends on the object of the research—if one is seeking a comprehensive review of affective symptoms, the Kiddie-SADS is recommended; if one is wanting a useful brief diagnostic questionnaire, the Newcastle Schema is as good as any. The attractiveness of the latter is that a mere 11 probes give rise to a low mis-classification rate (Kolvin *et al*, 1989).

# Factorial validity

## Method (a) Theoretical

*By factor and cluster analysis*: Factor analysis is designed to identify symptoms (and perhaps other features) which hang together in characteristic patterns (factor analysis); this view is consistent with the hypothesis that there is one general factor (or dimension) underlying all the symptoms, as well as additional differentiating or bipolar factors. The purpose of cluster analysis is to identify those sub-sets of features or individuals which cluster together, in the sense of having much in common within each cluster but little in common between the clusters. These methods not only summarise relationships between features, but may also highlight a new set of harmonies or structures (Cattell, 1965; Garside & Roth, 1978).

However, these multivariate techniques are not a classification panacea. The results of factor analysis may be considerably influenced by changes either in the size or composition of the subject sample or in the range of measures employed (Kendell, 1975). Another well-known limitation to the use of factor analysis for classification purposes is that in practice, only a minority of cases may be accommodated by the classification (Hewitt & Jenkins, 1946). There is also the question of whether it is legitimate to include variables which are binary in nature (Garside & Roth, 1978). These qualifications do not apply in the case of principal component analysis, which therefore appears to be a more robust technique for analysing clinical data.

On the other hand, while cluster analysis theoretically appears to be the most useful way of identifying relatively homogenous sub-sets of individuals, the validity and number of clusters identified are still open to debate. For instance, questions remain about how to establish the validity of the clusters generated; not only may differences emerge using different programmes of cluster analysis on the same population of patients, but different results are often obtained from a study of different samples of patients with the same diagnosis.

Despite such limitations, and provided that the pitfalls are constantly borne in mind, these techniques usefully complement the traditional clinical methods of identifying syndromes. In summary, multivariate techniques can either provide powerful statistical evidence in support of an already conceptualised classification or suggest new ways of categorising behaviour or classifying cases.

## Method (b) In practice

*Cluster analysis*: Clusters were identified using the "Clustan" package: the coefficients are of the dissimilarity type; there is iterative relocation with hierarchic fusion. Ward's method was employed which is designed to optimise (the minimum) variance within clusters (Ward, 1963) and tends to find clusters of relatively equal sizes and shapes.

The number of clusters is determined by examining the values of the fusion coefficients to discover sharp changes in their value (Aldenderfer & Blashfield, 1984). The number of clusters prior to these sharp changes was accepted as the most probable solution.

Clusters found by Ward's method can be ordered in terms of their overall organisation, that is, the elevation of their profile. In other words the solutions are much influenced by profile elevation. In our graphs we have presented the standard scores for the variables for each of the clusters derived from Ward's clustering technique.

## Findings

An important question is whether the concept of depression has factorial validity. This was explored by subjecting some of the data from the Goldberg *et al* (1970) standardised interview to Principal Component Analysis and to Cluster Analysis. For these purposes we included 12 items from the schema described in Fig. 1 and added one highly relevant variable, namely, school attendance over the previous month.

In a previous paper we studied the distinction between school phobia and depression when the cohort consisted of school phobic children (Kolvin *et al*, 1984). On this occasion the cohort consisted of 95 clinical cases who constituted a stratified sample of one in four of low scorers and one in two of the high scorers on the CDI. These were interviewed blind using the Goldberg standardised interview (1970); on this interview schedule the data are coded on 5 point ordinal scales. Principal component analysis was undertaken and only two factors were extracted which had an Eigen value greater than one: Varimax rotation of these factors was then undertaken. The first factor accounted for 41.6% of the variance and was a general factor of depression. The second factor accounted for 11.3% of the variance and on this the highest loadings were on days off school,

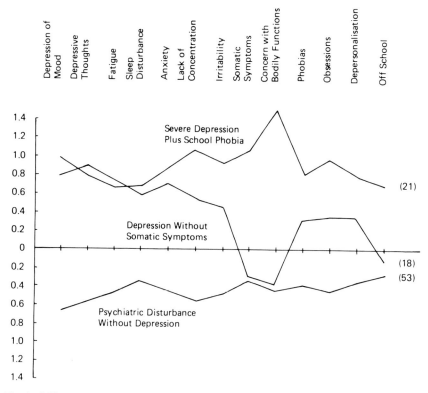

*Fig. 1. Goldberg standard interview*

somatic complaints, bodily function problems, phobias and anxiety and was labelled ''school phobia''. In addition, the data were subjected to cluster analysis and again a similar picture emerged. However, we prefer to present the findings in cluster analysis form because it locates individuals in categories, whereas Principal Component Analysis gives factors and loadings for each individual, but is not intended for categorisation.

Cluster analysis figures gave rise to three clusters (see Fig. 1)—a large group (*n* = 53) with a low profile on each of the variables included which was labelled general maladjustment—it is likely to represent an amalgam of neurotic, antisocial and attention-deficit disorders; a cluster of 18 individuals with a moderately high profile on most features representative of major depression with the exception of somatic symptoms. Finally, a cluster of 21 individuals with a high profile on somatic symptoms, affective symptoms, symptoms of phobic anxiety and also school attendance problems. The patterning of these clusters appears to confirm our original conception of a major syndrome of depression combined with school phobia (Kolvin *et al*, 1984); further, the analysis supports the notion of the 'masquerade syndrome': that is, school refusal may masquerade as an illness or complicate a genuine illness (Waller & Eisenberg, 1980).

On the basis of the above we draw two conclusions—that the clusters are distinguishable by severity of somatic and phobic symptoms. Thus there are likely to be two syndromes of depression in childhood, the first with severe and widespread anxiety and phobic symptoms and the second with equally severe depressive symptoms but with a de-emphasis of anxiety and phobic symptoms. The analysis thus allowed a distinction to emerge in behavioural terms but not in biological characteristics.

## Summary

A review is provided of some of the contributions of the Newcastle School of Child Psychiatry to the validation of childhood depression self-rating questionnaires and also of the United Kingdom and United States of America diagnostic schemata. It is concluded that the diagnostic schemata are equally valid provided duration and severity is taken into consideration.

Roth and colleagues (Kiloh & Garside, 1963; Carney *et al*, 1965) on the basis of multivariate analyses, asserted that two separate syndromes of depression can be distinguished—neurotic and psychotic but Kendell (1968) did not replicate these findings. In contrast our childhood data suggest clustering on the basis of behavioural severity especially of somatic and phobic symptoms. Perhaps the severe cluster can be perceived as resembling the major depression category of the DSM–III and the less severe remaining in that category rather than in the category of other specific affective disorders, simply because it is unlikely to have been present for the mandatory two years. In addition, it probably would fit better with the neurotic depression category of the ICD-9.

This paper describes how the use of multivariate analysis of symptoms occurring in childhood depression demonstrates the existence of different types of depression which are not readily recognisable by clinical means. Although the clinical value of this classification needs to be established in a larger sample, the contribution of such statistical techniques in enabling alternative categorical schemes for the classification of illness to be developed is evident.

## References

ALDENDERFER, M. S. & BLASHFIELD, R. K. (1984) *Cluster Analysis*. London: Sage Publications.

BIRLESON, P. (1981) The validity of depressive disorder in childhood and the development of a self-rating scale; a research report. *Journal of Child Psychology and Psychiatry*, **22**, 73–88.

CARNEY, M. W. P., ROTH, M. & GARSIDE, R. F. (1965) The diagnosis of depressive syndromes and the prediction of ECT response. *British Journal of Psychiatry*, **111**, 659–674.

CATTELL, R. B. (1965) The role of factor analysis in research. *Biometrics*, **21**, 405–435.

CHAMBERS, W. J., PUIG-ANTICH, J., HIRSCH, M., PAEZ, P., AMBROSINI, P., TABRIZI, M. & DAVIES, M. (1985) The assessment of affective disorders in children and adolescents by semistructured interview; test-retest reliablity of the K-SADS. *Archives of General Psychiatry*, **42**, 696–702.

FEIGHNER, J. F., ROBINS, E., GUZE, S. B., WOODRUFF, R. A. & WINOKUR, G. (1972) Diagnostic criteria for use in psychiatric research. *Archives of General Psychiatry*, **26**, 57–63.

FUNDUDIS, T., BERNEY, T. P., KOLVIN, I., FAMUYIWA, O. O., BARRETT, M. L., BHATE, S. R. & TYRER, S. (1989) *Childhood Depression: Reliability, Validity and Efficacy of Two Self Rating Measures on a Clinical Sample*. Awaiting publication.

GARSIDE, R. F. & ROTH, M. (1978) Multivariate statistical methods and problems of classification in psychiatry. *British Journal of Psychiatry*, **133**, 53–67.

GOLDBERG, D. P., COOPER, B., EASTWOOD, M. R., KEDWARD, H. B. & SHEPHERD, M. (1970) A standardized psychiatric interview suitable for use in community surveys, *British Journal and Preventive and Social Medicine*, **24**, 18–23.

HEWITT, L. E. & JENKINS, R. L. (1946) *Fundamental Patterns of Maladjustment, Dynamics of their Origin*. Springfield, Ill: Charles C. Thomas.

KENDELL, R. E. (1975) *The Role of Diagnosis in Psychiatry*. Oxford: Blackwell.
—— (1968) *The Classification of Depressive Illnesses*. London: Oxford University Press.
KILOH, L. G. & GARSIDE, R. F. (1963) The independence of neurotic depression and endogenous depression. *British Journal of Psychiatry*, **109**, 451–463.
KOLVIN, I., BERNEY, T. P. & BHATE, S. R. (1984) Classification and diagnosis of depression in school phobia. *British Journal of Psychiatry*, **145**, 347–357.
——, BARRETT, M. L., BHATE, S. R., BERNEY, T. P., FAMUYIWA, O. O., FUNDUDIS, T. & TYRER, S. *Major Depression in Childhood: Validation of Diagnostic Criteria* (1989). Awaiting publication.
KOVACS, M. (1978) *Children's Depression Inventory (CDI)*. University of Pittsburgh. Unpublished manuscript.
ORVASCHEL, H., PUIG-ANTICH, J., CHAMBERS, W. J., TABRIZI, M. A. & JOHNSON, R. (1982) Retrospective assessment of child psychopathology with the K-SADS-E. *Journal of the American Academy of Child Psychiatry*, **21**, 392–397.
PUIG-ANTICH, J. (1980) Affective disorders in childhood; A review and perspective. *Psychiatric Clinics of North America*, **3**, No. 3: 403–424.
SPITZER, R. L. & ENDICOTT, J. (1978) *The Schedule for Affective Disorders and Schizophrenia*. New York State Psychiatric Institute.
WALLER, D. & EISENBERG, L. (1980) School refusal in childhood: a psychiatric-paediatric perspective. In *Out of School: Modern Perspectives in School Refusal and Truancy* (eds L. Hersov & I. Berg). Chichester: Wiley.
WARD, J. H. (1963) Hierarchical grouping to optimize an objective function. *Journal of the American Statistical Association*, **58**, 236–244.
WEINBERG, W. A., RUTMAN, J., SULLIVAN, L., PENCIK, E. C. & DIETZ, S. G. (1973) Depression in children referred to an educational diagnostic center: diagnosis and treatment. *Journal of Paediatrics*, **83**, 1065–1072.

# 18 The classification of neurotic, anxiety and related disorders in light of ICD-10

## JUAN JOSÉ LÓPEZ-IBOR, JR.

The 10th version of the *International Classification of Diseases* of the World Health Organization is a new classification system which will be ready for use in 1992. Chapter F deals with mental and behavioural disorders and incorporates many of the advances of DSM–III and DSM–III-R, but it also takes into consideration perspectives from many different schools of thought throughout the world. Up to now a great number of experts, advisers, and consultants have worked intensively under the direction of the Mental Health Division of WHO in Geneva. In my opinion it is astonishing, in spite of such a diversity, how homogeneous, comprehensive and logical Chapter F is—something which has to do both with the efforts of the WHO Mental Health Division and the experts gathered, as well as with the scientific status of psychiatry itself.

ICD-10 will be used in many very different settings, including Third World countries and community medicine, where the opportunity for a well-trained staff and good working conditions are not always present. In order to achieve this goal Chapter F of ICD-10 will consist of four different classifications:

(a) one, called Definitions and Diagnostic Guidelines, for general clinical use
(b) another one which will include Research Diagnostic Criteria, which are stricter than the Diagnostic Guidelines in order to avoid possible false positive cases, which can severely contaminate the results of an investigation
(c) a multi-aspect system for the description of patients and their disorders
(d) a simpler classification with definitions appropriate for primary care use.

In the following I shall refer only to the Definitions and Diagnostic Guidelines, a draft of which is available and which has been subjected to extensive field trials in many countries. In comparison to DSM–III and DSM–III-R three general main differences are to be stressed (I shall focus later on a few more specific ones):

(a) The section to be considered in this paper is titled 'Neurotic, Stress-related and Somatoform Disorders' (Table I). Thus the term neurosis is still allowed, which is understandable because the psychoanalytical semantic loading that forced it to be withdrawn from DSM–III is weaker outside the USA, and, of course, almost absent in many Third World countries. Another reason to keep the name is that no other sound alternative is available. 'Emotional disorders' could be one, but if a section on affective disorders is also contained in Chapter F, who would be able to differentiate emotion from affect? (This question was raised by Strömgren at one of the WHO Geneva ICD-10 meetings).

TABLE I
*Neurotic and related disorders in ICD–10 Chapter F draft*

| F4 neurotic, stress-related and somatoform disorders |
|---|
| Phobic disorder |
| Other anxiety disorders |
| Obsessive-compulsive disorder |
| Reactions to severe stress and adjustment disorders |
| Dissociative disorder |
| Somatoform disorder |
|    Other |
|     Unidentified |

(b) The Section comprises the different neurotic disorders, together with those related to severe stress and those adopting somatic symptomatology. This approach is most welcome because of the strong relationships among them.

(c) The Definitions and Diagnostic Guidelines are less influenced by research criteria, and therefore in everyday use the number of diagnoses falling into residual categories might be much less significant.

## Historical backgrounds of classifications

A classification system is an instrument to describe reality to facilitate a specific goal (scientific exchange, basis for clinical decisions, data for epidemiological studies, and so on), be it only the one of order.

William Cullen in 1777 coined the term "neuroses" in his *First Lines of the Practice of Physic*, which he defined in the British tradition of nervous disorders as follows:

"almost all of the diseases of the human body might be called Nervous but there would be no use for such a general appellation; and on the other hand, it seems improper to limit the term, in the loose inaccurate manner in which it has hitherto applied to hysteria and hypochondriacal disorders, which are themselves hardly to be defined with sufficient precision. In this place I will propose to comprehend, under the title of Neuroses, all those preternatural affections of sense or motion, which are without pyrexia as a part of the primary disease; and all those which do not depend upon a topical affection of the organs, but upon a more general affection of the nervous system. . . ."

Preternatural means here "exceeding in degree or intensity what is natural or regular in nature" (*Webster's Dictionary*, 3rd edition), and therefore Cullen's concepts are extremely close to K. Schneider's (1967) concept of neuroses as "Abnorme Erlebniss Reaktionen" (Abnormal experiential reactions). Of course, some of Cullen's neuroses ended up in time in other categories once a "topical affection" of the brain was discovered (i.e., Parkinson's disease) or the disorder itself became better known. Anyhow, if we recognise that the brain is the functional support for emotions, memory, the ability to communicate with each other and the world and the whole realm of psychological life, Cullen's concepts can still be considered today as very modern.

Pichot (1983) has described the four main approaches to the classification of psychiatric disorders, which I am going to review briefly in their application to neurotic and anxiety disorders.

The first is *symptomatic* and was introduced by Pinel and his disciple Esquirol (DSM–III is less Kraepelinian than Pinelian, contrary to what is claimed by its authors). This kind of classification has many advantages: it is close to clinical reality and less prone to improper hypothesis, having a 'cleansing' or 'cathartic' effect leading to a return to the sources of the description of the disorders. Symptomatic classifications also pave the way for other approaches which usually follow, and so Esquirol himself in his lifetime developed a more psychopathological point of view of nosology. On the other hand, the greatest disadvantage of this approach is the dispersion of disorders that may be related or even unique. This method requires a hierarchical structure (as in DSM–III) unless one is willing to live with multiple diagnoses (as in DSM–III-R), which are useful for the retrieving of information and for future research, but pose the problem of co-morbidity. Therefore, I am inclined to see this approach as both transient and useful.

The second approach is *anatomic*, and was proposed for the first time by Bayle who described the "arachnitis chronique" of patients who died because of a general paresis of the insane. Of course, there is not much that can be done with this approach in the field of neurotic disorders, except to exclude them from the real psychiatric diseases (i.e., for K. Schneider, 1967, they belong to the abnormal modes of being).

A third approach is *syndromatic*, and was also initiated by Bayle because he not only described the movement and psychological symptoms of GPI, but also three stages in its evolution("délire monomaniaque", "délire maniaque", "démence"). The same method was applied by Kahlbaum and paved the way for Kraepelin's nosology. This approach is totally opposed to the symptomatic. It has the advantage of being fair to the natural history of the disorders, including several syndromes under the same diagnosis (i.e., manic-depressive disorders) but the knowledge of the natural history of most of the psychiatric disorders is still incomplete and many doubts can be raised in most of them. A good example is the Wolfman (Gardiner, 1971), the famous patient of Freud's, because we have the data from his treatments with Freud, with Muriel Gardiner and other psychoanalysts and also his own autobiography referring to his psychoanalytical experiences. In Table II we can see the diagnoses that could be given to the symptoms he suffered during the different episodes of his illness. Shall we

TABLE II
*The Wolfman's disorder(s)*

| Age | Symptoms/actual diagnosis | DSM–III |
|---|---|---|
| 3–6 | Temper tantrums<br>Phobias (wolves, . . .)<br>Obsessions (religious, . . .)<br>Infantile neurosis | Overanxious disorder |
| 10–17 | 'Periodic depressions almost every day' | ? |
| 19–23 | Obsessions, recurrent depressions, mild hypomanic state, neurasthenia | Atypical depression (bipolar II) |
| 36–39 | Depressions, asthenia, hypochondriasis, dysmorphophobic delusion, delusions | Atypical somatoform disorder (Dysmorphophobia) |
| 51–53 | Depression | Depressive episode (major?) |
| 60– | Mild depressive symptoms | Dysthymic disorder |
| Axis 3: | Compulsive personality | |

consider that Sergei P. (his real name) suffered one or several diseases during his lifetime?

The limits of our knowledge are the main limits to this approach, something which leads to the need to accept "formes frustres" (which became so important in Charcot's work) and of mixed atypical or "in-between" disorders so well described, for instance, by Scandinavian psychiatry.

The fourth model is *pathogenic*. A single cause explains the whole realm of nosology according to the degree of intensity of its presence. Morel was the first to propose it with his notion of "dégenerescence" which paved the way for the notion of endogenous disorders, and psychoanalysis is a good example of this kind of thought. Its advantages are that such a nosology is a good basis for the research of the pathogenic, psychopathological or somatic features of the disorder. But the disadvantages are great because of their trend towards non-specificity in nosology leading to the notions of "single psychosis" ["Einheitspsychose" as in Griesinger, in Janzarik (1959) or in Llopis (1954)] which, if sufficient scientific background is lacking, can lead to a negative attitude towards diagnosis [this approach was formulated in the USA by K. Menninger (1959) as: "No diagnosis at all"].

A fifth approach can be added to the four already described, which is *therapeutic*. Esquirol (1977) himself was influenced by it (he preferred the term mania to alienation because it was more medical, and therefore more able to be controlled by treatment). The concept of melancholia in DSM–III is a good example, and there is no need to expand on the comments of how much lithium has influenced the boundaries of bipolar disorders, the MAOI inhibitors the notion of atypical depressions, the neuroleptics the differentiation of positive and negative symptoms of schizophrenia, or the tricyclic antidepressants, the MAOI and the triazolobenzo-diazepines the isolation of panic disorders.

No diagnostic system is pure, and several of these approaches coincide in various of them according, not only to their general philosophy, but more importantly, to the specific kind of disorder being considered (the needs and the possibilities of classification are different for the organic mental disorders than for the personality disorders, for instance).

## Nosologic unspecificity of anxiety and depression

The words anxiety and depression refer to a disorder (sometimes a syndrome and sometimes a disease), to a symptom and to everyday feelings. A failure to make the distinction between these three meanings leads to nosological confusion. Response to treatment has a limited value in this area, probably because the physiological bases for these feelings have a lot in common; therefore, other external criteria for classification (clinical data including family history and so on), are needed. The struggle between the 'unitarists' and the 'dualists' is not over. The first place emphasis on the common features of affective and neurotic (emotional) disorders and the spectrum embracing one and the other. From the psychopathological point of view these concepts are adequate, and have led to, for instance, the research on the mechanism of action of psychotropic drugs in disorders which were previously considered as purely psychogenic. Also, the transition in the same patient from one end of the spectrum to the other has been described [i.e., "vitalisation", Weitbrecht (1968) "crystallisation", López Ibor Sr (1950, 1966)] or the opposite in the cases when a depressive disorder becomes chronic with residual symptoms that are of a neurotic nature, López-Ibor, Jr, 1982).

From the nosological point of view, it's another story. Sir Martin Roth (1982) and his co-workers and disciples have published a huge amount of evidence in favour of the nosological independence of anxiety disorders. Even during periods when new concepts, like atypical depression, emerged and when clinical experience showed how antidepressants, especially MAOI, were useful to treat "neurotic" disorders, these and other facts seem to tip the balance in favour of the "unitarists". It is interesting to mention that López-Ibor Sr (1950) developed the notion of an endogenous anxiety ("vital anxiety") which was as characteristic of neurotic disorders as vital sadness was of depression in K. Schneider's (1967) conception. Nevertheless, vital anxiety was different from vital sadness, therefore neurotic disorders were different from depressive disorders even though sometimes the same treatment could be applied to both; also in-between cases of difficult (or mixed) diagnosis cases could be found or evolution from one to the other could be present as previously mentioned.

The identification of a panic disorder as a different condition from other anxiety disorders has been the major advance in this field in the last years. Sir Martin Roth (personal communication) has criticised the approach of converting a symptom (panic attack) into a disorder but the trend from DSM–III to DSM–III-R paves the way for the notion of a "panic attack-anticipatory anxiety-agoraphobia complex". In DSM–III-R a single panic attack followed by significant anticipatory anxiety of one month's duration allows for the diagnosis. The main question in this field nowadays is if agoraphobia can present itself without previous panic attacks. In my opinion this is an artificial problem which has to do with the cutting point for the diagnostic criteria for panic attacks and the existence of 'sub-clinical', that is to say, 'sub-diagnostic' panic attacks.

This last problem leads to the question of normal v. morbid anxiety. Freud adopted Hecker's notion of neuroses as anxiety equivalents and raised the question of the why of their many forms (see Nunberg & Federn, 1962). In the early 1920s Freud reached the conclusion that anxiety was the primary phenomenon (not secondary to repression as described earlier) and neurotic symptoms became defence mechanisms or, better phrased, coping mechanisms of anxiety.

Bakan (1968) has stressed the strong parallelism between Freud's ideas and the concept of stress reaction as described by Selye. Briefly explained, living organisms are in equilibrium with their environment and possess mechanisms to maintain their homeostasis when external aggressions alter it or threaten to do so. The neurohumoral reactions induced by external aggression manifest themselves in Selye's (1956) General Adaptation Syndrome, which is the set of unspecific neurohumoral reactions to stress. The psychological response of individual human beings to external aggressions or threats (real or supposed) is anxiety—von Baeyer (1984) has defined anxiety as the experience of being threatened—which unchains several defence or coping mechanisms. Bakan (1968) has also called attention to the fact that in some circumstances the defence mechanisms put forward to face yet unidentified threats can become harmful to the individual organisms, and, in the end, can even become a risk to survival.

The notion of self-destructive mechanisms in individuals was recognised by Freud in the description of the death instinct or Thanatos and it is present in the concept of adaptation diseases. In my opinion, this bio-psychological model has to be expanded to become bio-psycho-social (López-Ibor, Jr, 1985, 1987) (Table III), including reactions to collective stresses as in disasters. Glass (1959) has described a series of phases in disasters and the psychological mechanisms involved in them (Table IV) which correspond very well with what happens at the biological and psychological levels of this model. Here, the external threat is overwhelming, and an individual vulnerability plays a much more minor role than it plays in the neurotic disorder.

This model takes into consideration the important fact that what takes place in the early phases has consequences for the advanced ones. The impact of an event for which an individual or the group is not prepared (he has not the protection of immunity, or denial has prevented the preparation of the individual or the group for action) unchains an exaggerated response that paves the way for the succeeding ones: exhaustion and the chronic stages. Defence mechanisms are coping mechanisms and every individual or social group is endowed with, or has been able to develop, particular coping styles. As Vaillant (1977) points out, some are healthy, such as anticipation, sublimation, humour and so on, while others are neurotic, immature or narcissistic. I believe that such mechanisms belong not only to the psychology of the individual but also to social psychology.

A disaster, due or not to natural causes, is an event that is not foreseen. At least, after it occurs reflections arise as to how it, or its consequences, could

TABLE III

*Phases of disasters and psychological reactions attached to them (Glass, 1959)*

| Period | Psychological reaction |
| --- | --- |
| Pre-impact | Denial, negation |
| Warning | Inefficient overactivity |
| Impact | None (too short duration) |
| Recoil | Underactivity, apathy |
| Post-impact | Hostility, anger, resentment |

TABLE IV

*Integrative model of stress; anxiety and (collective) panics*

| | Level | | |
| --- | --- | --- | --- |
| | Biological<br>General adaptation syndrome<br>(Selye) | Psychological<br>Post-traumatic stress disorders | Social<br>Disasters, catastrophes |
| 1 Pre-trauma: | | | |
| (a) positive defences | Immunology (congenital, acquired) | Anticipation, ability for sublimation . . . | Plans for emergencies |
| (b) negative or insufficient defenses | Lack of immunological barriers | Negation, lack of social lifestyles, lack of identity | Negation, lack of social identity and stability |
| 2 Acute response | (a) Ergotrophic (i.e. allergic diseases) | Warning period (overactivity) | Emergency measures (overreaction) |
| | (b) Trophotrophic | Recoil period (apathy . . .) | Underreactivity |
| 3 Chronic (mal)adaptation | Adaptation diseases (immunological) disease . . . | Post-impact period (anger, resentment) sickness . . . | Institutionalisation Illness |
| | as form and way of survival | | |

have been avoided or lessened. The word catastrophe bears an important nuance: in ancient Greece it meant the end of a tragedy, the unravelling of the plot. Very often the tragic climax is foreseen by the spectators, by the choir and a number of characters; but not by the hero, who arrogantly denies what is becoming evident for everybody else. The arrogant negation of the evidence in Oedipus is the expression of his madness and when, at the end of the play, he is forced to recognise his own origin, his reaction is extreme and severe. In every catastrophe, natural or man-made, the reactions that arise are directed at both the disaster itself or what made it or its consequences possible, and which was previously denied. Disasters or catastrophes bear a social dimension because the threat is overwhelming for the individual, and most of those affected will suffer from some consequences (individual vulnerability plays a secondary role here). In due time a minority group psychology develops in the survivors of a disaster (López-Ibor, Jr, 1987) even when single individuals are affected, as in rape or kidnapping, for instance.

The same concepts can be applied to depression. The question of 'normal v. morbid depression' is usually solved with some temporal criteria: grief due to loss becomes pathological grief or depression if it lasts too long. How long depends on the culture or the nosological system used, but this temporal criterion is not enough. Klerman (1983) has extensively described and revised the many aspects of this question.

In this context it is important to stress that feelings, emotions and affects are important for the survival of the individual. Sartre (1939) put forward the theory of emotions according to which they substitute (in the sense of the "Ersatzpsychologie") rationality when this is not possible any more, paving the way for a different world, magical and symbolic, where the individual finds new meanings. Bereavement is a way to survive a loss, withdrawn from a world where everyday life without the lost person is impossible. Isolation and retardation are the expression of withdrawal from the world of common reality where action and rationality are the norm. In the same way, the experience of an unidentified threat throws the anxious person into a world which is not safe any more and puts him in the situation of facing possible dangers.

Goldberg (1987) has recently put forward interesting evidence showing that, when facing stress, some individuals demonstrate psychological symptoms and some somatic ones. The somatisers have some initial advantages because their symptoms bear less stigma and they receive more attention from the health care system but, in the long run, these advantages become disadvantages because somatisers are more prone to becoming chronic patients than 'psychologisers'. These common links between the biological, psychological and social reactions to threats and the fact that some individuals tend more to 'psychologise' and others to 'somatise', justify the ICD–10 approach to have in the same section the neurotic disorders, those related to stress and the somatoform ones.

## Follow-up studies

As I mentioned above, López-Ibor Sr (1950) described vital anxiety. Initially he thought that the patients showing this feature were not really neurotic patients but a sub-category which he called "anxious thymopathy' (timopatía ansiosa).

As those patients were treated mainly with biological methods, what is described often as masking of symptoms in psychotherapy (see Alexander, French & Pollock, 1968) is absent from these patients, therefore allowing for follow-up studies. We are at present carrying out one in which we have included all the patients with the diagnoses of "timopatía ansiosa" having had the first visit to our clinic in the period from 1953 to 1963, and living in the Madrid area during the index episode. We have gathered data from the clinical records plus mail and telephone contacts, a visit to the clinic, psychological testing and visits to the first-degree relatives. With these data we have made retrospective DSM–III diagnoses and we have investigated how the different diagnoses are grouped among themselves in patients and the trends of changing diagnoses over the years. Table V shows the characteristics of the sample and Table VI the diagnoses at the index episode. The mean age of the index episode was 23.3 years for panic attacks and the mean follow-up was 35.9 years. Figure 1 shows the trends of evolution from which it is clear how one in two patients with

TABLE V
*Characteristics of the sample*

| | | |
|---|---|---|
| Diagnosis not confirmed | | 10 |
| Unable to be interviewed | | 161 |
| Cognitive impairment | 35 | |
| Physical disease | 7 | |
| Moved away | 119 | |
| Unwilling to be interviewed | | 107 |
| STUDY SAMPLE | | 102    (27%) |

TABLE VI
*Index episode diagnosis*

| | | |
|---|---|---|
| Panic attacks | | 72 |
| Uncomplicated anxiety disorder | 63 | |
| Anxiety disorder with limited phobic avoidance | 5 | |
| Anxiety disorder with extensive phobic avoidance | 4 | |
| Generalised anxiety disorders | | 30 |

TABLE VII
*The natural history of panic attacks versus generalised anxiety disorders*

| | Panic attacks (%) | Generalised anxiety (%) |
|---|---|---|
| Separation anxiety | 54 | 20 |
| Social phobia | 12.5 | 10 |
| Panic attacks | | |
| uncomplicated | 90.3 | — |
| with limited panic attacks | 40.3 | — |
| Generalised anxiety disorder | 40.3[a] | 100 |
| Somatoform disorder | 60 | 67 |
| Hypochondriasis | 45.8 | 25 |
| Major depression | 72 | 27 |
| with melancholia | 32 | — |
| Dysthymic disorder | 7 | — |
| Alcohol abuse | 8 | — |
| 'Chronic somatic complainers' | 48.6 | 50 |

[a]Patients with anticipatory anxiety might be included here

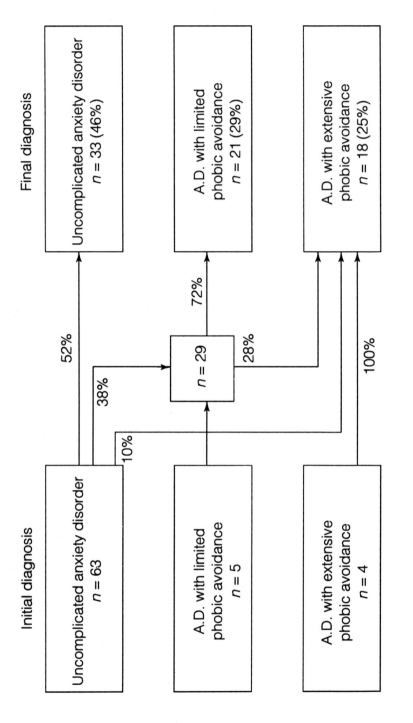

*Fig. 1.*

uncomplicated panic attacks developed some kind of phobic avoidance in the future and how limited phobic avoidance evolves in one out of four patients into extensive phobic avoidance.

The comparison of the natural history of the disorder of panic attacks with the generalised anxiety shows some interesting differences (Table VII). In both, separation anxiety during childhood is present, although much more evident in panic attacks. These data coincide with several others, something which leads to include separation anxiety with the "panic attack-anticipatory anxiety-agoraphobia complex". The patients with uncomplicated panic attacks frequently showed symptoms of generalised anxiety, although we are not able to differentiate this from separation anxiety. Patients with panic attacks also have more of a history of depressive disorders, both major and dysthymic disorder, and of alcoholism. Furthermore, both groups of patients show a high incidence of somatisation disorders, of hypochondriasis and of what we have called "chronic somatic complaints". Among these we include patients with symptoms not clearly identified as due to a somatic cause, but do not allow, because of insufficient data, a psychiatric diagnosis but lead to frequent visits to general practitioners or other physicians.

## *The ICD-10 approach on phobic and anxiety disorders*

The draft of ICD-10 used for field trials, which might still be changed slightly before its final version is approved, appears in Table VII. There, panic disorder is not only accepted as an independent disorder from generalised anxiety, but also from phobic disorders. After the field trials, two main modifications have been accepted: one is the sub-division of agoraphobia according to the presence or absence of panic attacks and the second is a clear acceptance of anticipatory anxiety in the description of panic attacks. In this last sense, ICD-10 is near to DSM-III-R and in the previous one (separation of panic disorders from agoraphobia) is nearer to DSM-III.

One of the most revolutionary categories of this section is the one called "Mixed anxiety and depressive disorder". In the definition, ICD-10 mentions that the patients included in this category demonstrate a mixture of mild to moderate degree of anxiety and depressive symptoms (the latter not fulfilling guidelines for mild depressive disorder or recurrent mild depressive disorder). It also mentions that these patients are very often seen in primary care and that many more exist in the population at large and never come to medical or psychiatric attention. This category will allow research into a very important and confused area where cultural aspects are important and where the distinction of the feeling of anxiety from the one of depression is not always possible.

In conclusion, over two centuries have elapsed since Cullen introduced the concept of neurosis. Most of his ideas are still valid today as the framework for the ICD-10 chapter on Neurosis, Stress-related and Somatoform Disorder. In it, a prototype is to be seen, the agoraphobia disorder which Sir Martin Roth has done so much to describe, its natural history and nosological identity. DSM-III, DSM-III-R and some research evidence which I have mentioned seem to identify a "separation anxiety-panic attack-anticipatory anxiety-agoraphobia complex". These disorders and some of those included in the

ICD-10 section on Neurotic, Stress-related and Somatoform Disorders can be understood as abnormal (preternatural) reactions to the experience of an external threat. This section also includes the psychopathological reactions to overwhelming stresses (those affecting most of the individuals involved and having therefore a social dimension) and other disorders such as obsessive-compulsive disorders and neurasthenia which remain outside the scope of the present paper.

# References

ALEXANDER, F., FRENCH, T. N. & POLLOCK, G. H. (1968) *Psychosomatic Specificity*. Chicago, London: University of Chicago Press.

BAEYER, W. VON (1984) Angst als erlebtes Becrohtsein. *Nervenarzt*, **55**, 349–357.

BAKAN, D. (1968) *Disease, Pain and Sacrifice. Towards a Psychology of Suffering*. Chicago: University of Chicago Press.

BAYLE, A. L. J.: see Pichot.

CHARCOT, J. M.: see Pichot.

CULLEN, W.: see LEIGH, D. (1961) *The Historical Development of British Psychiatry*. vol. 5. Oxford: Pergamon.

ESQUIROL, E. (1977) *De la hypomanie ou mélancholie* (Presentation par P. Fedida et J. Postel). Privat, Paris.

ESQUIROL, J. E. D.: see Pichot.

GARDINER, M. (ed.) (1971) *The Wolfman, by the Wolfman*. New York: Basic Books.

GLASS, A. J. (1959) Psychological aspects of disasters. *Journal of the American Medical Association*, **171**, 188–191.

GOLDBERG, D. P. & BRIDGES, K. (1987) The determinants of somatization. Presentation to the 9th World Congress of ICPM, Sydney, Aug–Sept 1987.

GRIESINGER, W.: see Pichot.

JANZARIK, W. (1959) *Dynamische Grundkonstellation in endogenen Psychosen*. Berlin: Springer.

KAHLBAUM, K. L.: see Pichot.

KLERMAN, G. L. (1983) The scope of depression. In *The Origin of Depression: Current Concepts and Approaches* (ed. J. Angst) pp. 5–25. Berlin: Springer.

KRAEPELIN, E.: see Pichot.

LLOPIS, B. (1954) La psicosis única. *Archivos de Neurobiología*, **17**, 1–39.

LÓPEZ IBOR, J. J. (1950, reprinted 1969) *La Angustia Vital*. Madrid: Paz Montalvo.

—— (1966) *Las Neurosis como Enfermedades del Ánimo*. Madrid: Gredos.

LÓPEZ-IBOR JR, J. J. (1982) Las neurosis. In *Psiquiatria*, vol. 2. (eds J. J. López-Ibor Jr, C. Ruiz Ogara & D. Barcia). pp. 741–787. Barcelona: Toray.

——, SORIA, J., CAÑAS, F. & RODRIGUEZ-GAMAZO, M. (1985) Psychological aspects of the toxic oil syndrome catastrophe. *British Journal of Psychiatry*, **147**, 352–365.

—— (1982) Las psicosis y los trastornos afectivos. In *Psiquiatria*, vol. 2. (eds J. J. López-Ibor Jr, C. Ruiz Ogara & D. Barcia). pp. 910–991. Barcelona: Toray.

—— & JIMENEZ ARRIERO, M. A. (1987) Psychosocial rehabilitation in disasters: experience of the Spanish toxic oil syndrome. *International Journal of Disability Studies*, **9**, 81–83.

MENNINGER, K. (1959) Towards a unitary concept of mental illness. In *A Psychiatrist's World* (by K. Menninger), vol. 2. pp. 516–528. New York: The Viking Press.

MOREL, B. A.: see Pichot.

NUNBERG, H. & FEDERN, E. (1962) *Minutes of the Vienna Psychoanalytic Society*. vol. 1 (1906–1908). New York: International University Press.

PICHOT, P. (1983) *Un Siècle de Psychiatrie*. Paris: Roche.

PINEL, Ph.: see Pichot.

ROTH, M. & MOUNTJOY, C. Q. (1982) The distinction between anxiety states and depressive disorders. In *Handbook of Affective Disorders*. (ed. E. S. Paykel). Edinburgh: Churchill-Livingstone.

SARTRE, J. P. (1939) *Esquisse d'une Théorie des Émotions*. Paris: Hermann.

SCHNEIDER, K. (1967) *Klinische Psychopathologie*. 8th edition. Stuttgart: Thieme.

SELYE, H. (1956) *The Stress of Life*. New York: McGraw Hill.

VAILLANT, G. (1977) *Adaptation to Life*. Boston: Little, Brown & Co.

WEITBRECHT, H. J. (1968) Psicopatología comparada de los estados depresivos. *Actas Luso-Espan olas de Neurologia y Psiquiatria*, **27**, 407–419.

# 19 Anxiety: does classification help?

**SYDNEY BRANDON**

The study of anxiety disorders has a long history. The term phobia, mentioned by Celsus (AD 30), has been used by physicians from the fifth century onwards, although with varying meanings, usually referring to irrational or disproportionate fear attached to objects and situations.

According to the *Oxford Companion for Medicine*, anxiety is an unpleasant mental state of foreboding, uneasiness and apprehension approaching fear which may be accompanied by signs of sympathetic overactivity such as tremor, sweating and tachycardia. When appropriate to the circumstances, such a state may be regarded as a physiological preparation for whatever ordeal or difficult task lies ahead. When inappropriate, excessive or prolonged, it is a symptom of mental disorder. Neither fear or panic are defined.

The *Oxford English Dictionary* lists under *anxiety* various definitions including: **1** The quality or state of being anxious; solicitude, concern; **3** (Path.) A condition of agitation and depression, with a sensation of tightness and distress in the praecordial region (1661).

*Fear* merits much longer entry including: **OE 2** The emotion of pain or uneasiness caused by the sense of impending danger, or by the apprehension of evil. In early use applied to the more violent extremes of emotion; **ME 3** A state of alarm or dread.

*Panic* also has an extensive entry which includes fear, terror etc: a contagious emotion such as was attributed to the action of the god Pan. A sudden excessive feeling of alarm or fear, usually affecting a body of persons, and leading to extravagant or injudicious efforts to secure safety. *Terror* is defined as ''The state of being terrified or greatly frightened; intense fear, fright or dread''.

Pinel (1801) described a number of syndromes of bodily complaints accompanied by 'une certaine anxieté'. In 1734 George Cheyne published *The English Malady or A Treatise on Nervous Diseases of All Kinds, as Spleen, Vapours, Lowness of Spirits, Hypochondriacal and Hysterical Distempers*. He claimed that neurotic behaviours were very common among the English and nothing to be ashamed of.

Robert Whytt (1714–1766) divided emotional disorders into hysteria, hypochondriasis and nervous exhaustion. The latter condition was called neurasthenia by George Beard (1839–1883) but it was William Cullen (1712–1790) who coined the term neurosis and also described in great detail the physical concomitants of what would now be described as an anxiety attack.

References to morbid anxiety or phobias in currently understandable terms came in the second half of the 19th century. Morel (1809–1873) identified phobia and other neuroses under the heading *délire emotif* thus introducing neuroses as a major component of a classification system. Theology and philosophy in the 19th century were concerned not only with guilt but with dread and Soren Kierkegaard (1813–1855), the Danish philosopher-theologian, described the pervasive psychological experience of anxiety, ascribing to it an exclusive ontological status in the sense of its being one of the basic attributes of man and a philosophical category necessary for the interpretation of human existence. Kierkegaard maintained that anxiety is the unavoidable companion of reflective consciousness in man arising from the recognition that a negation of being or a state of nothingness is both thinkable and possible. "The more conscious, the more intense the despair."

For Martin Heidegger, the state of being in the world "is in anxiety" and that is intrinsically linked to human freedom because only the acceptance of the terminality of existence and the experience of *Angst* (fear, anxiety or dread) makes that freedom possible. Under Jaspers and others, the study of anxiety came to occupy a central place in existentialist psychiatry and psychotherapy (Daseinsanalyse). There was emphasis upon the role of anxiety in enhancing the sense of being. Morbid anxiety was thought by May to be "cued off by a threat to some value the individual holds essential to his existence as a personality".

Thus, although anxiety is often differentiated from fear, and normal from morbid anxiety, both have elements of dread, some relationship to loss and there is no clear demarcation. Panic, apart from its use in describing a group phenomenon, appears to have been used largely as an indication of degree or severity of anxiety.

In 1870 Benedikt described dizziness occurring in open spaces and in 1871 Westphal published his classic monograph *Agoraphobie* in which he described three men unable to walk the streets without fear (or dreading that they would experience fear). One feared that he was going mad but all could venture out when supported by a companion or even a walking stick. The 'syndrome' and terminology were accepted from this date.

A 'syndrome' dominated by cardiac and respiratory symptoms was described among American Civil War soldiers by Da Costa in 1871. Although he adduced evidence that this condition had been recognised by military surgeons in conflicts during the preceeding 200 years, he regarded it as a functional disease of the heart exposed by military service rather than attributable to battle stress. In various forms it has been described in every campaign since, with 60 000 cases of "disordered action of the heart" during world war I in addition to many thousands of cases of "effort syndrome" (T. Lewis, 1919) and neurocirculatory asthenia (Oppenheimer & Rothschild, 1918). In the second world war, "effort phobia", "effort syndrome" and anxiety state were recognised as having a common core. It is noteworthy that many of those affected were not actually involved in combat.

Oppenheimer described "traumatic neurosis" in which anxiety was a morbid response to severe stress and this concept was adopted by Kraepelin as Schreckneurose (fright neurosis) in the 1896 edition of his textbook. Meanwhile Wernicke described a fear psychosis (Angst-psychose) which probably served as the prototype for the ''fear-happiness-psychosis'' (Angst-Gluck Psychose) later classified among the cycloid psychoses of the Kleist-Leonhard group.

Cannon (1871–1945), investigating rage and fear, demonstrated that emotions may activate physiological mechanisms in the ''fight-flight'' mechanism where expression of anger as aggression or relief of fear by flight would dissipate the response.

Freud (1895) was responsible for the recognition of anxiety neurosis as a separate entity. This he regarded as an ''actual neurosis'', i.e. a more or less somatic process devoid of symbolic value but due to dammed-up sexual (libidinal) energy. This is the so-called first theory, contrasting with the later metaphysical theory (1926) when he affirmed that the ego was ''the real locus of anxiety''. Under the second theory the concept of signal anxiety as an affective signal with regard to danger coming from within was developed. Thus both normal and neurotic anxiety could occur. His phenomenological descriptions are vivid and accurate and include descriptions of anxiety attacks closely resembling current descriptions of panic.

Pavlov (1849–1936) laid the foundations of the physiology of conditioning, but the natural experiment of the disastrous floods in Leningrad in 1924 suggested a basis for new conditioning procedures which resulted in the modelling of phobia. Pavlov proposed that it was the ''weak inhibitory'' or melancholic type of higher nervous activity which predisposed to pathological anxiety but he did not regard anxiety neurosis as a separate entity. Neurasthenia, psychasthenia (obsessional neurosis) and hysteria were his three categories of neurosis and each might include anxiety and phobias.

Following the first world war, the concept of psychoneurosis became firmly established and despite considerable variations a number of sub-types could be recognised—neurasthenia, anxiety neurosis, depressive neurosis, hysteria and obsessive compulsive disorder. Within anxiety neurosis somatic or psychic predominance was recognised but phobias were variously regarded as obsessional, hysterical or anxiety-based.

In the late 1950s Martin Roth began to formulate the concept of the phobic anxiety depersonalisation state (PADS), later known as the Calamity Syndrome. The 'illness' began abruptly in the majority of cases, often following some severe stress. In a substantial proportion of cases a mild or moderate anxiety state exists before the relatively abrupt development of the PADS. The 'agoraphobia' or PADS could be regarded as a simple anxiety state on which certain other specific symptoms are superimposed, those in particular that tend in their extreme form to give rise to the housebound housewife.

Roth emphasised that traits of dependence on other individuals are conspicuous and gave the early marriage of affected females as an example of their ''transfer of dependence''. Histrionic personality traits figure permanently in most clinical descriptions of phobic disorders.

In the summary he said ''A new form of neurotic illness is described. Its most consistent features are a combination of depersonalisation and a characteristic form of phobic anxiety, but in 40% of cases there are other features reminiscent of disturbances of temporal lobe function such as *déjà vu* phenomenon, metamorphopsia and panoramic memory and, in a higher proportion, more variable obsessional, hysterical, depressive features and vasomotor disturbances. In a few cases, short-lived episodes have been observed.

In a high proportion of cases the illness follows upon a calamity or acute physical illness'' (Roth, 1959).

Later, under his direction, a Newcastle group were grappling with the separation of anxiety, neurotic depression and endogenous depression (Gurney *et al*, 1972). Lewis, in 1936, maintained the tradition of Mapother and argued that there was no clear line between anxiety and depressive disorders and moreover depressive disorders were part of a continuum. Kendell (1968) and others continued to defend the Maudsley model while Roth shifted his ground only from Newcastle to Cambridge. Anxiety, it should be noted, consistently carried the worse prognosis.

Gelder & Marks (1966) argued persuasively for a distinction between encapsulated non-disabling monosymptomatic phobias, usually commencing early in life, and the more intricate phobic anxieties. Agoraphobic states commencing fairly suddenly in adult life in the decade between 25 and 35 years were more disabling with a different natural history and different response to treatment.

Both have gone on to demonstrate the efficacy of behavioural treatments. Marks now claims that computer-based programmes or self-instructional booklets are as effective as therapist-supervised treatments. His patients are, however, unusual in the duration of their illness and their powerful motivation to treatment. Gelder has continued to develop behavioural treatments but his group are now much concerned with cognitive therapies.

Speilberger and others have devoted much attention to the separation of state and trait anxiety but this has found little application in clinical practice, for there are few prospective studies of either normal or patient populations. Eysenck's efforts were also confounded by interactions between state and trait. Hamilton did not differentiate between clinical anxiety and panic, which makes the Hamilton Anxiety Scale difficult to interpret when distinct panic attacks occur.

Kelly (1973), Sargant (1962) and others in the 1960s described a group of phobic patients of "good personality" with or without overt depression who responded to monoamine oxidase inhibitors. They labelled this group "atypical depression", and although it enjoyed a period of popularity the term is now little used.

Panic attacks are mentioned by many authors where they appear to be regarded as variations in pattern or indices of severity of the underlying anxiety. Anxiety attacks may refer to distinct episodes lasting minutes, hours, days or even weeks. In 1964 Klein suggested that panic attacks indicate a distinct form of anxiety disorder and that they respond to treatment with imipramine whereas the background generalised anxiety does not. Many of the patients described showed avoidance behaviour or agoraphobia.

Since various authors (e.g. Clarke, 1986) have shown that exposure alone can reduce the panic attacks of agoraphobic patients, it is important to demonstrate whether panic attacks associated with generalised anxiety but not agoraphobia respond to antidepressants, but this has not yet been done.

There have also been reservations regarding the existence of frequent panic attacks without avoidance behaviour. Klein's view is that avoidance behaviour is secondary to the panic attacks. Others argue that the phobias have priority and panics arise from a fear of exposure to the feared situation.

It is of interest that in 1895 Freud wrote "In the case of agoraphobia . . . we often find the recollection of an anxiety attack; and what the patient actually fears is the occurrence of such an attack under the special conditions in which he believes he cannot escape it" and in *Studies in Hysteria* he describes Katharine whom he met during a mountain walk.

> "It suddenly comes upon me. There is first a pressure on my eyes. My head becomes so heavy and it hums so that I can hardly bear it, and then my chest begins to press together so that I cannot get my breath . . . the throat becomes laced together as if I choked . . . I always feel 'Now I must die' and I am otherwise courageous, I go everywhere alone, into the cellar and down over the whole mountain but on the day I have this attack, I do not trust myself anywhere. I always believe that someone stands behind me and suddenly grabs me."

The American Psychiatric Association *Diagnostic and Statistical Manual* (Third Edition) or DSM–III has taken a new approach to the classification of anxiety disorders and, in particular, distinguishes between 'panic' and generalised disorder.

Table I shows the diagnostic categories offered by DSM–III and the modifications proposed in the provisional revised version DSM–III-R.

The clear definition of panic attacks does not circumvent the difficulties of definition of panic disorder, which requires three distinct unprovoked panic attacks within the past three weeks each with at least four of the specified symptoms. This requirement inevitably requires an arbitrary cut-off point in what may be a continuum of disorder.

The recognition of obsessive-compulsive syndromes as clearly within the anxiety disorders gives recognition to the sterility of earlier attempts to explain and treat these disorders. Anxiety management training and specific behavioural manipulation are more effective than previously employed therapeutics.

In post-traumatic disorder the clearer conceptual definitions should increase the precision with which this diagnosis is made and accords better with the lessons from disasters and military psychiatry than previous categories. It is also interesting to note the light which this disorder brings to earlier concepts of compensation neurosis. In many cases of post-traumatic syndrome there is no element of financial reward and, in those cases where this is a factor, symptoms continue independently of financial settlement.

TABLE I
*Classification of anxiety disorders*

Simple phobia
Social phobia
Agoraphobia with panic attacks
Agoraphobia without panic attacks       } DSM–III
Panic disorder
    uncomplicated
    with limited phobic avoidance       } DSM–III-R
    with extensive phobic avoidance       (provisional)
    (agoraphobia with panic disorder)
Generalised anxiety disorder
Obsessive compulsive disorder
Post traumatic stress disorder
Atypical anxiety disorder

Diagnostic categories or syndromes are useful if they can be reliably applied, clarify aetiology or inform treatment or prognosis. Before considering whether panic disorder meets these requirements let us consider the *prevalence* of anxiety disorders.

Marks & Lader found surprising agreement among a series of studies conducted in the United States, United Kingdom and Sweden with current prevalence rates of 2.0–4.7% and more common in women, especially those aged between 16 and 40 years.

Weissman, Myers & Harding (1978) reported on a community survey in New Haven: 511 individuals were examined using SADS-L (Schedule for Schizophrenia and Affective Disorders—Lifetime Version) and, using Research Diagnostic Criteria, a diagnosis was made. They found 4.3/100 with anxiety disorders made up of 0.4 panic disorder, 2.4 generalised anxiety disorder, and 1.4 phobic disorder. Only 25% had sought psychiatric help in the previous year. Uhlenhuth *et al* (1983) and his group administered a symptom check test to over 3000 subjects. This is clearly not as reliable as a diagnostic interview and relied on one year prevalence whereas the New Haven structure used current rates. They reported 1.2/100 agoraphobia with panic attacks and 2.3/100 all other phobias. In a later review Weissman (1983) confirmed that anxiety states were distributed across the social and economic groups and confirmed the excess of females.

In 1985 Angst & Dobler-Mikola reported from Zurich a study of 3902 men aged 19 years and 2391 20 year-old women. Approximately half completed the SCL 90 and a 10% sample was selected for prospective interview study on the basis of high or low scores. There were 500 completed interviews, and diagnoses were derived from the checklist and the structured interview. The one year prevalences were generalised anxiety disorder 5.2%, panic 3.1%, agoraphobia 2.3%, (1.6 agoraphobia only, 0.7 agoraphobia and panic).

The Epidemiological Catchment Area Studies in the US on five sites used DSM–III criteria. Early reports from New Haven, Baltimore and St Louis report the following 6/12 prevalence

|                      | *New Haven* | *Baltimore* | *St Louis* |
|----------------------|-------------|-------------|------------|
| Panic disorder       | 0.6         | 1.0         | 0.9        |
| Agoraphobia          | 2.8         | 5.8         | 2.7        |
| Obsessive Compulsion | 1.4         | 2.0         | 1.3        |

In addition New Haven reported agoraphobia only 2.9 and agoraphobia plus panic 0.3.

In Leicester we have undertaken a community study using a large urban general practice and have been able to use the screening instruments and diagnostic criteria for panic disorder developed for the DSM–III-R reliably and without difficulty. Our first priority was to determine whether episodes of panic could be clearly identified and whether the operational criteria for the diagnosis of panic disorder were useful if practised. We also used the Marks Fear Phobia Questionnaire and the General Health Questionnaire but did not seek to make a comprehensive psychiatric diagnosis other than panic disorder and agoraphobia.

On the basis of this study we suggest one person in 10 experiences occasional panic attacks; one person in 20 has troublesome recurrent attacks; one person in 50 achieves the diagnostic criteria for panic disorder.

As an entity, panic disorder can be identified and reliably diagnosed according to the established operational criteria. The cut-off point between panic attacks and panic disorder is, however, entirely arbitrary. Some who do not achieve the frequency of attacks required for diagnosis achieve strategies of control which may involve limited avoidance or behavioural or cognitive techniques; others have a phobophobia, a fear of fear which limits their behaviour without or with few further attacks.

Turning to a larger population, we have documented 249 cases using the SCID-UP (Structured Clinical Interview DSM KKK Upjohn Version). Some were identified through the community survey and others referred to a panic disorder clinic advertised to general practitioners. All were offered an opportunity to participate in a controlled clinical trial of drug treatment, but only 45 completed the trial.

Of the 190 cases which met the criteria for DSM–III Panic Disorder, 47 were uncomplicated by any avoidance behaviour (Table II) and 51 were truly agoraphobic with extensive phobic avoidance (Table III). If these groups are examined separately quite marked differences are apparent (Table IV). The age of first attack is considerably lower in the phobic group and their duration of illness longer. Most striking, however, is the marked difference between male : female ratios, with men almost disappearing from the phobic group.

In Table IV a comparison between women with uncomplicated panic and those with extensive avoidance shows even more clearly the earlier onset, greater delay

TABLE II
*Uncomplicated panic disorder*

|  | Total | Current panic disorder | Panic disorder remission | Secondary panic disorder |
|---|---|---|---|---|
| Male | 20 | 9 | 7 | 4 |
| Female | 27 | 10 | 12 | 5 |
| Age at first attack | 30.2 | 30.4 | 28.7 | 33.0 |
|  | (11–57) | (14–51) | (11–51) | (21–57) |
| Age at onset of | 31.9 | 32.7 | 30.5 | 33.5 |
| panic disorder | (14–57) | (15–56) | (14–51) | (22–57) |
| Length of illness | 4.6 | 4.7 | 4.0 | 5.8 |
|  | (3/52–25) | (3/52–23) | (3/52–25) | (4/12–19) |

TABLE III
*Extensive phobic avoidance*

|  | Total | Current | In remission | Secondary* |
|---|---|---|---|---|
| Male | 2 | 2 | 0 | 0 |
| Female | 49 | 35 | 8 | 6 |
| Age at first attack | 26.7 | 25.0 | 27.3 | 36.2 |
|  | ( 4–58) | (4–58) | (10–48) | (22–55) |
| Age at onset of | 28.8 | 27.5 | 28.9 | 36.5 |
| panic disorder | (7–58) | (7–58) | (10–48) | (22–55) |
| Age at onset | 31.4 | 30.2 | 33.3 | 36.3 |
| of avoidance | (12–58) | (12–58) | (16–48) | (22–55) |
| Length of illness | 11.1 | 10.9 | 15.8 | 6.0 |
| (panic disorder) | (4/12–38) | (4/12–38) | (1–22) | (4/12–21) |

* mainly to primary depression

TABLE IV
*Panic disorder uncomplicated v. extensive avoidance (excluding secondary cases)*

|  | Uncomplicated (total) | Extensive (total) | Uncomplicated (male) | Uncomplicated (female) | Extensive (female) |
|---|---|---|---|---|---|
| Total | (n = 38) | (n = 45) | (n = 16) | (n = 22) | (n = 43) |
| Age at interview | 36.0 | 39.5 | 35.6 | 36.2 | 40.0 |
| Age at first panic attack | 29.6 | 25.4 | 27.7 | 30.8 | 25.4 |
| Age at onset of panic disorder | 31.6 | 27.8 | 30.3 | 32.5 | 27.8 |
| Age onset avoidance | — | 30.8 | — | — | 31.0 |
| Duration of panic disorder | 4.4 | 11.7 | 5.3 | 3.7 | 12.2 |

to panic disorder and long duration of illness in the latter. A surprising finding is the delay of 5.6 years to onset of avoidance behaviour.

What conclusions can be drawn from these data, which are virtually cross-sectional, not longitudinal, must be tentative?

We can say that, in the community, episodes of panic are common. Troublesome recurrent panic attacks are less so and panic disorder has a frequency of about one in 50, with a similar frequency in both sexes. Reliable scales are available for documenting these occurrences.

When we turn to the 249 cases, most have identified themselves as having a problem. We could either argue that those with uncomplicated panic and those with extensive phobic avoidance are drawn from different universes or that they come from a common pool. Given the latter assumption, we can say that of men who develop panic disorder only 9% (1 in 10) develop agoraphobia whereas 64.5% of women do so. Phobic developments are thus more likely in women, are associated with earlier onset, a prolonged interval to panic disorder and 4.7 years between first panic and phobic developments.

Can we offer any explanation for this? Much seems to lie in the cognitive appraisal of the consequences of panic. Can it be that men learn to cope with the panic by a variety of strategies associated with seeking support? Walking over to workmates, tackling a job which requires intense concentration and so on, thus learning to abort attacks; perhaps even adopting the walking stick or other prop as reported by Westphal. Many find it possible to reassure themselves that the feelings will pass off, and they do. Women, on the other hand, may have less access to support, they may be alone at home or in their office or engaged in a work task from which they can achieve disengagement only by "not feeling well"; they give in to the feeling rather than weather it.

In women the onset is earlier, the affected individual less mature and experiences a prolonged period of vulnerability before established panic disorder (2.4 years) and more than five and a half years before the onset of avoidance behaviour. Is it possible that during this lengthy period of uncertainty fear of further attacks produces nervousness, attention-seeking (needing) behaviour and excessive dependence. Could this be the explanation for the alleged neurotic dependency which is said to precede agoraphobia? One certainly sees more florid attention-seeking behaviour as agoraphobia progresses and it does last many years (15.8, range 1–22 years).

We can say with some confidence that panic disorder can be reliably diagnosed and that its study may cast light on the aetiology in this and related conditions.

Evidence not presented here suggests a differential response to treatment and the category has clear implications for prognosis. In other words, panic disorder is a useful addition to our diagnostic system and a syndrome well worth further study.

## References

AMERICAN PSYCHIATRIC ASSOCIATION (1980) *Diagnostic and Statistical Manual of Mental Disorders* (3rd edn.). Washington, DC: APA.

ANGST, J. & DOBLER-MIKOLA, A. (1985) The Zurich study of anxiety and phobia in young adults. *European Archives of Psychiatry and Neurological Science*, **253**, 171–178.

BEARD, G. (1880) *A Practical Treatise on Nervous Exhaustion (Neurasthenia)* Philadelphia: William Wood.

BECH, P., KASTRUP, M. & RAFAELSEN, O. J. (1986) Mini-compendium of rating scales of anxiety, depression, mania, schizophrenia with corresponding DSM–III syndromes. *Acta Psychiatrica Scandinavica*. Supplement 326, vol. 73.

BENEDIKT, V. (1870) Uber Platzschwindel. *Allgemeiner wiener Medizinische Zeitung*, **15**, 448.

BREUER, J. & FREUD, S. (1894) Studies on hysteria. In *The Standard Edition of the Complete Works of Sigmund Freud* (ed. J. Strachey). London: Hogarth Press (1961) vol. 3.

CANNON, W. B. (1932) *The Wisdom of the Body*. New York: Norton.

CHEYNE, G. (1734) *The English Malady or a Treatise of Nervous Diseases of all Kinds*. London: G. Strahan.

CLARKE, D. M. A. (1986) A cognitive approach to panic. *Behavioural Research and Therapy*, **24**, 461–470.

CULLEN, W. (1800) *Nosology: or, a Systematic Arrangement of Diseases, by Classes, Orders, Genera and Species; with the distinguishing characters of each, and outlines of the systems of Sauvages, Linnaes, Vogel, Sagor, and Macbride*. Edinburgh: Creech.

DA COSTA, J. M. (1871) On irritable heart: A clinical study of a form of functional cardiac disorder and its consequences. *American Journal of Medical Science*, **61**, 17.

FREUD, S. (1895) Obsessions and Phobias. In *The Standard Edition of the Complete Works of Sigmund Freud* (ed. J. Strachey). London: Hogarth Press. (1961) vol. 3.

GELDER, M. G. (1986) Panic attacks: new approaches to an old problem. *British Journal of Psychiatry*. **149**, 346–352.

—— & MARKS, I. M. (1966) Severe agoraphobias: A controlled prospective trial of behaviour therapy. *British Journal of Psychiatry*, **112**, 309–319.

GRAY, MELVIN (1978) *Neuroses: A Comprehensive and Critical View*. New York: Van Nostrand Reinhold.

GURNEY, C., ROTH, M., GARSIDE, R. F., KERR, T. A. & SCHAPIRA, K. (1972) Studies in the classification of depressive disorders. *British Journal of Psychiatry*, **121**, 162–166.

HEIDEGGER, M. (1968) *Existence and Being*. London: Vision Press.

JASPERS, K. (1913) *General Psychopathology*. Translated from 7th Edition by J. Hoenig and M. W. Hamilton, (1963) London: Manchester University Press.

KELLY, D. (1973) Phenelzine in phobic states. *Proceedings of the Royal Society of Medicine*, **66**, 949–950.

KENDELL, R. E. (1968) The problem of classification. In Recent Developments in Affective Disorder (eds A. Coppen & A. Walk). *British Journal of Psychiatry Special Publication No. 2*. Ashford: Headley Bros.

KIERKEGAARD, S. (1980) *The Concept of Anxiety*. (Edited and translated by R. Thomte). Princeton, USA: Princeton University Press.

KLEIN, D. F. (1964) Delineation of two drug responsive anxiety syndromes. *Psychopharmacologia*, **5**, 397–408.

KRAEPELIN, E. (1913) *Lectures on Clinical Psychiatry* (Translated by T. Johnstone) London: Baillière, Tindall & Cox.

LEWIS, A. J. (1936) Melancholia: prognostic study and case material. *Journal of Mental Science*, **82**, 488.

LEWIS, T. (1919) *The Soldier's Heart or the Effort Syndrome*. New York: P. B. Hoeber. (First published 1917).

MAPOTHER, E. (1936) Discussion on manic depressive psychosis. *British Medical Journal*, ii, 872.

MARKS, I. (1987) Behavioural psychotherapy in general psychiatry. *British Journal of Psychiatry*, **150**, 593–597.

—— & LADER, M. H. (1973) Anxiety states (anxiety neurosis) A review. *Journal of Nervous and Mental Disease*, **156**, 3–18.

OPPENHEIMER, B. S. & ROTHSCHILD, M. A. (1918) The psychoneurotic factors in the "irritable heart" of soldiers. *British Medical Journal*, **ii**, 29–31.

*OXFORD ENGLISH DICTIONARY* (1971) Oxford: Oxford University Press.

PAVLOV, I. P. (1941) *Conditioned Reflexes and Psychiatry*. New York: International Publishers.

PINEL, P. (1801) *Traité Medico-philosophique sur l'Alienation Mentale, ou la Manie*. (Translated by D. D. Davis). Facsimile of the London edition, 1806. New York: Hafner (1962).

ROTH, M. (1959) The phobic anxiety depersonalisation syndrome. *Proceedings of the Royal Society of Medicine*, **52**, 587–590.

SARGANT, W. (1962) The treatment of anxiety states and atypical depressions by the monoamine oxidase inhibitor drugs. *Neuropsychiatry*, **3** (suppl. 1), 96–103.

SLATER, E. & ROTH, M. (1969) *Mayer-Gross Slater and Roth Clinical Psychiatry (3rd Edition)*. London: Baillière, Tindall & Cassell.

UHLENHUTH, E. H., BALTER, M. B., MELLINGER, G. D., *et al* (1983) Symptom checklist syndromes in the general population. *Archives of General Psychiatry*, **40**, 1167–1173.

WALTON, J., BEESON, PAUL, B. & SCOTT, R. B. (1986) *The Oxford Companion to Medicine*. Oxford: Oxford University Press.

WESTPHAL, C. (1871) Die Agoraphobie: Eine neuropathische Erscheinung. *Archiv für Psychiatrie und Nervenkrankheiten*, **3**, 138–161.

WEISSMAN, M. M. (1983) The epidemiology of anxiety disorders. Rates, risks, familial patterns. Presented at the NIMH Conference on Anxiety and Anxiety Disorders, Sterling Forest Conference Center, Tuxedo, New York.

——, MYERS, J. K. & HARDING, P. S. (1978) Psychiatric disorders in a U.S. urban community 1975–76. *American Journal of Psychiatry*, **135**, 459–462.

WHYTT, R. (1765) *Observations on the Nature, Causes and Cure of those Disorders which have been called Nervous, Hypochondriac, or Hysteric, to which are prefixed some Remarks on the Sympathy of the Nerves*. Edinburgh: Becket & Du Hondt.

# 20 Agoraphobics and athletes: a personal account of Martin Roth's influence

## J. C. LITTLE

An account is given of my involvement in the earliest of the clinical studies of agoraphobia and depersonalisation at Newcastle. Some indication is given of our thoughts at that time about possible physical and psychological explanations of the clinical phenomena. There is passing comment on continuity of care, necessary conditions for clinical research, and the problem of objectivity.

There follows an outline of my subsequent work on physical prowess and neurosis, and of the manner in which the two studies, on female agoraphobics and on male athletic neurotics, are seen as being conceptually linked as demonstrations of specific stressor vulnerability

### Early efforts

Under the wartime conditions which prevailed when I was a student, very little, if any, research was undertaken in the medical school. Being at that stage of development which demands heroes, I was disappointed to find none immediately available, and turned for inspiration to the biography shelves of the medical library. Sir William Osler was the first hero and model I took on board, soon to be joined by the open-minded clinical observer Sir James McKenzie, William Pickles, the Wensleydale GP clinical epidemiologist, and Sir Thomas Lewis.

Thus primed I set out to do a bit of research on my own account, which on completion gained me a 'scholarship'; in reality a welcome, if modest, sum of money to spend on books.

For nearly a decade thereafter research was always put off until 'next year' when clinical demands would ease off and there would be no further examinations in prospect. It was not until the third year as senior registrar that I completed a clinical investigation and, having acquired the experience and qualifications then considered appropriate, began looking around for a consultant post.

At this climactic juncture I chose instead to apply for a further senior registrar post in what was then the impressively titled Joint Department of Psychological Medicine of the Royal Victoria Infirmary, Newcastle-upon-Tyne and the University of Durham. After weighing the pros and cons it seemed worth postponing the prospect of consultant status for a chance to work for a spell with the newly appointed Professor of Psychological Medicine, Martin Roth, whose qualities were already acclaimed in psychiatric circles and beyond. My application was successful and the decision to apply turned out to be the happiest I ever made in a career of ups and downs.

## Newcastle

I was surprised at first to find that this academic department in Newcastle made a significant contribution to the psychiatric services of the city, but soon realised that the heavy case load was of exceptional value for clinical research. I had a not too demanding standing commitment to the in-patient, out-patient and liaison services within the RVI, but was soon invited by the Professor to collect and study patients suffering from what he then called "phobic anxiety" (and later "agoraphobia") with depersonalisation—Roth's PAD syndrome—which had excited his curiosity before coming to Newcastle. For the first time I was being encouraged to pursue research opportunities arising from clinical experience.

### The PAD syndrome—observations and treatment.
### The problem of objectivity

Increasingly, patients were referred to me as cases, or possible cases, of PAD syndrome. There were limited psychiatric beds in the RVI and it became apparent that a good number of 'my' PAD patients would either have to be admitted elsewhere and pass out of my immediate care, or I would have to treat them as out-patients. It was in response to this dilemma that I first came to realise the value of continuity of medical care and to have reservations about the assumed advantages, for the patient, of admission to a hospital bed. In consequence I saddled myself with five more half-day out-patient consultation, therapy and follow-up sessions a week, for it soon became quite clear that patients cannot be adequately studied in depth for research in the absence of a personal medical commitment.

Just how one is to maintain a dedicated empathy throughout the course of a patient's illness while simultaneously functioning as detached observer is a question to which I was to give much attention later (Little 1968 & 1969(b); Little & McPhail, 1973; Little *et al*, 1977; McClelland *et al*, 1977). Meanwhile, untroubled by any such *folie de doute*, I continued to amass research data.

Martin Roth's ward rounds at the RVI were a delight. As it was his way to become so totally absorbed in whatever he was doing as to lose all sense of the passage of time, the team would assemble at the appointed hour, prepared if necessary for a long wait. Once the round did get under way we also forgot all about the clock. It was not unusual to arrive home from an 'afternoon' round to find the children fast asleep in bed, and a ruined dinner in the oven. Every patient would be most comprehensively interviewed until every point of possible relevance had been teased out and clarified. The subsequent exposition and discussion could last longer than the case presentation and interview combined. Roth's mental flexibility, allied to his extraordinary memory for the clinical detail of every patient he saw, surely lay at the root of his exceptional ability to identify recurrent associations and cause and effect relationships overlooked by those of us who tended to cling to perceptions more constrained by convention.

The research activities with the agoraphobic patients involved not only the assessment and recording of clinical features, premorbid characteristics, life experiences, inter-personal relationships and apparent precipitants, but also the patients' progress under treatment, which at that time meant out-patient intravenous thiopentone sessions twice or thrice a week. As more and more patients came into the study it was apparent that a high proportion of agoraphobic subjects also suffered degrees of unreality feelings, while most of those referred primarily on account of depersonalisation proved to be agoraphobic. Roth expressed a concept of depersonalisation as a "subtle abrogation" of consciousness mediated, if I remember rightly, via the reticular arousal system. (One can always spot those who have passed through the Newcastle Department by the way their professional discourse is larded with "Rothisms" of which the above, with "anxious self-scrutiny" and "the prurient curiosity of the hysteric" are but examples.)

What is yet to be explained is why for some people depersonalisation is pathologically alarming, for it is a well-nigh universal experience at some time or other in life which a majority recall as merely interesting, rather odd, or even slightly amusing.

## Clinical judgement, tests, and objectivity again

Psychological testing failed to show any difference between PAD patients and control subjects with respect to obsessionality. Nevertheless, I cling stubbornly to my judgement that these alert, well turned out pleasant young women, suffering an illness of startlingly sudden onset, typically precipitated by threats to health or a bereavement within the family circle, show a curious compounding of obsessional and histrionic traits which formal testing has not been able to detect. The foregoing will be recognised as a fair example of a clinician's attitude to test results: they are accepted if they confirm clinical judgement and rejected if they do not, which makes good sense despite the seductive, 'scientific' appeal of test procedures.

After cumulative exposure to agoraphobic subjects they can almost be identified by appearance and manner alone before the history has been elicited. Herein lies the 'Catch 22" of clinical judgement: if we wholeheartedly accept the argument of Popper (1972), after Whewell (1840), as elaborated by Medawar (1967), that we can only perceive what we already expect to perceive, then jumping to early conclusions is not going to alter the ultimate perceptually predetermined diagnosis one way or the other!

I bring in these unnerving considerations, with which I believe Professor Roth has little sympathy, only to warn other beginners with intellectual scruples that in a man-studies-man situation like psychiatric clinical research nothing is ever as straightforward as may at first appear. In practice, however, despite the philosophical doubts and reservations, one accepts the results and conclusions of well conceived and conducted clinical research projects as expressing something more than mere personal opinion made respectable by statistics.

The objective during the thiopentone treatment sessions was, with the needle *in situ*, to maintain the patient in a state of blunted awareness just this side of unconsciousness for 15 to 20 minutes. In this state, some spoke spontaneously and calmly about their agoraphobic and depersonalisation experiences, and some were persuaded, in the state of drug-induced calm, to visualise themselves in the anxiety-provoking real life situations. Yet others appeared to be so totally immersed in the thiopentone experience that they wished neither to talk nor to listen. The patients did not find the treatment distressing; a common verdict was "That was marvellous. I only wish I could feel like that all the time". The success rate was impressive and related neither to severity nor duration of illness. It was especially surprising that outcome was unrelated to the nature of the immediate response to the thiopentone-induced alteration of awareness.

### Seeking explanations

In our frequent discussions about the syndrome and the progress of the research the talk ranged from Wolpe's work in South Africa (Wolpe, 1961) to the observations of Kardiner from the battlefields of World War I (Kardiner, 1941). Roth eagerly expounded his views on the role of the reticular arousal system and other cerebral mechanisms in effecting the barbiturate-induced psychological changes. For my part, I diffidently pressed an alternative explanation of the drug effect as a deconditioning experience. So immersed did we become in elaborating our separate ideas that I do not think either was listening very closely to what the other was saying! In fairness I must concede the Professor was probably more attentive to my views than I thought, but I certainly have only a very vague recollection of the detail of the ideas he was then proposing, possibly because he was way ahead of me most of the time. Knowing what we do about mind/brain interactions there is no logical reason to think the psychological and physical explanations have to be incompatible. To think that way would be to stifle the prospect of expanding our understanding.

My notion was that the IV thiopentone invoked an alteration of consciousness sufficiently similar to depersonalisation, while simultaneously the sedating effect of the drug inhibited arousal of the anxiety which the patient had come to anticipate as an inevitable accompaniment. By repetition the linking of depersonalisation and anxiety was eroded. The explanation has the merit of allowing for the observed improvement in the subjects who, while under the influence of the barbiturate, neither spoke of their symptoms nor visualised themselves in the provocative situations.

## Leeds

In 1958 I moved from Newcastle to take up a consultant appointment at St James's Hospital in Leeds. Some time later Professor Roth presented an account of the PAD syndrome at the Royal Society of Medicine (Roth, 1959a), while I shared authorship of the preliminary report on the efficacy of the thiopentone treatment (King & Little, 1959). Not long after, the shattering news came through that all the research records I left in Newcastle—the original data on the 135 cases—had been taken out of the Department and somehow ended up on a bonfire. But further publications from Newcastle on the PAD syndrome appeared over the next few years (Roth, 1959b, and 1960; Harper & Roth, 1962; Roth & Harper, 1962; Roth, 1963; Roth *et al*, 1965), by which time I was involved in a different project altogether in Leeds, very much guided, however, by what

I had learned about clinical research from Martin Roth. Although I had lost the data from one research study I had gained the know-how for the next.

## Research opportunities. Roth's continuing influence

The project incorporated many of the progressive ideas expressed by Professor G. R. Hargreaves in the Heath Clark Lectures of the University of London (Hargreaves, 1957), and the service was so created as to encourage clinical research:

(a) until Hargreaves' untimely death St James's psychiatrists held part-time University posts, giving time for teaching and research
(b) the Leeds clinical experience was very rich—a euphemism for potentially overwhelming (Little *et al*, 1974)
(c) from Roth's department I handed on the unquestioned assumption that research was a natural component of training and practice
(d) over those years supporting medical staff were, almost without exception, enthusiastic and hard-working.

Many of the trainee medical staff who worked with me became involved in research despite, or possibly because of, the heavy case load: Basil James (James, 1964; Little & James, 1964), John Hughes (Hughes & Little, 1967), Alan Lloyd (Little *et al*, 1974), and Alan Kerr, *v. infra* (Little & Kerr, 1968).

Alone of all the vital requirements, the financing of projects was never adequately dealt with. In the rough world of academic and health service politics the set up was vulnerable. In a few years changes of policy seriously upset the balance and the party was over as far as research was concerned.

## The athletes' neurosis

While the golden era lasted I chose to study in greater depth the phenomenon of psychiatric breakdown in men who displayed excessive body pride—the narcissistic body builders we had observed on the general wards at Newcastle displaying what Roth dubbed the 'Mr Atlas' syndrome. The 'Atlas' patients at Leeds were different, however, possibly because the study included all male referrals, rather than a sample of general hospital in-patients as at Newcastle. It soon became clear that the Leeds patients were less preoccupied with the appearance and muscular development of their bodies than with the body's efficiency, strength and stamina in action. Their concern was with how the body functioned in heavy work or in sports.

It emerged that within the population of male neurotic patients there were two quite distinct groups, differing significantly with respect to a wide range of variables. There were the men characterised by extreme and well-nigh exclusive devotion to physical prowess—the athletic group—whose life stories had contained no hint of neurotic vulnerability. The neurotic illness occurred in the stage of waning powers on the threshold of middle age, and almost invariably followed immediately on a direct threat to physical well-being in the form of illness or accident, not infrequently the first ever experienced. In contrast were most of the remaining male neurotic subjects who turned out to have been quite uninterested in their own physical abilities. They were the non-athletic male neurotic patients whose life stories revealed many traditionally recognised neurotic markers. In very few had the illness followed any threat to physical well-being (Little, 1966; and 1969a)

## Controls

A collaborative study was then undertaken with Dr Alan Kerr, at that time a registrar at the St James's Unit, in an attempt to tighten up the conclusions. We set off at weekends or on weekday evenings to collect a control sample of males in the community. Armed with the case record of a male neurotic patient from the original cohort we approached that patient's general practitioner and together selected the GP record of the next same-aged male, as stacked alphabetically in the surgery filing cabinet. From there we went to the address where the GP introduced us and explained the purpose of the visit. Such is the attraction of the prospect of talking about oneself for an hour that none refused.

We prompted and listened to our male control subject, and often subsequently to the wife, for most of the men in the sample were married. An incidental but telling index of cooperation was the offer of refreshment in nearly 70% of the houses visited.

The resultant norms differed considerably from those established in authoritative publications but we felt they provided a better basis for comparison with our psychiatrically disturbed male subjects (Little & Kerr, 1968). After 15 years of confronting psychiatric patients in wards and out-patient clinics it was, for me, an eye-opening experience to encounter 'normal' people again in their own surroundings, a vital corrective which I would recommend for any long-term hospital-bound specialist, especially the academic psychiatrist deprived even of the albeit distorted insight to be gained by a visit to a psychiatric patient's home.

## The conceptual link: specific vulnerability and appropriate stressor

The Leeds studies of the athletes' neurosis link up conceptually with the earlier Newcastle work on agoraphobia and depersonalisation. Both studies demonstrate that for the ultimate manifestation of the neurosis a prior system of well-nigh exclusive overvaluation is a prerequisite. The overvaluation creates a vulnerability which remains dormant until a stressor appropriate to the vulnerability initiates the neurotic reaction. In general, the vulnerability is different in women and men, in ways which are not entirely unexpected. In the young women who develop agoraphobia and depersonalisation the vulnerability has lain in the overvaluation of the emotional bonds within the close family group. The trigger is a threat or disaster to someone within that circle; at its most typical it is the death of the mother.

In a significant proportion of males who develop neuroses the vulnerability has lain in exclusive devotion to physical prowess, a vulnerability which increases with the approach of middle age when the appropriate stressor of a threat to the man's own health and physical well being precipitates the neurosis.

## Neuroses of deprivation, and the 'surprise effect'

In both the women and the men we were seeing neuroses which were initiated by exposure to the appropriate stressor, usually for the first time in their lives.

The illness came like a bolt from the blue on persons not previously considered to be 'neurotic', a finding which calls into question the universality of Schneider's famous dictum: "there are no neuroses, only neurotics" (Schneider, 1923). The surprise effect created a crisis necessitating "reorganisations which do not belong to the arsenal of habitual adjustive responses" (Lindemann, 1944).

The two neurotic conditions studied are far from uncommon. A diagnostic breakdown of all new referrals over the three years 1964–66 (Little *et al*, 1974) showed agoraphobia/depersonalisation to have been prominent in 11.5% of all females, while the athlete's neurosis presented in 9% of all new males referred in 1964 (Little, 1969a). These are neuroses of deprivation and loss (Hill, 1960) rather than of conflict. "For where your treasure is, there will your heart be also". (Matthew 6.21 and Luke 12.34.)

## Martin Roth's lasting influence

It will, I trust, be appreciated by now that much of what I like to call 'my' researches and the contributions of those who later worked with me were inspired by the thinking and example of Martin Roth. No-one can take from us the joy of discovery but it is simply unconscious conceit not to admit one is a plagiarist (from an epigram by Goethe, quoted by Whyte (1979), and now plagiarised by me in 1987). Inevitably with the passage of time my personal contacts with Martin Roth lessened. In real time I worked with him for less than two years, and that was all of 30 years ago. Nevertheless, the influence of a good teacher bites deep. What I absorbed at Newcastle enriched my subsequent medical life profoundly, and at second hand must have affected the many trainee psychiatrists who subsequently worked with me.

*References*

HARGREAVES, G. R. (1957) *Psychiatry and the Public Health*. The Heath Clark Lectures, University of London, 1957.

HARPER, M. & ROTH, M. (1962) Temporal lobe epilepsy and the phobic anxiety/depersonalisation syndrome. Part I A comparative study. *Comprehensive Psychiatry*, **3**, 129–151.

HILL, D. (1960) In *Stress and Psychiatric Disorder* (ed. J. M. Tanner) Oxford: Blackwell.

HUGHES, J. S. & LITTLE, J. C. (1967) An appraisal of the continuing practice of prescribing tranquillising drugs for long-stay psychiatric patients. *British Journal of Psychiatry*, **113**, 867–873.

JAMES, B. (1964) A case of homosexuality treated by aversion therapy. *British Medical Journal*, i, 768–770.

KARDINER, A. (1941) *Psychosomatic Disease Monograph, II–III*, Washington.

KING, A. & LITTLE, J. C. (1959) Thiopentone treatment of the phobic anxiety/depersonalisation syndrome. *Proceedings of the Royal Society of Medicine*, **52**, 595–596.

LINDEMANN, E. (1944) Symptomatology and management of acute grief. *American Journal of Psychiatry*, **101**, 141–148.

LITTLE, J. C. (1966) *Physical Prowess and Neurosis*, MD thesis, University of Bristol, (unpublished).

—— (1968) Objectivity in clinical psychiatric research. *Lancet*, ii, 1072–1075.

—— (1969a) The athletes' neurosis—a deprivation crisis. *Acta Psychiatrica Scandinavica*, Fasc. **2**, 187–197.

—— (1969b) The evaluation of clinical phenomena in psychiatry. *Bristol Medico-Chirurgical Journal*, **84**, 191–196.

—— & JAMES, B. (1964) Abreaction of conditioned fear reaction after eighteen years. *Behavioural Research and Therapy*, **2**, 59–63.

——, COLWELL, J. J. K. & LLOYD, A. T. (1974) *Psychiatry in a General Hospital*. London: Butterworth.

—— & KERR, T. A. (1968) Some differences between published norms and data from matched controls as a basis for comparison with psychiatrically disturbed groups. *British Journal of Psychiatry*, **114**, 883–890.

—— & MCPHAIL, N. (1973) Measures of depressive mood at monthly intervals. *British Journal of Psychiatry*, **122**, 447–452.

——, MCCLELLAND, H. A. & KERR, T. A. (1977) Videotape techniques in assessing antidepressants. *British Journal of Clinical Pharmacology*, **4. Suppl. 2**, 227–232.

MCCLELLAND, H. A., KERR, T. A. & LITTLE, J. C. (1977) A clinical comparison of nomifensine and amitryptiline. *British Journal of Clinical Pharmacology*, **Suppl. 4**, 233–236.

MEDAWAR, P. B. (1967) Hypothesis and Imagination. In *The Art of the Soluble*, London: Methuen.

POPPER, K. (1972) *Conjectures and Refutations: the Growth of Scientific Knowledge*. 4th Edn. London: Routledge & Kegan Paul.

ROTH, M. (1959a) The phobic anxiety/depersonalisation syndrome. *Proceedings of the Royal Society of Medicine*, **52**, 587–595.

—— (1959b) The phenomenology of depressive states. *Canadian Medical Association Journal*, **4**, Special Supplement: McGill University Conference on Depression and Allied States, 32–54.

—— (1960) The phobic anxiety/depersonalisation syndrome and some general aetiological problems in psychiatry. *Journal of Neuropsychiatry*, **1**, 293–306.

—— (1963) Neurosis, psychosis and the concept of disease in psychiatry. *Acta Psychiatrica Scandinavica*, **39**, 128–145.

——, GARSIDE, R. F. & GURNEY, C. (1965) Clinical-statistical enquiries into the classification of anxiety states and depressive disorders. In *Proceedings of the Leeds Symposium on Behavioural Disorders* (ed. F. A. Jenner) Dagenham: May & Baker.

—— & HARPER, M. (1962) Temporal lobe epilepsy and the phobic anxiety/depersonalisation syndrome. Part II Practical and theoretical considerations. *Comprehensive Psychiatry*, **3**, 215–226.

SCHNEIDER, K. (1923) *Psychopathic Personalities*. Translated by M. W. Hamilton. London: Cassell (1958).

TANNER, J. M. (1951) Current advances in the study of physique. *Lancet*, **i**, 574–579.

WHEWELL, W. (1840) *The Philosophy of the Induction Sciences*, London.

WHYTE, L. L. (1979) *The Unconscious before Freud*. London: Friedmann.

WOLPE, J. (1961) The systematic desensitation treatment of neuroses. *Journal of Nervous and Mental Disease*, **132**, 189–203.

# 21 Cognitive pathology and cognitive treatment of depressive and anxiety disorder

**MICHAEL G. GELDER**

The development in recent years of cognitive therapy for anxiety and depressive disorders has been accompanied by a renewed interest in the psychopathology of the conditions. The focus of this new work has been on cognitive abnormalities, and the methods of investigation have been mainly those of experimental psychopathology. This approach to psychopathology is characterised by an attempt to relate studies of abnormal phenomena to investigations of normal psychological processes, using similar methods of enquiry and attempting to understand results within a common theoretical framework. Experimental psychopathology therefore supplements established methods of clinical investigation. Another importance of this approach to psychopathology is that it suggests new forms of treatment, and it is for this reason that this chapter is concerned with cognitive therapy as well as cognitive pathology.

It is because Sir Martin Roth has contributed in such an important way to the study of the clinical psychopathology of depressive and anxiety disorders that I have chosen this subject for my contribution to this volume.

The chapter is in five parts: an account of the cognitive abnormalities in depressive disorders; a brief review of the status of cognitive therapy for depression; an account of the cognitive abnormalities in anxiety disorders; a consideration of cognitive therapy for anxiety disorders; and a final summing up. However, before any of the subjects can be addressed, it is necessary to say something about the meaning of the word cognition. In psychology, cognitive means 'all forms of knowing': perceiving, attending, thinking, and memorising. In everyday clinical psychiatry, the term cognition is often used in a more restricted way, for example in describing the mental state, to refer to only two of these processes, attending and memorising. In the literature on cognitive therapy the term cognition is frequently used in another way, as if it were synonymous with thinking. In the present account the term will be used in the wider sense employed in psychology, and consideration will be given to all four aspects of cognition in depressive and anxiety disorders.

## Cognitions in depressive disorder

Interest in the cognitive abnormalities in depressive disorders can be said to have begun with the work of A. T. Beck. He published an important paper in which

185

he drew attention to certain features of the psychopathology of these disorders which, he suggested, had a role in causing and maintaining the conditions. The paper, which appeared in two parts, was called 'Thinking and Depression' (Beck, 1963; 1964). The first part contained a detailed account of the disordered thinking of 50 depressed patients. Many of the observations confirmed the classical descriptions of states of depression: low self-regard, self-criticism and self blame, the feeling that problems are overwhelming, and a preoccupation with suicide. Beck characterised these symptoms as features of a 'depressive triad' of negative ideas about that person's past, present, and future. Beck went on to describe two other features of depressive disorder which had not been widely recognised as important. First, he drew attention to the frequency and importance of intrusive thoughts with depressive themes (for example the sudden intrusive and distressing thought, 'I am a failure'). Second, he pointed out that the persistence of ideas about themes such as failure and hopelessness, in the presence of evidence to the contrary, must indicate an underlying disorder of logical thinking. He called this abnormal thinking 'paralogical', and described its characteristics. 'Arbitrary inference' was the process of drawing a conclusion from a limited set of evidence without considering other possibilities. 'Selective abstraction' was the process of focusing on one aspect of a complex situation, without giving appropriate consideration to others. 'Over generalisation' was drawing unreasonably wide conclusions from a single instance. Other features of paralogical thinking include 'magnification' which is the giving of undue importance to events; and 'absolutist thinking' which is using rigid dichotomies. It should be noted that Beck did not propose that these errors of logic were confined to depressive disorders: he drew attention in these early papers to the description by Kasanin (1944) of similar errors of reasoning in schizophrenia; and he proposed subsequently that similar logical errors occur in anxiety disorders (see Beck, Emery & Greenberg, 1985). It is also important to note that the same errors occur in normal thinking, though presumably to a lesser extent (see for example Kroglanski & Ajzen, 1983).

Beck went on to suggest that another psychological abnormality lay behind, and accounted for, the depressed patient's persistent misinterpretations of his past, present and future. To describe it, he used the term cognitive schema by which he meant "a structure used for screening, coding and evaluating impinging stimuli". A schema can determine the way in which information stored in memory is responded to, and it can influence the evaluation of interoceptive cues, or information about the external world. Beck suggested that automatic thoughts result from the impact of environmental events upon maladaptive schemata. He also proposed that abnormal schemata predispose to a depressive disorder and can prolong it. Finally, he suggested that these schemata can persist after recovery from the depressive disorder, though in a reduced or inactive form.

Schemata are hypothetical constructs, which have to be inferred from interpretations of experience, and from attitudes and expectations. In the 1964 account Beck also suggested that schemata could be identified from the analysis of dreams and free associations, though he did not develop this approach subsequently.

### Experimental studies of depressive cognitions

We have seen that Beck proposed four kinds of cognitive abnormality in depressive disorders: intrusive ('automatic') thoughts; depressive ideas such as self-blame and expectations of failure; distortions of logic; and abnormal schemata. What evidence is there to support these proposals?

Automatic thoughts have been quantified by the use of a questionnaire (Hollon & Kendall, 1980) which has confirmed that these thoughts are more frequent in depressive than in other psychiatric disorders (Hollon *et al*, 1986). Other studies have shown that the thoughts are more intrusive and more difficult to suppress in severely depressed patients than in patients with less severe depression (Teasdale & Rezin, 1978).

Of the ideas that make up the depressive triad, expectations of failure and helplessness have been studied most thoroughly. This is because helplessness is the central feature of an alternative account of the psychopathology of depression, suggested by Seligman (1975). His original account emphasised the role of 'learned helplessness', that is the failure to perceive any relationship between the actions and outcome. This account was unsatisfactory in several ways, and the theory was revised to take more account of cognitive factors (Abramson, Seligman & Teasdale, 1978). The revised theory introduced the idea of self blame: it supposes that depression occurs when a person thinks that he cannot control events, and that this is his own fault. Many experimental studies have demonstrated that depressed people are more likely than normal subjects to attribute failures in experimental tasks to themselves rather than external causes or chance; and that they evaluate their performance in more negative ways. In some experiments, however, mildly depressed subjects have been more accurate than the normal subjects in making these assessments (e.g. Alloy & Abramson, 1979). This finding suggests that it is not just that severely depressed people blame themselves inappropriately, but also that people who are clearly not depressed have a cognitive mechanism for protecting against the depressing effects of failure, and that this mechanism is less effective in states of depression. This change could exacerbate mood change arising from any cause, and set up a vicious circle of increasing depression.

Distortions of logic have not been investigated thoroughly. A cognitive error questionnaire has been developed by Le Febvre (1981) but it has proved difficult to distinguish reliably the various categories described by Beck (Kranz & Hammen, 1979).

The abnormal schemata proposed by Beck are difficult to investigate because their presence has to be inferred from other variables. The usual method has been to use a questionnaire (the Dysfunctional Attitudes Scale) to study attitudes that are assumed to reflect the schemata. In this procedure subjects are required to indicate how far they agree with statements such as: my value as a person depends greatly on what others think of me. Scores on this questionnaire are increased during a depressive disorder, returning to normal after recovery. Schemata can also be inferred from the way in which information is evaluated, and depressed people accept the validity of false negative feedback more readily than people who are not depressed (Rizley, 1978). The cognitive theory predicts that the persistence of high scores should be associated with relapse but there is no satisfactory evidence on this point.

Beck's description of the cognitive disorder of depressed patients does not take account of all cognitive functions: memory is the notable omission. There is strong evidence that normal subjects in temporary states of depression and patients with depressive disorders, recall more unpleasant and fewer pleasant events than do people in normal mood (Teasdale & Taylor, 1981; Teasdale & Fogarty, 1979; Lishman, 1972; Lloyd & Lishman, 1975). Moreover, among depressed patients, this effect is greater at times when mood is more depressed (Clark & Teasdale, 1982). This process is likely to be an important feature of the psychopathology of depressive disorders because it is capable of setting up a vicious spiral in which low mood leads to great recall of unhappy events which results, in turn, in further lowering of mood. Its significance in relation to cognitive therapy will be discussed later.

## Cognitive therapy for depressive disorder

Cognitive therapy was devised by Beck to put right the hypothesised cognitive abnormalities in depressive disorders. The procedures are based on two assumptions. The first is that depressive cognitions can be changed by psychological means. The second is that when cognitions change, alterations in mood and other features of the depressive disorder will follow. Beck decided that a broad approach would be required, and his treatment is a complicated assemblage of techniques directed to various aspects of the cognitive disorder. Some of the techniques are verbal, involving giving information and questioning attitudes and expectations. Other techniques are behavioural; they are used because attitudes and expectations often change more through new experiences than through reasoning. The techniques of cognitive therapy for depression, which are now well known, cannot be described in the space of this chapter [readers requiring an account of the procedure of cognitive therapy should consult Beck *et al*, (1979)]. The interest here is in the results of this treatment; and in whether its effects are brought about by altering depressive cognitions, and whether other kinds of treatment have similar effects.

There is good evidence that cognitive therapy produces substantial improvement in patients with major depressive disorders, and that this improvement is as great as that produced by antidepressant drugs (Rush *et al*, 1977). Also, Simons *et al*, (1986) reported lower relapse rates after cognitive therapy than drug treatment. Moreover, when cognitive therapy is added to the usual treatment for depressive disorders there is some speeding up of recovery, though the effect is modest and only apparent for a few weeks (Teasdale *et al*, 1984). To date, there is no convincing evidence that cognitive therapy is generally effective for depressed patients who have failed to respond to adequate drug treatment. There is, however, a clinical impression that some individuals do better with cognitive than with drug treatment, and Simons *et al*, (1985) reported different predictors of response to cognitive therapy and drugs.

The next question is whether improvement with cognitive therapy is due to a specific effect on depressive cognitions or to non-specific effects. Unfortunately, there is little direct evidence on this point. In one study (Teasdale & Fennell, 1982), the short-term effects of the full cognitive therapy procedure were compared with those of a procedure similar in all respects except that no attempt was made to alter cognitions. Only the effects within a single treatment session were studied: in this short period, the full cognitive therapy procedure led to greater change in cognitions, and to greater improvement in mood. However, this investigation did not demonstrate a change in cognition beyond the end of the single treatment session, nor was it established that the mood changes followed from the cognitive changes. In any case, even if it could be shown that changes in cognitions result from the specific cognitive therapy procedures, there may be other ways of bringing about the same changes. Thus cognitive change equivalent to that occurring in cognitive therapy has been found in depressed patients after treatment with antidepressant drugs (Simons *et al*, 1984).

In the absence of convincing direct evidence that changes in cognitive therapy are due to specific processes, indirect evidence has to be examined. One source of evidence concerns the effects of other treatments of depressive disorder. Interpersonal therapy is a highly structured form of counselling intended to treat depressive disorder by reducing problems in relationships. With major depressive disorder the results of this treatment appear to be about equivalent to those of cognitive therapy (Weissman *et al*, 1979). This finding could indicate that cognitive therapy has specific effects on cognitions, and interpersonal therapy has specific effects on social problems; and that change in cognitions and change in social relationships are alternative ways of bringing about improvement in major depressive disorders. However, it could also indicate that neither treatment is acting through the supposed specific mechanisms, but through non-specific therapeutic processes present in both. Such processes include the promotion of greater activity, which could improve mood by increasing pleasurable experiences and 'positive re-inforcement'; and the positive, structured approach which could reduce feelings of helplessness. Although it is not certain that these non-specific factors are sufficiently powerful to produce the improvements reported in the depressive disorders, it is important to remember that a large part of the effects of cognitive therapy could be non-specific. As Frank pointed out many years ago (Frank, 1961), most psychological treatments seem to act in this non-specific way however convincing their rationale.

Before leaving the subject of cognitive therapy for depressive disorders, its place in the management of depressed patients will be considered briefly. Several facts suggest that this place is of limited importance. First, antidepressant drugs are an effective treatment of depressive disorders, and it takes less time to treat with drugs than it does to use cognitive therapy. Although cognitive therapy seems to produce benefits equivalent to those of antidepressant drugs, and may have a lower drop out and relapse rate, the differences are not great enough to justify the routine use of so much additional professional time. Second, antidepressant drugs have recently been shown to be effective even in less severe depressive disorders for which the use of cognitive treatment might otherwise be recommended (Paykel, 1988). Third, the addition of cognitive therapy to the usual regime of antidepressant treatment does not produce any major benefit; at most there is only a slight speeding up of recovery in the first few weeks of treatment. Last, it has not been demonstrated that cognitive therapy is generally effective in patients who fail to respond to antidepressant drugs (though it is sometimes appropriate to try cognitive therapy in a particular case).

## Cognitions and anxiety disorders

Interest in the cognitive abnormalities of anxiety disorders began with the recognition of the limitations of an account of these disorders in terms of conditioning and learning, and of the shortcomings of simple behavioural treatments. It is, of course, widely recognised that anxious thoughts are part of the clinical picture of anxiety disorders. Until recently, however, there had been no systematic investigation of the cognitive processes of patients with anxiety disorders, and no clear theoretical framework in which to discuss the findings of such studies. A useful framework is the one that we have employed in discussing depressive disorders, with the four elements of perception, attention, memorising, and thinking; and there is some value in dividing the disorders of thinking into intrusive thoughts, anxious ideas, errors of logic, and schemata.

It is convenient to consider studies of perception and attention together. Compared with normal subjects, patients with anxiety disorders attend more selectively to threatening aspects of the environment. This selective attention has been shown, for example, by determining the speed at which a small target is detected on a screen when it is close to the position previously occupied by either a threatening word or a neutral word of equal length and frequency of use. In these circumstances, responses to the target are faster when it is near the position of the threatening stimulus than when it is near the neutral one (MacLeod *et al*, 1986). There is some evidence that this process of selective attention takes place outside conscious awareness. Thus, in one study, when information was presented to the attended ear in a dichotic listening task, there was slowing of the response to this information when threatening messages were presented to the unattended ear, but not when neutral messages were presented to this ear. This slowing occurred even though the person could not subsequently identify what had been presented in the unattended ear (Mathews & MacLeod, 1986). Normal subjects did not show these effects.

In contrast to the findings in states of depressed mood, studies have not shown an effect of anxiety on recall (Mogg *et al*, 1987). This difference between the two emotional states is consistent with the greater preoccupations with past events of depressed than of anxious people.

Of the disorders of thinking, intrusive thoughts seem to play a particularly important part in the maintenance of anxiety disorders. The content of the intrusive thoughts differs in a characteristic way in the different anxiety disorders. The most distinct abnormality is found in patients with panic attacks. They usually describe intrusive thoughts about heart disease, fainting, and dying. In social phobia, however, the intrusive thoughts are typically about embarrassment, and about criticism by other people. In generalised anxiety disorder, a wide variety of intrusive thoughts may be experienced, including thoughts about ill-health, social embarrassment, and the safety of others (Hibbert, 1984).

Beck has suggested that patients with anxiety disorders show the same illogical ways of thinking that he identified in depressed patients (see Beck *et al*, 1985). There is no direct evidence to support this assertion but as these ways of thinking are used by normal subjects it is not unlikely that they occur in states of anxiety as well.

The evidence for abnormal schemata in anxiety disorders is stronger than in states of depression. The best evidence is in patients with panic attacks where the schemata result in interpretations of information about bodily functions that ascribe to it more threat than is objectively present. This tendency has been investigated in relation to interpretations of the significance of changes in cardiac function. The evidence suggests that patients with panic attacks interpret benign changes in heart rate as evidence of impending heart disease. Thus when false feedback about heart rate is given to panic patients and to normal subjects, a false indication of rapid heart action leads to a greater increase of anxiety in patients than in normal subjects (Ehlers *et al*, 1988). Patients with panic attacks are also more likely than normal control subjects to interpret in a threatening way, ambiguous accounts of bodily sensations (Clark *et al*, 1988). For example, they are more likely to interpret palpitations as evidence of an impending heart attack rather than evidence of a benign process such as excitement. The results of a semantic priming experiment (Clark *et al*, 1988) provide further evidence of disordered schemata in panic patients. In this experiment the speed of response to a test word was measured under two conditions: after reading a neutral phrase, and after reading a phrase that was expected to activate the schema, namely a phrase concerned with cardiac function. Thus, after the phrase "if I had palpitations it could be", panic patients respond more rapidly to the word dying than to the word excited, suggesting that they were already primed to expect this outcome. After a neutral priming phrase the speed of their response to the two words was the same. Normal subjects do not show this effect of priming.

Little is known about the schemata in other kinds of anxiety disorders. Patients with social phobia report irrational expectations that other people will think unfavourably about them ('fear of negative evaluation'); and patients with agoraphobia describe fears about further episodes of anxiety. However, in neither case have there been experimental studies of the kind described above. Yet, as we shall see in the next section, experimental studies are the best basis for psychological treatment.

## Cognitive treatment for anxiety disorders

Cognitive treatment for anxiety disorders has developed in two main ways: as an adaption of Beck's cognitive therapy for depression, and as a series of new techniques intended to overcome specific shortcomings of behavioural treatments for anxiety disorders.

Beck's cognitive therapy for anxiety disorders attempts to modify automatic thoughts and schemata by using methods similar to those developed for the treatment of depression, combining them with exposure to anxiety-provoking situations, and with relaxation. This combination of procedures has the advantage that it can be used for a wide variety of anxiety disorders but it has the disadvantage that it is complex and time-consuming. To date, few clinical trials have been reported in which the value of this treatment has been assessed. Durham & Turvey (1987) found no differences in the treatment of anxiety disorders, between the end of treatment results of Beck's cognitive therapy and behaviour therapy; at six months follow-up, however, the cognitive therapy group had improved rather more. Clearly, further studies are required, including comparisons between Beck's cognitive therapy for anxiety, and the methods that are to be described next.

The alternative forms of cognitive therapy are less elaborate than Beck's. The distinguishing feature of these treatments is that they focus on a particular set of cognitions which are thought to be impeding natural recovery. One such cognition is the fear of further attacks of anxiety. This 'fear of fear' is usually approached by providing information about the physiology of anxiety, with the intention of making symptoms less frightening; and by teaching ways of coping with anxiety. The latter include distraction, relaxation, and the rehearsal of reassuring thoughts to counteract anxiety-producing intrusive thoughts. This combination of procedures is sometimes called anxiety management. For agoraphobia and social phobia, anxiety management is generally used in combination with a major component of exposure. For generalised anxiety disorder, anxiety management can be used alone, or combined with a component of exposure introduced to deal with the minor degrees of avoidance behaviour that are common in these disorders.

Patients with panic attacks respond quite well to this kind of treatment when the attacks are infrequent. When panic attacks are frequent, a different treatment is required. This treatment is focused on the specific cognitive abnormality of these patients, namely the misinterpretation of the significance of physical symptoms which was described above.

In the cognitive treatment of panic attacks, the feared somatic symptoms are induced in some harmless way, often by voluntary hyperventilation. At the same time the patient is encouraged to reconsider the significance of these symptoms and of similar ones arising during a panic attack, and encouraged to realise that the symptoms are harmless. This procedure, which is repeated several times, is combined with behavioural experiments in which the patient tests his new ideas in the course of daily life. This cognitive treatment leads to a rapid and substantial reduction of panic attacks which seems to last for more than a year after the treatment (Clark *et al*, 1985; Salkovskis *et al*, 1986).

Are these changes brought about by the specific procedures or by non-specific components of the treatment? So far, direct evidence on this point is lacking, but there is some indirect evidence pointing to specific effects. First, in a study of the treatment of social phobia, cognitive therapy had a greater effect than treatment which shared the same non-specific components and at the same time more change in the relevant cognitions took place with the cognitive therapy (Butler *et al*, 1984). Second, the specific cognitive changes identified in panic disorder change with cognitive treatment (Clark *et al*, 1988)—although it is not certain what changes occur with other treatments. Thus there is some indication that when the aims of cognitive treatment are linked to the findings of experimental psychopathology—as they have been with the anxiety disorders—they are more likely to act through specific mechanisms than when they are developed mainly from clinical observations—as they have been with depressive disorders.

Whether or not it is confirmed that the effects of cognitive therapy for anxiety disorder are due to specific mechanisms, the techniques are likely to continue to have a valuable place in clinical practice because drug treatment for these conditions is generally less satisfactory than that for depressive disorders. Unless novel drugs can be produced, pharmacological treatment will continue to have the dual problems of dependency and relapse.

## Conclusions

Beck made three important contributions to the understanding and treatment of depressive and anxiety disorders. First, he made careful clinical observations that drew attention to the importance of the cognitive abnormalities, and in suggesting ways in which they can be investigated. Third, he produced an effective treatment. These contributions are of the greatest significance, for they have established cognitive therapy as important in psychiatric research and practice. There are, however, some doubts whether Beck's cognitive therapy for depression acts specifically by changing abnormal cognitions, and some indications that to develop more specific forms of cognitive therapy it will be important to use the findings of experimental psychopathology to direct and fashion treatment techniques. The strongest support for this idea comes from work on panic disorder in which striking changes have followed a determined and focused attempt to change a limited set of cognitions that have been shown, in experimental studies, to characterise this condition. It is the difference between this intensive attack on a narrow therapeutic target and the wide-ranging approach to many targets, that distinguishes the cognitive techniques which originated from experimental studies of anxiety disorders from those which Beck developed from his clinical observations of depressive (and anxiety) disorders.

It is too early as yet to be confident that this experimental approach, and the targeted treatments that follow from it, will produce more effective psychological treatments than the numerous methods of therapy that have been developed as a result of clinical observations. Nevertheless, there are convincing reasons for testing this focused approach more thoroughly, and extending it to other disorders. Even if the experimental approach to psychopathology does not fulfil its promise as a basis for better treatment, it has already shown its value as a means of understanding the psychopathology of mood disorders, and of linking more closely work on normal and abnormal psychological processes.

If experimental studies of the psychopathology of anxiety and depressive disorders are to fulfil their potential, one further development is needed. There should be a closer relationship than has been achieved so far between psychological and 'biological' methods of investigation. Combined studies should be made, for example, of the nature and course of cognitive changes during drug treatments, and of changes in neurotransmitter systems during cognitive treatment. This combined approach to psychiatric disorders is one of the hallmarks of Sir Martin Roth's research. It is exemplified by his studies linking memory disorder and neuropathological changes in demented patients, and it is reflected in many other aspects of his research and scholarly writings. In Sir Martin Roth's hands this approach to the understanding and treatment of psychiatric disorders has led to important advances, and it is to be hoped that a combination of the new cognitive approaches with established 'biological' ones, will achieve similar success. Whatever the future of these cognitive methods, I hope that Sir Martin will accept this account of their past development and present position, as a tribute to his many achievements as a clinician, scholar, research worker, and statesman of psychiatry.

## References

ABRAMSON, L. Y., SELIGMAN, M. E. P. & TEASDALE, J. P. (1978) Learned helplessness in humans: critique and reformulation. *Journal of Abnormal Psychology*, **87**, 49–74.
ALLOY, L. B. & ABRAMSON, L. Y. (1979) Judgement of contingency in depressed and non-depressed students: sadder but wiser? *Journal of Experimental Psychology (General)*, **108**, 441–485.

BECK, A. T. (1963) Thinking and depression. I: idiosyncratic content and cognitive distortions. *Archives of General Psychiatry*, **9**, 324–333.
—— (1964) Thinking and depression. II: theory and therapy. *Archives of General Psychiatry*, **10**, 561–571.
——, RUSH, A. J., SHAW, B. F. & EMERY, G. (1979) *Cognitive Therapy for Depression*. New York: Guilford Press.
——, EMERY, G. & GREENBERG, R. (1985) *Anxiety Disorders and Phobias: A Cognitive Perspective*. New York: Basic Books.
BUTLER, G., CULLINGTON, A., MUNBY, M., AMIES, P. & GELDER, M. G. (1984) Exposure and anxiety management in the treatment of social phobia. *Journal of Consulting and Clinical Psychology*, **52**, 642–650.
CLARK, D. M. & TEASDALE, J. D. (1982) Diurnal variation in clinical depression and accessibility of memories of positive and negative experiences. *Journal of Abnormal Psychology*, **91**, 87–95.
——, SALKOVSKIS, P. M. & CHALKLEY, A. J. (1985) Respiratory control as a treatment for panic attacks. *Journal of Behaviour Therapy and Experimental Psychiatry*, **16**, 23–30.
——, ——, GELDER, M. G., KOEHLER, C., MARTIN, M., ANASTASIADES, P., HACKMAN, A., MIDDLETON, H. & JEAVONS, A. (1988) Test of a cognitive theory of panic. In *Panic and Phobia* (eds H. V. Wittchen & I. Hand), **2**, Munich: Springer-Verlag.
COYNE, J. C. & GOTLIB, I. H. (1983) The role of cognition in depression: a critical appraisal. *Psychological Bulletin*, **94**, 472–505.
DURHAM, R. C. & TURVEY, A. A. (1987) Cognitive therapy versus behaviour therapy in the treatment of chronic generalized anxiety. *Behaviour Research and Therapy*, **25**, 229–234.
EHLERS, A., MARGRAF, J., ROTH, W. T., TAYLOR, C. B. & BIRNBANNER, N. (1988) Anxiety produced by false heart rate feedback in patients with panic disorder. *Behaviour Research and Therapy*, **26**, 1–11.
FRANK, J. D. (1961) *Persuasion and Healing: A Comparative Study of Psychotherapy*. Baltimore: Johns Hopkins Press.
HIBBERT, G. A. (1984) Ideational components of anxiety: their origin and content. *British Journal of Psychiatry*, **144**, 618–624.
HOLLON, S. D. & KENDALL, P. C. (1980). Cognitive self-statements in depression: development of an automatic thoughts questionnaire. *Cognitive Therapy and Research*, **4**, 383–395.
——, —— & LUMRY, A. (1986) Specificity of depressogenic cognitions in clinical depression. *Journal of Abnormal Psychology*, **95**, 22–59.
KASANIN, J. S. (1944) *Language and thought in schizophrenia*. Berkeley: University of California Press.
KRANTZ, S. & HAMMEN, C. (1979) Assessment of cognitive bias in depression. *Journal of Abnormal Psychology*, **88**, 611–619.
KROGLANSKI, A. W. & AJZEN, I. (1983) Bias and error in human judgement. *European Journal of Social Psychology*, **13**, 1–44.
LE FEBVRE, M. F. (1981) Cognitive distortion and cognitive errors in depressed psychiatric and low back pain patients. *Journal of Consulting and Clinical Psychology*, **49**, 517–525.
LISHMAN, W. A. (1972) Selective factors in memory. II affective disorders. *Psychological Medicine*, **2**, 248–253.
LLOYD, C. G. & LISHMAN, W. A. (1975) Effect of depression on recall of pleasant and unpleasant experiences. *Psychological Medicine*, **5**, 173–180.
MACLEOD, C., MATHEWS, A. & TATA, P. (1986) Attentional bias in emotional disorders. *Journal of Abnormal Psychology*, **95**, 15–20.
MATHEWS, A. & MACLEOD, C. (1986) Discrimination of threat cues without awareness in anxiety states. *Journal of Abnormal Psychology*, **95**, 131–138.
MOGG, K., MATHEWS, A. & WEINMAN, J. (1987) Memory bias in clinical anxiety. *Journal of Abnormal Psychology*, **96**, 94–98.
PAYKEL, E. S., HOLLYMAN, J. A., FREELING, P. & SEDGWICK, P. (1987) Predictors of therapeutic benefit from amitriptyline in mild depression: a general practice placebo-controlled trial. *Journal of Affective Disorders*, **14**, 83–95.
——, ——, —— & —— (1988) Prediction of therapeutic benefit from amitriptyline in mild depression: a general practice placebo control trial. *Journal of Affective Disorders*, **14**, 83–95.
RIZLEY, R. (1978) Depression and distortion in the attribution of causality. *Journal of Abnormal Psychology*, **87**, 32–48.
RUSH, A. J., BECK, A. T., KOVACS, M. & HOLLON, S. (1977) Comparative efficacy of cognitive therapy and pharmacotherapy in the treatment of depressed out-patients. *Cognitive Therapy Research*, **1**, 17–38.
——, WEISSENBURGER, J. & EAVES, G. (1986) Do thinking patterns predict depressive symptoms? *Cognitive Therapy and Research*, **10**, 509–526.

SALKOVSKIS, P. M., JONES, D. R. O. & CLARK, D. M. (1986) Respiratory control in the treatment of panic attacks: replication and extension. *British Journal of Psychiatry*, **148**, 526–532.

SELIGMAN, M. E. P. (1975) *Helplessness: On Depression, Development, and Death*, San Francisco: Freeman.

SIMONS, A. D., GARFIELD, S. L. & MURPHY, G. E. (1984) The process of change in cognitive therapy and pharmacotherapy for depression. *Archives of General Psychiatry*, **41**, 45–51.

——, LUSTMAN, P. J., WETZEL, R. D. & MURPHY, G. E. (1985) Predicting response to cognitive therapy of depression: the role of learned resourcefulness. *Cognitive Therapy and Research*, **9**, 79–89.

——, MURPHY, G. E., LEVINE, J. L. & WETZEL, R. D. (1986) Cognitive therapy and pharmacotherapy for depression. *Archives of General Psychiatry*, **43**, 43–48.

TEASDALE, J. D. & FENNELL, M. J. V. (1982) Immediate effects on depression of cognitive therapy interventions. *Cognitive Therapy and Research*, **6**, 343–352.

——, ——, HIBBERT, G. A. & AMIES, P. L. (1984) Cognitive therapy for major depressive disorder in primary care. *British Journal of Psychiatry*, **144**, 400–406.

—— & FOGARTY, S. J. (1979) Differential effects of induced mood on retrieval of pleasant events and unpleasant events from episodic memory. *Journal of Abnormal Psychology*, **88**, 248–257.

—— & REZIN, V. (1978) The effects of reducing frequency of negative thoughts on the mood of depressed patients—tests of a cognitive model of depression. *British Journal of Social and Clinical Psychology*, **17**, 65–74.

—— & TAYLOR, R. (1981). Induced mood and accessibility of memories: an effect of mood state or of mood induction procedure? *British Journal of Clinical Psychology*, **20**, 39–48.

WEISMANN, M., PRUSOFF, B. A., DIMASCIO, A., NELL, C., GOKLANEY, M. & KLERMAN, G. L. (1979) The efficacy of drugs and psychotherapy in the treatment of acute depressive episodes. *American Journal of Psychiatry*, **136**, 555–558.

# 22 Research in the borderlands of neurosis

**MAX HARPER**

The observation that depersonalisation was frequently precipitated by a stressful event and conspicuously associated with phobic anxiety symptoms led Roth to the concept of the Phobic Anxiety-Depersonalisation Syndrome. Systematic enquiries in agoraphobic patients revealed a spectrum of episodic anxiety laden experiences generally regarded as supporting a diagnosis of temporal lobe epilepsy rather than a psychoneurosis. As part of a programme of research including psychophysiological and psychoendocrinological techniques, multivariate statistical analysis was used to explore the borderland between organic and functional in neurotic states, to improve diagnostic discrimination and to examine the hypothesis that disabling agoraphobia may involve temporal lobe dysfunction, prognostically and therapeutically distinct from temporal lobe epilepsy.

## Depersonalisation in anxiety states

The description of the phobic anxiety-depersonalisation syndrome (Roth, 1959) as a "new form of neurotic illness" generated considerable controversy, particularly about its status as an independent diagnostic entity. Roth documented the wide range of symptoms found in his study of 135 cases of phobic anxiety, drawing attention particularly to the parallels with the 'fright' neuroses seen following battle stress and to the evidence suggesting some "chronic derangement of the mechanism regulating awareness". The evidence showed, Roth asserted, that depersonalisation and phobic anxiety constituted "the essential core of the illness". As well as the symptoms of depersonalisation, other features reminiscent of temporal lobe dysfunction such as *déjà vu* phenomena, metamorphopsia and panoramic memory were found in 40% of the cases. These symptoms suggested that "a subtle sustained disturbance in the function of the temporal lobe or limbic system may be involved in the perpetuation of the phenomenon" (Roth, 1959), echoing Mayer-Gross' (1935) concept of depersonalisation as a "pre-formed functional response".

The importance of the temporal regions in phobic anxiety states was further supported by reference to cases where a focal abnormality was suggested by electroencephalographic, radiological or neuropathological evidence and particular parallels with the phenomena of temporal lobe epilepsy were considered.

As the description of precipitating factors and premorbid personality makes abundantly clear, this suggestion of cerebral localisation was not an example of reductionism but part of a general philosophy which seeks to use the overlap between organic and functional to shed light on the aetiology of syndromes on either side of the borderland. The arguments were fully considered by Roth in 1960, when he referred to studies on schizophrenia-like states in epilepsy, amphetamine psychosis and hysteria.

The close association between depersonalisation and anxiety had been described before by Mayer-Gross in 1935 who noted the onset of depersonalisation associated with acute anxiety in 10 of 26 cases, with a tendency to fainting which led to a suspicion of epilepsy in one case. Shorvon (1946), reviewing the organic disorders which were associated with depersonalisation, noted that this symptom was particularly associated with "fears of going out alone, and inability to travel. The initial onset is frequently accompanied by over-breathing or difficulty in breathing, a feeling of faintness without an actual faint and numerous somatic symptoms of anxiety". The relationship was also noted by Palmer (1941), and Oberndorf (1950) pointed out the value of studying symptoms associated with depersonalisation such as *déjà vu* experiences as part of the "depersonalising defence mechanism". Ackner (1954) reviewed the theories which regarded depersonalisation as a feature of cerebral dysfunction, citing the work of Penfield & Jasper (1947) on the results of stimulating the exposed temporal lobe during neurosurgery. Ackner concluded "there is no doubt that, if any one area of the brain is to be held more responsible than another, the organisation of the temporal lobe is such that it has the highest claim to consideration".

Further studies in Newcastle on the classification of affective disorders tended to confirm the earlier observations. A factorial analysis, (Roth *et al*, 1965) on 37 items drawn from a standard interview on 275 patients with neurotic disorders showed that features previously identified, i.e. situational phobias, panic attacks, depersonalisation, 'temporal lobe' features and attacks of unconsciousness tended to form a co-varying cluster. However, as Marks (1969), pointed out, it would be premature to conclude that the occurrence of 'temporal lobe' symptoms necessarily indicates a disturbance of temporal lobe function. Indeed, similar phenomena are found in otherwise normal subjects (Harper, 1969). The use of the term 'temporal lobe' may be misleading, although it was made clear that this was a convenient descriptive title incorporating the concept of depersonalisation as a pre-formed defence mechanism with the hypothesis that this may involve "a complex neuronal system closely interrelated both anatomically and physiologically" with the temporal lobe and adjacent regions (Harper & Roth, 1962).

## Neurosis and epilepsy

The prominence of 'temporal lobe features' such as *déjà vu* experiences, formed hallucinations and episodic depersonalisation in patients with phobic anxiety raises a diagnostic issue. Harper & Roth (1962) reviewed the significance of the non-convulsive forms of epilepsy described by Hughlings Jackson as 'epileptiform', of 'ictal' anxiety, paroxysmalness, 'reminiscence', and the ambiguities which arise from electroencephalographic evidence which falls short of the classical repetitive, unambiguous spike or spike and slow wave discharge with paroxysmal qualities recorded during a typical epileptic fit.

The diagnostic differentiation of epilepsy from other states, particularly neurotic disorders, presents many difficulties in spite of substantial developments in EEG technology. Mayer-Gross *et al* (1960) regarded it as "perhaps one of the most complex problems in medicine and one in which mistakes are frequent and may be fatal for the patient". Todd (1968), in a study of all referrals to an out-patient psychiatric service, showed that 19.4% of cases gave a history of recent 'blackouts'—a term of uncertain meaning (Nichols, 1963). Of 136 patients presenting with 'blackouts' 47% had psychogenic disorders and the next most common single diagnosis was epilepsy (12.5%). The dangers of over-interpreting the EEG have frequently been commented upon. It is now also recognised that the diagnosis and treatment of epilepsy increase the risk of pseudo-epileptic attacks. These issues have been fully reviewed by Riley & Roy (1982) where the relationship between epilepsy, hysteria, syncope, narcolepsy, migraine and a range of other episodic disorders including acute intermittent porphyria, paroxysmal symptoms in multiple sclerosis, paroxysmal choreo-athetosis etc are considered in terms of differential diagnosis. Jonas (1965) and Whitten (1969) suggested that a correct diagnosis of epilepsy was being missed by psychiatrically orientated practitioners. Collings (1958), Revitch (1964, 1966) and Toone & Roberts (1979) describe patients previously diagnosed as epileptic in whom the evidence on closer review favoured a non-epileptic diagnosis. Bergman & Green (1956) pointed out the problems of misinterpreting the EEG in patients with psychogenic disorder and Betts *et al* (1976) have reviewed related diagnostic issues.

A detailed comparative study of 30 phobic anxiety depersonalisation syndrome (PADS) cases, defined operationally, with 30 cases of temporal lobe epilepsy (TLE) drawn largely from out-patient neurological clinics, showed a considerable overlap in symptomatology as well as statistically significant differences (Harper & Roth, 1962; Roth & Harper, 1962). Acute episodes of anxiety, depersonalisation, *déjà vu* experiences and other phenomena often regarded as of special significance in the diagnosis of temporal lobe epilepsy occurred in patients with severe phobic anxiety states. Falling and loss of consciousness due to vaso-depressor syncope was confined to the neurotic group but did not wholly account for the overlap in symptomatology. In all the neurotic patients, attacks had occurred following emotional stress but these features, although positively related to the diagnosis of neurosis, were of less value in deciding whether or not a patient had epilepsy. The occurrence of phobic anxiety symptoms in patients with proven epilepsy illustrates the limitations of this approach. The points of similarity between the epileptic and neurotic groups had considerable significance. These comprised the occurrence in both groups of depersonalisation, *déjà vu* experiences, metamorphopsia, and other perceptual disturbances including formed hallucinations and memory disturbances. Paroxysmal attacks of fear, epigastric sensations progressing to attacks with disturbance or loss of consciousness and a history of anxiety and depressive symptoms precipitated by emotional stress occurred in both groups. Features considered central to the diagnosis of epilepsy—attacks with falling, loss of consciousness, incontinence and motor convulsions occurred occasionally in the neurotic patients, usually in association with syncopal features.

One way of resolving the diagnostic difficulties is to deny the validity of a sharp distinction between epilepsy and neurosis, i.e. the continuum hypothesis. Diethelm (1948) wrote, "In epilepsy the neurogenic and psychogenic are inseparably involved. Instead of accepting an either/or attitude one should look for quantitative differentiation". Barker & Barker (1950) suggested a spectrum, ranging from psychomotor convulsive equivalents through various manifestations described as neurotic to relatively appropriate expressions of thought, feeling and action and there have been a number of syndromes described, e.g. ictal neurosis, diacopal seizures, latent epilepsy, episodic behaviour disorders, episodic dyscontrol syndromes, etc. in which attempts have been made to categorise the interface between neurotic and epileptic conditions.

## The derivation of a diagnostic index

Part of the difficulty derives from the inability of any single feature within the clinical history to indicate a diagnosis unequivocally. Relative diagnostic values can, however, be conveniently expressed mathematically as the numerical weight assigned to each feature to maximise the possibility of diagnostic discrimination. To explore this further, data from the comparative study were submitted to multivariate statistical analysis and the results applied to a further group of 15 patients where the differential diagnosis had presented particular difficulties.

As an initial step, discriminant function analysis was applied to the original data. This procedure maximises the separation between pre-determined groups and provides weights which can be used to predict the classification of additional cases with the smallest possibility of error. The analysis requires an existing classification as its starting point. Hazards in the interpretation of the results of discriminant function analysis have been fully discussed (Hope, 1968; Grayson, 1987). The weight assigned to a particular feature cannot be regarded as an absolute measure of its diagnostic significance because features in any given analysis may interact in a complex fashion and much depends upon the selection of the items used in both the clinical and statistical analyses. Nevertheless, this procedure serves to quantify the symptomatology by giving each feature an explicit weight derived mathematically to contribute to a pre-determined classification. It demonstrates important steps in the complex process of making a clinical diagnosis and converts the clinical evaluation into what Bauer (1956) described as "that one tangible asset, a figure".

The potential application of a diagnostic index will be illustrated by reference to the 15 patients who were initially placed in an undiagnosed group and who shared the clinical features of both neurosis and epilepsy. These 15 patients were all referred for diagnosis and treatment; 13 were seen in the Department of Psychological Medicine in Newcastle and two further cases were seen in the Department of Psychological Medicine at the University of Queensland. Five were referred by general practitioners, eight by consultant neurologists and two by general physicians. All 15 patients had been suspected of having temporal lobe epilepsy and 12 had received anti-convulsant treatment. In addition, the 15 showed prominent neurotic features so that the diagnosis after careful initial interview remained equivocal.

The mean age of the undiagnosed group was 39.7 years, higher than the mean age of the two diagnosed groups, but not significantly so. The mean age of onset of illness was 33.5 years, significantly higher than the mean age of onset of the diagnosed groups ( $P < 0.05$ ). The undiagnosed group resembled the neurotic patients in being mostly women, four of whom gave a family history of neurotic illness. None had a family history of epilepsy. As in the diagnosed neurotic group, the illnesses had generally begun after stress and some of the individual attacks in the undiagnosed group appeared to be precipitated by emotional arousal. Attacks with a termination which was invariably sudden and attacks with a regular 'march' of symptoms were uncommon. In six of the group attacks of variable duration occurred. The undiagnosed group also resembled the neurotic group in that phobic anxiety, reactive depressive symptoms, sustained anxiety, a history of suicidal attempts or preoccupations and feelings of unsteadiness were common. Neurotic personality traits including mild chronic phobias, dependence, a low anxiety threshold and a history of phobias and other neurotic traits in childhood were also prominent. Attacks with syncopal features were identified in six of the undiagnosed group. Migraine had occurred in six patients, the same proportion as in the neurotic group.

As with the epileptic patients, a history of automatisms occurred in five cases with attacks of incontinence, self-injury, falling and a disturbance of consciousness followed by feelings of confusion being not uncommon. Three patients gave a history of illnesses likely to be associated with cerebral damage. Anxiety attacks with autonomic symptoms, episodic depersonalisation, episodic *déjà vu*

TABLE I

*Simplified weights derived from a discriminant function analysis of 20 items used for the calculation of patient scores*

| Clinical feature | Present | Absent |
|---|---|---|
| Family history of epilepsy | − 1 | − 2 |
| History of cerebral damage | 1 | 2 |
| History of infections | − 2 | − 4 |
| Situational phobias | 23 | 46 |
| Persistent anxiety | 20 | 40 |
| Stress at onset of illness | − 30 | − 15 |
| Emotional precipitation of attacks | − 6 | − 3 |
| Fixed 'march' in attacks | 6 | 3 |
| Termination of attacks, always sudden | 4 | 8 |
| Episodic speech disturbance | − 21 | − 42 |
| Automatisms | − 11 | − 22 |
| Episodic *déjà vu* | 7 | 14 |
| Episodic depersonalisation | 0 | 0 |
| Complete loss of awareness | − 16 | − 32 |
| Attacks with no change of awareness | − 6 | − 12 |
| Syncopal features | 17 | 34 |
| Self-injury in attacks | − 6 | − 12 |
| Incontinence in attacks | − 2 | − 4 |
| Convulsive movements | 4 | 8 |

| | Normal | Mild Non-specific | Abnormal | Epileptiform |
|---|---|---|---|---|
| EEG | − 48 | − 36 | − 24 | − 12 |

| *Patient scores on the 20 Item Scale* | | | | |
|---|---|---|---|---|
| 30 cases of PADS | | Mean | − 89.7 | S.D. 11.18 |
| | | Range | | − 109 to − 62 |
| 30 cases of TLE | | Mean | 3.5 | S.D. 10.92 |
| | | Range | | − 20 to 20 |
| PADS—TLE: | $t = -32.1312$, | | d.f. | 58, $P < 0.01$ |

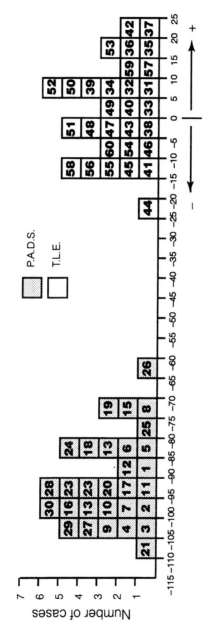

*Fig. 1. Distribution of diagnosed cases on a diagnostic index of 20 items*

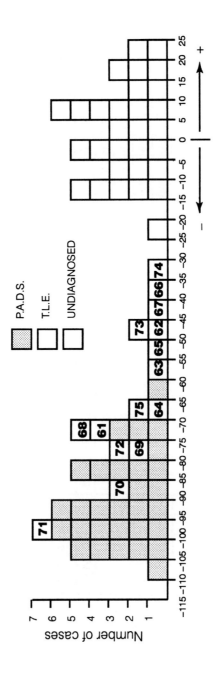

*Fig. 2. Distribution of 15 undiagnosed cases on a diagnostic index of 20 items*

experiences, attacks with loss of awareness, a history of convulsions and attacks precipitated by stress were found in proportionately more of these patients than in the neurotic group but proportionately less than in the epileptic group. Attacks with prominent mood change, disturbances of body image and formed hallucinations with insight occurred more commonly in the undiagnosed group than in either the diagnosed epileptic or neurotic patients. In none of the undiagnosed group was the EEG found to be diagnostic of epilepsy, although in six cases it was judged to be abnormal and in seven cases mild non-specific abnormalities had been found. In spite of the uncertainty in diagnosis, 12 of the 15 had received anti-convulsant therapy.

When the diagnosed patients' scores on the discriminant function analysis were plotted, complete separation into two groups corresponding to the original known groups of PADS and TLE was secured. Twenty items used to provide satisfactory discrimination are listed in Table I and Fig. 1 shows the distribution of cases on an index derived from these 20 items. The features included episodic depersonalisation, episodic *déjà vu*, precipitation of the illness by stress and a history that individual attacks were triggered by emotion. The scores of the 15 patients in the undiagnosed group were then calculated using this diagnostic index and plotted to show the distribution (Fig. 2). Eight of the 15 patients secured scores within the neurotic range whereas the remaining seven patients are distributed in the no man's land between the scores of epileptic and phobic patients. Thus on this index the undiagnosed group tended to resemble the neurotic patients rather than the epileptic patients in respect of the items included. Though some of the patients had histories highly suggestive of epilepsy they were distinguished from the epileptic subjects when only a small range of clinical symptomatology was sampled. This leaves open the question of whether these cases represent an intermediate form of disorder, a combination of both neurotic disorder and epilepsy or a diagnostic mixture of cases. The source of the clinical material and the criteria used to place patients in the undiagnosed group, i.e. having a clinical picture for which a diagnosis of either neurosis or epilepsy might be appropriate, made it inevitable that patients in this group would have some 'neurotic' features. If epilepsy is regarded as a categorical disorder, the issue then becomes whether these patients also have a form of epilepsy.

## Follow-up study

In the absence of unequivocal electroencephalographic data the only other procedure available for clarifying the diagnostic problem was a follow-up study with information on the further course of the patient's illness and its response to treatment. The 15 patients in the undiagnosed group and a few additional cases of interest were followed up with the help of their general practitioners and the records departments of the hospitals concerned. Thirteen of the 15 patients were seen personally and the information they supplied was supplemented by discussions with the family doctor and a review of their case records. Two patients were not seen personally in spite of visits to their homes. The home visit, however, resulted in helpful information from the patients' nearest relative which enabled a diagnostic conclusion to be reached for these two patients.

TABLE II
*Summary of follow-up results on 15 undiagnosed patients*

| Diagnostic conclusion | |
|---|---|
| Firm diagnosis of neurotic disorder | 11 |
| Neurotic disorder probable | 1 |
| Diagnosis equivocal | 2 |
| Neurotic state with barbiturate withdrawal fits | 1 |
| *Status at follow-up* | |
| Firm diagnosis of epilepsy | 0 |
| Continuing treatment from GP | 8 |
| Continuing treatment from psychiatrist | 3 |
| Receiving anti-convulsants | 6 |
| Receiving other drugs | 7 |
| Dependent on drugs | 8 |

The average duration of follow-up was 7.45 years with a range of three to nine years. Many patients records antedating the initial interview used for the clinical survey were also available for scrutiny. The final diagnoses for the undiagnosed group were made prior to and independently of the calculation of their scores on the diagnostic indices, the latter being based on data secured and coded at the time of initial interview. However, the diagnostic conclusions may have been influenced by the results of the earlier comparative study and by experience accumulated since the original information was collected. The follow-up information is summarised in Table II. On the evidence from the follow-up study it was concluded that 12 of the 15 patients had a neurotic illness without epilepsy. One patient was found after repeated study to have suffered from epileptic fits secondary to barbiturate dependence in the setting of a neurotic personality disorder. In two patients the diagnosis remained uncertain. Both patients continued to have attacks at the time of follow-up which could have been epileptic. In none of the patients had the possibility of temporal lobe epilepsy been confirmed by further observations. Nevertheless, six of the 15 were still receiving anti-convulsant therapy. There was evidence of dependence upon anti-convulsants in five of these cases. Six of the 15 patients were in good health and not troubled by continuing symptoms of any severity. Nine continued to have symptoms relevant to the study, although quasi-epileptic features were only conspicuous in three cases.

Discriminant function analysis has shown that separation of patients into neurotic and epileptic groups can be easily achieved without overlap using only a small amount of the clinical information available. This procedure does not explore alternative classifications of therapeutic or pathophysiological validity. The discriminant function analysis imposes a classification and the question of a continuum of disorders remains unresolved.

## Category or dimension?

This question can be further explored using a principal component analysis. This is a precise and convenient mathematical technique for describing a correlation matrix in terms of independent components which each account for a proportion of the total variance. These individual correlations may then be expressed as factor loadings or weights for each feature in respect of these components.

The components or factors in a principal component analysis do not necessarily correspond to fundamental properties of the subject matter. The procedure is "simply a means of reducing a cumbersome matrix of correlations to a more manageable size with the minimum loss of information" (Kendell, 1968). Nevertheless, components may relate to clinically relevant dimensions and, by multiplying the patient's score for a given feature against the factor loading for that feature, clinically significant groupings of patients may be suggested.

The correlation matrix on which the analysis was carried out included data from all the patients, including the undiagnosed group. Any grouping which emerges derives from the scores of the clinical features and not from the assigned diagnostic classification. Nevertheless this procedure does not exclude the possibility that halo effects from the attributed diagnosis contaminated the interpretation of symptoms and contributed to diagnostic groupings which emerge in the computer analysis. At least the diagnostic assumptions derived are made overt and explicit.

The analysis was carried out on a correlation matrix of 50 features using data from all 75 patients. Further analyses were carried out to produce independent dimensions. From those features which had a low loading on the first component of the principal component analysis a conspicuous co-varying cluster of 16 features was selected. An identical analysis was performed on 23 features with factor

TABLE III
*Simplified weights for the calculation of Ep scores from 16 features*

| If feature present or positive | Score |
| --- | --- |
| History of cerebral damage | 8 |
| History of cerebral infections | 6 |
| No stress at onset of illness | 9 |
| No precipitation of attacks | 10 |
| Termination of attacks, always sudden | 9 |
| Speech disturbance | 5 |
| Automatisms | 7 |
| Difficulty in recall | 8 |
| Total loss of awareness | 8 |
| Falling | 6 |
| Injury during attacks | 9 |
| Incontinence | 8 |
| Convulsions | 11 |
| Electroencephalographic data— | |
|     Epileptiform EEG | 10 |
|     Abnormal EEG | 6 |
|     Non-specific abnormalities | 3 |
|     Normal EEG | 0 |
| Age of onset | |
|     0–9 years | 12 |
|     10–19 years | 8 |
|     20–29 years | 6 |
|     30–39 years | 4 |
|     40–49 years | 2 |
|     Over 50 years | 0 |
| Duration of illness | |
|     Over 10 years | 10 |
|     6–10 years | 7 |
|     1–5 years | 3 |
|     Less than 1 year | 0 |

TABLE IV
*Simplified weights for the calculation of the N scores from 23 features*

| If feature is present or positive | Score |
|---|---|
| Migraine | 4 |
| Childhood phobias | 6 |
| Poor work record | 5 |
| Emotional instability | 7 |
| Mild chronic phobias | 7 |
| Emotional immaturity | 6 |
| Paranoid traits | 5 |
| Depersonalisation | 5 |
| Phobic anxiety | 9 |
| Persistent anxiety | 8 |
| Reactive Depression | 7 |
| Suicidal preoccupations | 6 |
| 'Hysterical' features | 7 |
| No regular 'march' | 6 |
| Episodic anxiety | 7 |
| Episodic autonomic symptoms | 4 |
| Formed hallucinations | 4 |
| Disturbances of perception | 4 |
| *Déjà vu* experiences | 3 |
| Episodic depersonalisation | 4 |
| Feelings of unsteadiness | 8 |
| Attacks preceded by tension | 3 |
| Syncopal features | 5 |

loadings at the opposite neurotic pole of the first component. The cluster of 16 items (Table III) were those relating to a diagnosis of epilepsy (Ep). The 23 features from the opposite pole of the first component (N) were largely those described in the phobic anxiety-depersonalisation syndrome (Table IV). The first component from the principal component analysis of the cluster of epileptic features represented 31.4% of the variance and the first component of the neurotic cluster 26.6% of the variance. Each of the 75 patients received two scores for components which represent the loading for the principal components of both symptom clusters. The patients' scores on these independently derived components were then plotted with the axes at right-angles. This procedure allowed the patients to be distributed in terms of the two syndromes identified by the original analysis. It allowed the neurotic symptoms in some epileptics and the quasi-epileptic features in patients with a phobic anxiety-depersonalisation syndrome to be scored separately.

The distribution of scores clarifies the diagnostic overlap and provides some quantification of the anxiety symptoms in epileptic patients. A high score on the Ep component does not prove that a patient is suffering from epilepsy but only that he/she tends to resemble epileptic subjects in respect of the 16 features involved. Those patients with the highest scores on the N factor also tended to have higher Ep scores. The N and Ep scores were positively correlated ($r = 0.467$, $P < 0.01$) whereas there was no significant correlation between the two scales for the 30 patients diagnosed as having temporal lobe epilepsy. This suggests that the quasi-epileptic features were more common in those neurotic patients with many of the 23 neurotic features than in those with few. This is confirmed by a re-examination of the clinical material. Those phobic patients who presented with attacks associated with loss of awareness and prominent 'temporal lobe'

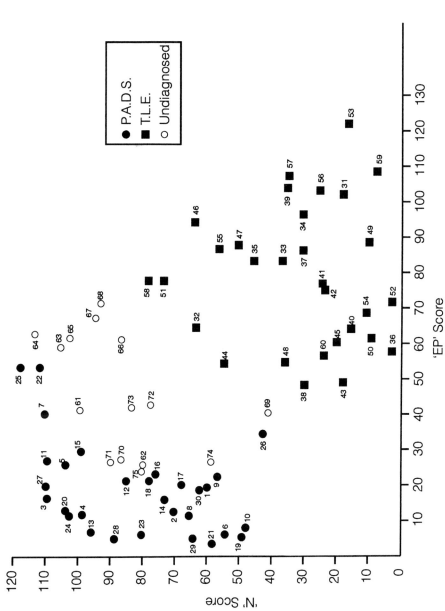

*Fig. 3. Distribution of 75 cases on 'Neurotic' and 'Epileptic' factors, derived from an analysis of symptom clusters, using simplified weights*

features tended to be those suffering from the more severe generalised anxiety states with multiple and severe neurotic personality traits.

The scores of the undiagnosed patients were also calculated on the Ep and N components. These patients had N factor scores within the range of the diagnosed neurotics. Six also had Ep factor scores within the range of the diagnosed epileptic patients. This procedure vividly illustrates the equivocal diagnostic status of many of the patients in this group. The two cases who remained undiagnosed after the period of follow-up both had high N and high Ep scores (Fig. 3).

The estimation of a patient's score on the separate Ep and N factors allows the strength of each component to be independently described. This procedure is helpful in arriving at an objective appraisal of symptomatology and in formulating a diagnosis by making a mathematical comparison between a new case and an existing population of known diagnosis. A score below the epileptic range on the Ep factor suggests that few features central to the clinical picture of epilepsy are present. If this had been interpreted as indicating insufficient evidence for a diagnosis of epilepsy nine of the 15 originally undiagnosed patients would have been correctly assigned to the neurotic group on the basis of their initial symptomatology, without the additional information from the long follow-up period and without the hazards of unnecessary anti-convulsant medication. A high Ep factor score when combined with a high N score suggests an alternative explanation for the quasi-epileptic features. The scores of the undiagnosed patients and the follow-up data suggest that these patients were mostly atypical and severely neurotic. It is parsimonious to conclude that a major part of the similarity between PADS and TLE relates to an overlap between such distinct conditions as psychogenic panic and ictal anxiety. It does not resolve the tantalising possibility originally raised by Roth that depersonalisation, *déjà vu* and other experiences arising in patients with agoraphobia demonstrate some functional disturbance of the temporal lobe or limbic system. This question can only be resolved by other lines of evidence.

The dichotomy agoraphobia/partial complex seizures represents only one of the many diagnostic conundrums which patients with 'funny turns' present to the clinician and this limits the general applicability of the Ep and N indices I have described. The early detection of treatable cerebral disease in patients presenting with symptoms suggestive of focal epilepsy of late onset is an important clinical priority. But costly, unnecessary and potentially harrowing investigations may be avoided in some cases by careful and informed evaluation of the history (including of course the history provided by observers) and a recognition of the frequency with which panic attacks and agoraphobic symptoms are combined with quasi-epileptic features suggestive of temporal lobe dysfunction. 'Temporal lobe symptoms' as part of an epileptic fit point to a focus in the temporal regions but similar symptoms in a neurotic disorder do not signal a diagnosis of epilepsy.

A premature diagnosis of epilepsy should be avoided. Trials of anti-convulsant treatment before a firm diagnosis has been reached are rarely indicated. Organic pathology can be identified by the use where appropriate of ambulatory EEG monitoring, 24 hour monitoring with video recording, and non-invasive radiological techniques such as computerised axial tomography. These procedures all permit the clinician to tolerate diagnostic uncertainty while providing support and awaiting developments which may place the diagnosis beyond doubt.

However, such techniques rest upon the validity of diagnostic entities. Roth (1960) explained the importance of 'simple nose-counting operations' as part of the judicious balance to be struck between sterile nosography and understanding based upon the dynamics of symptom formation—castigating Virchow who regarded pharyngeal and laryngeal diphtheria as unrelated examples of a membrane-forming order of inflammatory disease until bacteriological advances re-united diphtheria and croup as manifestations of a single entity.

The distinction between epileptic disorders and anxiety states in which quasi-epileptic features are prominent has heuristic value. The latter conditions are not associated with specifically epileptiform abnormalities in the EEG, there is little convincing evidence that anti-convulsant drugs are particularly beneficial, and they have a benign prognosis. However, there is still much to learn about the territories on either side of this borderland and 'more arithmetic' is an important precursor to further pathophysiological studies on the cerebral basis of neurotic disorder. Roth concluded his 1960 paper by quoting from an essay by Walshe: "It will be my submission, then, that the naturalist in medicine and his study which we call nosography is not an embryonic stage in the growth of modern medicine, but the very root and trunk of medicine upon which all else must be grafted, and by which alone the grafts can become fruitful."

## Acknowledgements

The work on which this study was based was begun during the tenure of a Mental Health Research Fund grant in the Department of Psychological Medicine, in the University of Newcastle, under the direction of Professor (Sir) Martin Roth. It was supported throughout by Professor Roth and it stems from his productive enthusiasm. Dr Roger Garside provided advice on the statistics and computer analysis with the practical help of Miss Eleanor Foster and Miss S. Allison. Mr J. W. Osselton and Dr Peter Leyburn assisted in the collection of the EEG data and the epilepsy cases were largely derived from the clinics of (the late) Dr Henry Miller and Dr (now Sir) John Walton. The discriminant function and principal component analyses and follow up studies were carried out in Newcastle, during a period of study leave from the University of Queensland and the material forms part of an MD thesis of the University of Queensland. My colleagues in both Departments, especially Professor F. A. Whitlock in Queensland and Dr D. W. Kay in Newcastle, provided much support and guidance. The mistakes are my own.

## References

ACKNER, B. (1954) Depersonalization. *Journal of Mental Science*, **100**, 838–872.

BARKER, W. & BARKER, S. (1950) Experimental production of human convulsive brain potentials by stress-induced effects upon normal integrative function: dynamics of the convulsive reaction to stress. In *Life stress and Bodily Diseases* (eds H. G. Wolff, S. G. Wolf & C. H. Hare). Baltimore: Williams & Wilkins.

BAUER, R. E. (1956) The present status of the diagnosis of hyper-thyroidism. *Annals of International Medicine*, **44**, 207–214.

BERGMAN, P. S. & GREEN, M. A. (1956) The use of electroencephalography in differentiating psychogenic disorders and organic brain diseases. *American Journal of Psychiatry*, **113**, 27–31.

BETTS, T. A., MERSKEY, H. & POND, D. A. (1976) Psychiatry. In *A Textbook of Epilepsy* (eds J. Laidlaw, A. Richens). Edinburgh: Churchill Livingstone.

COLLINGS, H. JR (1958) Recall with amobarbital (amytal) sodium in diagnosis of seizures. *Archives of Neurology & Psychiatry*, **80**, 408–413.

DIETHELM, O. (1948) Differential diagnosis of epilepsy. In *Epilepsy—Psychiatric Aspects of Convulsive Disorders*. (eds P. H. Hoch & R. P. Knight). New York: Grune & Stratton.

GRAYSON, D. A. (1987) Can categorical and dimensional views of psychiatric illness be distinguished? *British Journal of Psychiatry*, **151**, 355–361.

HARPER, M. & ROTH, M. (1962) Temporal lobe epilepsy and the phobic anxiety-depersonalization syndrome. *Comprehensive Psychiatry*, **3**, 129–151.

—— (1969) Déjà vu and depersonalization in normal subjects. *Australian and New Zealand Journal of Psychiatry*, **3**, 67–74.

HOPE, K. (1968) *Methods of Multivariate Analysis*. London: University of London Press.

JONAS, A. D. (1965) *Ictal and Subictal Neurosis: Diagnosis and Treatment*. Illinois: C. C. Thomas.

KENDELL, R. E. (1968) An important source of bias affecting ratings made by psychiatrists. *Journal of Psychiatric Research*, **6**, 135–141.

MARKS, I. M. (1969) *Fears and Phobias*. London: William Heinemann. p. 139.

MAYER-GROSS, W. (1935) On depersonalization. *British Journal of Medical Psychology*, **15**, 103–122.

——, SLATER, E. & ROTH, M. (1960) *Clinical Psychiatry*. London: Cassell.

NICHOLS, W. M. (1963) Funny turns. *Proceedings of the British Student Health Association*. **15**, 48–54.

OBERNDORF, C. P. (1950) The role of anxiety in depersonalization. *International Journal of Psycho-Analysis*, Vol. XXXI, Parts 1 & 2.

PALMER, H. A. (1941) A psycho-biological approach to the acute anxiety attack. *Journal of Mental Science*, **87**, 208.

PENFIELD, W. & JASPER, H. (1947) Highest level seizures. *Association for Research in Nervous and Mental Diseases Proceedings*. (Baltimore), **26**, 252.

REVITCH, E. (1964) Paroxymsal manifestations of non-epileptic origin. *Diseases of the Nervous System*, **25**, 662–670.

—— (1966) Episodes of inattention and perceptual alterations. *Diseases of the Nervous System*, **27**, 789–794.

RILEY, T. L. & ROY, A. (eds). (1982) *Pseudoseizures*. Baltimore: Williams & Wilkins.

ROTH, M. (1959) The phobic anxiety-depersonalization syndrome. *Proceedings of the Royal Society of Medicine*, **52**, 587–594.

—— (1960) The phobic anxiety-depersonalization syndrome and some general aetiological problems in psychiatry. *Journal of Neuropsychiatry*, **1**, 293–306.

——, GARSIDE, R. F. & GURNEY, C. (1965) Clinical-statistical enquiries into the classification of anxiety states and depressive disorders. In *Proceedings of the Leeds Symposium on Behavioural Disorders*. (ed. F. A. Jenner) Dagenham: May & Baker.

—— & HARPER, M. (1962) Temporal lobe epilepsy and the phobic anxiety-depersonalization syndrome. *Comprehensive Psychiatry*, **3**, 215–226.

SHORVON, H. J. (1946) The depersonalization syndrome. *Proceedings of the Royal Society of Medicine*, **39**, 779–792.

TODD, J. M. (1968) Blackouts. Unpublished PhD thesis: University of Aberdeen, 1968.

TOONE, B. K. & ROBERTS, J. (1979) Status Epilepticus: An uncommon hysterical conversion syndrome. *Journal of Nervous and Mental Disease*, **167**, 548–552.

WHITLOCK, F. A. (1967) The aetiology of hysteria. *Acta Psychiatrica Neurologica Scandinavica*, **43**, 144–162.

WHITTEN, J. R. (1969) Psychical seizures. *American Journal of Psychiatry*, **126**, 560–565.

# 23 Depression in general practice: The Newcastle connection

## THOMAS J. FAHY

In the 1960s, as a Mental Health Research Fund Fellow, I worked with David Kay, Roger Garside and Sydney Brandon on the Newcastle Depression Project. This project included comparative work on depression rating scales, (Fahy, 1969a) a comparison of phenelzine with amitriptyline in out-patients, (Kay, Garside & Fahy, 1973), the first controlled study of continuation therapy in ECT-treated depressives (Kay, Fahy & Garside, 1970), the prediction of ECT response (Fahy, Kay & Garside, 1969) and a general practice study described below (Fahy, Brandon & Garside, 1969). These were days of pondering the exact definition of symptoms and signs in conferences with Martin Roth.

Argument about symptoms on the points of psychopathological pins sometimes bordered on the medieval. Paper tape feed for the KDF 9 computer had to be punched by hand and the computerisation of psychiatric data was still the subject of merry derision among computer staff. There was a special atmosphere of the kind that can only be generated by a Department Head whose own enthusiasm for research is so transparently obvious as to be available to his colleagues by some kind of simple osmosis. Martin Roth was, and still is, like that.

The clinical-statistical approach of what has come to be known as the Newcastle School to problems of psychiatric nosology is well known. The essence of the approach developed by Martin Roth, Roger Garside, Leslie Kiloh and others was the careful definition of discrete items of psychopathology, and the application to their inter-correlations of multivariate statistical analysis. The results of this 'neo-Kraepelinian' method have been published widely throughout the 1960s and 1970s and will not be reviewed here. In the field of affective disorders one central finding was the demonstration of a categorical patient sub-type characterised by 'endogenous' symptoms, predictive of illness course and/or treatment response (Kiloh & Garside, 1963; Carney, Roth & Garside, 1965; Kiloh & Garside, 1977). The Newcastle view, that the endogenous sub-type exists, has been sometimes misinterpreted as a *dichotomous* position: that is, that the majority of depressives are either endogenous or 'neurotic'. In fact, nowhere in the Newcastle writings is there any statement to be found which might be interpreted to mean that there are any two depressive patient sub-types or syndromes which are mutually exclusive. This erroneous interpretation may owe something to bad communication but also stems from the vigorous opposition of those who support a dimensional model with endogenous and non-endogenous patients distributed fairly evenly along a continuum. Debates on these issues were conducted for the most part in esoteric statistical jargon (Kendell, 1976; Ni Bhrolchain, 1979; Roth, Garside, Gurney & Kerr, 1979) and many psychiatrists tired of following the argument. Findings supportive of the categorical (Newcastle) view were subject to two main criticisms. First, *bias* due to clinical preconception might have unduly influenced the results. The second, and perhaps the most telling criticism, was that the Newcastle work was confined to patients in hospital or specialty-service-associated patients who were not representative of the broad range of depressive subjects in the community. These criticisms apart, it seems likely now that the antagonists were arguing from different premises. In Newcastle, results depended on selection of items of psychopathology which were potentially discriminating: this was followed by sequential mathematical exclusion of non-discriminating items until a good discriminating dimension remained.

Other centres, and especially the Maudsley group exemplified by Kendell (1968), preferred check lists or case records to a specially constructed clinical interview as sources of data: this rather different approach did not yield convincing bimodal distributions of patients. Other studies also failed to replicate the Newcastle findings. Confirmation did, however, come from the US study by Sandifer, Wilson & Green (1966) whose approach was basically the same as that of the Newcastle workers. Ironically, further support from an unexpected quarter came from the demonstration of bimodality when Sir Aubrey Lewis's original data were analysed by Kiloh & Garside (1977).

The ensuing debates never reached any kind of closure. This is hardly surprising since there is little common ground between work based on information from clinical interview on the one hand and that based on possibly unbiased, but doubtfully relevant, data on the other. For a time the classification of affective disorders became unattractive as a subject for intensive investigation. More recently, however, some new developments have rekindled interest in this area. These include:

  (a) continued commercial interest in promoting drugs for depression—in particular, drugs for depression in general practice
  (b) the information explosion in neurochemistry opening up better opportunities for inter-disciplinary research
  (c) the belated recognition (Hoeper, Nycz, Cleary *et al*, 1979; Goldberg & Bridges, 1987) that mood disorders dominate the psychiatric morbidity of general practice which in turn has emerged as a public health problem of international proportions (Shepherd, Wilkinson & Williams, 1986)
  (d) a remarkable new trend (Williams & Clare, 1981; Mitchell, 1985; Strathdee & Williams, 1984) for British psychiatrists to spend more time in general practice liaison work
  (e) an accumulation of epidemiological evidence suggesting that melancholia in young people is on the increase (Klerman, 1987).
  (f) The sequential development of operational research criteria culminating in DSM–III–R and (imminently) ICD–10.

These were some of the influences which stimulated fresh interest in the classification of mood disorders outside the confines of psychiatric services. A number of fresh arguments have arisen. These include a seemingly endless debate on the issue of what constitutes a 'case' (Wing, Bebbington & Robins, 1981) and conflicting views as to whether affective disorders in the community are quantitatively or qualitatively different from the clinical material presenting to the hospital psychiatrist (Blacker & Clare, 1987). Other issues include a sociological approach to the aetiology of mood disorders (Brown & Harris, 1978, 1986; Henderson *et al*, 1981) and the complex associations between the latter and general somatic morbidity (Bridges & Goldberg, 1985). One net effect has been renewed concern about the clinical forms, natural history and outcome of psychiatric syndromes in extra-mural settings.

## The Newcastle general practice study

The present paper summarises one of the few attempts to extend the Newcastle approach to the study of depression in general practice. Much of the data presented is either unpublished (Fahy, 1969b; Fahy, Kay & Garside, 1969) or published obscurely (Fahy, 1969a, Fahy 1977). The paper concludes with a brief discussion placing these early observations in the context of more recent work.

### Material and methods

In 1966, eight general practitioners (seven in a group practice and the eighth in single handed private practice) identified, during a period of three months, 223 patients as being currently in need of treatment for depression and not suffering from schizophrenia, brain damage or mental subnormality. These cases comprised about 8 % of all attenders and included a slight excess of patients from middle social classes and under-representation of the aged from among those at risk. One hundred and thirty three consented to a research interview and were seen personally within one week of identification. Few referred patients failed to complete the research interview. The commonest cause of non-referral in 90 cases was the reluctance of the family doctor to suggest that his patient attend for psychiatric screening. No other major clinical or demographic characteristic distinguished the two groups.

At the research interview 52 pre-defined clinical features were recorded as present or absent and 43 of common occurrence were retained for subsequent analysis. A 30 % random sub-sample was given (at the same interview) a fully structured interview, Spitzer's Mental Status Schedule (Spitzer *et al*, 1966) and use was made of a number of standard psychiatric rating scales. At follow-up three to four months later, patients were rated for global outcome and change score on a number of rating scales. Unless otherwise stated, methods and results refer to 126 cases seen and followed up personally.

### Statistical methods

Using principal components analysis with varimax rotation, four clusters of clinical features were isolated each comprising five clinical features only. Factor analysis (unrotated) of the correlations within each cluster or syndrome yielded weighted *cluster scores*. Each of the 126 patients thus had four scores indicating the extent to which his or her clinical picture corresponded to that depicted in each of the four clusters. The distributions of scores were each subjected to the chi-square test for goodness of fit to normal.

**Results**

The clusters or *statistical syndromes* are depicted in Table I. They were interpreted as A: reactive depression; B: distinct quality-unvarying depression; C: phobic anxious depression; and D: severe suicidal depression. The distribution of patient scores for each of the syndromes (five variables) and the combined four syndromes (20 variables) are in Fig. 1.

*Cluster A (responsive reactive)* depicted a syndrome of depressed mood which could be temporarily alleviated. Other features included environmental precipitants, self-pity, a tendency to project and 'immature personality'. The generally normal distribution of cluster scores indicated that A was a *common trait* in the material and did not identify a distinct class of patient.

*Cluster B (distinct quality)* bore obvious resemblance to endogenous depression except for the absence of objective retardation which was virtually absent from this case material (Fahy, 1974a). B depicted a qualitatively distinct and constant depression syndrome, subjective retardation, regular morning exacerbation of symptoms and depressive loss of affect. Scores for B correlated − 0.63 with those for A. A bimodal and significantly abnormal distribution of scores for B confirmed the research hypothesis with the patients falling into two distinct groups according to whether they corresponded to B or were distinguished by an absence of B features (Fig. 1).

*Cluster C (neurotic/phobic)* was dominated by a history of maladaptive stress reaction ('neurotic'), situational phobias, circumscribed panic attacks, persistent anxiety and 'obsessional personality'. The distribution of scores for C was trimodal. This indicated that this syndrome discriminated three distinct groups: phobic anxious depressive patients (panic disorder?); non-phobic anxious depressive patients; and non-anxious (and non-phobic) depressive patients. There was a slight tendency for patients typical of Cluster C to possess the features of A in addition ($r = 0.22$, $P<0.05$), but not those of B ($r = -0.18$, $P<0.01$).

*Cluster D (severe/suicidal)* showed least conformity to any familiar depressive entity. Scores for D were of unimodal distribution and correlated strongly with scores

TABLE I
*'Statistical syndromes' (factor of origin)*

| Cluster A (I + ve) | | Cluster B (I − ve) | |
|---|---|---|---|
| (1) Blames others | 31% | (1) Distinct quality | 44% |
| (2) Self-pity | 65% | (2) Unvarying | 51% |
| (3) Psychological causes | 45% | (3) Feels slow | 68% |
| (4) Responsive mood | 69% | (4) Regularly worse a.m. | 38% |
| (5) 'Immature' | 12% | (5) Loss of feeling | 19% |
| Cluster C (II) | | Cluster D (III) | |
| (1) 'Neurotic' | 43% | (1) Sad affect (severity) | + |
| (2) Situational phobias | 24% | (2) Suicidal impulses | 14% |
| (3) Panic attacks | 22% | (3) Depersonalisation | 15% |
| (4) Diffuse anxiety | 59% | (4) Ideas of reference | 21% |
| (5) 'Obsessional' | 13% | (5) Global severity* | + |

*Independent rating by family doctor

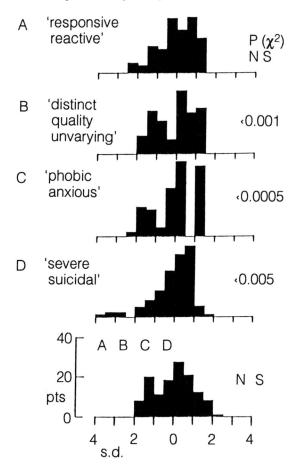

Fig. 1. Distribution of patient scores (n = 126)

on Hamilton's, Beck's and other scales of functional disability. D had dominated a general factor where most of the features had loadings of similiar sign suggesting it was a *trait of general severity*. D had negligible correlations with A ($r = -0.02$) and C ($r = 0.01$); correlation with B was 0.26 ($P<0.01$).

The last distribution profile at the bottom of Fig. 1 shows a slightly bimodal distribution when the 20 features of A + B + C + D were intercorrelated and factor analysed. The bimodality of factor scores, although apparent to the eye, just fails to reach statistical significance.

The overall pattern, therefore, was that endogenous depression (B) could be identified amongst general practice patients and, if other syndromes were ignored, this syndrome served to divide the case material into two overlapping groups without recourse to clinical diagnosis as a discriminating criterion. However, the endogenous depression syndrome in general practice was found to be singularly lacking in objective retardation and was independent of syndromes incorporating features of morbid anxiety. This was in contrast to observations of hospital patients where anxiety features and endogenous features tend to cluster at opposite poles of a bipolar factor. This finding fits in well with the now generally accepted notion that any clear dichotomy between endogenous and non-endogenous patients within psychiatric services owes much to nosocomial (hospital-related) influences whereby endogenous patients are frequently admitted together with the more severe and chronic neurotic patients. This concentration of endogenous and severe neurotic patients within hospitals makes it relatively simple to distinguish one from the other. One further inference is possible. Only by systematically jettisoning statistically irrelevant data did it prove possible to identify discrete patient sub-groups: when the number of variables was increased even to 20 (ABCD in Fig. 1) bimodality became statistically insignificant.

## Reliability and bias

The results described could hardly have arisen through lack of reliability since random errors favour unimodal and not multimodal distributions. The possibility that the abnormal distributions arose because of clinical preconception is more difficult to refute and further evidence on this question is desirable. A one in three sample (49 patients) was rated on a fully structured interview, Spitzer's Mental Status Schedule (Spitzer *et al*, 1966) which severely limited the opportunity for clinical cross examination and thus the operation of 'halo-effect'. Rater reliability was 0.92 (intra-class coefficient) before the study began.

A separate analysis of correlations between 22 features selected from the Mental Status Schedule for their resemblance to the 20 features retained from the Newcastle interview substantially reproduced the syndromes already described. This result encouraged the view that the original findings were not generated by clinical preconception alone. Furthermore, EPI scores (Eysenck & Eysenck, 1964) were self-rated at follow-up: their correlations validated the clinical judgements on 'neurotic personality' and 'obsessional personality' especially with regard to the anxious syndromes derived from Cluster C.

It was also possible to make a limited examination of *predictive validity* by correlating cluster scores with outcome recorded blind at three months. The results are in Table II. Neither reactive (A) nor endogenous (B) depression were, in this general practice setting, predictive of three month outcome. The trend was for Cluster C (phobic/anxious depression) to predict poor outcome. Severity (D) also predicted poor outcome, in contrast to hospital studies where high initial severity usually makes for substantial post-treatment reduction in symptom score. Finally, the notion that systematic omission of non-discriminating variables would favour bimodality was confirmed on a large separate sample of depressed hospital patients documented by other workers (Fahy, 1969b).

TABLE II
*Association of type of depressive syndrome with 3-month outcome ( n = 126 general practice depressed patients)*

| Syndrome | Correlation (r) with outcome |
| --- | --- |
| A (Reactive) | 0.07 Not significant |
| B (Endogenous) | 0.09 Not significant |
| C (Anxious) | 0.18 Almost significant |
| D (General severity) | 0.36 *P* < 0.01 (significant) |

Data from Fahy (1969) unpublished

### Three-month outcome

Short-term outcome was mixed. Of patients seen personally, 50% were recovered or greatly improved, 15% were slightly improved, and 30% were unchanged or worse. Outcome for those not seen personally was similar. Failure to improve was significantly related to increasing frequency of surgery contact and of recorded anti-depressant prescriptions. Duration of illness of over one year and chronicity of associated somatic conditions emerged as important predictors of chronicity. Adverse clinical predictors included phobias, hypochondriasis, depersonalisation and suicidal impulses and these were all significantly associated with chronicity of over one year.

### Referral rates

Specialist referral rates were uniformly low (Fahy, 1974). Psychiatric referrals were characteristically hopeless and difficult to reassure, diffusely anxious and subjectively retarded. Single men were selectively referred. An absence of hypochondriacal features characterised prompt referrals only. In general, patients referred to psychiatrists were obviously depressed in mood and had a wealth of psychiatric symptoms predominantly of endogenous type and not associated with overt physical stress at the onset of depressive symptoms. An equal number of patients was referred to non-psychiatric specialists and these were characterised by less obvious mood change and a previous history of having been referred to non-psychiatric specialists.

## *Discussion*

The work summarised here was done over 20 years ago, just as Shepherd's standard work on psychiatry in general practice first appeared (Shepherd, Cooper, Brown & Kalton, 1966). Since then research interest in psychiatric morbidity in the community has been spasmodic, although there have been significant advances in epidemiological method. Improved techniques of screening and case finding have successfully addressed the problem of depending on family doctors' judgements for case identification (Goldberg, 1978). The full extent of psychiatric morbidity in the community is finally being realised: epidemiological clinical and sociological investigations on a wide scale have yielded remarkably convergent findings, all pointing to a high prevalence of affective disorders in the community, much of it unrecognised and untreated and associated with significant somatic morbidity and mortality (Goldberg & Huxley, 1980; Freeling, Rao, Paykel *et al*, 1985; Murphy, Olivier, Sobol *et al*, 1986; Brown & Harris, 1986; Copeland, 1987). The complex pathways by which people suffering from depression seek and obtain care is much better understood (Paykel, Klerman & Prusoff, 1970; Fahy, 1974; Goldberg & Huxley, 1980).

Fully satisfactory efficacy studies of anti-depressant drugs in general practice have been slow to appear but early indications are that improved detection and appropriate treatment can improve the outlook for many patients (Ashcroft, 1986; Freeling, personal communication, 1987). Disputes about dimensions, categories and bimodal distributions have continued (Paykel, 1981; Grayson, 1987) and new statistical techniques such as latent trait analysis are helping to resolve inconsistencies between different diagnostic systems (Young, Scheftner, Klerman *et al*, 1986; Grayson, Bridges, Duncan-Jones & Goldberg, 1987). Most studies have continued to rely on epidemiological techniques and standard rating scales: few have used 'tailor-made' clinical interviews. In this quest for reliability and cross-national comparability of survey findings, it is perhaps understandable that the detailed study of the quality of suffering of the individual patient has been somewhat overlooked. Exceptions include a negected study by Cooke (1980) of the self-ratings of a general population sample and the recent examination by Williams & Skuse (1988) of the correlates of depressive thinking in elderly general practice attenders. At least two studies have suggested that, outside the confines of hospitals, endogenous depression may itself prove heterogenous (Cooke, 1980; Young *et al*, 1986). Bridges & Goldberg (1985), in their examination of the process of 'somatisation', also succeed in penetrating mere rating scale scores to the clinical reality beyond. Of the studies mentioned by Blacker & Clare (1987) in a recent review, few focused on problems of classification. Yet, Shepherd (1986), in summing up a symposium on mental illness in primary care settings has remarked: "Of all the topics that have been covered I agree that definition and classification are fundamental". The reference here is to the chasm of non-communication which persists between researcher and clinician, psychiatrist and family doctor, theory and practice and, finally, between family doctors themselves. Copeland (1987), speaking of untreated depression in the elderly on both sides of the Atlantic, asks: "How much longer is this suffering going to continue, which destroys so many potentially useful lives and is clearly associated with increased mortality? It is for epidemiologists to reveal the problem but it is up to general practitioners, particularly in academic departments of general practice, to investigate the causes and decide how the problem can be resolved in terms of the individual patient. Why has nothing been done? Could not the neglect in otherwise developed countries be described as a 20th century scandal?".

If progress has been as slow, as Shepherd and Copeland suggest, one reason may be the decline of phenomenology from a position of central importance in psychiatric training. It may be easier to sail into uncharted community waters bristling with rating scales rather than spend more time listening to fewer patients. A further reason why progress may have been slow is a reluctance of government funding agencies to support the evaluation of health policies predicated almost entirely on economic necessity. A final impediment to progress, and one which is more difficult to pin down, is that of mutual distrust between psychiatrists and primary care physicians, alluded to by Shepherd (1977). It is, therefore, encouraging to note that at least one psychiatrist/general practitioner group has taken up the challenge (Sireling, Paykel, Freeling *et al*, 1985; Sireling, Freeling, Paykel *et al*, 1985; Freeling, Rao, Paykel *et al*, 1985) and others will doubtless follow. A truly Kraepelinian task awaits the GP-psychiatrist of the future.

## References

ASHCROFT, G. W. (1986) In *Mental Illness in Primary Care Settings* (eds M. Shepherd, G. Wilkinson & P. Williams). London: Tavistock.

BLACKER, C. V. R. & CLARE, A. W. (1987) Depressive disorder in primary care. *British Journal of Psychiatry*, **150**, 737–751.

BRIDGES, K. & GOLDBERG, D. (1985) Somatic presentation of DSM III. Psychiatric disorders in primary care. *Journal of Psychosomatic Research*, **29**, 563–569.

BROWN, G. W. & HARRIS, T. (1978) *Social Origins of Depression: A Study of Psychiatric Disorder in Women*. London: Tavistock Publications.

—— & —— (1986) Stressor, vulnerability and depression: a question of replication, (editorial). *Psychological Medicine*, **16**, 739–744.

CARNEY, M. W. P., ROTH, M. & GARSIDE, R. F. (1965). The diagnosis of depressive syndromes and the prediction of ECT response. *British Journal of Psychiatry*, **111**, 659–665.

COOKE, D. J. (1980) The structure of depression found in the general population. *Psychological Medicine*, **10**, 455–463.

COPELAND, J. R. M. (1987) Prevalence of depressive illness in the elderly community. In *The Presentation of Depression: Current Approaches* (eds P. Freeling, L. J. Downey & J. C. Malkin). London: Royal College of General Practitioners.

EYSENCK, H. & EYSENCK, S. (1964) *Manual of the EPI*. London: University of London Press.

FAHY, T. J., BRANDON, S. & GARSIDE, R. F. (1969) Clinical syndromes in a sample of depressed patients: a general practice material. *Proceedings of the Royal Society of Medicine*, **62**, 331–335.

—— (1969a) Some problems in the assessment of current mental status of depressed patients. In *Das Depressiv Syndrom*, (eds H. Hippius & H. Selbach). Berlin: Urban und Schwarzenberg.

—— (1969b) The phenomenology of depression in hospital and in the community. Unpublished MD thesis, National University of Ireland, Dublin.

——, KAY, D. W. K. & GARSIDE, R. F. (1969) The prediction of ECT response. Paper read to the quarterly meeting of the Royal Medico-Psychological Association, Dublin. (Unpublished)

—— (1977) Some problems of method in the study of depression in general practice. In *Research and Clinical Investigation in Depression* (ed. J. Murphy). Northampton: Cambridge Medical Publications.

—— (1974) Pathways of specialist referral of depressed patients from general practice. *British Journal of Psychiatry*, **124**, 231–239.

—— (1974a) Hospital versus general practice depression: a direct clinical comparison. *British Journal of Psychiatry*, **124**, 240–242.

FREELING, P., RAO, B. M., PAYKEL, E. S., SIRELING, L. I. & BURTIN, R. H. (1985) Unrecognised depression in general practice. *British Medical Journal*, **290**, 1880–1883.

GOLDBERG, D. & BRIDGES, K. (1987) Screening for psychiatric illness in general practice: the general practitioner versus the screening questionnaire. *Journal of the Royal College of General Practitioners*, **37**, 15–18.

—— (1978) *Manual of the General Health Questionnaire*. Slough: National Foundation for Education Research.

—— & HUXLEY, P. (1980) *Mental Illness in the Community, the Pathways to Psychiatric Care*. London and New York: Tavistock.

GRAYSON, D. A. (1987) Can categorical and dimensional views of psychiatric illness be distinguished? *British Journal of Psychiatry*, **151**, 355–361.

——, BRIDGES, K., DUNCAN-JONES, P. & GOLDBERG, D. P. (1987) The relationship between symptoms and diagnosis of minor psychiatric syndromes in general practice. *Psychological Medicine*, **17**, 933–942.

HENDERSON, S., BYRNE, D. G. & DUNCAN-JONES, P. (1981) *Neurosis and the Social Environment*. Sydney: Academic Press.

HOEPER, E., NYCZ, G., CLEARY, P., *et al* (1979) Estimated prevalence of RDC. Mental disorder in primary medical care. *International Journal of Mental Health*, **8**, 6–15.

KAY, D. W. K., GARSIDE, R. F. & FAHY, T. J. (1973) A double blind trial of phenelzine and amitriptyline in depressed out-patients. A possible differential effect of the drugs on symptoms. *British Journal of Psychiatry*, **123**, 63–67.

——, FAHY, T. J. & GARSIDE, R. F. (1970) A seven month double blind trial of amitriptyline and diazepam in ECT treated depressed patients. *British Journal of Psychiatry*, **117**, 667–671.

KENDELL, R. E. (1968) *The Classification of Depressive Illness*. London: Maudsley Monograph, No. 18.

—— (1976) The classification of depression: a review of contemporary confusion. *British Journal of Psychiatry*, **129**, 15–28.

KILOH, L. & GARSIDE, R. F. (1963) The independence of neurotic and endogenous depression. *British Journal of Psychiatry*, **109**, 451–463.

—— & —— (1977) Depression: a multivariate study of Sir Aubrey Lewis's data on melancholia. *Australian and New Zealand Journal of Psychiatry*, **11**, 149–156.

KLERMAN, G. L. (1987) The current age of youthful melancholia: evidence for increase in depression in adolescents and young adults. *British Journal of Psychiatry*, **152**, 4–14.

MITCHELL, A. R. K. (1985) Psychiatrists in primary care settings. *British Journal of Psychiatry*, **147**, 371–379.

MURPHY, JANE, M., OLIVIER, D. C., SOBOL, A. N., MONSON, R. R. & LEIGHTON, A. H. (1986) Diagnosis and outcome: depression and anxiety in a general population. *Psychological Medicine*, **16**, 117–126.

NI BHROLCHAIN, M. (1979) Psychotic and neurotic depression: 1. some points of method. *British Journal of Psychiatry*, **134**, 87–93.

PAYKEL, E. S., KLERMAN, G. L. & PRUSOFF, B. A. (1970) Treatment setting and clinical depression. *Archives of General Psychiatry*, **22**, 11–21.

—— (1981) Have multivariate statistics contributed to classification? *British Journal of Psychiatry*, **139**, 357–362.

ROTH, M., GARSIDE, R. F., GURNEY, C. & KERR, T. A. (1979) Psychotic and neurotic depression: a reply on method. *British Journal of Psychiatry*, **135**, 94–96.

SANDIFER, M. G. (JR), WILSON, I. C. & GREEN, L. (1966) The two-type thesis of depressive disorders. *American Journal of Psychiatry*, **123**, Part 1, 93–97.

SHEPHERD, M., COOPER, B., BROWN, A. C. & KALTON, G. (1966) *Psychiatric Illness in General Practice*. London: Oxford University Press.

—— (1977) Mental illness and primary care (editorial). *American Journal of Public Health*, **77**, 12–13.

——, WILKINSON, G. & WILLIAMS, P. (ed.) (1986) *Mental Illness in Primary Care Settings*. London: Tavistock.

SIRELING, L. I., PAYKEL, E. S., FREELING, P., RAO, B. M. & PATEL, S. P. (1985) Depression in general practice: case thresholds and diagnosis. *British Journal of Psychiatry*, **147**, 113–118.

——, FREELING, P., PAYKEL, E. S. & RAO, B. M. (1985) Depression in general practice: clinical features and comparison with out-patients. *British Journal of Psychiatry*, **147**, 119–126.

SPITZER, R. L., FLEISS, J. L., ENDICOTT, J. & COHEN, J. (1966) The mental status schedule. *Archives of General Psychiatry*, **16**, 479–493.

STRATHDEE, G. & WILLIAMS, P. (1984) A survey of psychiatrists in primary care: the silent growth of a new service. *Journal of the Royal College of General Practitioners*, **34**, 615–618.

WILLIAMS, P. & SKUSE, D. (1988) Depressive thoughts in general practice attenders. *Psychological Medicine*, **18**, 469–475.

—— & CLARE, A. (1981) Changing patterns in psychiatric care. *British Medical Journal*, **282**, 375–377.

WING, J. K., BEBBINGTON, P. E. & ROBINS, L. N. (ed.) (1981) *What is a Case?* London: Grant McIntyre.

YOUNG, M. A., SCHEFTER, W. A., KLERMAN, G. L., ANDREASEN, N. C. & HIRSCHSFELD, R. M. A. (1986) The endogenous sub-type of depression: a study of its internal construct validity. *British Journal of Psychiatry*, **148**, 257–267.

# 24 Psychiatric services and primary care

## ALASDAIR A. McKECHNIE

Following graduation at Aberdeen in 1960 I decided that career options were either general practice or psychiatry. A desire to broaden general medicine, before deciding on a final pathway, included experience in geriatric medicine. This led to my first introduction to the work of Martin Roth and David Kay, which was held in some esteem even by physicians specialising in the care of the elderly! The decision to pursue a career in psychiatry was made and during my first years in the specialty the importance of the high academic standards of investigation set by Martin Roth became even more apparent. In 1966 I was fortunate enough to obtain a post at Newcastle upon Tyne as a senior research associate.

Armed with a DPM and with feelings, in fluctuating amounts, of determination and trepidation, Framlington Place became the base over the next few years for strenuous activity. As a research associate I was to be involved in extending earlier work into psychiatric illness in the elderly in a defined community sample. Published work (Kay, Beamish & Roth, 1964(a) and 1964(b)) had attracted DHSS funding to allow for a more detailed longitudinal study.

Prescribed reading was, of necessity, directed towards the work of those involved in general studies of psychiatric morbidity within defined populations. This was to include Essen-Möller et al (1956) and Shepherd et al (1966). The biased and small proportion of psychiatric morbidity with which psychiatrists were involved became all too obvious and this was true irrespective of age.

Another important aspect of this research experience was the strong emphasis on team work involving many disciplines. That the psychiatrist was paramount was far from obvious. Of great value too was involvement with general practitioners. For the first time in my professional experience time was spent in group practices, albeit with no active professional commitment to patient care.

This time in Newcastle had involved first-hand experience in the epidemiology of psychiatric illness in the elderly, but did not suggest, despite the opportunity and the challenge, furthering a career in the care of the elderly; rather it reinforced the field of general psychiatry, especially after a period as a senior registrar based at Newcastle General Hospital.

## Setting the scene

Would it be possible to get the best of both worlds—psychiatry and general practice? Such a possibility arose at Bangour Village Hospital, one-time pauper lunatic asylum for the City of Edinburgh. This was to be linked to the Livingston Scheme in anticipation of an integrated approach to health care based on health centres with primary care physicians having a part-time post within the specialty of their choice (SHS Studies, 1973, 1982).

Comprehensive patterns of psychiatric assessment, management and care have to accommodate two apparently polarised alternatives: the Victorian institution or the community orientated programme; the second claiming to be a more humane approach to serious disability, and able to cope with the consequences of abnormal reactions to stress, these reactions being of variable intensity. The district general hospital unit appears to be an alternative for short stay in-patient assessment and management. The community based programme has been identified with mental health centres, particularly in the USA. It is important to realise that the mental health centre should be 'a concept and not a building'.

The emphasis must be to develop an integrated service, a spectrum of care with, it is hoped, a balance between the various components necessary for such an approach. It is relevant to this review to state that the closer integration of primary care and psychiatry, with the emphasis on less disabling disorders, must be pursued along with other equally important areas of service.

A study of the long-stay cohort within the hospital helped to identify and follow-up the impact of rehabilitation on the hospital population (McKechnie, 1972; McKechnie *et al*, 1974). The results complied closely with others, e.g. Early & Nicholas (1971). A particular feature of the structure of the population, as in most Scottish psychiatric hospitals, was the high proportion of elderly. These were made up of two cohorts best considered separately: people who had grown old in hospital (functional psychoses) and those admitted later in life (predominantly with organic dementia).

Two separate psychogeriatric services were developed: one for part of Edinburgh and the other for West Lothian, a service model based on R. A. Robinson (1969). The development of a separate psychogeriatric assessment service was demonstrated to lead to considerably greater numbers of admissions and discharges (McKechnie & Corser, 1984)—the early influence of Sir Martin and Newcastle emerging again!

The relevance of these apparent digressions from the main theme of this review must be emphasised. A comprehensive integrated service is what is vital. Inevitably some aspects will take precedence but no part of such a service should be allowed to progress at the expense of less glamorous or fashionable elements.

Goldberg & Huxley (1980) have identified a logical approach to "mental illness in the community". They stated ". . . with the detection and management of psychiatric disorders by family doctors . . . the greatest share of the burden falls on their shoulders." They identified a simplified model with five levels representing different populations of subjects.

> "In order to pass from one level to another it is necessary to pass through a filter:
> 1. **Level 1** represents the community . . .

2. **Level 2** is represented by studies of psychiatric morbidity among patients attending primary care physicians *irrespective* (author's italics) of whether or not the physician has detected the 'illness behaviours' of the patient . . .
3. **Level 3** consists of those patients attending primary care physicians who are identified as psychiatrically sick by their doctor.
4. **Level 4** is represented by patients attending psychiatrists in out-patient clinics (and private offices). In the UK the primary care physician is critically placed to determine who will be referred—the third filter.
5. **Level 5** is represented by patients admitted to psychiatric hospitals and mental hospitals. They form the population most commonly referred to in national statistics of mental illness.''

However, (in whatever way) ''we choose to define a psychiatric illness in theory, in practice it is defined by the process of passing through the first three filters. Each of the filters is selectively permeable, so that some individuals are more likely to pass through than others. And we can already see that the key people deciding who shall pass through are the patient and the family doctor.''

The preceding paragraphs quoted verbatim provide an excellent framework against which to assess the current position and the future of the interaction between primary care and specialist psychiatric services.

The major consumers of health service resource remain children with their mothers, the elderly and those with conspicuous psychiatric morbidity especially in terms of perceived demand, by both clients and staff, middle-aged women.

In relation to **Levels 1** and **2**, epidemiological studies throughout various countries have identified very variable levels of morbidity. Taylor & Chave (1964) demonstrated a prevalence of about 35%. Goldberg (1972), and in subsequent papers using the General Health Questionnaire, has identified a prevalence of approximately 20%. Goldberg & Huxley (1980) have adopted the phrase ''conspicuous psychiatric morbidity''. This term was first applied by Kessel (1960). He used it to define all moderately disturbed people seen in a general practice setting and included those *undetected* by the general practitioner. Kessel estimated a rate of between 10% and 14%. Using the GHQ Corser & Philip (1978) reported on emotional disturbance in newly registered general practice patients in Livingston New Town. They, while accepting the GHQ as a survey instrument, commented ''whether what it measures is best considered as psychiatric illness or as a part of the normal range of emotional response to life events remains to be clarified''. These doubts are in keeping with the lower morbidity identified by Kessel.

Distress may be intense, for example, in bereavement reaction, but is likely to be time-limited. Illness might be in relation to severity or duration of symptoms, there is as yet no sure method of discriminating normal and abnormal reactions.

Mitchell (1983) has been a strong advocate of liaison psychiatry. He stated that liaison implies that each of the *partners* ''should work together in harmony and for mutual advantage. Of all the hospital specialists, the psychiatrist is probably the one who should find it most natural to have such a liaison with GPs because they have similar attitudes and philosophies''. He reviewed the published attempts to establish closer working links between psychiatrists and GPs.

McKechnie and colleagues (1981) showed that a multiprofessional team who saw patients and had regular discussions with GPs in NHS group practices, led to more people being referred with greater use of the multiple disciplines in psychiatry. These services were compared with a comparable service for patients referred through conventional channels, for example, out-patient clinics. These patients were more likely to have had previous contact with psychiatric services, were more likely to be admitted as in-patients and spent 70% more time as in-patients.

A further review over a six year period demonstrated that deployment of a specialist psychiatric team and closer integration with primary care physicians led to a greater proportion of first contact referrals being seen as out-patients compared with nationally derived data for both Scotland and England, with a relatively lower in-patient admission rate. The increase in out-patients was seen in health centres rather than traditional hospital based clinics (McKechnie, 1985). The inception rate for psychiatric illness referred to the specialist team was compared with the estimates from Camberwell/Salford data (Wing & Fryers, 1978). The first admission in-patient rate was lower but total contacts, mainly through health centre clinics and community psychiatric nurses, were higher.

This increase in first contacts is not reported in Nottingham (Tyrer *et al*, 1984). They found that the total referral increase was because of chronic cases. Their finding may reflect the greater sensitivity of a case register in defining first contacts. It would also be supported by earlier findings that the bulk of psychiatric disorder in the community is chronic or recurrent (Wilkinson *et al*, 1985).

Within this group are a range of affective disorders, the most common, but anxiety and personality disorders account for the highest proportion of severe disability (Regius *et al*, 1985). Where affective disorders are recognised by general practitioners, the profile of depressive illness is indistinguishable from hospital in-patients classified as endogenously depressed with a good treatment response to active pharmacological treatment (Thomson *et al*, 1982).

With the move towards community care, primary care, including that of physicians and health visitors, is central to this concept. It is estimated that 80% of those in the general community with psychiatric morbidity will attend their GP, although this will be actually recognised in a smaller proportion. It is likely that among those *failing* to make contact will be those discharged from hospital with chronic psychoses and this has been borne out by a number of studies, for example, Johnstone *et al* (1984). From this it is clear that more intensive follow-up by a multidisciplinary psychiatric team is vital.

Where community psychiatric nurses work closely with GPs (Robertson & Scott, 1985) outcome appears favourable. More specifically, in the treatment of chronic phobic and obsessive compulsive disorders behaviour therapy from a nurse therapist has been demonstrated to be more effective than routine treatment (Marks, 1985). This study was one of the few controlled trials of treatment conducted in a setting of primary care.

The value of behaviour therapy has been shown in a variety of circumstances and their techniques can be utilised by general practitioners as well as clinical psychologists and nurses (France & Robson, 1986). Their practical book identifies approaches useful in cognitive behavioural management of depression, the management of anxiety as well as a variety of other problems.

The value of self-help groups has also to be taken into consideration. These groups may divert those at work from inappropriate utilisation of scarce NHS resources and are very effective in their own right. These services may help to reduce morbidity before **Filter 1** (at primary care level). Those reviewed earlier improve general practice skills (**Filter 2**) and make specialist advice more readily acceptable (**Filter 3**). Most patients appear to prefer the treatment and management strategies to be made available in a primary care setting rather than the out-patient clinic. An intermediate and apparently acceptable (to client) step is the Mental Health Advice Centre, for example, Lewisham. This facility has tapped a large pool of untreated morbidity mainly from general practice sources. It has been developed along with a crisis intervention team (Boardman *et al*, 1987).

The economics of mental health services have been the subject of a recent leader (BMJ, 1987). Such studies as had been conducted demonstrated the cost benefits of community care. Published studies have demonstrated the value of social worker (Corney, 1984), clinical psychology services (McAllister & Philip, 1975) and community psychiatric nurses (Corser & Ryce, 1977) in relation to primary care. The makings of a team which can and will provide a better service are there.

The tools are there, better identification is feasible (Wing *et al*, 1978; Goldberg, 1972). Ways of increasing interviewing skills can be taught to all carers—including doctors (Maguire *et al*, 1978; Goldberg & Huxley, 1980). The social impact of life events can be identified (Brown & Harris, 1978).

The impact of physical illness in relation to psychological symptoms, very much a feature of Sir Martin Roth's researches, is being acknowledged. Even a description of "the importuning patient" (*ipse dixit*), the constellation of self-pitying and related factors independent of illness, physical or psychological has been recognised, not least in relation to demands for treatment.

It is painful to recall that the main reason for reorganisation of the National Health Service (England & Wales, 1973, Scotland, 1974) was to integrate primary health care with specialist services, mainly hospital based, working together within a defined coterminous general population of reasonable size. This worthy goal has become even more remote with successive administrative alterations. It seems that only one psychiatrist in five is actively involved in a primary care setting in England and Wales. In Scotland the proportion is higher, one in two. Perhaps the 80th anniversary of Sir Martin Roth's birth will be graced by his presence; and an integrated approach to psychiatric care the rule rather than the exception.

# *References*

BRITISH MEDICAL JOURNAL (1987), **4**, 793.

BOARDMAN, A. P., BOURAS, N. & CUNDY, J. (1987) *The Mental Health Advice Centre in Lewisham*. Research Department 3, National Unit for Psychiatric Research and Development, Lewisham Hospital, London.

BROWN, G. W. & HARRIS, T. (1978) *Social Origins of Depression*. London: Tavistock Publications.

CORNEY, R. H. (1984) The effectiveness of attached social workers in the management of depressed female patients in general practice. *Psychological Medicine Monograph Supplement 6*.

CORSER, C. M. & RYCE, S. W. (1977) Community mental health care: a model based on the primary care team. *British Medical Journal*, ii, 936–938.

—— & PHILIP, A. E. (1978) Emotional disturbance in newly registered general practice patients. *British Journal of Psychiatry*, 132, 172–176

EARLY, D. F. & NICHOLAS, M. (1971) The developing scene: ten year review of a psychiatric hospital population. *British Medical Journal*, iv, 793–795.

ESSEN-MÖLLER, E., LARSSON, H., UDDENBERG, C. E. & WHITE, G. (1956) Individual traits and morbidity in a Swedish rural population. *Acta Psychiatrica Neurologica Supplement*, 100, 1–160.

FRANCE, R. & ROBSON, M. (1986) *Behaviour Therapy in Primary Care*. London: Croom Helm.

GOLDBERG, D. (1972) The detection of psychiatric illness by questionnaire. *Maudsley Monograph*, No. 21, London: Oxford University Press.

—— & HUXLEY, P. (1980) *Mental Illness in the Community*. London: Tavistock Publications.

JOHNSTONE, E. C., OWENS, D. G. C., GOLD, A. & CROW, T. J. (1984) Schizophrenic patients discharged from hospital—a follow-up study. *British Journal of Psychiatry*, 145, 586–590.

KAY, D. W. K., BEAMISH, P. & ROTH, M. (1964(a)) Old age mental disorders in Newcastle-upon-Tyne: I—A study of prevalence. *British Journal of Psychiatry*, 110, 146–158.

——, —— & —— (1964(b)) Old age mental disorders in Newcastle-upon-Tyne: II—A study of possible social and medical causes. *British Journal of Psychiatry*, 110, 668–682.

KESSEL, N. (1960) Psychiatric morbidity in a London general practice. *British Journal of Preventive and Social Medicine*, 14, 16–22.

MAGUIRE, P., ROE, P., GOLDBERG, D., JONES, S., HYDE, C. & O'DOWD, T. (1978) The value of feedback in teaching interview skills to medical students. *Psychological Medicine*, 8, 695–705.

MARKS, I. (1985) Controlled trial of psychiatric nurse therapists in primary care. *British Medical Journal*, 290, 1181–1184.

MITCHELL, A. R. K. (1983) Liaison psychiatry in general practice. *British Journal of Hospital Medicine*, 30, 100–106.

MCALLISTER, T. A. & PHILIP, A. E. (1975) The clinical psychologist in a Health Centre: one year's work. *British Medical Journal*, iv, 513–514.

MCKECHNIE, A. A. (1972) A point prevalence study of a long term hospital population. *Scottish Health Bulletin*, 4, 250–258.

——, PHILIP, A. E., ROBERTSON, E. & SMITH, P. (1974) Follow-up of a long stay psychiatric population. *Scottish Health Bulletin*, 32, 1–4.

——, —— & RAMAGE, J. G. (1981) Psychiatric services in primary care: specialised or not? *Journal of Royal College of General Practitioners*, 31, 611–614.

—— & CORSER, C. M. (1984) The role of psychogeriatric assessment units in a comprehensive psychiatric service. *Scottish Health Bulletin*, 42, 25–35.

—— (1985) The development of an integrated psychiatric service in a Scottish community. *Acta Psychiatrica Scandinavica*, 72, 97–103.

REGIUS, D. A., BURKE, J. D., MANDERSCHEID, R. A. & BURNS, B. J. (1985) The chronically mentally ill in primary care. *Psychological Medicine*, 15, 265–273.

ROBERTSON, H. & SCOTT, D. J. (1985) Community psychiatric nursing: a survey of patients and problems. *Journal of Royal College of General Practitioners*, 35, 130–132.

ROBINSON, R. A. (1969) The prevention and rehabilitation of mental illness in the elderly. In *Interdisciplinary Topics in Gerontology*, 3, 89–102, (eds M. F. Lownthal & J. A. Zilli). Basel/New York: Karger.

SCOTTISH HEALTH SERVICE STUDIES (1973) *The Livingston Project—The First Five Years by Dr A. H. Duncan*, 29, Edinburgh: SHHD.

—— (1982) *The Livingston Scheme—A Ten Year Review*, 43, Edinburgh: SHHD.

SHEPHERD, M., COOPER, B., BROWN, A. C. & KALTON, G. W. (1966) *Psychiatric Illness in General Practice*. London: Oxford University Press.

TAYLOR, S. J. L. & CHAVE, S. (1964) *Mental Health and Environment*. London: Longmans.

THOMSON, J., RANKIN, H., ASHCROFT, G. W., YATES, C. M., McQUEEN, J. K. & CUMMINGS, S. W. (1982) The treatment of depression in general practice: a comparison of L-tryptophan, amitriptyline and a combination of L-tryptophan and amitriptyline with placebo. *Psychological Medicine*, 12, 741–751.

TYRER, P., SEIVEWRIGHT, N. & WOLLERTON, S. (1984) General practice psychiatric clinics: impact on psychiatric services. *British Journal of Psychiatry*, 145, 15–19.

WILKINSON, G., FALLOON, I. & BISWAJIT, S. E. N. (1985) Chronic mental disorders in general practice. *British Medical Journal*, 291, 1302–1304.

WING, J. K. & FRYERS, T. (1978) Statistics from the Camberwell and Salford psychiatric case registers 1964–74. MRC Social Psychiatry Unit, London, and Department of Community Medicine, University of Manchester.

——, MANN, S. A., LEFF, J. P. & NIXON, J. N. (1978) The concept of care in psychiatric population surveys *Psychological Medicine*, **8**, 203–219.

# IV.  Disorders of the elderly

# 25 Martin Roth and the 'Psychogeriatricians'

## TOM ARIE

Psychogeriatrics (the common but ungraceful title) was born as a service specialty in the 1960s. Until then interest in the mental disorders of old age had been largely clinical and neuropathological. Today special psychiatric services for old people are widely established, and the task of matching them to needs, and of studying their functioning and the issues that they pose, is preoccupying workers (and governments) not only in developed countries but also in the Third World.

Britain has led this movement, yet at the end of the 1960s there were less than half-a-dozen psychiatrists for whom this was their special interest. Now there are 250. Two-thirds of Health Districts have a special component of psychiatric services devoted to the aged, and the movement has the backing of professional bodies and of Government (Wattis, Wattis & Arie, 1981; and Wattis, 1988). How did it come about?

The origins are fivefold: first, pressure of the rapid increase in the number of the aged, particularly of the very aged, which in the 1960s was becoming evident in health and particularly in psychiatric services—it had been forecast by Aubrey Lewis just after the war, but few had then taken notice (Lewis, 1946); next, the growth in psychiatry's capacity to treat conditions previously regarded as hopeless (Post, 1978); third, the movement of psychiatry in the '50s and '60s away from mental hospitals towards shared responsibility for the treatment and care of people living at home; then, the successful development of geriatrics as a part of British medicine; and last, significantly, the writings and teaching of a small group of psychiatrists, of whom none were more eminent than Martin Roth and David Kay in Newcastle, and Felix Post in London. The work of such men has enhanced our understanding of the mental disorders of old age, but this chapter is not about those studies as such: it is about the 'psychogeriatricians', and Martin Roth's links with them as they have developed their services. Those wider studies, of course, form a crucial part of his influence on them, and have greatly enriched the field in which they work.

The prognostic studies from Graylingwell and the Newcastle studies, which described the epidemiology of the psycho-syndromes of old age, shed light on the distribution of mentally disordered old people between home and other compartments of care and the factors that determine their fate on follow-up. They are too well-known to need detailed citation here: they opened up the community psychiatry of the aged. The epidemiology of old age mental disorders as then measured in Newcastle is still quoted as the base for planning across the world. (That the rates found in Newcastle had wide confidence intervals was made clear in the original publications; more recent research workers are sometimes finding lower rates but the Newcastle figures continue to serve as a bench-mark.)

An important contribution in the present context was a paper published in the *British Medical Journal* (Kay *et al*, 1966) entitled 'Special problems of the aged and the organisation of hospital services'. The authors were David Kay, Martin Roth and, significantly, a local geriatrician, Michael Hall, later to become, in Southampton, one of the first professors of geriatric medicine. This paper was a landmark, for it focused attention on the needs for special arrangements for the growing numbers of old people with mental disorders. The question of sorting those old people who were at that stage often randomly being referred to almost every type of agency—psychiatric, general medical, geriatric and social— was then becoming a much debated issue (Kidd, 1962; Mezey, 1968), with concern about the extent and the possibly damaging effects of 'misplacement' of old people in units of the 'wrong' specialty. Among others drawing attention to the need for collaboration in the assessment of confused old people were Macmillan and his colleagues in Nottingham (Morton *et al*, 1968); Macmillan, a great psychiatric reformer, was much concerned with the special problems of the aged (Macmillan & Shaw, 1966).

The Kay, Roth & Hall paper was a firm statement of the need for specially focused collaborating services. The authors emphasised the intertwining of physical, mental and social factors in the psychosyndromes of old age, and called for meticulous assessment by all the disciplines concerned. Characteristically for Martin Roth, it was followed by action; a few years later the Brighton Clinic was established in Newcastle, a facility in which psychiatric and geriatric physicians collaborated in the investigation and treatment of old people in a general hospital. During the following years several of his papers (e.g. Roth, 1972) concerned questions about the development of such special services for old people.

## The 'psychogeriatric movement'

The 'psychogeriatricians', as they are known, often reluctantly, for it is an ugly name (but who can think of a better one?), have looked to Roth's writings as inspiration, and above all to Roth as the setter of a standard, rarely to be attained by others, of learning and of eloquence.

In 1973 Felix Post became the first Chairman of a Group for the Psychiatry of Old Age in the Royal College of Psychiatrists. Post was the father figure, Roth the distinguished godfather, an influential advocate in world fora, not least for some 30 years as a contributor to the initiatives of the World Health Organization (e.g. Roth, 1959).

In recent years there has been a happy series of encounters between Roth and the psychogeriatricians. On one occasion the psychogeriatricians travelled to Amsterdam for a relaxed meeting with Dutch colleagues, which is remembered not least for the companionship of Martin and Constance, Martin adorning the evenings with the after dinner speeches of which he is a master, and from which many are still quarrying their own anecdotes.

## The present scene in psychogeriatrics

Two reviews of the 'state of the art' in psychogeriatrics in the middle (Geigy, 1965) and at the end of the 1960s (Kay & Walk, 1971) stand as a statement of what had been achieved, and of the directions in which people were looking; significantly and appropriately, Roth's was the opening contribution to each (Roth, 1965 and 1971). At that time some half-a-dozen then younger psychiatrists were meeting at each others' hospitals as a 'coffee house group', sharing their early experiences of setting up local 'psychogeriatric' services. Most were based in London, but they were closely associated with others such as Robinson in Scotland (a pioneer almost alone in his generation, standing between Roth and Post, and the younger psychiatrists). Among them were Hemsi and Cockburn of Long Grove, MacDonald of Warlingham Park, Pitt then of Claybury, and Arie of Goodmayes; and in Newcastle, Bergmann and Blessed, in Colchester, Whitehead.

They met as a 'mutual support group', developing ideas and sharing problems. It was clear that, whereas each was working in different circumstances, they shared a common outlook and from their deliberations principles for the provision of psychiatric services for the elderly began to emerge. The group too, both collectively and individually, established contacts with government and with national bodies, aiming to draw attention to, and obtaining resources for, work with mentally disordered old people.

In 1973 they became an official Group within the College and in 1978 they acquired the full status of a Specialist Section. This Section, of whom subsequent Chairmen after Post have been Robinson, Arie, and currently Pitt, has formed the professional focus for the development of 'psychogeriatrics' in Britain. It has produced important documents of guidance on development of services and norms for staff and facilities, and responded to changing issues, most recently those posed by the sudden growth of the private sector of the care of the aged (Royal College of Psychiatrists, 1987). The Section now has some one thousand members—a measure of the interest in this field among psychiatrists in general, quite apart from those for whom it is their special concern.

Successive national surveys conducted from Nottingham and Leeds have revealed the remarkably rapid development of this new branch of the National Health Service (Wattis *et al*, 1981; Wattis & Arie, 1984; Arie *et al*, 1985; Wattis, 1988). Wattis estimates that in 1987 some 250 consultant psychiatrists were devoting their main professional interests to running well-defined local psychiatric services specifically for the aged, together with members of other relevant professions and in a wide variety of different styles, but again with a common philosophy; there have been many further reports describing such services (see, e.g., in Arie & Jolley, 1982, and Copeland, 1984).

During the late 1970s and early 1980s international networks began to be established in the field of old age psychiatry, with personal contacts through conferences, courses and through the Geriatric Psychiatry Section of the World Psychiatric Association, in close association with the World Health Organization, and the International Psychogeriatric Association. At the same time an apparatus of education has been established: the Royal College of Psychiatrists has defined standards both for specialist training in old age psychiatry, and for experience in this field for general psychiatrists. There are now four psychogeriatrician professors in England: Arie with a joint Department of Health Care of the Elderly in Nottingham (1977), Murphy (1983), Levy (1984) and Pitt (1986) in charge of divisions of old age psychiatry within departments of psychiatry in London University.

## A typical service (Arie, 1987)

The remainder of this chapter gives a description of the present shape of these services, the types of resources they deploy and some aspects of the styles in which they work. The principles for providing such services, and accounts of the staff and resources needed, have been the subject of a series of publications by individual workers, by the Royal College of Psychiatrists and by the Government (reviewed by e.g. Arie & Jolley, 1982, and by Copeland, 1984). There is also an important document from the Health Advisory Service entitled *The Rising Tide* (NHS Health Advisory Service, 1982); this body was established by Richard Crossman, the Secretary of State, in 1969 after a series of scandals in long-stay care. It is responsible to the Secretary of State and it visits services to review their activities and to disseminate good practice (Crossman, 1977). Some current issues of importance with which such services are concerned have been reviewed (Arie, 1986). Described here will be a typical service, though one of the virtues of these developments is the range of different styles of service which are to be found throughout the country (Glasscote *et al*, 1977; Norman, 1982).

Developments are likely to have taken place around a group of core workers and facilities, the latter often determined by what happened to be available in the locality; almost always a central figure, usually a psychiatrist, has been the moving spirit. One, and nowadays often two, psychiatrists will have special responsibility for the aged, and will work in close concert with nursing, psychology, remedial and social services staff, and managers; particularly collaborating with family doctors and their teams, and with geriatric medical services.

The facilities will include an admission unit. This is still too often in a single specialty mental hospital, but by universal agreement it should be, and in nearly 40% of services it now is, in the District General Hospital (Wattis, 1988). The mixed nature of the disorders of old people, and the complex inter-relationship between mental and physical components so often underlined by Martin Roth's work, demands that initial assessment and treatment should be in a setting where there is access to the full resources of a general hospital. Preferably such admission units will be near the (medical) geriatric admission unit so that a close working relationship can be established; in a few cases, especially where geriatrics and/or psychogeriatrics are on their own in single specialty hospitals remote from the district general hospital, joint patient units (sometimes called 'psychogeriatric assessment units') to which psychiatrists and geriatricians together admit, and in which they assess and treat patients, have been established; but the more common pattern is of collaboration between the psychogeriatric and geriatric services, rather than shared facilities.

In Nottingham a Department of Health Care of the Elderly based in the University Hospital brings together geriatricians, psychogeriatricians and the related staff as members of one team in one department, with a major educational programme (Arie *et al*, 1985); there is also a specialised orthopaedic geriatric unit, a stroke unit, and a continence service.

The longer-stay unit, offering also respite admissions, is usually in a peripheral hospital, and nowadays smaller units are favoured, as close as possible to their local communities. A wide range of experiment in regard to long-stay care is the subject of active debate; analogies with the nursing homes of other countries, but run by the National Health Service, are a small series of experimental long-stay units being specially funded by the Government. But, whether the unit is part of a large hospital or is free-standing, it should be small, domestic and uninstitutional, close to the local community, and it should be accepted that for most of the residents it is their permanent home. Much of long-stay care is now in the private sector, a development which raises problems of integration with statutory services in both operation and planning, and of quality control (Royal College of Psychiatrists, 1987).

The day hospital is an essential component. This is likely to be a small unit of perhaps 25 places, serving a locality, and offering the full range of psychiatric treatments (with the exception usually of electro-shock treatment, for which patients are likely to be taken to the hospital admitting unit). Patients attend for from one day to five days a week, a few units being able to offer care seven days a week. The unit is usually free-standing, but may be adjacent to another hospital unit, so that the day area is common to in-patients and day patients. The pattern of activity in a day hospital includes assessment, treatment and rehabilitation, though a few patients, particularly the demented, attend primarily for support.

A feature of day hospitals is that, often being independent units, staff roles can be deliberately blurred, emphasising more those aspects which staff have in common, or those personal attributes which do not derive from professional status, as much as specific professional skill. Close local networks are usually established by easy movement of staff between the day hospital and patients' homes and other facilities for the aged. In short, a day hospital often becomes a 'resource centre' for its locality.

But the main thrust of a service is towards maintaining independence, and even more important, choice for old people in their own homes. To achieve this there is close collaboration with extra-mural services—particularly the family doctor and his team and other nursing, social service, remedial and voluntary workers outside the hospital. Usually there will be a team of 'community psychiatric nurses' based either in the hospital or outside it, who act as a particularly effective bridge between the specialised service and the generality of old people and services for them.

## The 'style' of services

So much, in outline, for the personnel and 'plant'. Equally important is the 'style' in which these are deployed (Arie & Jolley, 1982). Thus, whenever they wish it, old people should be helped to remain at home, either by support there, or, where their condition may be improved this way, through a short stay in hospital or attendance at the day hospital. This primacy of domiciliary care derives from the assumption that people prefer wherever possible to remain in their own homes, and partly from necessity (since institutional resources are usually scarce).

In a good service virtually all referrals will first be seen at home, a senior psychiatrist, where necessary with other members of the team, being available to visit promptly. The psychiatrist will always accept shared responsibility, rather than merely giving a 'hit and run' opinion and then withdrawing. The building of confidence among patients, their carers and colleagues, obviously depends on the specialised service being willing tangibly to share responsibility, both for care and for the risk-taking which is an inevitable part of a system which gives primacy to helping often precariously functioning people to remain at home.

The service will set great store on collaboration with other agencies, statutory, voluntary and private, and to being readily available. It aims to be undefensive and unfussy, and must make it easy for those who seek help to reach it. The secretary to whom referrals and problems often first come is a key member of the team; her 'telephone manner' is likely to set the important first impression of the service.

## Voluntary organisations

Possibly the most important development of recent years in this field has been the growth of public awareness of the problems of mentally ill old people and of those who look after them. Voluntary bodies, of which the Alzheimer's Disease Societies (now active in many countries) are perhaps the best known, now form a vigorous alliance with the professions, each offering the other co-operation and a generally gingering critique. These bodies serve as pressure groups and in varying degrees provide education, raise research funds, and may themselves provide services.

## Education

The growing educational activities of those involved with providing psychiatric services for the aged overlap with programmes in the general field of ageing and geriatrics, and a common core curriculum, with differences of emphasis, is suitable for many of the different groups. Such a 'portable mini curriculum' covers the broad headings of: ageing of individuals; ageing in society; clinical practice; planning and provision of services; and the development of realistic and appropriate attitudes (Arie *et al*, 1985).

In addition to the demand for education from the lay public, there is growing demand for teaching and for practical experience by workers in almost all the health disciplines, many coming here from abroad; these matters now increasingly form part of the undergraduate education of most of the health professions. There is, too, great demand for short courses in these fields, and several are now available, most often based on university departments, in main centres in Britain for colleagues from abroad; a regular British Council course on 'psychogeriatrics' takes place in Nottingham (Martin Roth has been a distinguished contributor). The serious newspapers, radio and television nowadays generally tackle these matters with effectiveness and understanding.

## Research

This is not the place to attempt a summary of the research that is now moving fruitfully on a broad front. Reports of recent advances can be found in

Arie (1985), and Roth & Iversen (1986) have reviewed current research in Alzheimer's disease, to which they themselves have contributed with distinction. There is nowadays hardly a department of psychiatry, of geriatrics, or of social science or economics, which is not concerned in some measure with the mental disorders of old age; research in basic science departments has been particularly fruitful. International comparative studies also exist, though not yet on a large scale; these and the initiatives of the World Health Organization in this field have been described by Henderson & Macfadyen (1985). A significant area of study is concerned with the burden upon the supporters of the demented, and the ways in which professional inputs can be made more precisely effective (e.g. Gilleard, 1984; Challis & Davies, 1986). Useful descriptive reviews of services have been made by Alison Norman of the Centre for Policy on Ageing (Norman, 1982, 1987).

## Conclusions

Martin Roth, by his studies, his writings and his personal encouragement, has helped to foster a movement which is now established as an accepted part both of the National Health Service, and of academic and professional activity in psychiatry. Emphases and directions vary, but the vigour of the enterprise speaks for itself, and above all it is clear that this field has won the interest and energy of able and effective workers in all the health professions. This is not of its nature one of the 'glamour' specialties, but it has become respected as a legitimate and fruitful field of professional and academic activity, and as an essential component of the care of the aged. Its exponents acknowledge with enthusiasm and affection their debt to Martin Roth.

## References

ARIE, T. (1986) Some current issues in Old Age Psychiatry Services. In *The Provision of Mental Health Services in Britain* (eds G. Wilkinson & H. Freeman). London: Gaskell (Royal College of Psychiatrists).
—— (1987) 20 years of geriatric psychiatry in Britain. *Gerontopsychiatry* (Japan), **4**, 482–488. (The present chapter draws at some points, with permission, on this article.)
—— & JOLLEY, D. J. (1982) Making services work: Organisation and style of psychogeriatric services. In *Psychiatry of Late Life* (eds R. Levy & F. Post). Oxford: Blackwell. (This includes references to other work on services and to official memoranda.)
——, JONES, R. G. & SMITH, C. W. (1985) The educational potential of old age psychiatry services. In *Recent Advances in Psychogeriatrics in Britain* (ed. T. Arie). Edinburgh: Churchill Livingstone.
CHALLIS, D. & DAVIES, B. (1986) *Case Management in Community Care*. Aldershot: Gower.
COPELAND, J. R. M. (1984) Organisation of services for the elderly mentally ill. In *Handbook of Studies on Psychiatry and Old Age* (eds D. W. K. Kay & G. D. Burrows). Amsterdam: Elsevier.
CROSSMAN, R. H. S. (1977) *Diaries of a Cabinet Minister, vol. III*. London: Hamish Hamilton and Jonathan Cape.
GEIGY (1965) *Psychiatric Disorders in the Aged*: Report of a Symposium held by the World Psychiatric Association. Manchester: Geigy (UK) Ltd.
GILLEARD, C. J. (1984) *Living with Dementia: Community Care of the Elderly Mentally Infirm*. London: Croom Helm.
GLASSCOTE, R., GUDEMAN, J. E. & MILES, D. (1977) *Creative Mental Health Services for the Elderly*. Washington: American Psychiatric Association and Mental Health Association.
HENDERSON, J. H. & MACFADYEN, D. M. (1985) Psychogeriatrics in the programmes of the World Health Organization. In *Recent Advances in Psychogeriatrics* (ed. T. Arie). Edinburgh: Churchill Livingstone.

KAY, D. W. K., ROTH, M. & HALL, M. R. P. (1966) Special problems of the aged and the organisation of hospital services. *British Medical Journal, ii*, 967–972.

—— & WALK, A. (eds) (1971) *Recent Developments in Psychogeriatrics: A Symposium*. Royal Medico-Psychological Association. Ashford, Kent: Headley Brothers.

KIDD, C. B. (1962) Misplacement of the elderly in hospital. *British Medical Journal, ii*, 1491–1495.

LEWIS, A. (1946) Ageing and senility: a major problem of psychiatry. *Journal of Mental Science*, **92**, 150–170.

MACMILLAN, D. & SHAW, P. (1966) Senile breakdown in standards of personal and environmental cleanliness. *British Medical Journal, ii*, 967–972.

MEZEY, A. G., HODKINSON, H. M. & EVANS, G. J. (1968) The elderly in the wrong unit. *British Medical Journal, iii*, 16–18.

MORTON, E. V. B., BARKER, M. E. & MACMILLAN, D. (1968) The joint assessment and early treatment unit in psycho-geriatric care. *Gerontologia Clinica*, **10**, 65.

NHS HEALTH ADVISORY SERVICE (1982) *The Rising Tide*. Sutton, Surrey: Health Advisory Service.

NORMAN, A. (1982) *Mental Illness in Old Age: Meeting the Challenge*. London: Centre for Policy on Ageing.

—— (1987) *Senile Dementia*. London: Centre for Policy on Ageing.

POST, F. (1978) Then and now. *British Journal of Psychiatry*, **133**, 83–86.

ROTH, M. (1959) Mental health problems of ageing and the aged. *Bulletin of the World Health Organization*, **21**, 527–561.

—— (1965) Opening Address in Geigy (1965) *op. cit.* 3–10.

—— (1971) Classification and aetiology of mental disorders in old age: some recent developments. Chapter in D. W. K. Kay and A. Walk (eds) *op. cit.*

—— (1972) The psycho-geriatric problem with special reference to the needs of elderly people with progressive mental impairment. Chapter in *Approaches to Action* (ed. G. McLachlan). London: Oxford University Press, Nuffield Provincial Hospitals Trust.

—— & IVERSEN, L. L. (eds) (1986) Alzheimer's disease and related disorders. *British Medical Bulletin*, *1*, 42.

ROYAL COLLEGE OF PSYCHIATRISTS, SECTION ON THE PSYCHIATRY OF OLD AGE (1987) Private care for the elderly mentally ill. *Bulletin of the Royal College of Psychiatrists*, **11**, 278–282.

WATTIS, J. (1988) Geographical variations in the provision of psychiatric services for old people. *Age and Ageing*, **17**, 171–180.

—— & ARIE, T. (1984) Further developments in psychogeriatrics in Britain. *British Medical Journal*, **289**, 778.

——, WATTIS, L. & ARIE, T. (1981) Psychogeriatrics: A national survey of a new branch of psychiatry. *British Medical Journal* **282**, 1529–1533.

# 26 Roth's rules abroad:
## The genesis of a rational geriatric psychiatry in North America
### JOHN R. ROY

Martin Roth is the father of geriatric psychiatry in North America. His teachings on assessment, differential diagnosis and a neo-Kraepelinian organic psychiatry, consciously or unconsciously absorbed, inspired and determined the development of geriatric psychiatry services in Canada and the United States. It would be no exaggeration to claim also in the wider sphere of general psychiatry that Roth's concepts contributed significantly to the paradigm shift in North American psychiatry that sees well attended courses all over the continent on differential diagnosis, organic psychiatry and neurology for psychiatrists.

The early articles (Roth, 1955) that laid the foundations of modern geriatric psychiatry were slow to capture wide-spread attention, but from the publishing of the second edition of *Clinical Psychiatry* (Mayer-Gross, Slater & Roth, 1960) the nascent subspecialty of geriatric psychiatry had available at once an ideology, a science and methods of practical assessment in the Roth-Hopkins standardised Mental Information Test and in the later Blessed-Roth Dementia Rating Scale (Blessed *et al*, 1968). If you can measure something you have a science. The older false global concepts of 'senility' and 'hardening of the arteries' that had stultified development were replaced by the five operationally defined syndromes (Table I).

Gruenberg, an epidemiologist at Johns Hopkins University, published (1978) an influential article on the epidemiology of senile dementia, in which he characterises Roth's work as "more impressive than anything else in the literature" in linking presenting syndrome classifications with outcome.

From Roth's 1955 article, Gruenberg extracted in the following seven decision steps what he called Roth's Rules for the clinical assessment of newly presenting elderly patients with psychiatric symptoms:

(1) after completing the admission work-up, determine whether "mild memory impairment, partial disorientation (or) clouding of consciousness (or) evidence of impairment of intellect and personality . . . are part of an unequivocal progressive cerebral disease, symptoms of which have been present since the beginning of the illness." If so, proceed to step 4. Otherwise,

(2) if "the admission to hospital had been occasioned by a sustained depressive symptom complex (and) the affective symptoms were a prominent, consistent feature of the presenting illness", classify as *affective psychosis* (Ignore any intellectual or personality defects that did not lead to a positive determination in step 1.) Otherwise,

TABLE I
*Roth's five diagnostic categories*

| Original term | More familiar names in North America |
|---|---|
| 1. Senile psychosis | Senile dementia (of Alzheimer type) |
| 2. Arteriosclerotic psychosis | Multi-infarct dementia |
| 3. Acute confusion | Acute delirium |
| 4. Affective psychosis | Major primary depressive (and manic) disorder |
| 5. Late paraphrenia | Late onset paraphrenia |

(3) if "the most prominent feature of the illness is a well-organised system of paranoid delusions", classify as *late paraphrenia*. Otherwise,

(4) if the patient has a "history of (a) gradual and continually progressive failure in the common activities of life and (b) a clinical picture dominated by failure of memory and intellect and (c) disorganisation of personality", *and* if these three features are not "attributable to specific causes such as infection, neoplasm, chronic intoxication or cerebrovascular disease known to have produced infarction", classify as *senile dementia*. Otherwise,

(5) if the "dementia was associated with focal signs and symptoms indicative of cerebrovascular disease", classify as *arteriosclerotic psychosis*. Otherwise,

(6) "if remitting or markedly fluctuating course at some stage of the dementing process was combined with . . . emotional incontinence (or) preservation of insight (or) epileptiform seizures", classify as *arteriosclerotic psychosis*. Otherwise,

(7) "if there is any condition of rapidly evolving clouding of consciousness produced by some extraneous cause or appearing for no discoverable reason (not) occurring in a setting of definite dementia as could be judged from the patient's level of adjustment to the demands of daily life", classify as *acute confusion*. Otherwise, classify as *other*.

Gruenberg then went on to draw important lessons for the clinician, emphasising the place of Roth's work in the Hippocratic tradition and urging an optimistic, pragmatic attitude to clinical diagnosis and prognosis. The philosophy of the new geriatric psychiatry services that began to develop was well stated in Gruenberg's words:

> "Loss of brain substance and the associated decline in testable cognitive functioning will become more manifest if anemia is permitted to develop, if nutrition is neglected, and if fecal impactions are missed. While in the end the patient with senile dementia will die, the same is true of the clinician. The object of the care is not only to influence when the patient will die, but mainly to preserve comfort, a sense of dignity, and a maximum level of functioning for as long as possible."

Roth's natural history and outcome studies were replicated in Canada by Duckworth *et al* (1979), whose findings differed from the original only in the differing prognosis of senile dementia and paraphrenia, the result of the widespread use by the time of his study of neuroleptic drugs and a decline in mortality of senile dementia patients who thus tended to remain longer in treatment facilities.

Duckworth *et al* found that the Roth diagnostic categories had very significant validity in predicting outcome. The vast majority of patients diagnosed as suffering from functional disorders were discharged rapidly into the community. The best prognosis was displayed by patients suffering from mood disorders, with two thirds of these patients being discharged into the community by 90 days.

The prognosis of patients suffering from organic dementias, though better than two decades earlier, remained poor, with over half the patients dead at the end of four years. Only four of this group (11%) were ever discharged into the community.

Alexander B. Christie has also reported on changing patterns of mental illness in late life at Graylingwell Hospital, the site of Roth's original study 30 years previously (1982). Important changes were noted in the diagnostic distribution and outcome of cases admitted. As in Toronto, functional illness had given way to dementia, not as a proportion of patients admitted, but in the number of beds employed for their care six and 24 months after their index admission. Discharge rates for all diagnostic groups except acute confusional states had undergone considerable change and death rates had fallen. Christie found a four-fold increase in bed requirements for cases of dementia at two years, so that, despite a striking reduction in requirement for functional cases, there was an overall increase in bed requirement of 38% at the two-year mark.

In 1981 Blessed & Wilson (1982) used Roth's classification system to examine all (320) patients aged 65 and over admitted to St Nicholas Hospital, Newcastle-Upon-Tyne, during 1976. They found important differences in outcome at six months and two years in comparison with Roth's 1955 prognostic findings. The outlook for affective illness was nearly the same (at two years). For paranoid illnesses there was improvement in outcome in comparison with Roth's findings reported in 1955. Unlike Christie (1982), these authors did not find a further improvement in prognosis of affective disease since 1955. Nearly half of those surviving an acute confusional state had deteriorated or died between six months and two years and a similar prognosis was associated with diagnosis of senile and arteriosclerotic dementia, but there was an increased long-term survival rate in very old female patients with senile dementia compared to the 1955 publication. These authors' findings support the validity of Roth's rules as it was found possible "to allocate 90% of patients over 65 to one of the five clinical distinct and rarely over-lapping categories".

## Experience at McMaster University Medical School

When the opportunity arose at McMaster University to develop an academic geriatric psychiatry service, Roth's principles were used to develop the clinical assessment tools. At first funds were available only for the development of an out-patient clinic which was designed as follows, mindful of the clinical and epidemiological facts just discussed.

### An out-patient geriatric psychiatry service

Early referral was encouraged by educational programmes in the community.

The goal was to have patients referred at the earliest stage of neuropsychiatric symptomatology. All patients had a comprehensive assessment leading to a diagnostic formulation. This comprised a therapeutic plan—with special reference to potentially reversible conditions that might be contributing to functional, cognitive or psychiatric impairments and a management plan involving family supports and community resources. The likely prognosis and possible future needs were listed.

Training was provided to the clinic team and to community health professionals.

## Organisation of the clinic

The clinic staff functioned as a multi-disciplinary team, the members of which had developed skills beyond their traditional professional disciplines, focused upon the common aim of performing a comprehensive neuropsychiatric assessment. During the period of study, the team consisted of a psychiatrist, two social workers, a nurse, and an occupational therapist.

## The clinical assessment procedure

Patients were encouraged to attend the first clinic visit with their families or with someone who was familiar with the patient's functioning during the past six months. The patient spent approximately six hours in the clinic on the first visit, and during that time underwent the assessment procedures described later.

In order to collect a large amount of clinical and para-clinical data while preserving the patient's dignity in the midst of a complex and potentially frightening procedure, each patient was assigned a clinic member as case manager or prime therapist. The case manager's responsibilities included: explaining, supporting, encouraging and steering the patient through the clinic procedures and liaising with other health professionals and hospital departments on the patient's behalf. The case manager was also required to attend to any problems or needs that the patient had, and to observe and monitor behaviour, especially variations in the level of consciousness.

At the end of the first clinic visit, a case conference was held on each new patient. The information available at that point about the patient, including the detailed history of symptoms, mode of onset etc., and the findings on examination, was presented. A preliminary diagnostic formulation was made using Roth's criteria to give a primary and differential diagnosis. The need for further investigations or referrals to other physicians, possible therapeutic strategies, and needs for specific community care were listed. These components of the diagnostic formulation and the basic history data formed the basis of the initial report to the referring physician, which was sent within a few days.

The final (project) diagnosis utilising all the information available on the patient including EEG, CAT scan and a period of observation sometimes of several months at the clinic, was made in accordance with the definitions in the *International Classification of Disease* (1978) and with the principles in the long European psychiatry diagnostic tradition (Lishman, 1980; Roth, 1967; Post, 1971).

## Assessment methods

Each patient received a full neuropsychiatric history and examination. The criteria of Eisdorfer & Cohen (1980) were used in recording mode of onset and duration of symptoms.

All patients had an EEG and many had computerised axial tomography of head. A medical symptom checklist (Hall *et al*, 1978) was completed. Clinical and paraclinical items were entered in a computer data base in coded format.

*Cognitive assessment*

Assessment of cognitive function was performed using a battery of eight test groups derived primarily from the work of Strub & Black (1983). The order, method of presentation, and scoring criteria were that recommended by these authors. All tests were performed by the same person, an occupational therapist, who had received prior training on administration of the test. All sub-tests were scored on an ordinal scale: 0 = normal, no impairment; 1 = mild impairment; 2 = moderate impairment; 3 = moderate to severe impairment; 4 = severe impairment, unable to participate. The complete battery in order of presentation consisted of: a global estimate of consciousness, two tests of attention/concentration/vigilance, five tests of language and memory, three measures of construction, three tests of higher cortical function, seven tests of special cortical function, and a global estimate of judgment.

The Blessed-Roth Dementia Rating Scale (Blessed, Tomlinson & Roth, 1968) was used to assess the level of dementia and the Roth-Hopkins (1953) Mental Assessment score was recorded.

The EEG was recorded at the initial visit and described and interpreted by the same experienced neurologist, familiar with the electroencephalogram in advanced age, and blind to the clinical history, cognitive findings and CT scan results. The dominant background frequency was measured and recorded in Herz units, the degree site and/or distribution of slow activity were noted and recorded on an ordinal scale: 0 = no slowing, 2 = moderate (theta); 3 = severe (delta). The diagnostic opinion was recorded in the following categories: 1 = in keeping with neuronal degeneration, 2 = metabolic disturbance, 3 = suggestive of vascular disease, 4 = epileptic focus or dysrhythmia, 5 = no abnormality noted, 6 = medication effect, 7 = not otherwise specified. Nine standard CT scans of the brain were obtained using a Technicare Delta 2020 Ohio Nuclear CT Scanner and read by a neuroradiologist. Degree of atrophy was coded on an ordinal scale.

**Results**

The clinic has been very successful and it has proved possible to treat quite seriously ill, elderly, psychiatric patients totally in the community with very few requiring in-patient admission to general psychiatric wards.

The following are some clinical and demographic findings on 445 consecutive patients assessed during 1980–1982:

*Socio-demographic and clinical characteristics of 445 patients*

Socio-demographic characteristics are listed in Table II. Ninety-four per cent of the sample reported stable employment (homemaker included) during their employment years.

Thirty two per cent had had problems in marriage or sexual adjustment; 21% admitted to alcohol or drug abuse, and 42% had a family history of alcoholism.

TABLE II
*Socio-demographic characteristics of 445 patients*

| Marital status | | Socio-economic status | |
|---|---|---|---|
| Married | 168 (37.8%) | Lower | 94 (21.1%) |
| Widowed | 235 (52.8%) | Middle | 238 (53.5%) |
| Divorced/separated | 17 (3.8%) | Upper | 49 (11.0%) |
| Single | 25 (5.6%) | Not classifiable | 64 (14.4%) |
| *Living situation* | | *Education* | |
| Alone | 140 (31.5%) | No formal education | 10 (2.2%) |
| With spouse | 140 (31.5%) | Incomplete elementary school | 87 (19.6%) |
| With children | 53 (11.8%) | Primary/incomplete secondary | 266 (59.8%) |
| With others | 112 (25.2%) | Complete secondary | 30 (6.7%) |
| (e.g. lodging home) | | Post-secondary | 27 (6.0%) |
| | | Unclassifiable | 25 (5.6%) |

Forty-four per cent of patients had had symptoms from one week to 12 months, and 56% of patients had had symptoms for over one year. Over 70% of all patients had experienced psychiatric symptoms for six months or more prior to being seen at this clinic. For 51% of patients, referral was initiated by their family physician, 9% by another physician, 17% by a community worker, 5% came from other hospitals or clinics, and 12% came from miscellaneous sources.

From intake information, it was determined that 36% were referred for depression, 36% because of confusion and/or memory impairment; the remainder for disturbed behaviour (10%), anxiety (6%), and a number of miscellaneous, non-specific problems (8%).

Most patients complained of multiple symptoms. Seventy per cent had some degree of mood depression; 37% had persistent anxiety, 9% had anxiety attacks; 61% had a thinking disturbance, 30% had delusions, 20% had hallucinations, 35% had obsessive compulsive phenomena; 65% had sleep disturbance; 41% had a history of disorientation. At their first assessment, 82% had no suicidal thinking, urges or behaviour, 13% had suicidal ideation, 2% had suicidal urges, 1% were seen shortly after a suicide attempt, and a further 2% had a previous history of suicide attempts. Thirty-four per cent were thought to have inadequate food intake, and a further 5% had had prolonged anorexia; 43% had a history of weight loss. The mean weight at presentation was $59.4 \pm 14$ Kg (range 27 Kg to 125 Kg). The mean Blessed-Roth dementia score was 7.3, with a standard deviation of 4.75 (score range 0 to 21).

Of 445 patients, 216 reported a history of previous physical illness that affected choice of psychiatric therapy (12 had glaucoma). Eleven patients had had thyroidectomy; 100 had undergone other previous surgery. Seventy-six reported previous neurological disease, and 14 had a history of head injury. Eighty-two patients had a history of psychiatric illness, and 14 had previously received ECT.

The mean score on Hall *et al*'s medical symptom checklist was 10.9, with a standard deviation of 6.12 (range 0 to 48).

## Roth, DSM-III and project diagnostic categories

The prevalence of patients in each diagnostic group according to Roth and project diagnostic criteria is listed in Table III.

Table IV lists, for diagnosis of dementia and major depressive disorder,

TABLE III
*Roth and project diagnoses for 445 patients*

| Diagnosis | Roth | | Project | |
|---|---|---|---|---|
| | N | % | N | % |
| Primary depressive disorder | 103 | 23 | 120 | 27 |
| Senile dementia | 94 | 21 | 91 | 20 |
| Multi-infarct dementia | 29 | 6.5 | 19 | 4 |
| Delirium | 61 | 13.9 | 62 | 14 |
| Late onset paraphrenia | 5 | 1 | 5 | 1 |
| Functional psychiatric disorders* | 96 | 21.6 | | |
| Focal or diffuse organic cerebral syndromes[†] | 57 | 13 | | |
| Cerebrovascular disease | | | 35 | 8 |
| Anxiety/neurotic states | | | 30 | 7 |
| Normal pressure hydrocephalus | | | 1 | 0 |
| Other | | | 82 | 19 |

*Grief, neurosis, situational reactions
[†]Brain tumour, Huntington's chorea, progressive supernuclear palsy, other neurological syndromes

the McMaster findings with Roth criteria, Project Diagnosis and DSM–III (1980) in comparison with nine similar studies in the literature.

Notable is the closeness of the Roth operationally defined diagnostic groupings to the more elaborate, time-consuming and costly project diagnosis and the ability to perform very detailed geriatric psychiatry assessments in an out-patient setting.

TABLE IV
*Comparison with other samples*

| Authors | N | Service | Age Range ($\bar{x}$) | Males (%) | Females (%) | Diagnostic method | Dementia (%) | Depression (%) | Other (%) |
|---|---|---|---|---|---|---|---|---|---|
| Roy *et al*, 1989 | 445 | OP | 51–94 (75) | 28.0 | 72.0 | Roth | 21.0 | 23.0 | 56.0 |
| Roy *et al*, 1989 | | OP | 51–94 (75) | 28.0 | 72.0 | Project | 20.0 | 27.0 | 53.0 |
| Roy *et al*, 1989 | | OP | 51–94 (75) | 28.0 | 72.0 | DSM–III | 23.0 | 33.0 | 46.0 |
| Baribeau-Braun *et al*, 1979 | 83 | IP | 59–89 (73) | 27.0 | 73.0 | ICDA* | 22.9 | 19.3 | 57.8 |
| Barsa *et al*, 1985 | 185 | OP | Over 60 (na) + | na | na | DSM–III | 13.5 | 43.0 | 48.5 |
| Gilchrist *et al*, 1985 | 100 | IP | 55–90 (73) | 40.0 | 60.0 | DSM–III | 18.0 | 50.0 | 32.0 |
| Goldstein & Grant, 1974 | 148 | IP | Over 60 (na) | 41.0 | 59.0 | ICDA* | 21.6 | 27.7 | 50.7 |
| Kral *et al*, 1986 | 150 | OP | Over 60 (na) | 30.0 | 70.0 | na | 23.0 | 30.0 | 47.0 |
| Levy, 1985 | 176 | Home Visits | na (77) | 29.0 | 71.0 | DSM–III | 47.7 | 26.1 | 26.2 |
| Mei-Tal & Meyers, 1985/86 | 112 | IP | 60–76 (72) | 26.0 | 74.0 | DSM–III | 29.0 | 61.0 | 7.3 |
| Ruskin, 1985 | 67 | OP | Over 60 (na) | 36.0 | 64.0 | DSM–III | 19.0 | 24.0 | 57.0 |
| Spar *et al*, 1980 | 122 | IP | na (73.4) | 25.0 | 75.0 | DSM–III | 27.0 | 51.6 | 21.3 |

*International Classification of Diseases* adapted
+ na = not available

**Treatment given**

One hundred and twenty-three of the 445 required only out-patient assessment and advice, and a report to the referring source.

One hundred and two required anti-depressant medication. Twenty-nine were treated with anti-psychotic medication. Sixty-two received a course of formal psychotherapy. Seventy-six (17%) required immediate admission to a hospital facility (23 patients were admitted to in-patient psychiatry, and 53 went to other hospital units). Residential placement was arranged directly for 14 patients at the time of initial assessment. All patients received psychosocial management which included supportive psychotherapy and family therapy or family counselling. It was possible, with the support of excellent community nursing and social work services, to treat successfully severely depressed patients who lived alone on an out-patient basis.

## *Further research at McMaster using Roth rules*

The Mann-Whitney U test indicated good discrimination of the various ordinal scale cognitive, memory and cerebral function tests between Roth dementia and Roth depression groups (Table V).

TABLE V
*Mann-Whitney U test*
*Dementia/depression groups using ordinal cognitive and cerebral items*

| Variable | (N) | Dementia Median | Range | (N) | Depression Median | Range | Z Score | 1-tailed Probability |
|---|---|---|---|---|---|---|---|---|
| Level of consciousness | 91 | 0.0 | 2.0 | 102 | 0.0 | 3.0 | − 2.9719 | .0015 |
| Digits forwards | 88 | 5.0 | 7.0 | 99 | 5.0 | 7.0 | − 3.4970 | .0003 |
| Digits backwards | 88 | 3.0 | 5.0 | 99 | 3.0 | 6.0 | − 2.9418 | .0001 |
| Digit retention | 88 | 1.0 | 4.0 | 99 | 1.0 | 3.0 | − 2.7867 | .0027 |
| Vigilance | 87 | 1.0 | 4.0 | 94 | 1.0 | 4.0 | − 3.3744 | .0004 |
| Comprehension | 91 | 1.0 | 4.0 | 101 | 0.0 | 4.0 | − 5.2878 | .0000 |
| Repetition | 88 | 2.0 | 4.0 | 98 | 1.0 | 3.0 | − 3.9000 | .0001 |
| Naming | 87 | 1.0 | 4.0 | 100 | 0.0 | 2.0 | − 5.7128 | .0000 |
| Reading | 83 | 0.0 | 4.0 | 95 | 0.0 | 4.0 | − 2.7521 | .0001 |
| Writing | 88 | 0.0 | 4.0 | 98 | 0.0 | 4.0 | − 3.8441 | .0000 |
| Orientation | 90 | 2.0 | 4.0 | 101 | 0.0 | 3.0 | − 8.2822 | .0000 |
| Recent memory | 87 | 2.0 | 4.0 | 100 | 0.0 | 3.0 | − 7.8634 | .0000 |
| Remote memory | 85 | 1.0 | 4.0 | 101 | 0.0 | 3.0 | − 6.9694 | .0000 |
| New learning | 87 | 3.0 | 3.0 | 101 | 2.0 | 4.0 | − 6.6988 | .0000 |
| Memory for recent general events | 84 | 4.0 | 4.0 | 95 | 2.0 | 4.0 | − 5.6732 | .0000 |
| Copying | 86 | 2.0 | 4.0 | 95 | 1.0 | 4.0 | − 3.9000 | .0000 |
| Drawing to command | 77 | 3.0 | 4.0 | 95 | 1.0 | 4.0 | − 5.1868 | .0000 |
| Block design | 67 | 3.0 | 4.0 | 77 | 2.0 | 4.0 | − 2.6637 | .0038 |
| General knowledge | 82 | 2.0 | 4.0 | 100 | 0.5 | 4.0 | − 6.693 | .0000 |
| Verbal abstraction | 77 | 2.0 | 4.0 | 91 | 2.0 | 4.0 | − 3.5932 | .0002 |
| Calculation | 86 | 1.5 | 4.0 | 100 | 0.0 | 4.0 | − 5.9814 | .0000 |
| Apraxia | 87 | 1.0 | 4.0 | 99 | 0.0 | 2.0 | − 5.4822 | .0000 |
| Left-right orientation | 80 | 0.0 | 4.0 | 98 | 0.0 | 4.0 | − 3.6094 | .0002 |
| Finger agnosia | 76 | 0.0 | 4.0 | 96 | 0.0 | 2.0 | − 2.6072 | .0046 |
| Visual agnosia | 78 | 0.0 | 4.0 | 89 | 0.0 | 2.0 | − 5.6400 | .0000 |
| Geographic orientation | 88 | 2.0 | 4.0 | 99 | 0.0 | 4.0 | − 5.0279 | .0000 |
| Other parietal tests | 81 | 1.0 | 4.0 | 96 | 0.0 | 4.0 | − 4.4807 | .0000 |
| Judgement | 88 | 1.0 | 4.0 | 101 | 0.0 | 2.0 | − 4.3042 | .0000 |

TABLE VI
*Mann-Whitney U test on computed cognitive variables*

| Variable | Dementia n = 94 | | Depression n = 103 | | Z Score | 1-tailed Probability |
|---|---|---|---|---|---|---|
| | Median | Range | Median | Range | | |
| Attention tests | 1.0 | 2.0 | 0.0 | 2.0 | − 2.9236 | .0017 |
| Language tests | 1.0 | 5.0 | 0.0 | 4.0 | − 5.1327 | .000 |
| Memory tests | 4.0 | 5.0 | 2.0 | 5.0 | − 7.3286 | .000 |
| Construction tests | 2.0 | 3.0 | 1.0 | 3.0 | − 3.3719 | .0003 |
| Higher cognitive tests | 2.0 | 3.0 | 1.0 | 3.0 | − 4.5067 | .0000 |
| Special cerebral functions | 2.0 | 6.0 | 0.0 | 4.0 | − 5.8498 | .000 |
| Total battery score | 11.5 | 25.0 | 4.0 | 17.0 | − 6.9329 | .000 |

Table VI shows similar statistics for computed scores (sum of significant abnormality in sub-groups) for the cognitive functions. Of these new variables, only the total cognitive battery score approached normal distribution.

There was no significant difference in the ages or previous intelligence between the demented or depressed groups. The demented group had a mean 9.62 years of education, compared to 8.4 years for the depressed group; this difference was statistically significant when the values were compared using a Student's t-test ($t = 2.67$, $P = .008$).

Various items from history, assessment and paraclinical tests showed as clearly as the cognitive test battery items the ability of the Roth categorisation to discriminate among patients.

## Duration of symptoms

Of the demented elderly patients, 20.2% had symptoms for less than one year, and 56.9% of the depressed elderly had symptoms for less than one year. This difference in duration of symptoms was analysed between the two groups when the data were divided into greater or less than one year duration. The difference was significant ($X^2 = 26.7$, $P < .00005$).

## Mode of onset of symptoms

Of the demented group, 12.8% and of the depressed group, 35.9% reported sudden onset of symptoms; 87.2% of the demented group and 64.1% of the depressed group reported gradual or insidious onset of symptoms. This difference was significant for the two groups ($X^2 = 12.9$, $P < 0.0005$).

## EEG findings

There were significant differences between the two groups: 78% of the demented and 46% of the depressed had diffuse EEG slowing; 70% of the demented and 24% of the depressed had findings which were interpreted by a neurologist blind to clinical features as in keeping with neuronal degeneration.

The mean resting alpha was 7.899 for the dementia group and 8.163 for the depression group. This difference was statistically significant ($t = - 2.63$, $P < .005$).

## CT scan findings

Of demented patients, 65.8% and of depressed patients, 33.4% had cerebral atrophy.

## Dementia rating scale

The mean score on the Blessed Dementia Scale was 10.28 for the dementia group and 5.67 for the depression group. This difference was statistically significant ($t = 7.6$, $P < .0005$).

# Diagnosis of multi-infarct dementia

A further study examined the value of plasma high density lipoprotein cholesterol (HDLC) in predicting Roth-classified multi-infarct dementia versus Roth progressive idiopathic dementia (Muckle & Roy, 1985).

We studied 17 consecutive men who presented at the Geriatric Psychiatry Service, Chedoke Hospital Division of Chedoke-McMaster Hospitals. On the basis of Roth criteria, I diagnosed SDAT in 12 patients and MID in five patients. The means and ranges of HDLC levels were significantly ($P < 0.001$) lower in the MID group (mean = 0.94 mmol/l, range = 0.88–0.98 mmol/l, SEM = 0.02 mmol/l) to the extent that there was no overlap with the SDAT group (mean = 1.37 mmol/l, range = 1.11–1.68 mmol/l, SEM = 0.06 mmol/l).

# A memory clinic at McMaster University

With the advent of drugs putatively able to enhance memory function it became apparent that it was essential to detect and differentiate cognitive disorders long before a clinical diagnosis of dementia could be made and a memory clinic was developed as a component of the Geriatric Psychiatry Service at McMaster. The aims of this clinic are to carry out thorough assessments in patients presenting with early cognitive or cerebral function impairment in an endeavour, firstly, to explore the possible clinical and neurotransmitter heterogeneity of those cases that ultimately could be classified as Alzheimer's disease or progressive idiopathic dementia and, on the other hand, to develop the principles of a neuropsychopharmacology of memory and cognitive function, both in respect to the causation of memory and cognitive impairments by side-effects of pharmacological agents and in the amelioration of cognitive deficits by pharmacological or neuropharmacological means.

Though using various high technological procedures such as CT scan, spectral analysis of EEG, PET scan, computerised presentation of neuropsychological tests, neuropharmacological probes and neuroendocrinological challenge tests, the actual theoretical underpinnings of research in the memory clinic are essentially a neo-Rothian approach (Roth, 1967) that seeks to relate clinical phenomenology, mode of development of history and prospective natural history with paraclinical measures in order to delineate homogeneous subgroups with clusters of clinical phenomenology and paraclinical findings that would be predictive of specific neurotransmitter or neuromodulator-based separate individual syndromes each ultimately with a specific pharmacological therapy.

These clinical and research initiatives of the Department of Geriatric Psychiatry at McMaster have now attracted generous clinical funding from the Ontario Health Ministry for a Comprehensive Geriatric Psychiatry Regional Service including a 20-bed in-patient research geriatric psychiatry ward which will be used for special assessments of dementia and cognitive impairments, an expanded memory and psychopharmacology out-patient clinic and a consultation outreach team. Funding is also imminent for a geriatric psychopharmacology research centre which will mainly be evaluating, at clinical and basic science levels, the efficacy and modes of action of drugs on cognitive function.

## Conclusion

Those of us who have been influenced in our careers in psychiatry by contact with Martin Roth in our formative years have a great deal for which to be grateful. Martin's wide interests in psychiatry and his cultured, humanist outlook have influenced many branches and aspects of psychiatry as a profession and as an academic discipline. Specifically in the new subspecialty of geriatric psychiatry his inspiration has been of crucial importance in several ways. He laid the foundations of a science of diagnosis leading to a rational use of therapy in late life psychiatry. He has shown us that the assessment and treatment of elderly persons with psychiatric illness is at once a privilege and a challenge. In the encounter with the ageing human being we are faced with our own ageing and with questions about the meaning and purpose of existence. From his firm base in the European tradition, Martin has taught us how to bring to the ageing patient with neuropsychiatric disturbances the best of modern technology, delivered in a context of respect for the individual, his humanity and his right to contribute to decision-making, but always at a level of meticulous psychiatric assessment and effective therapy that is not inferior to that available to the younger person with psychiatric symptoms. At a time when psychiatry is under attack from outside and suffering still from dissensions within, when psychiatry as a profession is at risk of losing large components to other disciplines such as behavioural neurology, neuropsychology and cognitive science, it is no little thing to be reminded of our history within the main stream of European neuropsychiatry and our duty to pass on to new generations of psychiatrists the essence of a psychiatry worth saving.

## References

BARIBEAU-BRAUN, J., GOLDSTEIN, S. & BRAUN, C. (1979) A multi-variate study of psychogeriatric patients. *Journal of Gerontology*, **34**, 351–357.

BARSA, J. J., KASS, F., BEELS, C. C., *et al* (1985) Development of a cost-efficient psychogeriatrics service. *The American Journal of Psychiatry*, **142**, 238–241.

BLESSED, G., TOMLINSON, B. E. & ROTH, M. (1968) The association between quantitative measures of dementia and of senile change in the grey matter of elderly subjects. *British Journal of Psychiatry*, **114**, 797–811.

—— & WILSON, I. D. (1982) The contemporary natural history of mental disorder in old age. *British Journal of Psychiatry*, **141**, 59–67.

CHRISTIE, A. B. (1982) Changing patterns in mental illness in the elderly. *British Journal of Psychiatry*, **140**, 154–159.

*DIAGNOSTIC AND STATISTICAL MANUAL OF MENTAL DISORDERS (3rd edn)* (1980) Washington: American Psychiatric Association.

DUCKWORTH, G. S., KEDWARD, H. B. & BAILEY, W. F. (1979) Prognosis of mental illness in old age. A Four Year Follow-up Study. *Canadian Journal of Psychiatry*, **24**, 674–682.

EISDORFER, C. & COHEN, D. (1980) Diagnostic criteria for primary neuronal degeneration of the Alzheimer's Type. *Journal of Family Practice*, **4**, 533–557.

GILCHRIST, P. N., ROZENBILDS, U. Y., MARTIN, E., *et al* (1985) A study of 100 consecutive admissions to a psychogeriatric unit. *The Medical Journal of Australia*, **143**, 236–237.

GOLDSTEIN, S. & GRANT, A. (1974) The psychogeriatric patient in hospital. *The Canadian Medical Association Journal*, **111**, 329–332.

GRUENBERG, E. M. (1978) Epidemiology of senile dementia. In *Advances in Neurology* (ed. B. S. Schoenberg). New York: Raven Press.

HALL, R. C. W., POPKIN, M. K., DEVAUL, R. A., *et al* (1978) Physical illness presenting as psychiatric disease. *Archives of General Psychiatry*, **35**, 1315–1320.

INTERNATIONAL CLASSIFICATION OF DISEASES (revision 9) (1978) Clinical Modification (vol. 2). Ann Arbor, Commission of Professional and Hospital Activities.

KRAL, V. A., PALMER, R. B. & YAKOVISHIN, V. (1986) A psychogeriatric out-patient service in a general hospital: Is it medically worthwhile? *The Psychiatric Journal of the University of Ottawa*, **11**, 140–142.

LEVY, M. T. (1985) Psychiatric assessment of elderly patients in the home: A survey of 176 cases. *Journal of the American Geriatric Society*, **33**, 9–12.

LISHMAN, W. A. (1980) *Organic Psychiatry: The Psychological Consequences of Cerebral Disorder*. Boston: Blackwell Scientific Publications.

MAYER-GROSS, W., SLATER, E. & ROTH, M. (1960) *Clinical Psychiatry (2nd edn)*. London: Baillière.

MEI-TAL, V. & MEYERS, B. S. (1985–86) Empirical study on an inpatient psychogeriatric unit: Diagnostic complexities. *The International Journal of Psychological Medicine*, **15**, 91–109.

MUCKLE, T. J. & ROY, J. R. (1985) High-Density lipoprotein cholesterol in differential diagnosis of senile dementia. *The Lancet*, **i**, 1191–1193.

POST, F. (1971) The diagnostic process. In *Recent Developments in Psychogeriatrics* (Royal College of Psychiatrists, Special Publications No. 6), (eds D. W. K. Kay & A. Walk) Ashford: Headley Brothers.

ROTH, M. (1955) The natural history of mental disorder in old age. *Journal of Mental Science*, **101**, 281–301.

—— (1967) The clinical interview and psychiatric diagnosis, have they a future in psychiatric practice? *Comprehensive Psychiatry*, **8**, 427–438.

—— & HOPKINS, B. (1953) Psychological test performance in patients over 60. I Senile psychosis and the affective disorders of old age. *Journal of Mental Science*, **99**, 439–450.

ROY, J. R., ROBERTS, R. S., MOLLOY, D. W. & MUNROE-BLUM, H. (1989) Outpatient neuropsychiatric assessment in late life. I. Concepts and methods; II. Epidemiological and clinical profile of 445 consecutive patients. (In press).

RUSKIN, P. E. (1985) Geropsychiatric consultation in a university hospital: A report on 67 referrals. *The American Journal of Psychiatry*, **142**, 333–336.

SPAR, J. E., FORD, C. V. & LISTON, E. H. (1980) Hospital treatment of elderly neuropsychiatric patients. II Statistical profile of the first 122 patients in a new teaching ward. *Journal of the American Geriatric Society*, **28**, 539–543.

STRUB, R. L. & BLACK, F. W. (1983) *The Mental Status Examination in Neurology*. Philadelphia: F. A. Davis.

# 27 The normal elderly—
# the by-product of a survey

**KLAUS BERGMANN**

I am honoured to be asked to contribute to the tribute to Sir Martin Roth's 70th year. Sir Martin's public contributions will be well chronicled and I would like to make my acknowledgement a more personal one.

When I arrived at Newcastle upon Tyne in 1964 to begin full-time research under the direction of Sir Martin and the supervision of David Kay, I was frightened and amazed at the considerable freedom that I was given. Initiation into the mysteries of epidemiological work came gradually and, sometimes painfully and slowly, I realised the large amount of strategic and tactical planning that had already gone into the whole operation, which gave me the framework within which to operate. Also, I learnt how to ask the kind of questions that could be answered and to create categories, make comparisons and generate testable hypotheses. Sir Martin's refusal to fudge the issue by setting up universally applicable satisfying philosophical generalisations constituted a lesson in scientific thinking which benefits me today.

Another great lesson which illuminated community studies was the clearly defined diagnostic categories, derived from the Graylingwell studies and prognostically validated in hospital studies, which allowed us to examine the effects of psychiatric disorder on survival and social need in the community. Generally, the rewards of a reductionist rather than a holistic approach were clearly shown. Even today, when there is talk about the problems of the elderly in general as opposed to discussion of particular problems of older people, pessimistic inaction seems to be the fruit of such discourse.

However, as we ploughed through nearly 800 community respondents to our survey of the elderly, the normal elderly seemed like useless chaff obscuring our precious 'organics' and 'psychotics' and even our more common 'neurotics', fit only to be candidates for various matched control groups. Looking back on the survey, the normal elderly became more important and their achievements more impressive and, although they could not be defined as a categorical group, contact with them was valuable and instructive.

When an older relative or friend functions well, shows flexibility, energy and enterprise, we pay them the dubious 'ageist' compliment of saying that they are not really old at all! The professional investigating the aged relies heavily on the deficit model for investigating changes in later life, perhaps because most professionals work with the dependent elderly either in institutions or at least with those seeking help.

Psychologists measuring age-related decline cross-sectionally have found an inexorable downward progression which must have filled most middle-aged people with fear, let alone the elderly (Wechsler, 1958). This view has been challenged by those like Schaie (1967) who have demonstrated cultural cohort effects. Experimental psychology, while moving away from a psychometric approach, still takes a decremental view of information processing and problem solving in the elderly, related often to a reduction of the speed of information processing (Botwinnick, 1977; Rabbitt, 1977). Personality studies generally do not take such a decremental view of ageing, mostly demonstrating a stability of personality traits, though increasing introversion is a common observation. Neugarten (1977) reviewed a number of aspects of personality function investigated in older populations and divided these into negative, neutral and positive aspects of personality in relation to old age (Table I). Positive aspects of personality were less commonly studied than the others.

The tendency to stereotype the elderly seems to work in a negative direction. Harris *et al* (1975) examined the view that the public expressed about the "very serious problems of the elderly" concerning matters such as fear of crime, poor health, not feeling needed, poor housing etc. In all cases the elderly held less negative views than those ascribed to them (Table II).

Have such negative views of old age always obtained? Looking for quotations can lead to equivocal results. Shakespeare said, "Crabbed age and youth cannot

TABLE I
*Personality: various aspects investigated in relation to ageing*

| 'Negative' | 'Neutral' | 'Positive' |
|---|---|---|
| Egocentricity | Risk taking | Happiness |
| Dependency | Perceived locus of control | Morale |
| Dogmatism | Self concept | Reminiscence |
| Rigidity | Self image | Dreams and day dreams |
| Cautiousness | Attitudes to ageing | |

TABLE II
*Differences between personal experiences of Americans aged 65 and over, and expectations held by other adults about those experiences*

| | Very serious problems experienced by the elderly themselves (Percentage) | Very serious problems the public expects the elderly to experience (Percentage) | Net difference |
|---|---|---|---|
| Fear of crime | 23 | 50 | + 27 |
| Poor health | 21 | 51 | + 30 |
| Not having enough money to live on | 15 | 62 | + 47 |
| Loneliness | 12 | 60 | + 48 |
| Not having enough medical care | 10 | 44 | + 34 |
| Not having enough education | 8 | 20 | + 12 |
| Not feeling needed | 7 | 54 | + 47 |
| Not having enough to do to keep busy | 6 | 37 | + 31 |
| Not having enough friends | 5 | 28 | + 23 |
| Not having enough job opportunities | 5 | 45 | + 40 |
| Poor housing | 4 | 35 | + 31 |
| Not having enough clothing | 3 | 16 | + 13 |

Source: L. Harris and Associates. *The Myth and Reality of Aging in America* (Washington, D.C.: The National Council on the Ageing, Inc., 1975), p. 31.

live together, youth is full of pleasance, age is full of care.'' On the other hand, Stevenson took a more developmental view of ageing, ''To love playthings as well as a child, to lead an adventurous and honourable youth and to settle, when the time comes, into a green and smiling age, is to be a good artist in life and to deserve well of your neighbour''. Perhaps the great art of the past can give some indications of positive virtues seen in the aged. The portraitist mirrors the attitudes and views of his society; for example, the wisdom, power and authority in Raphael's portrait of the old white-bearded Pope Julius II. In the secular world philosophers such as Hobbes, who lived to the age of 91 years, transmits his power and authority through the portrait by Joseph Wright. Rembrandt's portrait of an old lady does not suggest the kind of person who would meekly accept the offer of meals on wheels or of a nice day centre!

What, then, can be said about the normal elderly in our survey? The majority of them seemed to enjoy life and to cope well with its vicissitudes, adapting to sometimes quite dramatic change, and to be happy with their remaining family and friends. It was difficult to define the 'normal subjects', either on a statistical basis or even according to an ideal norm. Mental health is to be devoutly wished for but desperately difficult to define!

A definition by exclusion was attempted in order to define a group of normal subjects to study vis-à-vis 'neurotic' subjects. Normal subjects were not demented, not psychotic and not exhibiting more than a minimal number of neurotic symptoms. Subjects with grossly deviant personalities were also excluded. Such normal subjects might almost merit the term 'supernormal' although they did comprise about half the sample (Table III). This group did not conform to the stereotype of older people: their greater health concern, hypochondriasis, complaints of loneliness, the presence of disability, poor self care, and limited mobility (see Table IV): 93% were not lonely, a similar number were not hypochondriacal, and nearly 80% considered that their health was good and cared for themselves well. However, only 70% had no disability and unlimited mobility. Our survey subjects compared well with normal survey subjects of all ages rated for excessive health concern on the Cornell Medical Index (Shepherd *et al*, 1966). A picture of the normal older person can be constructed by examining the negative correlations of various psychopathological features associated with those subjects placed in the normal group (Table V). They seem to have been more secure as children and more likely to have experienced harmonious family life. In adult life their own marriages are more secure and their children reveal less evidence of psychiatric disturbance. A positive attitude to their health, satisfaction with social relationships and human contacts characterises their attitudes in old age.

What can be learnt from this, perhaps artificially selected but substantial, group of elderly people? The first lesson that the clinician accustomed to patients learns is that these are independent people, who have high expectations of themselves, see themselves as useful and coping and able to determine their own fates. For the psychiatrist, working with elderly neurotic and disturbed elderly patients without brain damage, such normal old people remind him that there is the possibility of 'adjustment', and give a glimpse of a normative ideal to be detected among the elderly in the community, well hidden from helping agencies and health care professionals. The concept of sick role behaviour (Parsons, 1950) includes the idea that there is a valid excuse for not meeting normal social

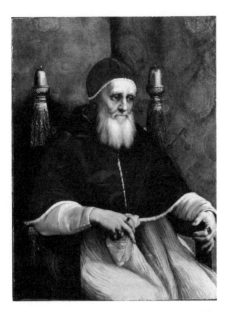

*Fig. 1. Pope Julius II.* (Raphael). *Reproduced by courtesy of the Trustees, The National Gallery, London.*

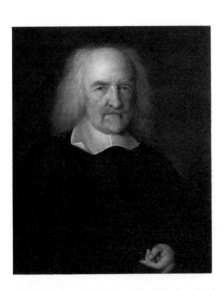

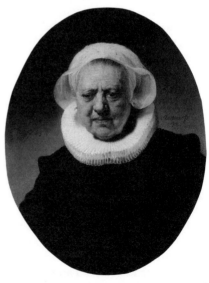

*Fig. 2. Thomas Hobbes.* (J. M. Wright). *Reproduced by courtesy of the Trustees, National Portrait Gallery, London.*

*Fig. 3. Portrait of an 83 year-old Woman* (Rembrandt van Rijn). *Reproduced by courtesy of the Trustees, The National Gallery, London.*

TABLE III
*Distribution of sample by age, sex and diagnosis*

| | Normal | | Late onset neurotic | | Chronic neurotic | | Deviant personality | |
|---|---|---|---|---|---|---|---|---|
| | M | F | M | F | M | F | M | F |
| 65–69 yrs | 27(9.0) | 24(8.0) | 10(3.3) | 21(7.0) | 4(1.3) | 18(6.0) | 4(1.3) | 4(1.3) |
| 70–74 yrs | 35(11.7) | 29(9.7) | 5(1.7) | 20(6.7) | 11(3.7) | 15(5.0) | 3(1.0) | 4(1.3) |
| 75 + yrs | 18(6.0) | 15(5.0) | 2(0.7) | 14(4.7) | 2(0.7) | 11(3.7) | 2(0.7) | 2(0.7) |
| Total | 80(26.7) | 68(22.7) | 17(5.7) | 55(18.4) | 17(5.7) | 44(14.7) | 9(3.0) | 10(3.3) |
| | 148(49.4) | | 72(24.0) | | 61(20.4) | | 19(6.3) | |

| | Total by sex | | Grand total |
|---|---|---|---|
| | M | F | |
| 65–69 yrs | 45(15.0) | 67(22.3) | 112(37.3) |
| 70–74 yrs | 54(14.7) | 68(22.7) | 122(40.7) |
| 75 + yrs | 24(8.0) | 42(14.0) | 66(22.0) |
| Total | 123(41.0) | 177(59.0) | 300(100.0) |
| | 300(100.0) | | |

(percentages in parentheses)

TABLE IV
*Normal subjects: morale and physical status*

| Morale | |
|---|---|
| Own health good (and good with qualifications) | 78% |
| Not lonely | 93% |
| Not hypochondriacal | 93% |
| *Physical capacity* | |
| Disability absent or mild | 69% |
| Unlimited mobility | 71% |
| Good self care | 79% |

TABLE V
*The normal elderly person: a random sample survey*

| | |
|---|---|
| *Early life* | |
| No report of childhood neurotic traits, | 0.30 P<.001 |
| Poor family relationships not reported, | 0.18 P<.01 |
| *Family* | |
| No evidence of marital disharmony | 0.18 P<.01 |
| No history of psychiatric disorder in children, | 0.17 P<.01 |
| *Attitudes* | |
| Does not see himself as unduly worrying, unsociable, prone to mood swings, | 0.45 P<.001 |
| Not hypochondriacal, | 0.34 P<.001 |
| Sees own health as good, | 0.34 P<.001 |
| Not lonely, | 0.25 P<.001 |
| *Personality ratings* | |
| Not anxiety prone, | 0.46 P<.001 |
| Not insecure and rigid, | 0.30 P<.001 |
| Not neuraesthenic, | 0.19 P<.01 |
| *Physical health* | |
| No gastro-intestinal disorder, | 0.23 P<.001 |
| No physical disability, | 0.19 P<.01 |
| *Social measures* | |
| Many daily contacts, | 0.19 P<.01 |
| No loss of children in the last five years, | 0.17 P<.01 |

obligations. The neurotic person may often come to be defined as sick as an alternative to suffering sanctions for his failure. However, the role expectations of the elderly are so low that it is not surprising that only the most gross psychosis or dementia brings them for treatment. Their role seems to be not to be a noticeable nuisance. Until we can make more stringent demands of the older person there seems little hope of developing a psychotherapeutic approach to suit their needs. The normal elderly person seems to undertake many tasks in order to maintain what Erikson (1959) describes as 'ego integrity' and avoid despair. In trying to define the social obligations of the elderly, and implicitly the kind of expectations we might have of their role, an intuitive and subjective guess may be all that is possible at present. The aims for an 'ideal' adjustment to old age might be listed as follows:

(a) having a satisfying occupation
(b) the maintenance of a good and satisfying relationship with family, friends, neighbours and helpers
(c) coping with losses both of other people and of self-esteem
(d) adjustment to and coping with pain and disability
(e) evaluating realistically one's own need for help, while maintaining maximum choice and independence
(f) accepting the imminence of death and completing one's 'life review'.

Armed with high expectations of the elderly and the feeling that old age gives a chance to develop new strengths, perhaps society can learn to put more demands on its older citizens and offer more help when their experience of life, previous deprivation and current stresses and vicissitudes make it difficult to meet such demands.

## References

BOTWINNICK, J. (1977) Intellectual abilities. In *Handbook of the Psychology of Aging* (eds J. E. Birren & K. W. Schaie). Cincinatti: Van Nostrand Reinold.

ERIKSON, E. H. (1959) Identity and the life cycle. In *Selected Papers, Psychological Issues, vol. 1*, No. 1, Monograph 1. New York: International Universities Press.

HARRIS, L. AND ASSOCIATES. (1975) *The Myth and Reality of Aging in America*. Washington, DC: The National Council on Aging.

NEUGARTEN, B. L. (1977) Personality and Aging. In *Handbook of the Psychology of Aging* (eds J. E. Birren & K. W. Schaie). Cincinatti: Van Nostrand Reinold.

PARSONS, T. (1950) Illness and the role of the physician. *American Journal of Orthopsychiatry*, **21**, 452–460.

RABBITT, P. (1977) Changes in problem solving ability in old age. In *Handbook of the Psychology of Aging* (eds J. E. Birren & K. W. Schaie). Cincinatti: Van Nostrand Reinold.

SCHAIE, K. W. (1967) Age changes and age differences. *Gerontologist*, **7**, 128–132.

SHEPHERD, M., COOPER, B., BROWN, A. C. & KALTON, G. W. (1966) *Psychiatric Illness in General Practice*. London: Oxford University Press.

WECHSLER, D. (1958) *The Measurement and Appraisal of Adult Intelligence*. Baltimore: Williams & Wilkins.

# 28  Psychiatric aspects of sensory deficits in the elderly

## ALEXANDER F. COOPER

"Deformities and imperfections of our bodies, as lamenesse, crookednesse, deafnesse, blindness, be they innate or accidentall, torture many men: yet this may comfort them, that those imperfections of the body doe not a whit blemish the soule or hinder the operations of it, but rather help and much increase it".

Burton (1621)

My interest in this field was initially stimulated by Martin Roth when he handed me a copy of a paper by Silverman (1964). After reviewing various studies of perception in schizophrenia, including his own findings of attentional dysfunction in these illnesses, Silverman proposed a process of 'ideational gating' in paranoid patients which ensures that only stimuli acceptable to the patient's thinking are allowed to enter consciousness. These observations had obvious relevance to the high prevalence of deafness in paraphrenic subjects previously reported by Kay & Roth (1961), and it was suggested that I should carry out a re-examination of the prevalence and nature of sensory deficits in a series of these patients. Professor Roth gave me the impression that the project would take just a few weeks, after which I would be participating in another large-scale study going on in the Department. Little did he or I then realise that over three years would pass before the research could be completed!

In recent years the frequent association of physical illness and psychological disturbance has become well established, and Lloyd (1977) has suggested various mechanisms that might account for the relationship. Apart from coincidental occurrences, physical and psychiatric illness may occur together in clusters during stressful periods of life (Hinkle & Wolff, 1957). Psychiatric disorders, such as severe depression and anorexia nervosa and also psychotropic drug therapy, may lead to somatic complications, and alterations of cerebral metabolism during the course of physical illness or its treatment may cause a variety of psychiatric manifestations. However, psychological problems associated with physical illness or disability may also be a consequence of the non-specific stress or the developmental or psycho-social implications of the disorder. Taking the quotation from Robert Burton as our 'null hypothesis', this article will, therefore, consider to what extent defects of hearing and vision in the elderly contribute to the functional psychological abnormalities that may be associated with them.

There are many psychological consequences of impaired hearing and a satisfactory understanding of such problems is complicated by the fact that the word 'deafness' is a blanket expression, including all types of hearing difficulty (Denmark, 1969). Probably the two most important variables that should be considered are the degree of hearing loss and the age of onset of deafness. When deafness is profound, it is important to differentiate between those who are congenitally deaf or became deaf prior to the acquisition of speech and language (the early profound or prelingually deaf) and those whose deafness came later in life (the postlingually deaf).

## Early profound deafness

Early profound deafness is present in about 1 in 1000 of the population. In the growing child it leads to developmental retardation by depriving the affected person of a wide range of general knowledge and experience from an early age (Altshuler, 1971). Most significant is the inability to appreciate the spoken word, leading to failure of normal development of verbal (auditory) language. Thus, the majority of profoundly deaf people have severe linguistic and literacy problems and tend to rely on manual methods of communication. They are also deprived of the experience of emotionality which is communicated through verbal interchange and which is so essential to normal personality development (Denmark, 1969; Altshuler, 1971). The deaf person, therefore, may suffer retardation of his emotional and personality development as well as linguistic and cognitive deficiencies.

Reviewing extensive research into the psychiatric problems of the prelingually deaf carried out in various centres over the previous 20 years (Rainer *et al*, 1963; Denmark & Eldridge, 1969), Altshuler (1971) drew attention to the impulsive-aggressive behaviour which occurs so frequently in these patients, irrespective of the primary psychiatric diagnosis. Indeed, in most series, problems of behaviour and maladjustment apparently related to deafness were by far the commonest disorders encountered. Altshuler contrasted these findings with the remarkably low incidence of severe depression and obsessional symptoms and the smaller prevalence of schizophrenia in the deaf, compared with the normally hearing.

### The profoundly deaf in later life

Although there have been many psychiatric studies of deaf children (Meadow, 1981) and adults (Altshuler & Abdullah, 1981) little attention has been focused on the psycho-social problems of the elderly deaf. However, Becker (1980) and Becker & Nadler (1980) have begun to remedy this deficiency by reporting an anthropological study of elderly deaf people in the San Francisco Bay area. They point out that prelingual deafness is not only a sensory deficit; it also has social, emotional, and cultural implications which are unique to communities of deaf people. The majority of the aged deaf have had hearing parents with whom they could not communicate adequately, so that they were unable to acquire the language and cultural attitudes of the deaf until the school years. During that period strong identification was created within the group, producing group cohesiveness akin to that of an ethnic minority. In adulthood, the majority of deaf people marry deaf partners so that the 'deaf identity' is maintained throughout the life course. Deafness defines their relationship to the rest of society and in old age results in a high level of peer interaction which is particularly important to the individual's adaptation to ageing.

Older deaf people, therefore, have developed the basis for a strong system of social support over their lifetime. However, a major disadvantage is a tendency for the deaf to segregate themselves from hearing organisations. In old age, Social Services are not readily available to the deaf on account of communication difficulties and the agencies serving the general population of deaf people are unfamiliar with the needs of the aged. However, Becker & Nadler (1980) show how these difficulties can be overcome by integrating deaf people into an agency serving the elderly in general, by recognising the importance of the deaf identity, yet providing deaf people with opportunities to interact with their hearing peers. Although this study provides no information on the levels of psychiatric morbidity among elderly deaf people, Becker (1981) suggests that the combination of deaf identity and strong systems of social support sustain the elderly deaf against isolation and loss of self-esteem. A climate is created which enables them to adapt to their own disability in old age and it might be that, compared with the hearing, the elderly deaf are relatively protected from psychosocial trauma such as bereavement (Becker, 1980).

## The hard of hearing

In contrast to early profound deafness, there have been very few studies which have attempted to investigate systematically the psychiatric problems of the hard of hearing. Denmark (1969) has appealed for a greater awareness among psychiatrists of the profound implications of this form of deafness and Rawson (1973) has drawn attention to the dearth of sociological, psychological and psychiatric research on the problems of hard of hearing and deafened adults. This concern is particularly relevant in the case of the elderly, in whom the prevalence of deafness is much higher than among younger people and increases rapidly with age. Studies of prevalence in the community using self-ratings or observer-ratings of hearing impairment have consistently produced results suggesting a prevalence of 30–40% (Wilkins, 1948; Townsend & Wedderburn, 1965). However, the use of audiometric techniques has yielded estimates almost twice that level (Gilhome Herbst & Humphrey, 1980). Using as a measure of deafness the degree at which a hearing aid is normally considered to be necessary, these authors found that 60% of a sample aged 70 years or over living in their own homes had significant impairment of hearing when tested by pure-tone audiometry. Over 40% were substantially or severely deaf according to these criteria, including 70% of those aged 80 years or over. Corbin *et al* (1984) reported similar findings.

### Psychiatric illness in the hard of hearing

Various clinical observations and research studies of the hard of hearing are in agreement that depression appears to be the most common reaction encountered (Knapp, 1948; Ramsdell, 1962; Denmark, 1969; Mahapatra, 1974). This can be severe and associated with suicidal behaviour, especially if the onset is sudden.

There has been less agreement on the incidence of paranoid reactions. Some authors (Ramsdell, 1962: Denmark, 1969; Rousey, 1971) have commented on the morbid suspiciousness and hostility in these patients, some of whom were frankly psychotic, while others (Ingals, 1946; Knapp, 1948) have found such reactions to be rare. Mahapatra (1974), in a controlled study, demonstrated that psychological disturbance was significantly commoner in a group of middle-aged patients with bilateral conductive deafness due to otosclerosis than in a group of similar age with unilateral deafness from the same cause. The neurotic form of depression was the commonest syndrome in the bilateral group (35%), but the prevalence of paranoid schizophrenia (10%) was also much higher than expected.

Thomas (1984) has recently reported a large-scale study of psychological disturbance in samples of non-geriatric patients, drawn from NHS clinics, suffering from various forms of hearing impairment. The results showed that at least one in five of hearing-impaired patients experienced a high level of psychological disturbance long after acquiring a hearing aid and receiving available rehabilitation. The problems consisted of minor affective symptoms such as anxiety, depression, and listlessness; the author was forced to conclude that in the present state of knowledge, large numbers of the hearing-impaired people will continue to suffer residual handicap even after they have received a hearing aid.

In their investigation of hearing impairment and mental state in the elderly, Gilhome Herbst & Humphrey (1980) found that 35% of their sample were suffering from at least 'limited' depression on the screening procedure used and 11% could be regarded as having 'pervasive' depression. Sixty-nine per cent of the sample who were depressed were also deaf, and this relationship remained significant when both age and socio-economic status were taken into account. Eastwood *et al* (1985) reported similar findings from a study of hearing impairment and mental disorders in a home for the elderly. Sixty-six per cent of the sample had clinically significant hearing loss, 53% were found to have a diagnosable psychiatric illness, and over 60% of those with severe-to-profound hearing impairment had a psychiatric disorder.

## Hearing disorders in the functional psychoses of the elderly

As long ago as 1915, Emil Kraepelin described the occurrence of persecutory delusions in the hard of hearing and since his time an association between deafness and paranoid symptoms in schizophrenic patients has occasionally been noted (Pritzker, 1938; Houston & Royse, 1954). More recently, reports have appeared showing an increased prevalence of hearing impairment in patients suffering from schizophrenic and paranoid psychoses compared with control groups suffering from other illnesses, particularly those developing for the first time in old age.

Kay & Roth (1961) studied two series of patients suffering from 'late paraphrenia' admitted to two hospitals in England (Graylingwell) and Sweden (Stockholm). They used 'late paraphrenia' as a suitable descriptive term, without prejudice as to aetiology, for all patients with a paranoid symptom-complex in which signs of organic dementia or sustained confusion were absent and in which the condition was judged, from the content of the delusions and hallucinations,

cognitive impairment in this group compared with non-symptomatic subjects. Reviewing the whole subject, Corbin & Eastwood (1986) concluded that given the existing evidence, there is little support for a causal relationship between acquired sensory deficit and the mental disorders of old age. However, they acknowledge two possible exceptions: first, the onset of nonpsychotic depression following sensory loss which is seen by the sufferer as handicapping or disabling (Gilhome Herbst & Humphrey, 1980); secondly, referring to their own and the Newcastle studies, the catalysis or exacerbation of psychotic illness in individuals with a predisposition to develop schizophrenic illness.

## The role of hearing loss in paranoid psychosis

The mode of action of deafness in the genesis of paranoid psychosis in later life is not clear but there are a number of ways in which the disturbances associated with long-standing hearing loss might be implicated. Although it has long been accepted that chronic deafness is commonly associated with suspiciousness and paranoid attitudes, both Myklebust (1964) and Thomas (1984) failed to demonstrate the presence of significant paranoid personality traits among the deaf and hard of hearing.

It seems likely, however, that other forms of psychological reaction and social maladjustment to this form of disability might play a part. There is little doubt that a considerable social stigma attaches to deafness in contrast to blindness (Barker, 1953) and Heider & Heider (1941) have put forward interesting suggestions to account for the more favourable reactions to the blind. Unlike deafness, blindness is a handicap that is visible to all so that, by contrast, the behavioural abnormalities and communication problems of the deaf, whose disability is not so apparent, are often wrongly attributed to personality idiosyncracy and lend themselves easily to humour and ridicule. Roth & McClelland (1971) suggest that the psycho-social sequelae of physical deformity and sensory defects may have a common explanation. Both may increase sensitivity, social withdrawal and feelings of inferiority and interfere with interpersonal relationships; these factors may aggravate any premorbid personality traits predisposing to illness. The role of deafness in the aetiology of paranoid disorders, therefore, may be related to the psycho-social reactions it produces as one form of chronic physical disability.

Another possible mode of action is one which lends support to a general theory of schizophrenia. Kirk (1968) proposed that perceptual disturbances should be regarded as primary factors in the aetiology of schizophrenia rather than as symptoms of the disease and illustrated how the clinical manifestations of schizophrenia might develop, as a perceptually impaired individual interacts with his social environment. Although Kirk postulated central nervous dysfunction as the basis of the perceptual defect in schizophrenia, it is reasonable to suggest that lesions of the peripheral nervous system directly involved in perception, such as hearing loss, could also be implicated. By demonstrating that deafness may play a crucial role in the aetiology of paranoid psychosis as it occurs in the elderly (Cooper *et al*, 1974; Cooper *et al*, 1976), these studies may have provided further support for the theory that disturbances of auditory perception, notably that of speech, may be of particular importance in the aetiology of schizophrenia (Lawson *et al*, 1964; Chapman, 1966).

## *The blind and visually impaired*

In contrast to prelingual deafness, the main conclusion to emerge from studies of the blind is that, although visual defect introduces considerable practical problems of daily living in areas such as travel, eating and personal care, of itself it appears not to lead to abnormal social adjustment in later life. Lowenfeld (1955) considered that the only 'real limitations' for the blind child are derived from the physical aspects of the disability, leading to lack of visual experience and restricted mobility. Provided the blind child is afforded favourable educational opportunities and an understanding psycho-social environment, relatively normal psychological development into adulthood and old age should be a realistic aim (Raskin, 1962).

### The prevalence of visual impairment in the elderly

There have been relatively few epidemiological studies of visual impairment in the elderly and wide variations in prevalence have been reported depending on the methods of sampling and the criteria of visual loss employed. One of the most comprehensive surveys in recent years was that of Milne & Williamson (1972) who measured the visual acuity of a random sample of 487 elderly people aged 62 to 90 years living in a defined area of Edinburgh. They found that when subjects were wearing distance glasses if appropriate, 42% of the sample had visual acuity of 6/18 or worse in the better eye, there being no difference between the sexes.

What seems to be well established and agreed by most authors is that visual acuity, like hearing ability, diminishes significantly with age. Milne & Williamson (1972) found that 11% of men under 70 years had visual acuity of 6/24 or worse compared with 34% of men of 70 years and over. The corresponding figures for women were 13% and 32% Cataract was found in 19% of men and 32% of women and its prevalence was significantly associated both with increasing age and with diminishing visual acuity.

### Psycho-social reactions to visual impairment and blindness

It is now well documented that surgery to the eye followed by patching and immobilisation is an important cause of post-operative behaviour disturbances ranging from restlessness and irritability to frank delirium (Heiman, 1977). The majority of patients are elderly and have undergone cataract extraction but ageing is not thought to be the major cause, as similar episodes can occur in younger patients undergoing treatment for retinal detachment. Probably the most significant factor is sensory deprivation which is aggravated by immobilisation, social isolation in a strange environment and, in older patients, the presence of cerebral disease, hearing impairment and systemic illness. The most important approach to the problem must be prevention and Weisman & Hackett (1958) have discussed how the alleviation of pre-operative anxiety, investigation and treatment of physical illness and the reduction of social isolation, may contribute to the lessening of this particular complication of eye surgery, especially in the elderly.

Although blindness is a disability which drastically alters the life-style of the formerly sighted person, there have been relatively few systematic investigations of the psychological sequelae of loss of vision in the middle aged or elderly. Fitzgerald (1970) studied the reaction to loss of sight of all 66 newly blinded adults who had been registered as blind in London during the course of one year. The ages of the patients ranged from 21 to 65 years, and two thirds were over the age of 45. The onset of blindness was gradual over a period of two weeks or more in two thirds of cases and although only 1.5% were totally blind, the remainder were severely visually handicapped and all functionally blind.

At the onset of blindness, a major dysphoric reaction to loss of vision occurred in the vast majority of subjects, many reporting initial total disbelief that they were losing their sight. Although others ostensibly acknowledged their handicap, their subsequent behaviour frequently demonstrated partial denial or protest in that they sought second opinions, resisted using a white cane or attempted to continue work for which sight was essential. Eventually disbelief was replaced by emotional states ranging from moderate upset to severe depression and finally they passed through a recovery phase which in most cases did not begin until many months after the onset of blindness.

At the time of interview which, on average, was 1.5 years after the onset of blindness, there was much continuing disability, even among those who claimed to have recovered from their distress. Two thirds complained of continuing depression and one third or more of persisting anxiety, feelings of anger and insomnia. A substantial minority showed evidence of heightened suspiciousness and paranoid ideation. Only one half were willing to use a white cane for travel and identification which is a sensitive index of poor acceptance of the loss.

Fitzgerald *et al*, (1987) have recently reported a follow-up study of the same group of subjects who were re-examined after a period of four years. There was only a slight increase in the acquisition of blind skills while more than 50% of the group were still experiencing depression and anxiety. One third or more were continuing to report insomnia, crying, anger and irritability. Multivariate statistical analysis of the data from both studies gave predictors of outcome which indicated that young married males, older non-Protestants (in a predominantly Protestant community) the foreign born and those without family histories of blindness, were at highest risk of poor adjustment to blindness.

In a similar study, Keegan *et al*, (1976) investigated a randomly chosen sample of 114 subjects who had been declared legally blind and registered with the Canadian National Institute for the Blind (CNIB). The age range was 13–70 and 55% of the sample were over the age of 55 years. From the psychological viewpoint, the most vulnerable groups were the middle-aged and elderly, those with low incomes, those who did not accept visual loss as permanent, those who declined offers of rehabilitation and those who were 'humble, shy and expedient' on personality test profiles. The best level of functioning was found in those who had given up false hopes of regaining their vision. Acceptance of blindness occurred most frequently at the onset and, later, at the time they were declared legally blind. However, the authors noted that 80% of their subjects experienced their greatest psycho-social distress following the onset of visual loss while, at a later stage, declaration of blindness in itself led to no particular crisis or diminished social or psychological adjustment. They point out that physicians and ophthalmologists, who are available at times of greatest crisis when acceptance should be encouraged, are often not interested or are not informed of the major psycho-social crisis taking place. The CNIB cannot offer assistance at onset because of the legal definition of blindness and the authors suggest that earlier recognition of the psycho-social sequelae of severe visual loss and earlier involvement of the CNIB and other helping agencies is imperative. They also urge that ways must be found of promoting more understanding of the problems of acceptance of visual loss and how it can be encouraged so that the associated psycho-social morbidity can therefore be minimised.

Although various authors (Cholden, 1958; Schulz 1977) have written accounts of the psychiatric and social problems experienced by the blind and visually impaired, these studies by Fitzgerald (1970), Fitzgerald *et al*, (1987) and Keegan *et al*, (1976) represent the most recent attempts to investigate these phenomena in a systematic way. Although it is known that impairment of visual acuity is much commoner in old age, little attention has been paid to the psycho-social morbidity that might be associated with loss of vision in this age group.

## Visual impairment in the functional psychoses of the elderly

Reference has already been made to the significance of hearing loss as a factor in the aetiology of the paranoid psychoses of later life (Kay & Roth, 1961; Cooper *et al*, 1974; Kay *et al*, 1976). Mayer-Gross *et al*, (1969) have pointed out that the blind do not seem to be particularly liable to become paranoid and suggest that deafness may have a more disturbing effect because it constitutes a greater barrier between man and man; whereas blindness chiefly intervenes between man and the inanimate world.

Although Kay & Roth (1961) noted that visual defects in patients with 'late paraphrenia' were no more frequent than in control groups of the same age, other authors have reported a high prevalence of impaired vision in these illnesses. Herbert & Jacobson (1967) detected significant abnormalities of vision in 47% of their series of patients with 'late paraphrenia'. McClelland *et al*, (1968) and Roth & McClelland (1971) reported visual findings similar to those they obtained for hearing impairment. The overall prevalence of visual defects such as cataract, glaucoma, myopia and squints in the schizophrenic group was 6.7% compared with 3.0% among the affective; and in the over 60 age group the rates were 25.5% and 10.4% respectively.

In the study of hearing loss in elderly patients with paranoid and affective psychoses (Cooper *et al*, 1974) the visual acuity and ocular pathology of the patients were also examined (Cooper & Porter, 1976). The basic uncorrected visual acuity showed no significant association with diagnosis in either eye but when the optimum visual acuity was examined (i.e. the acuity when spectacles were habitually worn or the uncorrected acuity if they were not) a highly significant association was found betwen paranoid illness and visual acuity in the eyes with poorer vision. Taking both eyes into account, the optimum visual acuity in the paranoid group of patients was considerably worse than in the affective group. Furthermore, in the paranoid group, 52% of patients had an optimum visual acuity of 6/24 or worse in one or both eyes compared with 26% in the affective group and this difference was significant. On the basis of a screening test, ocular pathology was detected in 56% of the paranoid group and in 37% of the affective group; significantly more cataract was found in the better eyes of the paranoid group.

Although the findings of this study indicated that impaired visual acuity and ocular pathology were more common in paranoid than in affective illnesses in later life, the authors considered that only tentative conclusions could be drawn regarding their aetiological significance since retrospective judgements as to their prevalence at the onset of illness could not be made as reliably, as in the case of deafness. The finding of significantly impaired vision in one eye in the paranoid group was unlikely to have been associated with any serious social handicap compared with the control group but it is possible that unilateral visual impairment might produce adverse psychological effects in susceptible individuals through interference with visual perception. However, the authors considered that such an effect would be minimal and of less importance than hearing impairment in the aetiology of paranoid illnesses.

The role of cataract is difficult to account for, especially in the absence of any significant effect on visual acuity. There are, however, obvious psychological links between sensory defect and physical disfigurement since both may increase sensitivity, social withdrawal and paranoid tendencies (Roth & McClelland, 1971). It is possible, therefore, that factors such as these may have operated in some of the paranoid patients with visual defects in this series.

## Conclusions

This review has demonstrated that although defects of the special senses are associated with substantial psycho-social morbidity, whatever the modality, research in this area has so far concentrated largely on the problems of the young and middle-aged. Despite the fact that the prevalence of both hearing and visual impairment is much higher among the elderly and increases rapidly as age advances, comparatively little attention has been given to the psychiatric sequelae of sensory deficits in old age. Furthermore, although various studies of physical illness associated with functional psychosis have indicated that sensory impairment particularly hearing loss is of aetiological importance in the paranoid psychoses of later life, the role of these deficits is not clear. There is, therefore, ample scope for further enquiries in this field of study, and urgent calls for further research (Rawson, 1973; Keegan, 1976) should not go unheeded.

## References

ALTSHULER, K. Z. (1971) Studies of the deaf: relevance to psychiatric theory. *American Journal of Psychiatry*, **127**, 1521–1526.

ALTSHULER, K. & ABDULLAH, S. (1981) Mental health and the deaf adult. In *Deafness and Mental Health* (eds L. K. Stein, E. D. Mindel & T. Jabaley). New York: Grune & Stratton.

BARKER, R. G. (1953) *Adjustment to Physical Handicap and Illness: A Survey of the Social Psychology of Physique and Disability*. New York: Social Science Research Council.

BECKER, G. (1980) *Growing Old in Silence*. Berkeley: University of California Press.

—— (1981) Coping with stigma: lifelong adaption of deaf people. *Social Science and Medicine*, **15B**, 21–24.

—— & NADLER, G. (1980) The aged deaf: integration of a disabled group into an agency serving elderly people. *Gerontologist*, **20**, 214–221.

BURTON, R. (1621) *The Anatomy of Melancholy*. 1st Ed., Part 2, Sect. 3, Memb. 2. Oxford: Cripps.

CHAPMAN, J. (1966) The early symptoms of schizophrenia. *British Journal of Psychiatry*, **112**, 225–251.

CHOLDEN, L. S. (1958) *A Psychiatrist Works with Blindness*. New York: American Foundation for the Blind.

CHRISTENSON, R. & BLAZER, D. (1984) Epidemiology of persecutory ideation in an elderly population in the community. *American Journal of Psychiatry*, **141**, 1088–1091.

COOPER, A. F. & CURRY, A. R. (1976) The pathology of deafness in the paranoid and affective psychoses of later life. *Journal of Psychosomatic Research*, **20**, 97–105.

——, ——, KAY, D. W. K., GARSIDE, R. F. & ROTH, M. (1974) Hearing loss in paranoid and affective psychoses of the elderly. *Lancet*, ii, 851–854.

——, GARSIDE, R. F. & KAY, D. W. K. (1976) A comparison of deaf and non-deaf patients with paranoid and affective psychoses. *British Journal of Psychiatry*, **129**, 532–538.

—— & PORTER, R. (1976) Visual acuity and ocular pathology in the paranoid and affective psychoses of later life. *Journal of Psychosomatic Research*, **20**, 107–114.

CORBIN, S., REED, M., NOBBS, H., EASTWOOD, K. & EASTWOOD, M. R. (1984) Hearing assessment in homes for the aged: A comparison of audiometric and self-report methods. *Journal of the American Geriatrics Society*, **32**, 396–400.

—— & EASTWOOD, M. R. (1986) Sensory deficits and mental disorders of old age: causal or coincidental associations? *Psychological Medicine*, **16**, 251–256.

DENMARK, J. C. (1969) Management of severe deafness in adults. The psychiatrist's contribution. *Proceedings of the Royal Society of Medicine*, **62**, 965–967.

DENMARK, J. C. & ELDRIDGE, R. W. (1969) Psychiatric services for the deaf. *Lancet*, ii, 259–262.

EASTWOOD, M. R., CORBIN, S. L., REED, M., NOBBS, H. & KEDWARD, H. B. (1985) Acquired hearing loss and psychiatric illness: an estimate of prevalence and co-morbidity in a geriatric setting. *British Journal of Psychiatry*, **147**, 552–556.

FITZGERALD, R. G. (1970) Reactions to blindness. *Archives of General Psychiatry*, **22**, 370–379.

——, EBERT, J. N. & CHAMBERS, M. (1987) Reactions to blindness: a four-year follow-up study. *Perceptual and Motor Skills*, **64**, 363–378.

GILHOME HERBST, K. & HUMPHREY, C. (1980) Hearing impairment and mental state in the elderly living at home. *British Medical Journal*, **281**, 903–905.

HEIDER, F. & HEIDER, G. M. (1941) Studies in the Psychology of the Deaf No. 2. *Psychological Monographs*, **53**, No. 242.

HEIMAN, J. (1977) Psychiatric experience associated with eye surgery and trauma requiring patching. In *Psychiatric Problems in Ophthalmology* (eds J. T. Pearlman, G. L. Adams & S. H. Sloan). Illinois: Charles C. Thomas.

HERBERT, M. E. & JACOBSON, S. (1967) Late paraphrenia. *British Journal of Psychiatry*, **113**, 461–469.

HINKLE, L. E. & WOLFF, H. G. (1957) The nature of man's adaptation to his total environment and the relation of this to illness. *Archives of Internal Medicine*, **99**, 442–460.

HOUSTON, F. & ROYSE, A. B. (1954) Relationship between deafness and psychotic illness. *Journal of Mental Science*, **100**, 990–993.

INGALLS, G. S. (1946) Some psychiatric observations on patients with hearing defect. *Occupational Therapy and Rehabilitation*, **25**, 62–66.

KAY, D. W. K., COOPER, A. F., GARSIDE, R. F. & ROTH, M. (1976) The differentiation of paranoid from affective psychoses by patients' premorbid characteristics. *British Journal of Psychiatry*, **129**, 207–215.

—— & ROTH, M. (1961) Environmental and hereditary factors in the schizophrenia of old age. *Journal of Mental Science*, **107**, 649–686.

KEEGAN, D. L., ASH, D. D. G. & GREENOUGH, T. (1976) Blindness: some psychological and social implications. *Canadian Psychiatric Association Journal*, **21**, 333–340.

KIRK, R. V. (1968) Perceptual defect and role handicap: Missing links in explaining the aetiology of schizophrenia. *British Journal of Psychiatry*, **114**, 1509–1521.

KNAPP, P. H. (1948) Emotional aspects of hearing loss. *Psychosomatic Medicine*, **10**, 203–222.

KRAEPELIN, E. (1915) Der Verfolgungswahn der Schwerhörigen. In *Psychiatrie, Ein Lehrbuch für Studierende und Artze*. Leipzig: Barth, Auflage 8, Band IV.

LAWSON, J. S., McGHIE, A. & CHAPMAN, J. (1964) Perception of speech in schizophrenia. *British Journal of Psychiatry*, **110**, 375–380.

LLOYD, G. G. (1977) Psychological reactions to physical illness. *British Journal of Hospital Medicine*, **18**, 352–356.

LOWENFELD, B. (1955) Psychological problems of children with impaired vision. In *Psychology of Exceptional Children and Youth* (ed. W. M. Cruickshank). Englewood-Cliffs, NJ.: Prentice Hall.

MAHAPATRA, S. B. (1974) Deafness and mental health: psychiatric and psychosomatic illness in the deaf. *Acta Psychiatrica Scandinavica*, **50**, 596–611.

MAYER-GROSS, W., SLATER, E. & ROTH, M. (1969) *Clinical Psychiatry*, 3rd Edn, London: Baillière, Tindall and Cassell.

McCLELLAND, H. A., ROTH, M., NEUBAUER, H. & GARSIDE, R. F. (1968) Some observations on a case material based on patients with common schizophrenic symptoms. In *Proceedings of the Fourth World Congress of Psychiatry*, 1966. London: Excerpta Medica Foundation.

MEADOW, K. P. (1981) Studies of behaviour problems of deaf children. In *Deafness and Mental Health* (eds L. K. Stein, E. D. Mindel & T. Jabaley). New York: Grune and Stratton.

MILNE, J. S. & WILLIAMSON, J. (1972) Visual acuity in older people. *Gerontologica Clinica*, **14**, 249–256.

MOORE, N. C. (1981) Is paranoid illness associated with sensory defects in the elderly? *Journal of Psychosomatic Research*, **25**, 69–74.

MYKLEBUST, H. R. (1964) *The Psychology of Deafness*, 2nd Edn, New York: Grune and Stratton.

POST, F. (1962) *The Significance of Affective Symptoms in Old Age*. Maudsley Monograph No. 10. London: Oxford University Press.

—— (1966) *Persistent Persecutory States of the Elderly*. London: Pergamon.

PRITZKER, B. (1938) Paranoia und Schwerhörigkeit. *Schweizerische Medizinische Wochenschrift*, **7**, 165–166.

RAINER, J. D., ALTSHULER, K. Z., KALLMAN, F. J. & DEMING, W. E. (1963) *Family and Mental Health Problems in a Deaf Population*. New York: Columbia University Press.

RAMSDELL, D. A. (1962) The psychology of the hard-of-hearing and the deafened adult. In *Hearing and Deafness* (eds H. Davis & R. Silverman). New York: Holt, Rinehart and Winston.

RASKIN, N. J. (1962) Visual disability. In *Psychological Practices with the Physically Disabled* (eds J. F. Garret & E. S. Levine). New York: Columbia University Press.

RAWSON, A. (1973) *Deafness: Report of a Departmental Enquiry into the Promotion of Research*. DHSS Reports on Health and Social Subjects No. 4. London: HMSO.

ROTH, M. & McCLELLAND, H. A. (1971) Sensory defects, physical deformity and somatic illness in schizophrenia. In *Vestnik Academicheskikh Nauk SSSR*, Meditsina, **5**, 77–79.

ROUSEY, C. L. (1971) Psychological reactions to hearing loss. *Journal of Speech and Hearing Disorders*, **36**, 382–389.

SCHULZ, P. J. (1977) Reaction to the loss of sight. In *Psychiatric Problems in Ophthalmology* (eds J. T. Pearlman, G. L. Adams & S. H. Sloan). Illinois: Charles C. Thomas.

SILVERMAN, J. (1964) The problem of attention in research and theory in schizophrenia. *Psychological Review*, **71**, 352–379.

SJÖGREN, H. (1964) Paraphrenic, melancholic and psychoneurotic states in the presenile-senile period of life. *Acta Psychiatrica Scandinavica*, **40**, Supplement 176.

THOMAS, A. J. (1984) *Acquired Hearing Loss: Psychological and Psycho-Social Implications*. London: Academic Press.

TOWNSEND, P. & WEDDERBURN, D. (1965) *The Aged in the Welfare State*. Occasional Papers on Social Administration No. 14. London: Bell.

WEISMAN, A. D. & HACKETT, T. P. (1958) Psychosis after eye surgery. *New England Journal of Medicine*, **258**, 1284–1289.

WILKINS, L. T. (1948) *The Prevalence of Deafness in the Population of England, Scotland and Wales*. London: Central Office of Information.

# 29 What became of late paraphrenia?

## DAVID W. K. KAY

*Abstract*

Roth's (1955) hypothesis concerning late paraphrenia (LP) is recalled and subsequent developments noted. Its distinctness from the dementias of old age and its affinity to paranoid schizophrenia are confirmed, but careful clinical description of subtypes and related conditions is desirable, in view of the advent of the new brain imaging and genetic techniques.

Thirty-three years ago, Sir Martin Roth published *The Natural History of Mental Disorders in Old Age* (Roth, 1955) in which he differentiated five groups of disorders by symptomatology and outcome. He wrote: "Most of the classical accounts of mental disorder of old age confine themselves to the pre-senile, senile and arteriosclerotic psychoses . . . cases with a predominantly depressive or paranoid picture or with clouding of consciousness alone were described . . . but were attributed to an underlying cerebral illness . . . Consequently, weight was given to neurological findings of a quite subtle character . . .". Roth & Morrisey (1952) had already drawn attention to the high rate of suicide in old age and its relation to depression. This and the recent successes of ECT in some elderly patients made it necessary to re-evaluate the old system of classification. Moreover, the specificity of some of the neuropathological lesions traditionally associated with mental illness in the old had been cast in doubt by some recent findings (Rothschild, 1956) and this question required re-examining in the light of the new evidence.

Roth & Morrisey (1952) surveyed the geriatric population in Graylingwell Hospital and found schizophrenic patients whose illness had begun after the age of 60 and whose symptoms were paraphrenic in character. After preliminary studies of outcome and of psychological test performances (Roth & Hopkins, 1953; Hopkins & Roth, 1953), patients whose illnesses presented with predominantly affective symptoms and patients with a steadily progressive disorganisation of intellect and personality were provisionally assigned to distinct nosological groups. The paraphrenic group and two other diagnostic categories, arteriosclerotic psychosis and acute confusion, had contained too few patients for any clear pattern in their natural history to emerge, and the investigation was extended to a larger material (Roth, 1955).

The term late paraphrenia (LP) distinguished the illness from the chronic schizophrenias found in mental hospital patients and emphasised the clinical similarities to the illness of this name described by Kraepelin and later shown to be a relatively late form of schizophrenia. The working hypothesis was that LP would follow a course distinct from that of the organic psychoses.

In the event, the pattern of outcome of each of the five groups was distinctive in terms of the percentages discharged from hospital, remaining as in-patients, or dead: patients with LP characteristically were alive, unchanged and in hospital after two years. The differences were not accounted for by age. When the case-records were studied for evidence of clinical overlap, no organic case with a history of well-integrated paranoid delusions or presenting with paraphrenic features could be found.

Kay & Roth (1961) found LP in about 10% of first admissions aged 60 years or over to the Graylingwell (UK) and Stockholm (Sweden) hospitals. The main features were marked female predominance, social isolation, deafness, and abnormalities of personality, Clinically, there were many schizophrenia-like disorders of thought, mood and volition, good preservation of personality and memory and, except in one subgroup, conspicuous hallucinations.

The association of LP with cerebral disease was considered in some detail. Focal brain disease was found in some patients, but the history and absence of progression during long-term follow-up suggested that its role in LP was at most a minor one. New onsets of cerebrovascular disease had been related to the onset of LP in not more than 5% of cases.

Unequivocal organic mental syndromes at onset of illness had already been excluded, but in 9% of the cases some doubt remained. Of these only two or possibly three progressed during follow-up; in the remainder the symptoms were thought to have been secondary to the psychosis. Features suggestive of senile dementia had eventually developed in 12% of all cases before death, but were difficult to evaluate owing to the unavoidable reliance on records and the inaccessible state of many of the patients due to psychosis, deafness, blindness, or extreme age. Moreover, the long interval before these features had appeared (over ten years in 80% of the cases) and the patients' normal lifespan argued against an organic contribution to the aetiology of LP. The incidence of cerebral disease was thought to be in keeping with neuropathological observations on functional groups (Corsellis, 1962) and with the expectation in the general population.

Neuropathological studies in Newcastle-upon-Tyne showed that senile plaques and neurofibrillary tangles in LP were significantly fewer than in senile or arteriosclerotic dementia and no more common than in elderly patients with affective disorder, acute confusion without dementia or uncomplicated physical illness (Blessed *et al*, 1966). Roth (1971) pointed out that the term "senile paranoid psychosis" imputed a predominantly organic aetiology to the schizophrenias of late life which was not justified by the data. However, in fact, only five paraphrenic brains had been examined, and there was some overlap with the organic dementias.

### Subgroups and the relationship of LP to schizophrenia

Three subgroups were proposed: lifelong paranoid personalities without hallucinations (20%); patients with delusions and hallucinations that were intelligible, i.e. not bizarre, considering the actual circumstances (25%); and patients with bizarre or erotic delusions and numerous schizophrenic features. It was, however, doubtful to what extent any demarcation between cases really existed (Kay & Roth, 1961).

Descriptively, LP was a form of schizophrenia; but its aetiology was a matter for further investigation. Family studies suggested that patients with LP might be susceptible to schizophrenia-like illnesses, and that the differences from schizophrenia were of a quantitative kind. However, there were several instances of patients having relatives with LP, as noted also by Herbert & Jacobson (1967), which suggests the possibility of a more specific predisposition.

## Developments

The purpose of the remainder of this paper is to review progress. Despite the opinion of Bridge & Wyatt (1980a, b) that it was imperative to undertake the investigation of elderly patients with LP who had been too long ignored by the research community, there has been relatively little in the English language literature. Dementia and depression have monopolised attention. Recently, however, there have been signs of a revival of interest.

### Hospital studies

Standard interviews such as the *Geriatric Mental Status (GMS)* schedule of Gurland *et al* (1976a) have improved the reliability of diagnoses. In the US/UK Diagnostic Project, schizophrenia was diagnosed by the project team in 14–19% of elderly patients consecutively admitted to the psychiatric hospitals in Queens County, New York City and Camberwell, London (Copeland *et al*, 1975). The percentages are higher than the hospital diagnoses of schizophrenia; and patients with paranoid delusions were specifically likely to be misdiagnosed as organic (Gurland *et al*, 1976a).

Blessed & Wilson (1982) found that 90% of their psychogeriatric patients in Newcastle fitted clinically into the five groups described by Roth (1955), including 6% with LP beginning after 65. The proportion of elderly patients with LP admitted to hospital may be falling despite more referrals, admissions with dementia apparently being maintained at the expense of patients with functional disorders (Christie & Wood, 1987). The subsequent history of patients who are referred but not admitted is not clear.

Blessed & Wilson (1982) reported that the outcome in LP had strikingly improved in that the majority of patients were discharged by six months. This may have been in part due to more effective treatment. However, by two years about 20% were in residential care. Christie (1982) made similar observations in Scotland.

### Community studies

In community studies the diagnosis of schizophrenia still presents difficulties in the absence of an informant. In the Epidemiological Catchment Area (ECA) studies the prevalence of schizophrenia in community residents aged 60 or over was one to three per 1000 (Weissman *et al*, 1985; Kramer *et al*, 1985), compared with 14 per 1000 between 18 and 64, and was four times higher in women than in men. However, the proportion of late onset cases was not reported in the ECA studies. Copeland *et al* (1987a,b) were not able to diagnose schizophrenia among 841 elderly community residents in New York and London, and there was only one case among 1070 residents aged 65 or over in Liverpool; this may be compared with 56 organic cases and 121 depressive cases.

## Incidence

Schizophrenia or paranoia was diagnosed in 4.4% of all first admissions aged 65 and over to mental hospitals in England and Wales (1983), but ages of onset are not available. The age-specific first admission rate for schizophrenia was 8.7 per 100 000 in the 65–74 age group and rose to 14.5 in the 75 + age group (DHSS, 1985). The Camberwell Psychiatric Register also shows a modest rise in first-ever contacts with schizophrenia after 65 (Wing & Der, 1984). Holden (1987) estimated the annual incidence of LP in Camberwell to be 17–26 per 100 000 depending on whether or not cases thought to be of organic aetiology were included.

## LP and cerebral diseases

Several observations are relevant to Roth's (1955) hypothesis that LP is distinct from the organic dementias.
(a) Delusions and hallucinations are reported by relatives in nearly 50% of cases (Rabins *et al*, 1982); suspiciousness and false accusations are even commoner. However, in most cases these symptoms are transient and clearly due to loss of memory and grasp. They give rise to no diagnostic difficulty in the presence of symptoms of dementia (Fish, 1960).

Of greater interest is the diagnosis and classification of paranoid psychoses closely resembling LP when they immediately precede or accompany the onset of dementia. Roth (1955) could find no examples at Graylingwell. However, Larsson *et al* (1963) found 18% of their cases of senile dementia were of paranoid type. Post (1966) studied cases with proven or suspected brain disease, mainly senile or vascular, and found psychoses that were indistinguishable in paranoid symptoms and subtypes from functional cases of LP. He was therefore unable to define a paranoid syndrome specific to organic paranoid psychosis. However, Holden (1987) did find certain differences: organic cases were older, female preponderance was less, childhood was less often disturbed, and precipitants at onset were fewer. For discriminating between organic and functional cases, first rank symptoms were not very useful; but visual hallucinations had discriminatory value (Holden, 1987). A case with delusions of infidelity associated with Alzheimer's disease was described by Shepherd (1961). Cummings (1985) found delusions without hallucinations in 15% of cases of SDAT at an early or mid-phase of development, their complexity decreasing with the degree of impairment.

Irrespective of the paranoid symptoms, the presence of dementia is associated with a high mortality, poor response to treatment, short survival at home and prolonged institutionalisation (Holden, 1987), not merely due to lapsing from therapy (Post, 1966). Holden (1987) believed that organic factors could play a substantial role in the paraphrenic psychoses of late life. It would be interesting to know more about the premorbid personality of patients with organic paraphrenias.

(b) Psychoses resembling LP may also occur as a result of a cerebral disease or intoxication in the complete absence of symptoms of organic type. Such cases would be diagnosed as organic delusional disorder or organic hallucinosis, if DSM–III criteria were used. Holden (1987) found 10% of his cases were symptomatic due to syphilis, myeloproliferative disease, carcinoma of the prostate, chronic heart disease or pernicious anaemia, although it is not clear on what grounds these were regarded as the cause of the LP. However, the occurrence of paranoid-hallucinatory states accompanying syphilis and pernicious anaemia is well established (Whitehead & Chohan, 1972; Davison & Bagley, 1969), and a LP syndrome should alert the physician to the possibility of covert physical disease, including occult B12 deficiency and hypothyroidism. Diseases affecting the temporo-limbic and subcortical systems are perhaps the most likely to give rise to psychoses with prominent delusions and hallucinations (Davison & Bagley, 1969; Cummings, 1985).

(c) In cases in which evidence of organic or symptomatic aetiology at onset is lacking, long-term follow-up has shown that the lifespan of patients is almost normal and that the incidence of organic disease is probably no more than is to be expected in elderly persons (Post, 1966; Kay, 1962). In a recent study, only 8% of non-demented patients with LP eventually developed dementia after 10 years' follow up (Holden, 1987). These studies support Roth's original observations.

### Relationship to schizophrenia

The resemblance to paranoid schizophrenia is often striking. Fish (1960) noted that with increasing age at onset schizophrenia took on a paraphrenic character with prominent auditory hallucinations. In several studies the incidence of first rank symptoms (FRS) of Schneider in patients with LP has been reported to be 40–60% (Post, 1966; Grahame, 1984; Holden, 1987) which may be compared with about 50% (range 28–72%) found in schizophrenic subjects (Mellor, 1982). Characteristic auditory hallucinations were the commonest type of FRS, whereas thought insertion and thought withdrawal did not occur (Grahame, 1984). The reasons for this are speculative, but Levine *et al* (1982) found that FRS did not hang together as a cluster but tended to be associated with comparable second rank symptoms. Thought insertion, for instance, is associated with formal thought disorder (Mellor, 1980), which is not a feature of LP.

Grahame (1984) also compared his cases with various research criteria for the diagnosis of schizophrenia. Despite failure to fulfil Langfeldt's (1960) criteria, due perhaps to an emphasis on negative symptoms not characteristic of LP, Grahame concluded that LP belongs to the group of schizophrenias. This accords with the response to phenothiazine drugs, which is usually excellent provided that the patient is compliant (Post, 1966). Raskind *et al* (1979) found fluphenazine enanthate given intramuscularly in small doses every two weeks rapidly improved 11 of 13 out-patients with LP; significant adverse side effects were uncommon. The presence of mild or moderate dementia need not necessarily exclude the use of neuroleptic drugs (Whitehead, 1975). The chances of successful maintenance in the community are improved if a therapeutic relationship can be established (Post, 1966; Berger & Zarit, 1978).

## Subtypes of LP

Organic paraphrenias are discussed above. Fish (1960) also recognised psychogenic reactions and affect-laden paraphrenias. About half the non-organic patients, those with FRS, appear to be suffering from paranoid schizophrenia, the remainder may be regarded as suffering from schizophrenia-like illnesses or simple paranoid psychoses (Post, 1966; Grahame, 1984). Kendler & Davis (1981) reviewed the biochemistry and concluded that there might be a higher level of brain noradrenaline in paranoid than in non-paranoid schizophrenia (Kendler & Davis, 1981), but there were no data on paranoid psychosis; and there are none on LP. Surprisingly, systematic comparisons of LP with chronic paranoid schizophrenia have never been undertaken. Recently Naguib *et al* (1987) reported that the HLA antigens in LP differ from the markers usually associated with paranoid schizophrenia, suggesting that LP may be distinct from this disorder.

Several studies of LP refer to cases of paranoid psychosis (Grahame, 1984; Post, 1966; Holden, 1987), which is also known as delusional disorder (DD). The characteristic features are non-bizarre delusions without prominent hallucinations (Winokur, 1977). DD is probably distinct from schizophrenia and affective disorder (Kendler, 1982). Admissions peak in the fifth and sixth decades, but continue into the eighth decade, and women predominate. Prognosis is poor. Hallucinosis is absent in simple DD or paranoia (Kendler, 1980), as it was in 20% of the Graylingwell-Stockholm cases. Several studies have found DD not to be genetically related to schizophrenia (Watt *et al*, 1980; Kendler & Hays, 1981; Kendler *et al*, 1981; Kendler *et al*, 1985).

Holden (1987) studied elderly patients diagnosed as suffering from "functional paranoid psychoses" in the Camberwell Register and Maudsley Hospital Case Register. In addition to 20% of affective and symptomatic cases, and a small group with schizo-affective disorder, Holden recognised schizophreniform and paranoid subgroups distinguished by the presence or absence of FRS. Reactive, endogenous and organic elements seemed to be present, a preponderance of one element being balanced by less of the others. LP seemed to consist of a spectrum of overlapping conditions, with differing mortality and response to treatment. The number of cases in each sub-group was, however, small and prospective studies, including brain scans to measure brain density and ventricular-brain ratios, were desirable (Holden, 1987). In one study, patients with LP had significantly larger lateral cerebral ventricles and greater cognitive deficits than aged-matched volunteers (Naguib & Levy, 1987). As in some younger schizophrenic subjects, the ventricular enlargement may have preceded the onset of the psychosis and constituted a risk factor. High resolution CT and PET scans were recommended in future work (Naguib & Levy, 1987).

### Sensory deficits and co-morbidity

Corbin & Eastwood (1986) pointed to the difficulty of evaluating hearing from either self-reports or physicians' observations. Cooper (1976) described the sensory deficits found in elderly patients with paranoid or affective psychoses, when objective measures of auditory and visual loss were employed. Acquired partial deafness usually due to middle ear disease contracted early in life was found to be commoner in patients with paranoid psychosis, possibly because it had created psychological and social difficulties. A connection between deafness and auditory hallucinations is postulated (Berger & Zarit, 1978) but has not been proven. Premorbid traits of solitariness, sensitivity and suspicion, family history, and fewer surviving children were other features that differentiated paranoid from affective patients (Kay *et al*, 1976).

Moore (1981) rightly emphasised the importance of controlling for age, seeing that the prevalence of deafness (and blindness) rises steeply with age in the general population. Moore examined the Item Sheets at the Bethlem Royal and Maudsley Hospitals, 1970–72, and selected patients described as "deaf or blind (complete or partial)" for study. Deafness was found to be relatively uncommon in patients with affective psychoses and Moore suggested that it was inappropriate to use affective patients as controls. However, Eastwood *et al*, (1985), in an audiometric study of residents of nursing homes, found the percentages of psychiatric normals, affectives and paraphrenics *without* hearing loss to be 37%, 40% and 17% respectively, and Mahapatra (1974) diagnosed depression in 34% of bilaterally deaf patients aged 15–65 admitted to an ENT unit with otosclerosis. Paranoid schizophrenia was diagnosed in 10%, which seems extraordinarily high.

The effect of treating deafness in paranoid illness has seldom been reported, but a case of a 75 year old woman with LP who benefited by being provided with a hearing aid for her chronic bilateral conductive hearing loss was described by Eastwood *et al* (1981).

The role of visual defects in paranoid illness is harder to assess (Cooper, 1976). Complex visual hallucinations may occur during the course of progressive eye disease without loss of insight (White, 1980), but could be the basis for psychotic experience in susceptible persons.

Some physical diseases, such as untreated pernicious anaemia (Whitehead & Chohan, 1972), are reported to be associated with a high incidence of paraphrenia-like illness but correction of the physical disorder does not always cure the psychosis (Davison & Bagley, 1969).

**Classification**

Further progress in studying the varieties of LP may depend on the availability of reliable and widely used systems of clinical classification. The ICD and DSM–III both offer considerable choice. In ICD–9, LP is referred to in the section on Paranoid States 297.2, where it is equivalent to involutional or senile paranoid state. Schizophrenia, paranoid type, 295.3, specifically excludes paraphrenia. Paranoid states associated with senile dementia are included in 290.2, Senile Dementia, depressed or paranoid type. Paranoid states associated with alcoholism are included in section 291, while non-alcoholic paranoid states associated with other conditions may be coded in section 294.8 as Mixed Paranoid and Affective Organic Psychotic States; the physical disease is coded separately. A diagnosis of Paranoid Schizophrenia specifically excludes LP, on the grounds that thought disorder and affective flattening are more prominent and personality less well preserved in the former.

LP is not mentioned in DSM–III (R) (1987) but is no longer automatically excluded from the schizophrenias by an upper age limit as it was in DSM–III

(1980). Late onset of schizophrenia may be specified if the disorder, including the prodromal phase, develops after age 45.

The newer categories, Organic Delusional Syndrome 293.81, and Organic Hallucinosis 293.82, define disorders due to organic or metabolic brain disease that lack specific cognitive features and resemble affective, paranoid or schizophrenic disorders (Lipowski, 1984). These categories were criticised by Roth (1981) for implying knowledge about causation that ought first to be established by further research. However, they seem to be intended for cases where there is already a measure of agreement about the connection between the psychosis and the physical condition (Lipowski, 1984); for example, psychotic states in temporal lobe epilepsy and Huntington's disease (Davison, 1987). When the psychosis is due to medical use of a drug, such as L–DOPA, the appropriate section is 292.11, Other or Unspecified Psychoactive Substance-induced Organic Mental Disorder. The specific factor is noted on Axis III, but when hallucinosis is due to alcohol it is presumably entered under Alcoholic Hallucinosis 291.30.

Paranoid states associated with senile dementia are recorded in section 290.20, Primary Cerebral Degeneration with delusions, Alzheimer's disease being coded on Axis III when the diagnosis is confirmed by autopsy. Paranoid states accompanying multi-infarct dementia are coded as Multi-infarct Dementia with delusions 290.42, and the cerebrovascular disease noted on Axis III.

In DSM–III (R) terms, many cases of LP would probably be entered as Paranoid Schizophrenia 295.3, with late onset, or as Schizophreniform Psychosis 295.4. A few cases may fulfil criteria for Schizoaffective Disorder 295.7. It has already been suggested that some cases may be found to conform to Delusional Disorder 297.1. The differential diagnosis would include Major Depression with mood-incongruent psychotic features 296.24, and Senile Dementia with delusions, referred to above. Organic Hallucinosis and Organic Delusional Disorder should be considered only if a specific organic or toxic factor known to be capable of causing psychotic symptoms has been demonstrated.

## Conclusions

Roth's concept of late paraphrenia gave a new identity to a disorder that was previously regarded as a form of senile dementia in which the presence of delusions was part of the intellectual failure. However, the occurrence of a psychosis with onset late in life, distinct from mania or depression, but responsive to neuroleptic treatment and with a normal lifespan, has been confirmed, and the resemblance of many of the cases to schizophrenia of the paranoid type is striking. It is of interest, therefore, that work on genetic markers suggests that LP may be distinct from paranoid schizophrenia.

In addition, psychoses indistinguishable from LP may accompany senile or vascular or occasionally other types of dementia. In general, a role for the pathological (or normal) changes of ageing in the majority of cases of LP is difficult to sustain in view of the progressive increase in dementia but not of LP in the older age groups. However, recent observations, that ventricular size is increased in LP, raise questions about organic factors which are similar to those that occur in schizophrenia.

Compared with the earlier studies, discharge rates have much improved. However, very few cases of LP are identified in community surveys of the elderly population, and the whereabouts, conditions and long-term outcome of patients with this disorder is currently not well documented.

## References

AMERICAN PSYCHIATRIC ASSOCIATION (1980) *Diagnostic and Statistical Manual of Mental Disorders, III.* Washington, DC: APA.
—— III Revised (1987) Washington, DC: APA.
BERGER, K. S. & ZARIT, S. N. (1978) Late-life paranoid states: assessment and treatment. *American Journal of Orthopsychiatry,* **48**, 528–538.
BLESSED, G., TOMLINSON, B. E. & ROTH, M. (1966) The association between quantitative measures of dementia and of senile change in the cerebral grey matter of elderly subjects *British Journal of Psychiatry,* **114**, 797–811.
—— & WILSON, I. D. (1982) The contemporary natural history of mental disorder in old age. *British Journal of Psychiatry,* **141**, 59–67.
BRIDGE, T. P. & WYATT, R. J. (1980a) Paraphrenia: paranoid states in late life. I. European research. *Journal of the American Geriatrics Society,* **28**, 193–200.
—— & —— (1980b) Paraphrenia: paranoid states in late life. II. American research. *Journal of the American Geriatrics Society,* **28**, 201–205.
CHRISTIE, A. B. (1982) Changing patterns in mental illness in the elderly. *British Journal of Psychiatry,* **140**, 154–159.
—— & WOOD, E. R. M. (1987) Psychogeriatrics 1974 to 1984: expanding problems and fixed resources. *British Journal of Psychiatry,* **151**, 813–817.
COOPER, A. F. (1976) Deafness and psychiatric illness. *British Journal of Psychiatry,* **129**, 216–226.
COPELAND, J. R. M., KELLEHER, M. J., KELLETT, J. M., GOURLAY, A. J., COWAN, D. W., BARRON, G. & DE GRUHY, J. and GURLAND, B. J., SHARPE, L., SIMON, R., KURIANSKY, J. & STILLER, P. (1975) Cross-national study of diagnosis of the mental disorders: a comparison of the diagnoses of elderly psychiatric patients admitted to mental hospitals serving Queens County, New York, and the former Borough of Camberwell, London. *British Journal of Psychiatry,* **126**, 11–20.
——, GURLAND, B. J., DEWEY, M. E., KELLEHER, M. J., SMITH, A. M. R. & DAVIDSON, I. A. (1987a) Is there more dementia, depression and neurosis in New York? A comparative study of the elderly in New York and London using the computer diagnosis AGECAT. *British Journal of Psychiatry,* **151**, 466–473.
——, DEWEY, M. E., WOOD, N., SEARLE, R., DAVIDSON, I. A. & MCWILLIAM, C. (1987b) Range of mental illness among the elderly in the community: prevalence in Liverpool using the GMS–AGECAT package. *British Journal of Psychiatry,* **150**, 815–823.
CORBIN, S. L. & EASTWOOD, M. E. (1986) Sensory deficits and mental disorders of old age: causal or coincidental associations? *Psychological Medicine,* **16**, 251–256.
CORSELLIS, J. A. N. (1962) *Mental Illness and the Ageing Brain.* Maudsley Monograph No. 9. London: Oxford University Press.
CUMMINGS, J. L. (1985) Organic delusions: phenomenology, anatomical correlations, and review. *British Journal of Psychiatry,* **146**, 184–197.
DAVISON, K. (1987) Organic and toxic concomitants of schizophrenia: association or chance? In *Biological Perspectives of Schizophrenia* (eds H. Helmchen & F. A. Henn). London: Wiley.
—— & BAGLEY, C. R. (1969) Schizophrenia-like psychoses associated with organic disorders of the central nervous system: a review of the literature. *British Journal of Psychiatry (Special Issue No. 4),* 113–184.
DEPARTMENT OF HEALTH & SOCIAL SECURITY (1985) *Mental Health Statistics,* London: HMSO.
EASTWOOD, R., CORBIN, S. & REED, M. (1981) Hearing impairment and paraphrenia. *Journal of Otolaryngology,* **10**, 306–308.
——, ——, ——, HOBBS, N. & KEDWARD, H. B. (1985) Acquired hearing loss and psychiatric illness: an estimate of prevalence and co-morbidity in a geriatric setting. *British Journal of Psychiatry,* **147**, 552–556.
FISH, F. (1960) Senile schizophrenia. *Journal of Mental Science,* **106**, 938–946.
GRAHAME, P. S (1984) Schizophrenia in old age (late paraphrenia). *British Journal of Psychiatry,* **145**, 493–495.

GURLAND, B. J., FLEISS, J. L., GOLDBERG, K. & SHARPE, L. with COPELAND, J. R. M., KELLEHER, M. J. & KELLETT, J. M. (1976a) A semistructured clinical interview for the assessment of diagnosis and mental state in the elderly: the Geriatric Mental Status Schedule. II. A factor analysis. *Psychological Medicine*, 6, 451–459.

HERBERT, M. E. & JACOBSON, S. (1967) Late paraphrenia. *British Journal of Psychiatry*, 113, 461–469.

HOLDEN, N. L. (1987) Late paraphrenia or the paraphrenias? A descriptive study with a 10-year follow-up. *British Journal of Psychiatry*, 150, 635–639.

HOPKINS, B. & ROTH, M. (1953) Psychological test performance in patients over 60. II. Paraphrenia, arteriosclerotic psychosis, acute confusion. *Journal of Mental Science*, 99, 695–701.

INTERNATIONAL CLASSIFICATION OF DISEASES, 9th edition. (1977) Geneva: World Health Organization.

KAY, D. W. K. (1962) Outcome and cause of death in mental disorders of old age: a long-term follow-up of functional and organic psychoses. *Acta Psychiatrica Scandinavica*, 38, 249–276.

—— & ROTH, M. (1961) Environmental and hereditary factors in the schizophrenias of old age ("late paraphrenia") and their bearing on the general problem of causation in schizophrenia. *Journal of Mental Science*, 107, 649–686.

——, COOPER, A. F., GARSIDE, R. F. & ROTH, M. (1976) The differentiation of paranoid from affective psychoses by patients' premorbid characteristics. *British Journal of Psychiatry*, 129, 207–215.

KENDLER, K. S. (1980) The nosological validity of paranoia (simple delusional disorder). *Archives of General Psychiatry*, 37, 699–706.

—— (1982) Demography of paranoid psychosis (delusional disorder). *Archives of General Psychiatry*, 39, 890–902.

—— & DAVIS, K. L. (1981) The genetics and biochemistry of paranoid psychoses, *Schizophrenia Bulletin*, 7, 689–709.

—— & HAYS, P. (1981) Paranoid psychosis (delusional disorder) and schizophrenia: a family history study. *Archives of General Psychiatry*, 38, 547–551.

——, GRUENBERG, A. M. & STRAUSS, J. S. (1981) An indepdendent analysis of the Copenhagen sample of the Danish adoption study of schizophrenia: III. The relationship between paranoid psychosis (delusional disorder) and the schizophrenic spectrum disorders. *Archives of General Psychiatry*, 38, 985–987.

——, MASTERSON, C. C. & DAVIS, K. L. (1985) Psychiatric illness in first-degree relatives of patients with paranoid psychosis, schizophrenia and medical illness. *British Journal of Psychiatry*, 147, 524–531.

KRAMER, M., GERMAN, P., ANTHONY, J. C., VON KORFF, M. & SKINNER, E. A. (1985) Patterns of mental disorders among the elderly residents of Eastern Baltimore. *Journal of the American Geriatrics Society*, 33, 236–245.

LANGFELDT, G. (1960) Diagnosis and prognosis in schizophrenia. *Proceedings of the Royal Society of Medicine*, 53, 1047–1052.

LARSSON, T., SJÖGREN, T. & JACOBSON, G. (1963) Senile dementia. A clinical, sociomedical and genetic study. *Acta Psychiatrica Scandinavica*, Supplement 167.

LEVINE, R., RENDERS, B., KIRCHHOFER, M., MONSOUR, A. & WATT, N. (1982) The empirical heterogeneity of first rank symptoms in schizophrenia. *British Journal of Psychiatry*, 140, 498–502.

LIPOWSKI, Z. J. (1984) Organic mental disorders—an American perspective. *British Journal of Psychiatry*, 144, 542–546.

MAHAPATRA, S. B. (1974) Deafness and mental health: psychiatric and psychosomatic illness in the deaf. *Acta Psychiatrica Scandinavica*, 50, 596–611.

MELLOR, C. S. (1980) First rank symptoms of schizophrenia. *British Journal of Psychiatry*, 117, 15–23.

—— (1982) The present status of first rank symptoms. *British Journal of Psychiatry*, 140, 423–424.

MOORE, N. C. (1981) Is paranoid illness associated with sensory defects in the elderly? *Journal of Psychosomatic Research*, 25, 69–74.

NAGUIB, M. & LEVY, R. (1987) Late paraphrenia: neuropsychological impairment and structural brain abnormalities on computed tomography. *International Journal of Geriatric Psychiatry*, 2, 83–90.

——, McGUFFIN, P., LEVY, R., FESTENSTEIN, H. & ALONSO, A. (1987) Genetic markers in late paraphrenia: a study of HLA antigens. *British Journal of Psychiatry*, 150, 124–127.

POST, F. (1966) *Persistent Persecutory States of the Elderly*. Oxford: Pergamon Press.

RABINS, P. V., MASE, N. L. & LUCAS, M. J. (1982) The impact of dementia on the family. *Journal of the American Medical Association*, 248, 333–335.

RASKIND, M., ALVAREZ, C. & HERLIN, S. (1979) Fluphenazine enanthate in the out-patient treatment of late paraphrenia. *Journal of the American Geriatrics Society*, 27, 451–473.

ROTH, M. (1955) The natural history of mental disorder in old age. *Journal of Mental Science*, 101, 281–301.

—— (1971) Classification and aetiology in mental disorders of old age: some recent developments. In *Recent Developments in Psychogeriatrics* (eds D. W. Kay & A. Walk). *British Journal of Psychiatry*, Special Publication No. 6. Ashford: Headley Brothers.

—— (1981) Discussion of paper on classification of late life organic states and the DSM–III. In *Clinical Aspects of Alzheimer's Disease and Senile Dementia. Aging, vol. 15* (eds N. E. Miller & G. D. Cohen). New York: Raven Press.

—— & HOPKINS, B. (1953) Psychological test performance in patients over 60. I. Senile psychosis and the affective disorders of old age. *Journal of Mental Science*, **99**, 439–450.

—— & MORRISEY, J. D. (1952) Problems in the diagnosis and classification of mental disorders in old age. *Journal of Mental Science*, **98**, 66–80.

ROTHSCHILD, D. (1956) Senile psychoses and psychoses with cerebral arteriosclerosis. In *Mental Disorders in Later Life*, 2nd. edn (ed. O. J. Kaplan). California: Stanford University Press.

SHEPHERD, M. (1961) Morbid jealousy: some clinical and social aspects of a psychiatric problem. *Journal of Mental Science*, **107**, 687–753.

WATT, J. A. G., HALL, D. J., OLLEY, P. C., HUNTER, D. & GARDINER, A. Q. (1980) Paranoid states of middle life: familial occurrence and relationship to schizophrenia. *Acta Psychiatrica Scandinavica*, **61**, 413–426.

WEISSMAN, M. M., MYERS, J. K., TISCH, G. L., HOLZER, C. E., LEAF, P. J., ORVASCHEF, H. & BRODY, J. A. (1985) Psychiatric disorders (DSM–III) and cognitive impairment among the elderly in a U.S. urban community. *Acta Psychiatrica Scandinavica*, **71**, 366–379.

WHITE, N. J. (1980) Complex visual hallucinations in partial blindness due to eye disease. *British Journal of Psychiatry*, **136**, 284–286.

WHITEHEAD, T. (1975) Long-acting phenothiazines. *British Medical Journal*, **2**, 502.

WHITEHEAD, J. & CHOHAN, M. (1972) Paraphrenia and pernicious anaemia. *Geriatrics*, **27**, 148–158.

WING, J. K. & DER, G. (1984) *Report of the Camberwell Psychiatric Register 1964–1984*. London: Institute of Psychiatry.

WINOKUR, G. (1977) Delusional disorder (Paranoia). *Comprehensive Psychiatry*, **18**, 511–521.

# 30 Mental disorder and criminal behaviour in the elderly

**STEPHEN J. HUCKER**

With the increasing numbers of elderly people in the population, much attention has been directed towards the plight of those in that age group who become victims of criminal behaviour. Far less interest has been shown in old people who themselves commit crimes. Perhaps this is not surprising: all countries which report their statistics show that antisocial behaviour is associated with youth and declines dramatically with advancing years (Pollak, 1941, p. 213; Moberg, 1953, p. 768). Nevertheless, in the United States at least, reports that crime is increasing among the elderly population (Shichor & Kobrin, 1978; Malinchak, 1980; Shichor, 1984) have appeared, to the extent that the popular press began to publish provocative articles suggesting an imminent "elderly crime wave" (Harper, 1982). Whether or not this is the case, the phenomenon of criminal behaviour by old people was first discussed as long ago as 1899 at a conference in Budapest (Pollak, 1941).

## The prevalence of crime committed by the elderly

A number of authors have attempted to establish the extent of crime committed by the elderly. These studies have usually involved scrutiny of official arrest or conviction statistics, such as the Uniform Crime Reports issued by the Federal Bureau of Investigation in the United States. Earlier reports indicated that the commonest crimes of old age were fraud and embezzlement, sex offences (Pollak, 1941) and drunkenness (Moberg, 1953) and were committed typically by first time offenders. Keller & Vedder (1968) noted that drunkenness and disorderly conduct were, in fact, the commonest two offences for all age groups but that vagrancy, minor assaults, sex offences and, unexpectedly perhaps, vandalism, were commoner in older age groups.

However, Shichor & Kobrin (1978), using data from the Uniform Crime Reports for the years 1964 to 1976, noted a 224% increase in serious crimes committed by persons aged 55 years and over, a substantially greater increase than the 43% for all age groups. Also, a large proportion of arrests of the elderly were for violent crimes such as serious assaults. Compared to earlier reports, vagrancy and drunkenness had declined substantially although arrests for driving while intoxicated had increased. In a subsequent study Shichor (1984) found these trends in crime committed by the elderly had continued. Using Uniform

Crime Reports for 1970 to 1980, but using a different methodology to Shichor, Wilbanks (1984) found a decrease in the total number of arrests of the elderly over this period, but with a disproportionate increase in minor sex offences and a sharp increase in drunkenness, vagrancy and gambling.

Epstein, Mills & Simon (1970) studied all those aged 60 years and over who were arrested in San Francisco over a four month period in 1967–68, a sample of 722 individuals. Typically, the elderly arrestee was male, white and arrested for drunkenness though apprehensions for gambling, disturbing the peace and aggravated assault were also common.

Burnett & Ortega (1984) also studied arrests of an older age group (in this case those 50 years and over) but found a decline in the total number of arrests between 1962 to 1967 and 1970 to 1980. Petty theft, fraud and embezzlement dramatically increased over the time period but arrests for drunkenness, minor sex crimes and other minor offences declined. However, the authors caution that the number of elderly persons involved in these offences was small.

Recently a British study (Taylor & Parrott, 1988) has been published of male prisoners custodially remanded to Brixton Prison in London between 1979 to 1980. Of these, only 3% (63 men) were aged 55 and over.

Thus, although there are some differences of opinion among writers on this subject, it is clear that the elderly make a minute contribution to the total amount of crime committed and there is very little support for the notion that an "elderly crime wave" is sweeping western societies.

## *Crimes in old age of special psychiatric interest*

Compared with the findings based on studies of official criminal statistics contributions to the psychiatric literature on crime in old age have tended to focus on sexual and violent crimes.

### (a) Sex offences

Although sexual offences have been considered the commonest crimes of the elderly (Abrahamsen, 1944; Bergman & Amir, 1973; Devon, 1930; Fox, 1946; Schroeder, 1936), Roth (1968) noted that according to British official statistics, sex offences constituted only about 12% of all offences in this age group. Similarly, Keller & Vedder (1968) found that sex offences occupied 12th position among the 'top 20' crimes in those aged 60 years and older according to the FBI's Official Crime Reports. In the study by Epstein *et al* (1970) referred to earlier, there were only four sex offenders among their 722 arrestees aged 60 years and older. It is also noteworthy that in most of the widely quoted studies of sex offenders (for example, Gebhard, Gagnon, Pomeroy & Christensen, 1965; Mohr, Turner & Jerry, 1964; Radzinowicz, 1957) elderly perpetrators were uncommon. Therefore, it seems likely that the frequency of sex offences by the elderly has been exaggerated by the sources of data employed. The concept of the 'dirty old man' is evidently mythological.

Among sexual offences committed by the elderly, those involving child victims are generally considered the most frequent (Ellis, 1933; Pollak, 1941; Whiskin, 1967, 1968; Zeegers, 1966, 1978). Hucker & Ben-Aron (1985) studied

70 individuals referred to the Forensic Clinic of the Clarke Institute of Psychiatry in Toronto and found 43 of these were sex offenders, 67% involving victims under age 12 years and a further 14% aged 13 to 15 years.

East (1944) proposed that elderly sex offenders most frequently select child victims because they themselves are unattractive to adult females and fear rejection by them. He argued that "fantasy and desire have outlived potency" so that they are capable only of "partial sexual acts" short of intercourse (Whiskin, 1968). The crime may also represent an attempt to boost a flagging sense of masculinity (Whiskin, 1968). Roth (1968) suggested that children tend to trust "grandfather" figures. Others have, less charitably, argued that children are chosen as victims because they are less able than adults to defend themselves, easier to bribe, more amenable to threats, and less likely to report the incident (Henninger, 1939).

Most elderly offenders are said to be first-time offenders with no previous record of sexual or any other type of offence (Moberg, 1953; Roth, 1968; Zeegers, 1968, 1978) and they are often described as being of previously "blameless character" (Pollak, 1941; Slater & Roth, 1969). However, about a quarter of Hucker & Ben-Aron's (1985) and Zeegers' (1966, 1978) cases had previous convictions for sexual offences.

According to Hucker & Ben-Aron's (1985) data, the elderly sex offender is typically involved in non-violent sexual activities with the child victim, such as exposing, touching or occasionally oral sex. Violent sexual attacks by the elderly are very rare but not totally unknown (Whiskin, 1968).

The most popular theory advanced to explain why elderly men might commit sexual crimes has been that they are suffering from dementia (East, 1944; Ellis, 1933; Henninger, 1939; Rollin, 1973; Rose, 1970; Rothschild, 1945; Ruskin, 1941; Storr, 1964; Sutherland, 1924; von Krafft-Ebing, 1965; Whiskin, 1968; Zeegers, 1966, 1978). However, others have disputed this (Allersma, 1971; Brancale, MacNeil & Vuocolo, 1965; Groth, Burgess, Birnbaum & Gary, 1978; Hirschmann, 1962) although some who argue for the importance of organic deterioration concede that the offence itself may be the "first sign of senile change" (Henninger, 1939). Others have acknowledged that the more typical features of dementia may be lacking (Ellis, 1933; Roth, 1968). Pollak (1941) claimed that sex crimes by the elderly often lack planning and caution although Roth (1968) noted that sometimes the degree of circumspection shown by the offender is surprising.

Hucker & Ben-Aron (1985) found that 14% of their elderly sex offenders were suffering from dementia of some degree. However, comparison with community surveys of the prevalence of organic mental disorders in the elderly population indicates that they are rather similar to this figure. For example, Essen-Möller (1956) found 15.8%, Kay, Beamish & Roth (1964), 11.3%, Nielsen (1963), 18.5% and Sheldon (1948) found 15.6% suffering from "mild mental deterioration" to severe organic brain syndrome. Although Hucker & Ben-Aron's data would therefore suggest that elderly sex offenders do not suffer from dementia to any greater degree than elderly people in the general population, the obvious question which arises is why authorities such as Whiskin (1967, 1968) and Zeegers (1966, 1978) found much higher percentages in their studies. Whiskin (1967, 1968) diagnosed nine out of his 15 cases as suffering from organic brain disease but admitted that his diagnostic criteria were imprecise, using the term "pseudo-organic syndrome" to refer to cases where "social isolation and attempts at regressive solutions'' contributed to the clinical picture. Zeegers (1978) used existential criteria such as a ''restriction of their 'being-in-the-world' rather than memory impairment or intellectual incapacity'' and it seems likely that the nearly 50% of his cases to whom this applied would not satisfy currently accepted criteria for dementia.

Alternative explanations for the elderly sex offender's behaviour have included unspecified ''changes in the prostate'' (Sutherland, 1924) and ''regression'' due to emotional factors (Revitch & Weiss, 1962). It certainly seems that longstanding emotional problems are not uncommon among elderly sex offenders. Although Hirschmann (1962) considered that most elderly sex offenders were previously well adjusted sexually, Zeegers (1966, 1978) found that, although many had been married, a substantial number were divorced or had experienced marital difficulties; an impression shared by Roth (1968). Hucker & Ben-Aron (1985) found that while 86% of their elderly sex offenders had been married at some time, 70% of these relationships were judged to have been ''below average'' in quality, many of them having ended in divorce.

Similarly, the social problems that accompany old age, such as loneliness and isolation following death of friends and separation from family, together with reduced income, are prominent factors found among elderly sex offenders (Allersma, 1971; Hucker & Ben-Aron, 1984; Law, 1979; Meyers, 1965; Mohr, Turner & Jerry, 1964; Revitch & Weiss, 1962). These factors might be thought to contribute to the offence by drawing the elderly person to the company of children in settings such as public parks. However, Hucker & Ben-Aron (1985) found that while most of their elderly sex offenders, though perhaps no more than other elderly people, had very limited social contacts, about half of their offences occurred in the home of the offender or the victim, the relationship often being that of a relative, friend or acquaintance.

Pollak (1941) believed that many elderly sex offenders were committed in a state of drunkenness. Hucker & Ben-Aron (1985), however, found that only 14% had been intoxicated at the time of their offences, although 21% of the sample were diagnosed as ''alcoholic''. Many authors have supported the view often provided by offenders that they were themselves the victim of seduction by a child (Allersma, 1971; Henninger, 1939; Meyers, 1965; Pollak, 1941; Slater & Roth, 1969; Virkkunen, 1975; Zeegers 1966, 1978), although most current workers in the field of child sexual abuse repudiate such claims as one of the typical rationalisations verbalised by sex offenders of any age (Stermac & Segal, 1987).

Most elderly sex offenders, if convicted, are given non-custodial sentences such as a fine, caution or suspended sentence with probation, and their recidivism rate is low at about 7% (Hucker & Ben-Aron, 1985).

Presumably, though firm evidence based on laboratory testing (Freund, 1981) is so far lacking, many of these men have a sustained erotic preference for children rather than adult partners but have either usually kept their impulses under control and acted out only infrequently, or simply escaped detection throughout most of their lives.

### (b)  Violent offences

Typically, the elderly are viewed as victims rather than perpetrators of violent crime. Certainly violent crimes by members of this age group are uncommon

(Epstein, *et al*, 1970; Wilbanks & Murphy, 1984). This is probably one reason why violent behaviour by the elderly has been little studied (Petrie *et al*, 1982). However, Tardiff & Sweillam (1979, 1980) found that assaultive behaviour by elderly people, often in association with organic brain disease, is a frequent reason for admission to a public psychiatric hospital in the United States.

Available psychiatric studies of murderers contain few references to elderly offenders. MacDonald (1986) suggests that in this age group disinhibition due to organic brain changes may contribute to violence and observes that "paranoid ideas or delusions frequently underlie homicidal assaults". Gillies (1976) in a study of 400 Scottish murderers found only three, all diagnosed as "psychotic", over 65 years of age. In his survey of 150 murders at Matteawan State Hospital in New York, Lanzkron (1963) reports 17 cases aged 60 years and older and in an earlier paper (Lanzkron, 1961) emphasised the occurrence of paranoid syndromes, especially delusional jealousy, in this group. In this context it is notable that among a series of 110 morbidly jealous murderers at Broadmoor Hospital in the United Kingdom, Mowat (1966) found nine elderly men. Häffner & Böker (1982), in a substantial psychiatric and epidemiological study of mentally abnormal offenders, found that 34 out of a sample of 533 (6.4%) were aged over 60.

Rosner, Wiederlight & Schneider (1985) reported on 25 "geriatric felons" referred to their forensic psychiatry clinic in New York City. Of these, 22 had been charged with violent offences, six for murder and six for manslaughter. Of these, seven were diagnosed as having organic mental syndromes, six as suffering from schizophrenia, two affective disorders and one atypical paranoid disorder. Paranoid ideation was a feature in 13 cases "regardless of their major diagnostic category".

Taylor & Parrott (1988) reported on the characteristics of a sample of 63 individuals aged 55 and over remanded to Brixton Prison in London. About half of these men showed active psychiatric symptoms, 37% having a functional psychosis and 27% were alchoholics. None of these men had been charged with homicide and violent offences were uncommon in this particular prison sample.

Hucker & Ben-Aron (1984) conducted a controlled investigation of 16 elderly offenders charged with violent crimes, mainly homicide and attempted homicide, referred to the Forensic Service of the Clarke Institute of Psychiatry in Toronto. It was striking that half of the elderly violent defendants suffered from some kind of functional mental disorder. These, together with organic mental disorders, accounted for 75% of the whole group (11 out of 16 cases). Also of interest was the number (44%) who displayed paranoid symptoms, irrespective of the basic diagnosis, a feature that was noted previously by Rosner *et al* (1985) and also by Taylor & Parrott (1988). Young violent men, in contrast, were diagnosed most often (in 63% of cases) as having features of antisocial personality disorder. Only 13% of the elderly violent individuals were given this diagnosis. Alcoholism was present in 50% of the violent elderly, although this was not different to a statistically significant extent than the two control groups (young violent and elderly non-violent offenders).

While there were no statistically significant differences between elderly and young violent offenders with respect to the relationship between offender and victim, slightly more (69% versus 44%) in the elderly violent group were family members or close friends of the assailant. Most (88%) of the elderly violent offenders committed their offences in their own homes. Domestic quarrels were the context for 44% (compare 6% in the young men) of the elderly violent incidents among whom delusional motives predominated (38% versus 6%). Of the elderly group, 56% had harboured hostile feelings towards their victim before the crime though this did not differ statistically from the younger violent group.

Roth (1968) mentions that in rare cases a suicidal elderly person's violence may extend towards others in the vicinity. It was his impression that murderous violence in the absence of suicidal tendencies is very rare in the elderly. Hucker & Ben-Aron (1984) found that only small numbers of either the elderly or young violent individuals were suicidal after their crimes. Only one elderly subject, the only female in either group, actually succeeded in killing herself before she came to trial.

In many important respects, therefore, according to Hucker & Ben-Aron's study, elderly violent offenders resembled their youthful counterparts; they are as likely to be a relative or friend of the victim, as likely to have harboured hostile feelings towards the victim, as likely to be under the influence of alcohol and no more prone to suicidal behaviour after the crime.

The finding of a large number of serious mental disorders in Hucker & Ben-Aron's elderly violent patients is similar to that of Rosner *et al* (1985) which derived from a similar group of subjects. Much the same was found in a study by Petrie *et al* (1982) of 222 patients admitted to a geriatric psychiatry unit in a state mental hospital in the United States. Eighteen of them had been involved in acts of violence. Organic brain syndrome occurred in only 17% whereas the rest suffered from serious mental disorders such as paraphrenia, manic depressive psychosis, schizophrenia or atypical paranoid disorder.

## (c) Shoplifting

In younger individuals shoplifting, especially by women, may be associated with mental disorder (Gibbens & Prince, 1962). In men, these authors showed that shoplifting was often the final phase in the career of recidivists previously convicted for a wide range of offences. Feinberg (1984), however, found that in his elderly sample from Miami, Florida, where 6.7% of the elderly in the USA reside, men and women were equally represented and in Curran's (1984) study 60% were male. Feinberg's offenders appeared mainly to steal luxury items while Curren's group typically stole household items or personal goods. From both studies it is clear that financial hardship was not the reason for the thefts. Feinberg believed that the thefts were usually intentional and not a result of memory impairment. Indeed three quarters of them admitted feeling guilty about the behaviour. However, surprisingly, most did not in fact view themselves as offenders at all. Shoplifting by the elderly has often been viewed as a strategy to gain attention and perhaps overcome feelings of isolation and loneliness. In fact, most of Feinberg's and Curran's elderly shoplifters were married and had good social contacts. Although shoplifting may be associated with minor mental disorders, such as depression, especially in middle-aged women, there seemed to be other factors at work in elderly people convicted or arrested for this offence. It seems unlikely that psychiatric disorder plays any significant part in shoplifting behaviour in this older age group.

In his thoughtful paper Feinberg (1984) notes similarities between the status, role obligations and expectations of the elderly and the young. Although there are also important differences he suggests that theories derived from the study of juvenile delinquency might help understand better the involvement of the elderly in certain types of crime, including shoplifting.

## (d) Alcohol-related offences

It has been noted earlier in this survey that a number of authors have indicated an association between alcohol use and criminal behaviour by the elderly (Epstein, *et al*, 1970; Shichor & Kobrin, 1978 and Shichor, 1984). Of Taylor & Parrott's (1988) remanded elderly offenders 27% were diagnosed "alcoholic". In Hucker & Ben-Aron's (1985) study of elderly sex offenders alcoholism was present in 21% and in their study of violent elderly offenders (Hucker & Ben-Aron, 1984) 50% were diagnosed as alcoholic.

Alcoholism is, in fact, a serious problem among the elderly in general. The average annual death rate from alcoholic disorders for white males aged 60 to 69 years in the United States in 1965 was 52%, dropping to 27% for those 70 or over (Simon, Epstein & Reynolds, 1968). In 100 consecutive admissions to a psychiatric screening ward for those 60 years or older, 44% were diagnosed as having alcoholism (Giatz & Baer, 1971). Elderly alcoholics were also less well tolerated in the home and had generally been admitted to institutions at an earlier age than elderly non-alcoholics.

While the correlation between alcoholism and violent and sexual offences has been established in the elderly, the fact that fewer numbers of them were actually intoxicated at the times of their offences indicates that alcohol is not the only factor in the commission of the offences. Predisposing tendencies in the case of sex offences and, in elderly violent offenders, mental illness together with interpersonal tensions noted in homicides at all ages may be more important.

## *Conclusions*

The evidence is that, despite some concern over an apparent increase in the numbers of elderly offenders, this age group contributes relatively little to the overall problem of crime in the community. Most studies of arrests indicate that old people are involved usually in alcohol-related offences, assaults, minor sex crimes, embezzlement, fraud and thefts. Studies conducted of referrals to forensic clinics are obviously and necessarily an unrepresentative group but among these sex crimes, especially involving child molestations, and serious crimes of violence predominate. The former may well be paedophiles who have acted upon their sexual inclinations towards children only infrequently or, at least, have usually avoided detection and arrest in the past. Their recidivism rate appears to be low and this, together with the typically non-violent nature of their behaviour, seems to justify the sympathetic manner in which they are usually handled by the courts. Violent elderly offenders on the other hand, at least those referred for psychiatric evaluation, in most cases are found to suffer from a major mental illness often with a strong paranoid element in their clinical presentation. Such individuals need specialised medical and psychiatric care.

As the numbers of elderly people in the community increase, it can be expected that the criminal justice system will need to accommodate to the needs of this special group. Some jurisdictions, such as Florida in the United States (Fry, 1984; Newman & Newman, 1984), have already developed diversion programmes for elderly offenders and similar experimental approaches have been attempted in the United Kingdom (Taylor & Parrott, 1988).

As the foregoing review has tried to show, elderly offenders, although not a large group at the present time, do manifest significant social and psychiatric problems and will probably be studied increasingly more closely in the future.

## References

ABRAHAMSEN, D. (1944) *Crime and the Human Mind*. New York: Columbia University Press.

ALLERSMA, J. (1971) Ouderdom en criminaliteit. *Nederlands Tijdschrift Voor Gerontologie*, **2**, 285–293.

BERGMAN, S. & AMIR, M. (1973) Crime and delinquency among the aged in Israel. *Geriatrics*, **28**, 149–157.

BRANCALE, R., MACNEIL, D. & VUOCOLO, A. (1965) Profile of the New Jersey sex offender: A statistical study of 1,206 male sex offenders. *Welfare Reporter*, **16**, 3–9.

BURNETT, C. & ORTEGA, S. (1984) Elderly offenders: A descriptive analysis. In *Elderly Criminals* (eds W. Wilbanks & P. K. H. Kim). Maryland: The University Press of America.

CURRAN, D. (1984) Characteristics of the elderly shoplifter and the effect of sanctions on recidivism. In *Elderly Criminals* (eds W. Wilbanks & P. K. H. Kim). Maryland: The University Press of America.

DEVON, J. (1930) Age and crime. *Police Journal*, **3**, 118–126.

EAST, W. N. (1944) Crime, senescence and senility. *Journal of Mental Science*, **90**, 836–849.

ELLIS, H. (1933) *Psychology of Sex*. London: W. Heinemann.

EPSTEIN, L. H., MILLS, C. & SIMON, A. (1970) Antisocial behaviour of the elderly. *Comprehensive Psychiatry*, **11**, 36–42.

ESSEN-MÖLLER, E. (1956) Individual traits and morbidity in a Swedish rural population. *Acta Psychiatrica et Neurologica Scandinavica*, Suppl. 100.

FEINBERG, G. (1984) Profile of the elderly shoplifter. In *Elderly Criminals* (eds D. Newman, E. Newman & M. Gewirtz). Massachusetts: Oelgeschlager, Gunn & Hain.

FOX, V. (1946) Intelligence, race and age as selective factors in crime. *Journal of Criminal Law*, **37**, 141–152.

FREUND, K. (1981) Assessment of pedophilia. In *Adult Sexual Interest in Children* (eds M. Cook & K. Howells). Toronto: Academic Press.

FRY, L. J. (1984) The implications of diversion for older offenders. In *Elderly Offenders* (eds W. Wilbanks & P. K. M. Kim). Maryland: The University Press of America.

GEBHARD, P., GAGNON, J. H., POMEROY, W. B. & CHRISTENSON, C. V. (1965) *Sex Offenders: An analysis of types*. New York: Harper & Row.

GIATZ, C. M. & BAER, P. E. (1971) Characteristics of elderly patients with alcoholism. *Archives of General Psychiatry*, **24**, 372–378.

GIBBENS, T. C. N. & PRINCE, J. (1962) *Shoplifting*. London: Institute for the Study and Treatment of Delinquency.

GILLIES, H. (1976) Homicide in the West of Scotland. *British Journal of Psychiatry*, **128**, 105–127.

GROTH, A. N., BURGESS, A. W., BIRNBAUM, H. J. & GARY, T. S. (1978) A study of the child molester: Myths and realities. *Journal of the American Criminal Justice Association*, **41**, 17–22.

HÄFFNER, H. & BÖKER, W. (1982) *Crimes of Violence by Mentally Abnormal Offenders*. Cambridge: University Press.

HARPER, T. (1982) An elderly crime wave? Aged offenders tax criminal justice system. *National Law Journal*, **4**, (15 June), 1.

HENNINGER, J. M. (1939) The senile sex offender. *Mental Hygiene*, **23**, 436–444.

HIRSCHMANN, J. (1962) Zur Kriminologie der Sexualdelikte des alternden Mannes. *Gerontologica Clinica*, **4**, 115–119.

HUCKER, S. J. & BEN-ARON, M. H. (1984) Violent elderly offenders: A comparative study. In *Elderly Criminals* (eds W. Wilbanks & P. K. M. Kim). Maryland: The University Press of America.

—— & —— (1985) Elderly sex offenders. In *Erotic Preference, Gender Identity and Aggression in Men* (ed. R. Langevin). New Jersey: L. Erlbaum Associates.

KAY, D. W. K., BEAMISH, P. & ROTH M. (1964) Old age mental disorder in Newcastle-upon-Tyne. Part I. A study of prevalence. *British Journal of Psychiatry*, **110**, 146–158.

KELLER, O. J. & VEDDER, C. B. (1968) The crimes that old people commit. *The Gerontologist*, **8**, 43–50.

KRAFFT-EBING, R. VON (1965) *Psychopathia Sexualis*. English trans. by H. E. Wedeck. New York: Putnams Sons.

LANZKRON, J. (1961) Murder as a reaction to paranoid delusions in involutional psychosis and its prevention. *American Journal of Psychiatry*, **118**, 426–427.

—— (1963) Murder and insanity: A survey. *American Journal of Psychiatry*, **119**, 754–758.

LAW, S. K. (1979) Child molestation: A comparison of Hong Kong and Western findings. *Medicine, Science and the Law*, **19**, 55–60.

MACDONALD, J. M. (1986) *The Murderer and His Victim*. 2nd edn. Springfield, Illinois: C. C. Thomas.

MALINCHAK, A. (1980) *Crime and Gerontology*. New Jersey: Prentice-Hall.

MEYERS, T. J. (1965) Psychiatric examination of the sexual psychopath. *Journal of Criminal Law*, **56**, 31.

MOBERG, D. (1953) Old age and crime. *Journal of Criminal Law, Criminology and Police Science*, **43**, 764–776.

MOHR, J. W., TURNER, R. E. & JERRY, M. B. (1964) *Pedophilia and Exhibitionism*. Toronto: University of Toronto Press.

MOWAT, R. R. (1966) *Morbid Jealousy and Murder*. London: Tavistock.

NEWMAN, E. S. & NEWMAN, D. J. (1984) Policy implications of elderly crime. In *Elderly Criminals* (eds E. S. Newman, D. J. Newman & M. Gewirtz). Massachusetts: Oelgeschlager, Gunn & Hain.

NIELSEN, J. (1963) Geronto-psychiatric period-prevalence investigation in a geographically delimited population. *Acta Psychiatrica et Neurologica Scandinavica*, **38**, 307–330.

PETRIE, W. M., LAWSON, E. C. & HOLLENDER, M. H. (1982) Violence in geriatric patients. *Journal of the American Medical Association*, **248**, 443–444.

POLLAK, O. (1941) The criminality of old age. *Journal of Criminal Psychopathology*, **3**, 213–235.

RADZINOWICZ, L. (1957) *Sexual Offences*. London: MacMillan.

REVITCH, E. & WEISS, R. (1962) The pedophiliac offender. *Diseases of the Nervous System*, **23**, 1–6.

ROLLIN, H. (1973) Deviant behavior in relation to mental disorder. *Proceedings of the Royal Society of Medicine*, **66**, 99–103.

ROSE, E. F. (1970) Criminal responsibility and competency as influenced by organic disease. *Missouri Law Review*, **35**, 326–348.

ROSNER, R., WIEDERLIGHT, M. & SCHNEIDER, M. (1985) Geriatric felons examined at a Forensic Psychiatry Clinic. *Journal of Forensic Sciences*, **30**, 730–740.

ROTH, M. (1968) Cerebral disease and mental disorders of old age as causes of antisocial behavior. In *The Mentally Abnormal Offender* (eds V. S. de Rueck & R. Porter). London: J. & A. Churchill.

ROTHSCHILD, D. (1945) Senile psychoses and cerebral arteriosclerosis. In *Mental Disorder in Later Life* (ed. O. Kaplan). Stanford: Stanford University Press.

RUSKIN, S. H. (1941) Analysis of sex offences among male psychiatric patients. *American Journal of Psychiatry*, **97**, 955–968.

SCHROEDER, P. L. (1936) Criminal behavior in the later period of life. *American Journal of Psychiatry*, **92**, 915–924.

SHELDON, J. H. (1948) *The Social Medicine of Old Age*. London: Nuffield Foundation.

SHICHOR, D. & KOBRIN, S. (1978) Note: Criminal behavior among the elderly. *The Gerontologist*, **18**, 213.

—— (1984) The extent and nature of lawbreaking by the elderly: A review of arrest statistics. In *Elderly Criminals* (eds E. Newman, D. Newman, & M. Gewirtz). Massachusetts: Oelgeschlager, Gunn & Hain.

SIMON, A., EPSTEIN, L. & REYNOLDS, L. (1968) Alcoholism in the geriatric mentally ill. *Geriatrics*, **23**, 125–131.

SLATER, E. & ROTH, M. (1969) *Clinical Psychiatry*. 3rd edn. London: Baillière, Tindall & Cassell.

STERMAC, L. & SEGAL, Z. (1987) Cognitive distortions among child molesters. Paper presented at the Annual Meeting of the American Psychological Association, New York, August.

STORR, A. (1964) *Sexual Deviation*. Harmondsworth, Middlesex: Penguin Books.

SUTHERLAND, E. H. (1924) *Principles of Criminology*. Chicago: Lippincott.

TARDIFF, K. & SWEILLAM, A. (1979) The relation of age to assaultive behavior in mental patients. *Hospital and Community Psychiatry*, **30**, 709–711.

—— & —— (1980) Assault, suicide and mental illness. *Archives of General Psychiatry*, **37**, 164–169.

TAYLOR, P. J. & PARROTT, J. M. (1988) Elderly offenders: A study of age-related factors among custodially remanded prisoners. *British Journal of Psychiatry*, **152**, 340–346.

VIRKKUNEN, M. (1975) Victim-precipitated pedophilia offences. *British Journal of Criminology*, **15**, 175–180.

WHISKIN, F. E. (1967) The geriatric sex offender. *Geriatrics*, **22**, 168–172.

—— (1968) Delinquency in the aged. *Journal of Geriatric Psychiatry*, **1**, 242–262.

WILBANKS, W. (1984) The elderly offender: Placing the problem in perspective. In *Elderly Criminals* (eds W. Wilbanks & P. K. H. Kim). Maryland: The University Press of America.

—— & MURPHY, D. (1984). The elderly homicide offender. In *Elderly Criminals* (eds E. Newman, D. Newman & M. Gerwitz). Massachusetts: Oelgeschlager, Gunn and Hain.

ZEEGERS, M. (1966) Dementie in Verband Met Het Delict Ontucht. *Tijdschrift voor Strafrecht*, **75**, 265.

—— (1978) Sexual delinquency in men over 60 years old. (Personal communication.)

# 31 Clinical psychology with the elderly: Aspects of intellectual functioning, personality and adjustment

## PETER G. BRITTON

This brief review attempts to outline some of the contributions which have been made over a period of almost 40 years by clinical psychologists working with Sir Martin Roth. Their work has covered a greater understanding of the basic processes of ageing in terms of intellect and personality and the application of this knowledge to the care of those affected by the abnormalities of ageing.

We can get some perspective on the developments of these years from a consideration of the baseline of awareness in the early 1950s. While there had been some psychological research into the ageing process, there was little evidence of methodological sophistication. Many studies lacked appropriate control for the confounding effects which cohort differences in maturational experiences produce in inference from studies. Much was made of extrapolation to the elderly from research with so-called ageing groups. Sometimes these 'ageing' groups were as young as 40 to 60 years of age. One of the best reviews of the work of this period is that by Shock (1951), who emphasised the above issues and reflected on the poverty of systematic work with the aged in both theory and methodology.

In the United Kingdom Martin Roth was one of three crucial figures in bringing about a change in both quality and quantity of psychological research in the 1950s. He established a group around him at Graylingwell, Chichester, some of whose members transferred to Newcastle in the mid-1950s and formed the nucleus of workers in the major Newcastle studies, which were at their peak in the mid-1960s. The momentum gained in terms of psychological research was carried forward by those remaining at Newcastle and by the many who passed through the Department to posts elsewhere. This picture has considerable similarity to the catalytic effect of the other major psychological research groups of the period; that of Welford at Cambridge, which concentrated on the experimental psychology of ageing (Welford, 1968) and that of Heron at Liverpool (Heron & Chown, 1967) which focused on research into the relationships between social and psychological functioning.

A fundamental contribution of Martin Roth was to integrate the study of psychological aspects of ageing within individuals from both community and hospital or other long-term care settings. The Newcastle studies were, and still are in many respects, unique in their presentation of psychological data from representative samples which fully reflected the whole population. Much published work at that time, and this happens even today, used volunteer samples which may not have represented their underlying populations and which certainly did not usually include those people in hospital for whatever reason. To realise the value of the Newcastle work from the 1960s to the late 1980s, it is worth looking at the citations of baseline comparative data in the currently published studies of the 1980s; Newcastle studies are well represented.

Let us then overview some of the psychological studies of this period. We will look at work on the psychology of intellect and the more diffuse area of personality and adjustment. We will attempt to trace development of thought and application, the influence on both models of understanding of process and their implications for care.

## Intellectual functioning

The 1950s were a period when the widely held view of normal intellectual change with advancing age was that of relative stability from 20 to 60 years, with a gradual decline into old age (see Wechsler, 1958). In abnormal states the decline was held to be similar in nature, but accelerated. The Graylingwell studies (Hopkins & Roth, 1953) showed that this simplistic picture was not one that could be readily held, and pioneered innovations in both assessment techniques and theoretical models.

The assessment techniques used in these studies drew heavily on psychological models of memory functioning. This link between experimental and applied research has been a constant theme in relation to rapidly advancing knowledge of basic memory processes. Hopkins & Roth also used user-friendly test items, which were easy to administer to confused elderly subjects. From these studies may be traced the 'memory processes' content of many scales for the assessment of the elderly in the psychiatric context; through the Dementia Scale of Blessed *et al* (1968) to the CAMDEX of the 1980s (Roth *et al*, 1986).

In the late 1950s and early 1960s the major Newcastle surveys of the elderly were initiated. These covered medical, psychiatric, social and psychological functions, and their representative samples formed the basis for the work carried out by psychologists over the period to the mid-1970s. The psychological input to this work was co-ordinated by Savage, and the initial work, carried out by Bolton and Britton in 1963 to 1967. Their target groups were elderly hospital patients (and those in care) and elderly people in the community respectively. This work was reported in detail in Savage *et al* (1973).

Bolton concentrated on those individuals who had been admitted to hospital or taken into care with the psychiatric disorders of old age. His primary remit was to explore the theoretical and methodological basis of the psychological assessment of these individuals and to contribute to the efficiency of their diagnosis and care. In this context there were two central issues. Firstly, the adequacy of global intellectual measures such as the Wechsler Adult Intelligence Scale (WAIS) as an assessment and diagnostic tool and, secondly, the utility of the newly emerging tests of memory such as the Inglis Paired Associate Learning Test and the Walton-Black Modified Word Learning Test.

The WAIS was found to have some major problems when used in this context. The range of items available and their difficulty level were not appropriate for elderly people with dementia. Indeed, the results obtained cast considerable doubt on the, then extensive, use of WAIS-derived diagnostic indices of dementia (Bolton, Britton & Savage, 1966). In contrast, the Modified Word Learning Test was found to be extremely useful as a discriminator of intellectual deficit, although requiring modification to render it more 'user-friendly' (Bolton, Savage & Roth, 1967).

In the community context, the task was to validate the WAIS as an intellectual test and to develop a short and reliable version as a tool for the screening of elderly people. In general, the WAIS was found to be a useful test for this group. Although there were difficulties caused by the relatively high 'floor' of the test (few easy items), in general it performed well and the normative data provided proved appropriate to the UK as well as the USA. A short form produced for use specifically with the elderly (Britton & Savage, 1966a) was extensively used in the UK in clinical practice and research in the 1970s. This work also suggested that there were some subtle and interesting variations in intellectual functioning in the elderly with functional psychiatric disorders.

The themes which emerged from these two major projects were carried on in further research through the late 1960s and into the 1970s. Hall followed up both the hospital and community samples in a developmental study of intellect. She found a general stability of intellect in the people over 70 over an approximately five to seven year time span *unless* physical or psychiatric illness had intervened. From this work emerged an early test of performance learning (Savage & Hall, 1973) which is interesting in that it anticipates the many attempts to produce usable tests in this area which were published in the late 1970s and early 1980s. The earlier findings of inter-relationships between intellect and functional illness were followed up by Nunn (Nunn *et al*, 1974) who found changes clearly related to severity of functional illness.

These studies have had a substantial effect on the nature of investigations into intellectual functioning in the aged. The past ten years have seen considerable advances in the understanding of basic cognitive processes, particularly those of memory. The explosion of interest in Alzheimer's disease and in investigations into its pyschological consequences in the 1980s has had a consistent representation of those who have worked at, or been influenced by, the Newcastle models and methods of the 1960s and 1970s.

Much of this work has been reviewed in a book by two psychologists much influenced by Martin Roth (Woods & Britton, 1985). It is significant that this book, the first UK text on clinical psychology with the elderly, was written by two people who had been trained and worked within the Newcastle elderly group.

## Personality and adjustment

During the 1950s there was a noticeable increase in the number of research studies attempting to obtain a clearer understanding of personality changes in the elderly and their effects on adjustment. The phenomenon of ageism, a negative evaluation of the elderly and of their potential common in Western societies leads to distorted appraisal. Among the common misconceptions are assumptions of increasing withdrawal from social and environmental contacts, an increase in instability and increasing introversion.

The psychological component of the Newcastle studies incorporated assessment of personality, using standard psychometric measures of personality. The purpose was to assess the validity and reliability of these measures when used with the elderly and to attempt to identify any changes in personality structure which may occur in the group. A wide variety of measures was used and this work, fully reported in Savage *et al* (1977), remains amongst the most comprehensive to date.

The initial investigations with the Newcastle community aged concentrated on using a major international personality measure, the Minnesota Multiphasic Personality Inventory (MMPI), in order to assess its utility (Britton & Savage, 1966b). It was found that this scale could be given to the elderly and that reliability and validity were acceptable. However, the subtest scores showed considerable differences from the normative data for younger subjects, suggesting that extreme caution should be exercised in the use of this measure without the provision of more extensive and appropriate normative data.

One of the more interesting findings from this work was that the MMPI subscales distinguished those within the community sample who showed evidence of mild functional mental illness from the normal group. The identification of this subgroup, consisting primarily of those not under active treatment, is important and led to the development of an MMPI derived short scale (15 items) for the identification of this group (Britton & Savage, 1967). This scale was successfully used in a number of studies in the 1970s and, as with some of the cognitive scales mentioned earlier, traces of it are apparent in some current routine psychogeriatric questionnaires.

The study of the personality characteristics of the Newcastle community group developed with the use of the Cattell Sixteen Personality Factor Questionnaire (16PF). This factor-based personality measure had been extensively used at the time in the USA with British versions appearing in the 1960s. Again, it was found that the scales could be applied to the community elderly, although not those with sensory or concentration difficulties. The results obtained showed that the elderly were as a whole more introverted and socially withdrawn than the younger groups in the test standardisation samples. The adjustment of the community group was investigated by Savage *et al* (1977), who evaluated the use of both Self Concept and Life Satisfaction scales. These scales were again found to be of potential value in clinical work with the elderly provided that attention was paid to appropriate age-related normative data.

One of the most important contributions made by the Newcastle studies as a whole was to the understanding of the structure of personality in the elderly. The MMPI data were subjected to factor analyses which suggested that there was a first, strong component of general overall adjustment. This focused on stable and controlled personality change linked to a preservation of intellectual functioning and an absence of psychopathology. A further significant factor linked functional illness to increased 'sensitivity' in personality change, particularly those concerned with internal 'somatic' variables. A third factor associated the relationship of the individual to his/her external and social environment with a decrement in intellectual functioning and, possibly, organic illness (Britton & Savage, 1969).

A comparable comprehensive analysis of the Cattell 16PF structure of the community group (Gaber, 1983) has provided one of the best insights into the structure of personality in the elderly. Gaber used cluster analysis in an attempt to identify and distinguish groups within the overall sample. Four groups emerged: those in Group 1 were the normal group (54% of the sample) who managed to cope with changes in themselves and their environment. They could, however, be intolerant of excessive change and were quite shrewd and calculating in their interactions with others on a social basis. Those in Group 2 (20% of the sample) were noticeably more reserved and introverted, with actions and ideas clearly internally based, keeping themselves to themselves. Those in Group 3 (11% of the sample) were markedly unstable—'perturbed and disturbed'—with many problems of interaction on a social basis and with family and professionals. They were tense, anxious, emotionally unstable and uncontrolled. Those in Group 4 (16% of the sample) seemed exceptionally well-adapted. Their intellect was well preserved and they were noticeably in control of their personal and social lives.

These four groups, which also reflect some of the dimensions extracted from the MMPI findings, are interesting in their implications for a structure of personality in the elderly. It would certainly seem that there is a possible distinction between the 'copers', those who are relatively stable, and those who are less stable with a sensitive personality. The latter carries an implication of less adequate adjustment and coping when faced with the demands of the ageing process. These features are of value as we are increasingly faced with responsibility for the elderly who may have to care for their relatives, and need to know whether they retain adequate coping mechanisms.

This group of studies utilised the community sample; similar but smaller investigations looked at the personality of the aged hospital patients from the Newcastle studies. This task was much more difficult since the measures used are far less appropriate when the cognitive loss and concentration problems characteristic of the psychiatric disorders of the elderly become a major influence. In general it was found, not surprisingly, that the standard measures of personality were subject to major problems of reliability and validity with these elderly patients, and that their routine use was not recommended.

This work on personality and adjustment represents the only comprehensive attempt in the UK to use global measures of assessment with an aged sample. They did reflect many of the difficulties of using personality measures devised on another continent in a vastly different cultural setting. It might now be argued that these psychometric approaches are unsatisfactory, indeed they are little used in practice. Some questions may appear quite irrelevant to the older person, the models of personality reflected in the tests may be firmly rooted in younger persons (even in childhood). However, following the general moves away from using such tests which seemed to characterise the 1970s and early 1980s we may see newly developed measures which are based on age appropriate theory and methodology.

It seems that the Newcastle studies did show that there were aspects of the nature of and change in personality structure in old age which were 'face valid' and useful to practitioners. If such findings could be obtained from tests developed for other age ranges, and subject to the flaws inherent in their theoretical bases, we might be able to produce far more relevant, reliable and valid measures of those essential functions, given appropriate application of the psychology and methodology of the late 1980s. It seems a pity that advances in these areas lie well behind those in intellectual assessment.

## Consolidation and development

In retrospect, the period of Sir Martin Roth at Newcastle can be seen as one in which the psychologists working with the elderly were laying the groundwork for more detailed investigation of many of the general psychological processes investigated in the earlier studies. It is difficult to put oneself back into the days of the early 1960s when decisions were made concerning the phenomena to be investigated and the tests to be used. I am fortunate in this respect to have notes and minutes from the monthly meetings of the early to mid-sixties when both the general plans for the projects were discussed and the aims and methods of specific participants were examined in great detail.

From these sources emerges the driving force of Sir Martin with the strength of intellect and purpose to keep what was a very complex organisation on a considered path. In day to day terms David Kay kept the various threads of the project—medical, psychiatric, social, psychological—in sequence and, for most of the time, in harmony. As the supervisor of the psychologists, Savage attempted to keep an unruly bunch on target. Yes, we all got our PhDs and publications and jobs, thanks to the whole team.

The value of any research group must be judged by its impact on their subject. The overall contribution of the many psychologists involved was to obtain firm UK baseline information on aspects of the functioning of the normal and abnormal elderly from a unique representative community sample. Much was added by their ability to combine and collate this information with the medical and social data. The psychological material was published in the two books already referred to in this paper (Savage *et al*, 1973, 1977) which are classic baseline books.

The latter part of Sir Martin's time at Newcastle saw psychological research moving in two directions, both of which had been predicted in the PhDs of the late 1960s. One was the investigation of specific psychological processes of learning and memory, the other the application of psychological theory to the care of the elderly and their relatives.

The paper by Woods & Britton (1977) summarised a considerable amount of work in Newcastle in the early 1970s on the application of the newly evolving psychological therapies to the care of the elderly. This work had not had the high profile of the Newcastle Old Age Projects but was, in contrast, a low profile attempt to extend the use of techniques then common in the care of the adult mentally ill to the elderly. Much to the surprise of the authors the paper provoked considerable interest and activity. It was heavily cited during the 1980s as a source of ideas in other papers. One further outcome was an invitation to write what is the only current UK text on clinical psychology with the elderly (Woods & Britton, 1985). These publications, and more especially the work of Woods at Newcastle and the Institute of Psychiatry, have done much to establish a role and purpose for the clinical psychologist in the care of the elderly.

The investigation of the basic psychological processes underlying the mental health problems of the elderly has also continued until the present. In an internal paper to Sir Martin Roth written in 1967 the need was stressed for the investigation of defined clinical groups using detailed specific tests of learning and memory appropriate to the patient groups. It is interesting that it is only in the explosion of research in Alzheimer's disease in the 1980s that these expectations are beginning to be fulfilled. Much is now known about the processes of memory which has implications for the diagnosis and care of the elderly with abnormalities of learning and memory (Britton, 1988).

In this respect it is interesting to look at the work of Morris on the relationship between memory process and disorders of the elderly. This work combines a basis of the Newcastle ethos of the 1960s and 1970s with the clear insights into memory process of the Cambridge MRC Applied Psychology Unit of the 1980s.

The initial study, carried out in Newcastle (Morris *et al*, 1983), showed that, in the long-term memory disorders in senile dementia, cued recall was able substantially to ameliorate the deficit. This implied that the memory was still available for access, but retrieval mechanisms were ineffective. Moving to short-term memory, (Morris, 1984, 1986) found that the short-term memory deficit of senile dementia is a combination of reduced capacity of the short-term store and an increased rate of forgetting or loss from this store. The sophistication of this work is at a level far removed from that of two decades before in the early Newcastle studies!

We then have an impression of the impact of psychologists working with Sir Martin. The early years saw much effort put into the study of basic psychological processes in the elderly and a successful outcome in publications. The later years have seen a consolidation of this work and its applications to the care of the elderly. Many research and clinical psychologists trained in the Department under his influence have spread around the country and the world and have had a significant impact on knowledge and practice.

## References

BLESSED, G., TOMLINSON, B. E. & ROTH, M. (1968) The association between quantitative measures of dementia and of senile change in the cerebral grey matter of elderly subjects. *British Journal of Psychiatry*, **114**, 797–811.

BOLTON, N., BRITTON, P. G. & SAVAGE, R. D. (1966) Some normative data on the WAIS and its indices in an aged population. *Journal of Clinical Psychology*, **22**, 184–188.

——, SAVAGE, R. D. & ROTH, M. (1967) The MWLT on an aged psychiatric population. *British Journal of Psychiatry*, **113**, 1139–1140.

BRITTON, P. G. & SAVAGE, R. D. (1966a) A short form of the WAIS for use with the aged. *British Journal of Psychiatry*, **112**, 417–418.

—— —— (1966b) The MMPI and the aged: some normative data from a community sample. *British Journal of Psychiatry*, **112**, 941–943.

—— —— (1967) A short scale for the assessment of mental health in the community aged. *British Journal of Psychiatry*, **113**, 521–523.

—— —— (1969) The factional structure of the Minnesota Multiphasic Personality Inventory from an aged sample. *Journal of Genetic Psychology*, **114**, 13–17.

—— (1988) Abnormalities in the elderly. In *Adult Abnormal Psychology* (eds E. Miller & P. Cooper). Edinburgh: Churchill-Livingstone.

GABER, L. (1983) Activity vs engagement revisited: personality types in the aged. *British Journal of Psychiatry*, **143**, 140–149.

HERON, A. & CHOWN, S. M. (1967) *Age and Function*. London: Churchill.

HOPKINS, B. & ROTH, M. (1953) Psychological test performance in patients over sixty: II, paraphrenics, arteriosclerotic psychosis and acute confusion. *Journal of Mental Science*, **99**, 451–463.

MORRIS, R. G. (1984) Dementia and the functioning of the articulatory loop system. *Cognitive Neuropsychology*, **1**, 143–157.

——, WHEATLEY, J. & BRITTON, P. G. (1983) Retrieval from long-term memory in senile dementia: cued recall revisited. *British Journal of Clinical Psychology*, **22**, 141–142.

—— (1986) Short-term forgetting in senile dementia of the Alzheimer type. *Cognitive Neuropsychology*, **3**, 77–97.

NUNN, C., BERGMANN, K., BRITTON, P. G., FOSTER, E. M., HALL, E. H. & KAY, D. W. K. (1974).Intelligence and neurosis in old age. *British Journal of Psychiatry*, **124**, 446–452.

ROTH, M., TYM, E., MOUNTJOY, C. Q., HUPPERT, F. A., HENDRIE, H., VERMA, S. & GODDARD, R. (1986) CAMDEX: A standardised instrument for the diagnosis of mental disorder in the elderly with special reference to the early detection of dementia. *British Journal of Psychiatry*, **149**, 698–709.

SAVAGE, R. D., BRITTON, P. G., BOLTON, N. & HALL, E. H. (1973) *Intellectual Functioning in the Aged*. London: Methuen.

—— & HALL, E. H. (1973) A performance learning measure for the aged. *British Journal of Psychiatry*, **122**, 721–723.

——, GABER, L. B., BRITTON, P. G., BOLTON, N. & COOPER, A. (1977) *Personality and Adjustment in the Aged*. London: Academic Press.

SHOCK, N. W. (1951) Gerontology. *Annual Review of Psychology*, **2**, 353–370.

WECHSLER, D. (1958) *The Measurement and Appraisal of Adult Intelligence*. Baltimore: Williams & Wilkins.

WELFORD, A. T. (1968) *Fundamentals of Skill*. London: Methuen.

WOODS, R. T. & BRITTON, P. G. (1977) Psychological approaches to the treatment of the elderly. *Age and Ageing*, **6**, 104–112.

—— & —— (1985) *Clinical Psychology with the Elderly*. London: Croom-Helm.

# 32 Psychiatric and medical aspects of ageing in mental handicap

**KENNETH DAY**

I little thought when I came to Newcastle as a young registrar in the mid 1960s that I would find my psychiatric career in the field of mental handicap. Then, as sadly all too often now, the specialty was regarded as an uninteresting backwater and a refuge for those who didn't make the grade in mainstream psychiatry. Nothing, of course, can be further from the truth: it is a most fascinating, challenging and stimulating field in which to work, as many young psychiatrists are now finding out. I have Sir Martin to thank, not so much for encouraging me to enter the field, but rather for not discouraging me from doing so, and for his continuing advice and support once I had made the move. It was he who encouraged and facilitated my first venture into research, obtaining the grant which enabled me, together with Steve Hucker and Sandra George, to produce the most scientific study yet of psychotic disorder in the adult mentally handicapped (Hucker *et al*, 1979).

Changing and improving services was the main concern in my early days as a consultant—a vast task in which the ageing and elderly mentally handicapped were scarcely noticeable. It is only during this decade that the implications of the much improved increased life expectancy of mentally handicapped people have come to be recognised (WHO, 1985). This paper reviews currently available studies on psychiatric and medical aspects of ageing in the mentally handicapped. That some of the first papers on this topic should have come from the Newcastle stable (Day, 1985, 1987) is not perhaps so surprising.

## Life expectancy and demography

A trend towards increased life expectancy in mentally handicapped people was first noted in the 1960s (Primrose, 1966; Heaton-Ward, 1968; Richards, 1969; Richards & Sylvester, 1969) and confirmed by all subsequent studies. In the UK, Richards & Siddiqui (1980) showed that the mean age for both sexes in a large institutionalised population had risen significantly during the 25 year period from 1953 to 1978, and that the percentage of patients over the age of 55 years had increased from 15.9% to 24.7% for males and from 23.4% to 40.9% for females; Carter & Jancar (1983) reported an increase in the average age of death from 14.9 years to 58.3 years for males and from 22 years to 59.8 years for females between 1930 and 1980 for patients in Stoke Park Hospital, Bristol;

TABLE I

Surveys of the elderly mentally handicapped (from Day 1987)

| Source | Northgate Hospital | Strathmartine Hospital | Meanwood Park Hospital | England National Statistics | Western States USA | Northern Ireland | New York State USA | USA National Survey Selected Sample |
|---|---|---|---|---|---|---|---|---|
| | Day (1987) | Ballinger (1978) | Spencer (1978) | DHSS (1984a) | O'Connor et al (1970) | Mackay & Elliot (1975)* | Janicki & MacEachron (1984)* | Hauber et al (1985) |
| Survey date | 1984 | 1977 | 1978 | 1979 | 1968 | 1971 | 1978–82 | 1982 |
| Population surveyed | hospital | hospital | hospital | hospitals | 19 State institutions | community & hospital | community & institutions | community & institutions |
| Lower age limit | 65 years | 65 years | 65 years | 65 years | 60 years | 65 years | 63 years | 63 years |
| No. of patients | 99 | 38 | 64 | 6315 | 463 | 209 (77% in hospital) | 3896 (62% in institutions) | 77 |
| % Mentally handicapped population | 19% | 6.5% | 11.6% | 13.9% | — | 4.4% (7.3% hosp popn) | 7.8% | 4.7% |
| F : M ratio | 2 : 1 | 2 : 1 | 2 : 1 | 14% excess F 2 : 1 over 70s | 1 : 1 | 1 : 1 (hospital) 1.2 : 1 (comm) | 1 : 1 (63–72 years) 1.5 : 1 (73 years & over) | 1.8 : 1 (institutions) 1 : 1 (community) |
| Mod/mild mental handicap | 65% (IQ 35–70) | 82% (IQ 36–85) | 56% (IQ 40–69) | — | 54%† | 35% hospital 44% comm (IQ 50–75) | 30% institutions† 52% community | 38% institutions 81% community (IQ 36–84) |
| 65–74 years | 68% | 79% | — | 70% | 81% (60–74 years) | 55% (65–69) | 60% institutions 70% community 63–72 years | — |
| Duration hosp/ institution care | 94% over 10 years | 95% over 6 years | 85% over 20 years | 93% over 5 years | 87% over 10 years | — | — | — |

*Derived from
†Definition not specified

and Tait (1983) reported a life expectancy similar to that of the general population in a 12 year follow-up study of 222 patients in hospital with an IQ of 50 or below and an age of 57 years or over at follow-up. A similar picture has emerged from studies in other developed countries (Balakrishnan & Wolf, 1976; McCurley *et al*, 1972; Miller & Eyman, 1978).

The life expectancy of Down's syndrome individuals has also increased dramatically from a mean life expectancy of 9 years in 1929 (Penrose, 1949) to the mid 50s, with some living beyond 60 years (Masaki *et al*, 1981; Fryers, 1984; Carter & Jancar, 1983; Dupont *et al*, 1986). Sadly, this has exposed a predisposition to premature senility and dementia.

The majority of elderly mentally handicapped people are in their mid 60s to mid 70s—even today comparatively few reach their 80s, and are functioning in the mild to moderate mental handicap range: the sex distribution is equal in the predominant age band with a female lead emerging in people over 75, but not to the extent of that in the general population (Table I). Life expectancy is much lower in the severely mentally handicapped than in the mildly handicapped with far fewer surviving into old age (Tarjan *et al*, 1969; Balakrishnan & Wolf, 1976): those who do are relatively free from brain damage and associated physical disabilities (Janicki & MacEachron, 1984; Day, 1987).

## Psychiatric disorder

There are few specific studies of psychiatric disorder in this age group (Reid & Aungle, 1974; Reid *et al*, 1978; Ballinger, 1978; Day, 1985, 1987): some data are also available from more general studies of psychiatric morbidity in the mentally handicapped (Table II). This indicates prevalence rates of around 30% for psychiatric disorder in the middle-aged and elderly mentally handicapped, and 20% in the over 65s. Minor psychiatric symptoms not amounting to psychiatric illness have also been reported in a quarter to a half of over 65 year olds (Day, 1987; Ballinger, 1978). In the general population, increasing age is associated with an increasing prevalence of psychiatric illness but Day (1985) found a progressive fall in the proportion of hospital residents affected by any form of psychiatric disorder from 48.7% in the 40 to 49 year old age group to 16.7% in the over 70s; this trend held true for behaviour disorders, psychoses (apart from a slight peak in the 60s) and the neuroses, but was reversed in dementia when the highest incidence was in the over 70s. A similar trend was demonstrated by Lund (1985), who also found an increase in dementia in the over 65s, and Jacobson *et al* (1985). Hogg *et al* (1988) have argued that this is due principally to a progressive decline in the incidence and severity of behaviour disorders with age. There were no significant differences between the under and over 60 year-olds in Corbett's (1979) study, and Hauber *et al* (1985) found an increase in all forms of psychiatric disorder from 3.7% in the 40 to 62 year-olds to 6.3% in the 63 year-olds and over.

The disease pattern is similar to that for psychiatric disorder in the mentally handicapped as a whole but differs significantly from a comparable non-handicapped population (Fig. 1). **Behaviour and personality disorders** comprise the largest diagnostic category, accounting for between a third and a half of presentations in all studies (Table II). Using normative data, Day (1985)

TABLE II
Psychiatric illness in ageing and elderly mentally handicapped people

| Author & study details | Day 1985 Hospital residents 40 years & over n = 357 | Day 1985 Psychiatric admissions 40 years & over n = 43 | Day 1987 Hospital residents 65 years & over n = 99 | Corbett 1979* Epidemiological sample 45 years & over n = 119 | Memolascino et al* 1987 Psychiatric admissions 36 years & over n = 101 | Lund 1985* Epidemiological sample 45–64 yrs n = 94 | Lund 1985* Epidemiological sample 65 yrs & over n = 94 |
|---|---|---|---|---|---|---|---|
| Overall prevalence** | 30% | 20% | 20% | 37.6% | 18.6% | 29.9% | 25.9% |
| **Diagnostic breakdown*** | | | | | | | |
| Schizophrenia | 27.5% | 21.5% | 35% | 12.8% | 26% | 3.1% | 3.7% |
| Affective psychosis | 9.2% | — | 5% | 4% | 8% | 6% | — |
| ? Psychoses | | | 5% | 7.9% | 14% | 3% | — |
| Dementia | 9.2% | 9.5% | 30% | — | 17.8% | 6% | 22.2% |
| Neurosis | 3.7% | 33.3% | 5% | 3% | 6% | 1.5% | — |
| Behaviour/personality disorder | 50.5% | 35.7% | 25% | 41.5% | 19% | 10.4% | — |
| Other | — | — | — | — | 8% | — | — |

\* Derived from
\*\* % Total sample
\*\*\* % Total psych. disorder

calculated that this represents a three to five times greater prevalence than in the non-handicapped if drug and alcohol dependency are included, and a ten to fifteen times greater prevalence if they are not. This massive over-representation is principally due to the many unique behaviour problems occurring in the severely mentally handicapped, and in part to the fact that antisocial behaviour in the mildly mentally handicapped is much more likely to lead to admittance to hospital than it is in the non-handicapped. Behaviour and personality disorders are commoner in males and there is a marked association with organic brain damage; explosive behaviour disorders are the main problem in the severely mentally handicapped, while antisocial conduct is the main presenting problem in the mildly mentally handicapped (Day, 1985). In the severely mentally handicapped, behaviour disorders tend to be long-standing and persistent, often dating from adolescence, and do not show the usual amelioration with ageing found in the non-handicapped (Reid *et al*, 1984), suggesting that brain damage and failure of maturation as well as environmental influences are important sustaining factors (Day, 1985).

The **psychoses** are the second largest group of disorders in this age group, but show a reduced prevalence compared to the general population. This is almost certainly due to the fact that despite an improved life expectancy, comparatively few mentally handicapped people survive into their 60s and 70s, decades in which there is a massive rise in this group of disorders in the general population. The difficulty of making an accurate diagnosis in the severely mentally handicapped (Reid, 1972; Hucker *et al*, 1979) may also be a factor. As in the general population, **affective psychosis** is a disease of the middle years (Heaton-Ward, 1977; Day, 1985), although there is some evidence for a somewhat lower age of onset in the mentally handicapped (Reid, 1972; Hucker *et al*, 1979), and it is more common in females (Reid, 1972; Hucker *et al*, 1979; Wright, 1982; Day, 1985). It follows a typical recurring course, and bipolar illnesses are common. Out of 24 cases of affective psychosis in mentally handicapped people aged 40 years and over, Day (1985) found that 21 (88%) had suffered recurrent illnesses with up to eight episodes in a 10 year period, and in 15 (63%) the illness was bipolar. Fourteen (60%) of Carlson's (1979) 23 cases collected from the literature suffered a bipolar illness, and in 14 (88%) of Hucker *et al*'s 16 cases the illness was recurrent with up to ten episodes over a period of 11 to 20 years and bipolar in seven (44%).

**Paranoid psychosis** is the other common illness and accounted for nine (56%) of the 16 cases of schizophrenia in the 40s described by Day (1985). As in the non-handicapped, the onset is invariably in the fifth, sixth and seventh decades (Reid, 1972; Heaton-Ward, 1977; Hucker *et al*, 1979; Day, 1985) and an association with TLE, severe disorders of vision and hearing and interpersonal difficulties has been reported (Reid, 1972; Day, 1985). A third important group are the '**adult autists**'—a term coined by Forrest & Oguremni (1974) to describe those individuals who take the autistic features displayed in childhood with them into adulthood and who are apt to be mis-classified as psychotic, and who account for between 5% and 14% of cases. Day (1985) also described a small group of ? psychotics who exhibit periodic behaviour disturbance with bizarre features strongly suggestive of a psychosis but where the diagnosis cannot be firmly established.

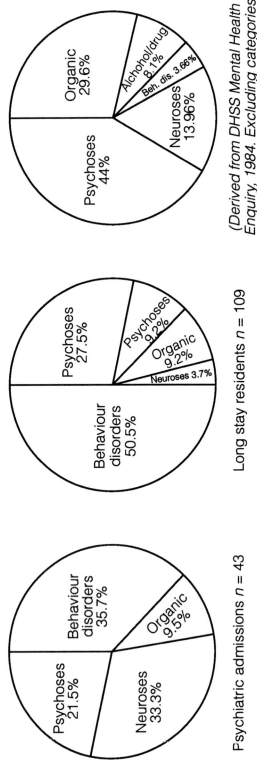

Psychiatric admissions *n* = 43

Long stay residents *n* = 109

(*Derived from DHSS Mental Health Enquiry, 1984. Excluding categories 'other' and 'mental'*)

First admissions to mental illness hospitals and units in England 1979 aged 45 years and over

*Fig. 1. Pattern of psychiatric illness in ageing and elderly mentally handicapped hospital residents, admission from the community and the general population (From Day, 1985)*

A low or nil prevalence of **neurotic disorder** is reported in most studies (Leck *et al*, 1967; Williams, 1971; Forrest & Oguremni, 1974; Heaton-Ward, 1977; Ballinger & Reid, 1977; Corbett, 1979; Lund, 1985; Gostatson, 1985). Possible reasons include a generally sheltered lifestyle which insulates against external and internal stresses and the greater likelihood of behavioural or psychotic rather than neurotic reactions to stress, particularly in the more severely mentally handicapped (Reid, 1982; Day, 1985). However, in a recent study of over 200 mentally handicapped children followed from birth to 22 years of age, Richardson *et al* (1979) considered that 26% displayed neurotic problems. Day (1985) also found a high prevalence of neurotic disorder in admissions from the community. Reactive depression and anxiety states were the main illnesses, there was a female to male ratio of two to one and evidence of constitutional predisposition. Precipitating factors included domestic disputes, interpersonal problems and deteriorating health, but the death or serious illness of the last caring relative and its dramatic consequences for the life of the individual was the most common and potent stress (Day, 1985) and is a major cause of long-term stays in hospital in this age group (Carter, 1984).

Reported rates for **dementia** in the ageing and elderly mentally handicapped are comparable to those for the general population. In a study of 155 hospital in-patients aged 45 years and over, Reid & Aungle (1974) recorded an overall prevalence of 7.1% and a prevalence of 13.6% in the over 65s. Tait (1983) gives similar figures of 7% for overall prevalence and 12.3% in the over 65s in a survey of 137 hospital in-patients aged 55 years and over, while Day (1987) found a prevalence of 6% for definite dementia and a further 6% with signs of early dementia in 99 long-stay hospital residents aged 65 years and over. A decline in intellectual functioning after late middle age, which became significant and was accompanied by loss of self care skills and physical deterioration in 18%, was reported by Hewitt *et al* (1986) in a study of 148 hospital residents aged 65–88 years psychologically tested over a period of 50 years. Both senile dementia and cerebral arteriosclerotic dementia have been reported, the latter being associated with a history of hypertension and cerebrovascular accidents (Reid & Aungle, 1974; Reid *et al*, 1978; Tait, 1983). Late onset epilepsy and other neurological symptoms occur, particularly in association with arteriosclerotic dementia, and serial EEG recordings may reveal progressive deterioration (Reid & Aungle, 1974; Tait, 1983; Day, 1985).

## Down's syndrome and Alzheimer's disease

The characteristic senile plaques of Alzheimer's disease were first described in the brain of a Down's individual by Struwe (1929). There have since been many studies, all of which have demonstrated Alzheimer's changes in practically 100% of the brains of Down's individuals aged 35 years or over at death and an increase in the magnitude of change with age (Malamud, 1964; Solitaire & Lamarche, 1966; Haberland, 1969; Olson & Shaw, 1969; Burger & Vogel, 1973; Liss *et al*, 1980; Roper & Williams, 1980; Sylvester, 1984; Wisniewski *et al*, 1985).

Despite the almost universal nature of the neuropathological changes, only a proportion of Down's individuals aged 40 years and over show the clinical features of dementia, and there is a lack of correlation between clinical symptoms and pathology. The following prevalence rates have been reported: 6% (Day, 1985);

12.5% (Roper & Williams, 1980); 25% (Reid & Aungle, 1974); and 45% (Thase, 1982). Age-related cognitive change including intellectual deterioration (Nakamura, 1961; Hewitt, *et al*, 1985); orientation problems (Wisniewski *et al*, 1978; Thase *et al*, 1982, 1984); and short-term memory deficits (Dalton *et al*, 1974; Dalton & Crapper, 1977) have been shown to occur significantly more frequently in older than younger Down's individuals, and in a longitudinal study of 23 Down's individuals aged 50 years or over, Hewitt *et al* (1985) found that 39% showed significant intellectual deterioration over an average retest interval of 3.7 years, although none showed clinical signs of dementia. An increase in the prevalence of epilepsy (Sourander & Sjögren, 1970; Veall, 1974); EEG abnormalities (Tangye, 1979; St Clair & Blackwood, 1985); and abnormal reflexes (Owens *et al*, 1971; Wisniewski *et al*, 1978; Thase *et al*, 1982, 1984; Sand *et al*, 1983) with age have also been reported: the diagnostic value of late onset epilepsy has been emphasised by Reid *et al* (1978).

Miniszek (1983) has suggested that intellectual impairment, additional physical complications and the protected situation of the individual may mask the early manifestations of the disease and modify its later features, thus creating diagnostic difficulties. But there may be discrete differences between those who develop clinical dementia and those who do not: some researchers, for example, have found a significant association between intellectual deterioration and macrocytosis (Eastham & Jancar, 1983; Hewitt *et al*, 1985). Elucidation will hopefully come from longitudinal clinico-psychological-pathological studies now in progress.

The basis of the association between Down's syndrome and Alzheimer's disease is not known. A number of hypotheses have been advanced, including a disordered immunological system, a general syndrome of premature ageing and Down's syndrome as a progressive condition (Oliver & Holland, 1986; Corbett, 1985; Wright & Whalley, 1984) but the possibility of an inherited predisposition to both non-dysjunction of chromosome 21 and Alzheimer's disease is the most favoured by recent research. Family studies have revealed a significant excess of Down's individuals in the probands of sufferers from familial Alzheimer's disease (Heston *et al*, 1981; Heyman *et al*, 1983), and the genes for beta-amyloid protein, which occurs as deposits in the brains of individuals with Alzheimer's disease, and for familial Alzheimer's disease have recently been detected and located in the same region on chromosome 21. These findings strongly implicate a defect in a gene on chromosome 21 or its regulation in Alzheimer's disease, and raise the possibility of amyloid protein as the causal agent and suggest that increased susceptibility to Alzheimer's disease in Down's syndrome is a consequence of extra gene dosage causing premature amyloid deposition (*Lancet*, 1987). Interestingly, the gene for the enzyme superoxide dismutase (SOD) is also located on chromosome 21 in the same region: the activity of this enzyme has been shown to be increased in the brains of Down's individuals (Brooksbank & Balazs, 1983) and Sinet (1982) has postulated that excess SOD activity leads to oxidative damage within the brain cells thus causing the ageing process.

## Physical health: morbidity and mortality

The mentally handicapped surviving into old age enjoy a generally more favourable health status than the mentally handicapped population as a whole.

TABLE III
*Major medical problems in the ageing and elderly mentally handicapped*

| Source | Day 1987 *Hospital residents 65 years & over* *n* = 99 | | | | Hogg et al 1988 *Hospital residents 50 years & over* *n* = 501 | DHSS 1972 *Hospital residents 65 years & over* *National Statistics* | Jacobson et al 1985* *Population survey 65 years & over* *n* = unknown | Hauber et al 1985 *National sample 63 years & over* *n* = 210 | Janicki & MacEachron 1984 *Population survey 63 years & over* *n* = 2856 | |
|---|---|---|---|---|---|---|---|---|---|---|
| Survey details | 65–69 years | 70–74 years | 75 years & over | Total | | | | | 63–72 years | 73 years & over |
| Mobility problems | 21% | 31% | 57% | 34% | 24.6 | 13% | 22% | — | — | — |
| Fractures | 0% | 8% | 27% | 12% | — | — | — | — | — | — |
| Visual impairment | 18% | 17% | 37% | 24% | 8.2 | — | 21% | 6.7% | 32% | 45% |
| Hearing impairment | 12% | 17% | 37% | 22% | 9.3 | — | 26% | 15.6% | | |
| Incontinence | 12% | 14% | 10% | 12% | — | 11% | — | — | — | — |
| Cardio-respiratory disease | 6% | 34% | 33% | 24% | 7% | — | 29% | 30.7% | 36% | 63% |

*Derived from

In a study of 38 mentally handicapped patients aged 65 years and over, Ballinger (1978) found that 42% had no health problems and only 21% needed geriatric care. Hauber *et al* (1985) examined a national sample of mentally handicapped people aged 63 years and over in the USA and found that 69% of those living in the community and 51% of those living in institutions displayed no chronic health disorders, 25% suffered from one condition and less than 5% from three or more. Day (1987) found that 23% of mentally handicapped hospital residents aged 65 years and over had no medical or surgical problems, 33% had one condition, 26% two conditions and 17% three or more conditions with an average of 1.92 for those affected, and that 87% of those aged 75 years and over had one or more conditions compared to 50% of the 65 to 69 year age group.

The main problems are those associated with the progressive physical deterioration expected in old age with loss of mobility, an increased proneness to falls and accidental injuries, deterioration in vision and hearing, and incontinence (Table III). All show a progressive increase with age and a marked increase in the mid 70s (Janicki & MacEachron, 1984; Jacobson *et al*, 1985; Day, 1987; Hogg *et al*, 1988). Thus, the health problems of the elderly mentally handicapped are comparable to those of the elderly population as a whole, and although dependency levels are higher in the former, this is essentially due to the underlying mental handicap; it is only in the over 75s that dependency increases as a direct consequence of deteriorating physical and mental health (Day, 1987).

Increased life expectancy coupled with improved medical treatment has resulted in marked changes in causes of death. There has been a progressive decline in deaths from tuberculosis and status epilepticus, formerly common killers in institutionalised populations (Carter & Jancar, 1983), and a corresponding increase in deaths from age related conditions—non-tubercular respiratory tract infection, cardiovascular and cerebrovascular disease and carcinoma (Primrose, 1966; Richards & Sylvester, 1969; McCurley *et al*, 1972; Jancar & Jancar, 1977; Carter & Jancar, 1983). Non-tubercular respiratory tract infection has become the major cause of death, accounting for between 35% and 60% of recorded deaths (Richards & Sylvester, 1969; McCurley *et al*, 1972; Carter & Jancar, 1983; Tait, 1983), the risk of death from this cause being four to ten times greater in the mentally handicapped than in the general population (Richards & Sylvester, 1969; Carter & Jancar, 1983). Resistant strains of bacteria and poor coughing and sneezing reflexes have been implicated, but so far no satisfactory explanation has been forthcoming (Blackwell, 1979). Vascular disease (cerebrovascular accidents and heart disease), which accounts for around 30% of deaths (Tait, 1983), has shown a four to five fold increase since the 1950s (Carter & Jancar, 1983) but is still well below that for the general population. Carter & Jancar (1983) found that deaths due to carcinoma had risen from 2.3% during the 1930 to 1955 period to 13% during the 1956 to 1980 period and that the average age of death from carcinoma for both sexes had risen progressively to 65 years in 1970–80. Deaths from cancer of the gastrointestinal tract were much higher than expected, which they suggest may reflect factors other than increasing longevity alone.

## Service needs

The high prevalence of psychiatric disorder found in all studies must be taken into account in planning the specialist psychiatric services required as long-stay hospitals run down and care in the community develops. While treatment in community residential settings will be possible for many, a substantial number will require to be managed on a short to medium, and in some cases a long-term basis, in specialised treatment units (Day, 1983). The high prevalence of behaviour disorders and their persistence into old age is particularly noteworthy; the specialist requirements in terms of facilities and staff needed to manage these disorders have been insufficiently appreciated in some of the more idealistic proposals for the development of community care. Neurotic disorder is also a significant problem and its incidence is likely to rise as new approaches to care and changing lifestyles increasingly expose ageing and elderly mentally handicapped people to the stresses and strains of every day life. The death of a parent or caring relative is a particularly potent stress in this age group and more attention needs to be given to bereavement counselling (Oswin, 1985).

The vast majority of ageing and elderly mentally handicapped are mildly handicapped, 'young' and fit, and have few major health problems. Their requirement is for 'structured retirement programmes' within the mental handicap services. Regular health screening is essential to detect newly arising medical, surgical and psychiatric problems—mentally handicapped people are particularly poor at self reporting illness (McDonald, 1985). Detection should lead to appropriate treatment, but as Day (1985) has shown, there may be reluctance to treat some conditions, for example, cataracts, and some individuals, for example, the severely mentally handicapped, because of real or perceived problems of co-operation and management. The small group of people who show significant physical and mental deterioration with age have care and nursing needs indistinguishable from other geriatric patients. Their geriatric problems completely overshadow their mental handicap and there is a strong argument for caring for them within the generic geriatric services.

Of elderly mentally handicapped people in the UK, 90% are living in mental handicap hospitals where they have spent most of their lives (DHSS, 1984a). It is essential that their capacity to adjust to and benefit from any radical changes in the pattern of their lives is properly evaluated before they are automatically included in large scale deinstitutionalisation and resettlement programmes. But whatever the policy intentions, the reality is that many will remain in hospital where they already constitute a substantial and increasing proportion of the population. Urgent attention therefore needs to be given to the development of special facilities for them within the hospital setting. Some hospitals have made a start by grouping the elderly together, developing special accommodation, improving regular health screening and providing special occupational and recreational activities (DHSS, 1984b; Jancar, 1987). But there is still much to be done: all too often, elderly mentally handicapped people are still to be found inappropriately placed on wards with much younger, overactive or behaviourally disturbed residents and without any form of occupation for most of the day (Day, 1987).

## Conclusion

The growing population of elderly and ageing mentally handicapped people poses an increasing problem to service providers. More research is needed into their characteristics. Age related mental and physical health problems, which can crucially influence care needs, occur with the same frequency as in the elderly general population and there are special problems in Down's syndrome. It is essential that adequate account is taken of these in future service planning.

## References

BALAKRISHNAN, T. R. & WOLF, L. C. (1976) Life expectancy of mentally retarded persons in Canadian institutions. *American Journal of Mental Deficiency*, **80**, 650–662.

BALLINGER, B. R. (1978) The elderly in a mental subnormality hospital: A comparison with elderly psychiatric patients. *Social Psychiatry*, **13**, 37–40.

—— & REID, A. H. (1977) Psychiatric disorder in an Adult Training Centre and a hospital for the mentally handicapped. *Psychological Medicine*, **7**, 525–528.

BLACKWELL, M. W. (1979) *Care of the Mentally Retarded*. Boston: Little Brown.

BROOKSBANK, B. W. L. & BALAZS, R. (1983) Superoxide Dismutase and lipoperoxidation in Down's syndrome foetal brain. *Lancet*, **i**, 881–882.

BURGER, P. C. & VOGEL, F. S. (1973) The development of pathologic changes of Alzheimer's disease and senile dementia in patients with Down's syndrome. *American Journal of Pathology*, **73**, 457–468.

CARLSON, G. (1979) Affective psychosis in mental retardates. *Psychiatric Clinics of North America*, **2**, 525–533.

CARTER, G. & JANCAR, J. (1983) Mortality in the mentally handicapped: A 50 year survey at Stoke Park Group of Hospitals (1930–1980). *Journal of Mental Deficiency Research*, **27**, 143–156.

—— (1984) Why are the mentally handicapped admitted to hospital? *British Journal of Psychiatry*, **145**, 283–288.

CORBETT, J. (1979) Psychiatric morbidity and mental retardation. In *Psychiatric Illness in Mental Handicap* (eds F. E. James & R. P. Snaith). Special publication of the Royal College of Psychiatrists. Ashford, Kent: Headley Brothers.

—— (1985) Is Down's syndrome a progressive condition? *Journal of The Royal Society of Medicine*, **78**, 499–502.

DALTON, A. L., CRAPPER, D. R. & SCHLOTTERER, G. R. (1974) Alzheimer's disease in Down's syndrome: visual retention deficits. *Cortex*, **10**, 366–367.

—— & —— (1977) Down's syndrome and ageing of the brain. In *Research to Practice in Mental Retardation, vol. 3. Biomedical Aspects* (ed. P. Mittler), 391–400. Baltimore: University Park Press.

DAY, K. A. (1983) A hospital based psychiatric unit for mentally handicapped adults. *Mental Handicap*, **11**, 137–140.

—— (1985) Psychiatric disorder in the middle aged and elderly mentally handicapped. *British Journal of Psychiatry*, **147**, 660–667.

—— (1987) The elderly mentally handicapped in hospital: A clinical study. *Journal of Mental Deficiency Research*. **31**, 131–146.

DHSS (1972) *Census of Mentally Handicapped Patients in Hospital in England and Wales at the End of 1970*. Statistical and Research Report Series No. 3, London: HMSO.

—— (1984a) *Inpatient Statistics from the Mental Health Enquiry for England (1979)*. Statistical and Research Reports Series No. 25.

—— (1984b) *Helping Mentally Handicapped People with Special Problems: Report of a DHSS Study Tecm*. London: HMSO.

DUPONT, A., VAETH, M. & VIDEBECH, P. (1986) Mortality and life expectancy of Down's syndrome in Denmark. *Journal of Mental Deficiency Research*, **30**, 111–120.

EASTHAM, R. D. & JANCAR, J. (1983) Macrocytosis and Down's syndrome. *British Journal of Psychiatry*, **143**, 203–204.

FORREST, A. D. & OGUREMNI, O. O. (1974) The prevalence of psychiatric illness in a hospital for the mentally handicapped. *Health Bulletin*, **32**, 199–202.

FRYERS, T. (1984) *The Epidemiology of Severe Intellectual Impairment*. London: Academic Press.

GOSTATSON, R. (1985) Psychiatric illness amongst the mentally retarded. Supplement No. 318. *Acta Psychiatrica Scandinavica*.

HABERLAND, C. (1969) Alzheimer's disease in Down's syndrome: Clinico-neurological observations. *Acta Neurologica Belgica*, **69**, 369–380.

HAUBER, F. A., ROTEGARD, L. L. & BRUININKS, R. H. (1985) Characteristics of residential services for older/elderly mentally retarded persons. In *Ageing and Developmental Disabilities: Issues and Approaches* (eds M. P. Janicki & H. M. Wisniewski), 327–350. Baltimore: Paul Brookes Publishing.

HEATON-WARD, W. A. (1968) The life expectation of mentally subnormal patients in hospital. *British Journal of Psychiatry*, **114**, 1591–1592.

—— (1977) Psychosis in mental handicap. (The Blake Marsh Lecture 1976) *British Journal of Psychiatry*, **130**, 525–533.

HESTON, L. L., MASTRI, A. R., ANDERSON, E. & WHITE, J. (1981) Dementia of the Alzheimer type: clinical genetics, natural history and associated conditions. *Archives of General Psychiatry*, **38**, 1085–1090.

HEWITT, K. E., CARTER, G. & JANCAR, J. (1985) Ageing in Down's syndrome. *British Journal of Psychiatry*, **147**, 58–62.

——, FENNER, M. E. & TORPY, D. (1986) Cognitive and behavioural profiles of the elderly mentally handicapped. *Journal of Mental Deficiency Research*, **30**, 217–225.

HEYMAN, A., WILKINSON, W. E., HURWITZ, B. J., SCHMECHEL, D., SIGMON, A. H., WEINBERG, T., HELMS, M. J. & SWIFT, M. (1983) Alzheimer's disease; genetic aspects and associated clinical disorders. *Annals of Neurology*, **14**, 507–516.

HOGG, J., MOSS, S. & COOKE, D. (1988) *Ageing and Mental Handicap*. London: Chapman & Hall.

HUCKER, S. J., DAY, K. A., GEORGE, S. & ROTH, M. (1979) Psychosis in mentally handicapped adults. In *Psychiatric Illness and Mental Handicap* (eds F. E. James & R. P. Snaith). Special publication of the Royal College of Psychiatrists.

JACOBSON, J. W., SUTTON, M. S. & JANICKI, M. P. (1985) Demography and characteristics of ageing and aged mentally retarded persons. In *Ageing and Developmental Disabilities: Issues and Approaches* (eds M. P. Janicki & H. M. Wisniewski). Baltimore: Paul Brookes Publishing.

JANCAR, J. (1987) *Monograph on Medical Aspects of Ageing in the Mentally Handicapped*. Stoke Park Hospital, Bristol.

JANCAR, M. P. & JANCAR, J. (1977) Cancer and mental retardation (a forty year review). *Bristol Medico-Chirurgical Journal*, **92**, 3–7.

JANICKI, M. P. & MACEACHRON, A. E. (1984) Residential, health and social service needs of elderly developmentally disabled persons. *The Gerontologist*, **24**, 128–137.

*LANCET* (1987) Editorial: Alzheimer's disease, Down's syndrome and chromosome 21, *i*, 1011–1012.

LECK, I., GORDON, W. L. & McKEOWN, T. (1967) Medical and social needs of mentally subnormal patients. *British Journal of Preventative and Social Medicine*, **21**, 115–121.

LISS, L., SHIM, C., THASE, M., SMELTZER, D., MALOONE, J. & COURI, D. (1980) The relationship between Down's syndrome and dementia, Alzheimer's type. *Journal of Neuropathology and Experimental Neurology*, **39**, 371.

LUND, J. (1985) The prevalence of psychiatric morbidity in mentally retarded adults. *Acta Psychiatrica Scandinavica*, **7**, 563–570.

MALAMUD, N. (1964) Neuropathology. In *Mental Retardation* (eds H. A. Stevens & R. Heber). Chicago: University of Chicago Press.

MASAKI, J., HIGURASHI, M., IIJIMA, K., ISHIKAWA, N., TANAKA, F., FUJII, T., KUROKI, Y., INNUMA, K., MATUSO, H., TAKESHITA, K. & HASHIMOTO, S. (1981) Mortality and survival for Down's syndrome in Japan. *American Journal of Human Genetics*, **33**, 629–639.

McCURLEY, R., MACKAY, D. N. & SCALLY, B. G. (1972) The life expectation of the mentally subnormal under community and hospital care. *Journal of Mental Deficiency Research*, **16**, 57–66.

McDONALD, E. P. (1985) Medical needs of severely developmentally disabled persons residing in the community. *American Journal of Mental Deficiency*, **90**, 171–176.

MACKAY, D. N. & ELLIOTT, R. (1975) Subnormals under community and hospital care. *Journal of Mental Deficiency Research*, **19**, 21–28.

MENOLASCINO, F. J., LEVITAS, A. & GREINER, C. (1987) The nature and types of mental illness in the mentally retarded. *Psychopharmacology Bulletin*, **22**, 1060–1071.

MILLER, C. & EYMAN, R. (1978) Hospital and community mortality rates among the retarded. *Journal of Mental Deficiency Research*, **22**, 137–145.

MINISZEK, N. A. (1983) Development of Alzheimer's disease in Down's syndrome individuals. *American Journal of Mental Deficiency*, **87**, 377–385.

NAKAMURA, H. (1961) Nature of institutionalised adult mongoloid intelligence. *American Journal of Mental Deficiency*, **66**, 456–458.

O'CONNOR, G., JUSTICE, R. S. & WARREN, N. (1970) The aged mentally retarded: institution or community care? *American Journal of Mental Deficiency*, **75**, 354–360.

OLIVER, C. & HOLLAND, A. J. (1986) Down's syndrome and Alzheimer's disease: A review. *Psychological Medicine*, **16**, 307–322.

OLSON, M. I. & SHAW, C. M. (1969) Pre-senile dementia and Alzheimer's disease in mongolism. *Brain*, **92**, 147–156.

OSWIN, M. (1985) Bereavement. In *Mental Handicap* (eds M. Craft, J. Bicknell & S. Hollins). London: Baillière Tindall.

OWENS, D., DAWSON, J. C. & LOSIN, S. (1971) Alzheimer's disease in Down's syndrome. *American Journal of Mental Deficiency*, **75**, 606–612.

PENROSE, L. S. (1949) The incidence of mongolism in the general population. *Journal of Mental Science*, **95**, 685–688.

PRIMROSE, D. A. (1966) Natural history of mental deficiency in a hospital group and in the community it serves. *Journal of Mental Deficiency Research*, **10**, 159.

REID, A. H. (1972) Psychoses in adult mental defectives: (i) Manic depressive psychosis. (ii) Schizophrenic and paranoid psychoses. *British Journal of Psychiatry*, **120**, 205–218.

—— (1982) The Psychiatry of Mental Handicap. Oxford: Blackwell Scientific Publications.

—— & AUNGLE, P. G. (1974) Dementia in ageing mental defectives: A clinical psychiatric study. *Journal of Mental Deficiency Research*, **18**, 15–23.

——, MALONEY, A. F. J. & AUNGLE, P. G. (1978) Dementia in mental ageing defectives: a clinical and neuropathological study. *Journal of Mental Deficiency Research*, **22**, 233–241.

——, BALLINGER, B. R., HEATHER, B. B. & MELVINS, S. J. (1984) The natural history of behavioural symptoms among severely and profoundly mentally retarded patients. *British Journal of Psychiatry*, **145**, 289–293.

RICHARDS, B. W. (1969) Age trends in mental deficiency institutions. *Journal of Mental Deficiency Research*, **13**, 171.

—— & SYLVESTER, B. E. (1969) Mortality trends in mental deficiency institutions. *Journal of Mental Deficiency Research*, **13**, 276–292.

—— & SIDDIQUI, A. Q. (1980) Age and mortality trends in residents of an institution for the mentally handicapped. *Journal of Mental Deficiency Research*, **24**, 99–105.

RICHARDSON, S. A., KATZ, M., KOLLER, H., McLAREN, L. & RUBINSTEIN, B. (1979) Some characteristics of a population of mentally retarded young adults in a British city: A basis for estimating some service needs. *Journal of Mental Deficiency Research*, **23**, 275–283.

ROPER, A. H. & WILLIAMS, R. S. (1980) Relationship between plaques, tangles and dementia in Down's syndrome. *Neurology*, **30**, 639–644.

SAND, T., MELLGREN, S. I. & HESTNES, A. (1983) Primitive reflexes in Down's syndrome. *Journal of Mental Deficiency Research*, **27**, 39–44.

SINET, P. M. (1982) Metabolism of oxygen derivatives in Down's syndrome. *Annals of the New York Academy of Sciences*, **396**, 83–94.

SOLITAIRE, G. B. & LAMARCHE, J. B. (1966) Alzheimer's disease in senile dementia as seen in mongoloids: neuropathological observations. *American Journal of Mental Deficiency*, **70**, 840–848.

SOURANDER, P. & SJÖGREN, H. (1970) The concept of Alzheimer's disease and its clinical manifestations. In *Ciba Foundation Symposium: Alzheimer's Disease and Related Conditions* (eds G. E. W. Wolstenholme & M. O'Connor), 11–16. London: Churchill.

SPENCER, D. A. (1978) The elderly mentally handicapped in hospital. *Apex: Journal of the Institute of Mental Subnormality*, **5**, 24.

STRUWE, F. (1929) Histopathologische Untersuchungen über Entstehung und Wesen der senilen Plaques. *Zeitschrift für die gesamte Neurologie und Psychiatrie*, **122**, 291–307.

ST CLAIR, D. & BLACKWOOD, D. (1985) Premature senility in Down's syndrome. *Lancet*, ii, 34.

SYLVESTER, P. E. (1984) Nutritional aspects of Down's syndrome. *British Journal of Psychiatry*, **145**, 115–120.

TAIT, D. (1983) Mortality and dementia among ageing defectives. *Journal of Mental Deficiency Research*, **27**, 133–142.

TANGYE, S. R. (1979) The EEG and incidents of epilepsy in Down's syndrome. *The Journal of Mental Deficiency Research*, **23**, 17–24.

TARJAN, E., EYMAN, R. K. & MILLER, C. R. (1969) Natural history of mental retardation in a state hospital revisited. *American Journal of Disturbed Children*, **117**, 609–620.

THASE, M. E. (1982) Longevity and mortality in Down's syndrome. *Journal of Mental Deficiency Research*, **26**, 177–192.

——, LISS, L., SMELTZER, D. & MALOONE, J. (1982) Clinical evaluation of dementia in Down's syndrome: preliminary report. *Journal of Mental Deficiency Research*, **26**, 239–244.

——, TIGNER, R., SMELTZER, D. & LISS, L. (1984) Age related neuropsychological deficits in Down's syndrome. *Biological Psychiatry*, **4**, 571–585.

VEALL, R. M. (1974) The prevalence of epilepsy among mongols related to age. *Journal of Mental Deficiency Research*, **19**, 99–106.

WILLIAMS, C. E. (1971) A study of the patients in a group of mental subnormality hospitals. *British Journal of Mental Subnormality*, **17**, 29–41.

WISNIEWSKI, A. E., HOWE, J., GWYN-WILLIAMS, D. & WISNIEWSKI, H. M. (1978) Precocious ageing and dementia in patients with Down's syndrome. *Biological Psychiatry*, **13**, 619–627.

WISNIEWSKI, K. E., WISNIEWSKI, H. M. & WEN, G. Y. (1985) Occurrence of neuropathological changes and dementia of Alzheimer's disease in Down's syndrome. *Annals of Neurology*, **17**, 278–282.

WORLD HEALTH ORGANISATION (1985) *Mental Retardation: Meeting the Challenge. WHO Offset Publications. No. 86, Geneva.*

WRIGHT, E. C. (1982) *The presentation of mental illness in mentally retarded adults. British Journal of Psychiatry*, **141**, 496–502.

WRIGHT, A. F. & WHALLEY, L. J. (1984) Genetics, ageing and dementia. *British Journal of Psychiatry*, **145**, 20–38.

# 33 Clinicopathological studies in mental disorder in old age: The Newcastle studies 1963–1977

**GARRY BLESSED**

No tribute to Sir Martin Roth's contribution to psychiatry would be complete without reference to the clinicopathological studies conducted under his direction in Newcastle in the 1960s and 1970s.

Studies on the classification of psychiatric disorder of later life (Roth, 1955) had revealed five clinically distinct categories of illness which accounted for 95% of all cases admitted to Graylingwell Hospital. Overlap of symptomatology between cases was uncommon, and differing patterns of outcome could be distinguished. It was unusual for cases initially diagnosed as depression to develop dementia later. Work in collaboration with Barbara Hopkins revealed differences in mean levels of cognitive skill displayed by patients allotted to the above categories, with patients suffering from dementia obtaining the lowest scores on the Roth Hopkins test of orientation and information (Roth & Hopkins, 1953; Hopkins & Roth, 1953).

The above findings paved the way for a clinicopathological study, for they disproved the then popular 'unitary' theory for the development of mental disorder in later life; namely that mild forms of senile cerebral degeneration would produce affective disorder or paranoia, while severe forms would lead to dementia, with in many cases a progression from functional to a predominantly organic pattern of psychiatric symptomatology.

Roth attempted to establish post-mortem studies of the patients assessed at Graylingwell, but few results were obtained before his transfer to Newcastle in 1956. It was to be nearly seven years before he obtained funding and recruited a neuropathologist to carry out the Newcastle studies, and his determination to embark on those was undoubtedly enhanced by the investigations carried out by Corsellis in the early 1960s. He performed over 300 autopsies on patients from Runwell Hospital and had related post-mortem findings to clinical diagnoses allocated during life. He found that 75% of those with functional diagnoses had relatively normal brains, compared with 75% of cases of dementia, where brain pathology was of moderate or great degree of severity (Corsellis, 1962).

Roth identified three weaknesses in this otherwise important study. Firstly, there had often been a long interval between the diagnostic formulation recorded in the case notes and the post-mortem examinations; secondly, no attempt had been made to assess cognitive function during life; and thirdly, the ordinate measure of severity of the pathological processes utilised by Corsellis lacked precision.

# Method

The Newcastle study, which began in 1963, involved the clinical examination of a cohort of hospital in-patients who each received a psychiatric assessment aimed at providing a clinical diagnosis utilising the categories previously defined by Roth in the Graylingwell studies. A 'control' group of medically ill in-patients, free from detectable mental disorder, was also established. All cases were further assessed for cognitive ability using a modification of the Roth Hopkins test incorporating additional material suggested by the studies of Shapiro and others (1956). This allowed the assignment of a *test score* which could be related to psychiatric diagnosis and correlated with brain changes at post mortem. Again, relatives and carers of patients were asked to report on cognitive, personality, habitual and behavioural handicaps according to a schedule devised by Blessed (Blessed *et al*, 1968) and on the basis of their responses, a *dementia score* was assigned. When patients survived greater than six months, both tests were repeated, and any significant changes in the clinical picture were also recorded.

Tomlinson carried out the pathological study, and developed quantitative assessments which contributed the following measures:

(a) brain weight in grammes

(b) ventricular size in millilitres

(c) mean senile plaque counts (average of 60 fields)

(d) percentage of hippocampal cells affected by glomerulo-vacuolar degeneration (GVD) (Simchovicz, 1910)

(e) neurofibrillary tangle density in the hippocampus

(f) neurofibrillary tangle density in the neocortex

(g) volume of infarction in the cerebral hemispheres.

A pathological diagnosis which described the major structural abnormalities found was also made.

# Results

The more important findings of the studies were as follows:

(a) *Prevalence of the main types of dementias*

Alzheimer change alone was the pathological basis for dementia in 64% and made an important contribution to the pathological picture in a further

TABLE I
*Prevalence of the main types of dementias*

| Pathological diagnoses | n | % | % |
|---|---|---|---|
| Alzheimer's disease | 61 | 50.4 | 64.4 |
| Probable Alzheimer's disease | 17 | 14.0 | |
| Multiple cerebral infarction | 10 | 8.2 | 10.7 |
| Probable multiple CI | 3 | 2.5 | |
| Alzheimer's + multiple infarction | 7 | 5.8 | 11.6 |
| Probable AD + MI | 7 | 5.8 | |
| Special brain lesions | 4 | 3.3 | |
| No significant pathology | 12 | 9.9 | |
| Totals | 121 | 99.9 | |

11%, so that over 75% of the cases showed Alzheimer pathology of at least moderate severity.

(b) *Relationship between pathological measures and clinical diagnoses*
These are shown in summary in Table II. Patients with senile dementia had significantly higher mean plaque counts, tangle density and GVD counts than all other categories. Patients with multiple infarction dementia had significantly higher mean volumes of hemispheric infarction. Brain weights tended to be low in the Alzheimer cases, and 80 to 100 grammes higher in functionally ill, arteriosclerotic and acutely confused cases, but the differences were not significant. Curiously, the numerically small group of patients dying on geriatric wards also had low brain weights—close to those recorded for Alzheimer patients.

TABLE II
*Neuropathological measures v. psychiatric diagnosis*

|    | Clinical category | Brain weight | Senile plaques | NFTs (C)** | NFTs (H)*** | GVD**** | Infarction |
|----|-------------------|--------------|----------------|------------|-------------|---------|------------|
| n  |                   |              |                |            |             |         |            |
| 51 | Senile dementia | 1200 (147)* | 19.1 (4.15) | 1.84 (1.2) | 1.94 (1.0) | 14.9 (10.4) | 11.9 (58) |
| 21 | Multiple infarct dementia | 1284 (122)* | 5.8 (7.8) | 0.47 (.87) | 0.8 (1.1) | 2.75 (6.2) | 73.6 (68.7) |
| 18 | Acute confusion | 1294 (75)* | 5.6 (6.2) | 0.05 (.76) | 1.0 (1.4) | 2.9 (7.2) | 7.0 (14.3) |
| 19 | Affective illness | 1280 (184)* | 1.9 (2.5) | 0.10 (.33) | 0.66 (.85) | 1.9 (4.9) | 5.1 (12.6) |
| 9 | Paranoid illness | 1299 (129)* | 5.7 (8.9) | 0.10 (.95) | 0.9 (1.0) | 5.2 (7.4) | 4.1 (4.4) |
| 9 | Geriatric patients | 1220 (42)* | 4.5 (3.9) | 0.2 (1.0) | 1.1 (1.3) | 1.9 (1.9) | 16.5 (31.6) |

*Standard deviations
**Neurofibrillary tangles (C) Cortex
***Neurofibrillary tangles (H) Hippocampus
****Glomerulo-vacuolar degeneration

(c) *Relationship between clinical diagnosis and pathological diagnosis*
This is shown in Table III; where a patient had clinical evidence for senile dementia plus parietal lobe features (aphasia, agnosia, apraxia) the diagnosis of Alzheimer's disease was confirmed in every case save one. Those with senile dementia alone mainly had Alzheimer's disease, but approximately one in five cases either had mixed pathology or little evidence for major pathological damage to the brain. A clinical diagnosis of multi-infarct dementia (MID) was confirmed in 50% of cases, found to be due to mixed pathology in 30%, and unconfirmed in 20% (5% Alzheimer and 15% no detected change). In nine cases, the clinical aetiology of the dementia was uncertain, often because it arose in patients with severe medical illnesses who were nevertheless free from evidence for clouded consciousness or delirium. All cases proved to have Alzheimer pathology. Six of 17 cases with combined depression and dementia had normal brains, and are likely to have been cases of pseudo-dementia—further confirmation of the need, identified by Ron *et al* (1979), for caution in assigning a diagnosis of dementia to a cognitively impaired patient with significant depression. The diagnosis of dementia in the clouded patient often presents clinical difficulties. Such patients should be regarded as having potentially reversible cognitive disorders, yet all the cases followed to autopsy had pathological changes of at least moderate severity.

Clinical dementia without confirmatory pathological change proved to be commoner than the absence of dementia in cases with clear pathological damage,

TABLE III

*Clinical versus neuropathological diagnoses*

| Clinical diagnosis | Pathological diagnosis | | | | | | | | Total clinical cases |
|---|---|---|---|---|---|---|---|---|---|
| | Alzheimer | Probable Alzheimer | Multiple cerebral infarction | Less severe multiple cerebral infarctions | Mixed AD + multiple infarctions | Less severe mixed disease | Special lesions | Normal brain | |
| Senile dementia | 20 (69.0)* | 3 (10.3) | — | — | — | 3 (10.3) | — | 3 (10.3) | 29 |
| SDAT | 13 (93.0) | 1 (7.1) | — | — | — | — | — | — | 14 |
| Alzheimer's disease | 6 (85.7) | — | 1 (14.3) | — | — | — | — | — | 7 |
| MID | — | 1 (5.0) | 8 (40.0) | 2 (10.0) | 3 (15.0) | 3 (15.0) | — | 3 (15.0) | 20 |
| Mixed dementia | 5 (62.5) | 2 (25.0) | — | — | 1 (12.5) | — | — | — | 8 |
| Dementia (uncertain aetiology) | 8 (88.9) | 1 (11.1) | — | — | — | — | — | — | 9 |
| Dementia (special brain disorder) | — | — | — | — | — | — | 4 | — | 4 |
| Dementia + affective disorder | 5 (29.4) | 4 (23.5) | — | — | 2 (11.8) | — | — | 6 (35.3) | 17 |
| Acute confusion + dementia | 4 (30.7) | 5 (38.5) | 1 (7.7) | 1 (7.7) | 1 (7.7) | 1 (7.7) | — | — | 13 |
| Not demented | 1 (1.8) | 3 (5.4) | — | — | — | 1 (1.8) | 1 (1.8) | 50 (89.3) | 56 |
| Total (pathological categories) | 62 | 20 | 10 | 3 | 7 | 8 | 5 | 62 | 177 |

*Numbers in brackets are percentages of total clinical cases

Table IV

*Cognitive ability in 244 elderly people*

| Diagnosis | n | Mental test score (Mean)* | Standard deviation |
|---|---|---|---|
| Senile dementia | 45 | 10.7 | 8.85 |
| Arteriosclerotic dementia | 37 | 13.9 | 7.78 |
| Affective illness | 47 | 29.7 | 5.63 |
| Paraphrenia | 34 | 26.6 | 10.71 |
| Acute confusion | 35 | 20.3 | 7.50 |
| Geriatric in-patients | 46 | 33.3 | 3.59 |

*Maximum possible MTS = 37

but the latter cases did arise. Severe pathological change in such cases was a very unusual finding and was confined to a single chronic schizophrenic patient who scored full marks on the memory, information and concentration test six months before her sudden death when autopsy revealed good, but probably not unequivocal, evidence for Alzheimer's disease.

(d) *Relationship of performance on mental testing to psychiatric diagnosis*
The results are shown in Table IV. Geriatric in-patients judged to be free from significant mental illness on psychiatric assessment scored higher than those assigned to the mental illness categories. Of the latter, patients with affective illness or paraphrenia obtained the highest scores, and differences in mean scores between those two categories did not differ significantly. Lowest scores were assigned to cases of senile and arterio-sclerotic dementia, again with no significant difference between the mean scores in the two groups. Patients with acute confusion showed cognitive skills significantly better than the demented patients, but worse than the functionally ill cases. (All statements refer to '$t$' test results, $P < .05$ being regarded as significant.)

e) *Correlation between measures of daily functional ability and cognitive ability and pathological changes*
These results have been extensively reported elsewhere and will not be repeated here in detail. Suffice to say that relatives' assessments of the presence of disabilities typical of dementia and calculated as a 'dementia score' correlated positively to a highly significant degree with both Alzheimer change and volumes of hemisphere infarction. Scores allocated for performance on the Newcastle version of the Roth Hopkins Test (Blessed *et al*, 1968) were again significantly correlated (negatively of course) with measures of brain damage of both types.

## Neurochemical and histochemical changes, plus pathological studies of the tectal forebrain

E. K. Perry and R. H. Perry joined the team in 1975 and undertook additional neurochemical, histochemical and neuropathological studies of cases coming to post mortem. The cholinergic system was examined first and after it had been shown that choline acetyl transferase (CAT) and acetyl choline esterase (ACE) were valid markers for the integrity of the system, that levels declined relatively slowly after death in the refrigerated cadaver, and that treatment prior to death with neuroleptic drugs did not greatly affect levels found at post-mortem, it was possible to look at the relationships between: clinical diagnosis and mean levels; measures of the severity of pathological change and mean levels; and measures of the severity of cognitive impairment during life and mean levels of these 'markers'.

CAT levels were significantly reduced below normal in the neocortex, mammillary bodies, caudate nucleus and amygdaloid nucleus in senile dementia Alzheimer type (SDAT) cases alone (Perry & Perry, 1980). Levels were reduced in hippocampus in SDAT ( $P<.001$) multiple infarction dementia ( $P<.01$) and depression ( $P<.05$). No significant reduction was found in the substantia nigra or the cerebellum.

CAT levels were reduced to the greatest extent in those areas of the brain most affected by Alzheimer pathology, and when the severity of Alzheimer change was related to the reductions in CAT or ACE, significant correlations between mean plaque count and CAT ( $r = -0.82$, $P<.001$) and between neurofibrillary tangle formation (NFT) and ACE ( $P<.01$ between mean levels in cases with no tangle formation and those with extensive NFT) were found.

When CAT levels were related to cognitive performance, using the Mental Test Score as a measure of the latter, a highly significant correlation ( $r = 0.81$, $P<.001$) was confirmed (Perry, E. K. *et al*, 1978).

Histochemical studies confirmed that ACE virtually disappears from the hippocampus in cases of SDAT, and other observations revealed that extensive reductions also occur in the subiculum, entorhinal and neocortex, but not in the spinal cord or caudate nucleus.

By contrast, other transmitter systems were found to be much less severely or specifically affected in Alzheimer brains. Glutamic acid D-carboxylase (GAD) was reduced in SDAT and in unipolar depression, but reductions did not appear to be localised to any specific region of the brain (Perry, E. K. *et al*, 1977). Reductions could also be found in cases of multiple infarction dementia and dialysis dementia, and GAD reduction was not apparently related to the density of senile plaque formation ( $r = -.21$, NS).

The striking reduction in choline acetyl transferase activity led R. H. Perry to examine the nucleus of Meynert for evidence of neuronal loss. In six SDAT cases examined (Perry *et al*, 1982) CAT activity in the nucleus was reduced by at least 90%, while on average the neurone count was reduced by only 33%. These observations were thought to be consistent with a 'down regulation' of transmitter specific enzyme production in cholinergic neurones, and that neurone loss might be a secondary feature of the disease.

Reports that the serotonergic and non-adrenergic systems might also be affected in Alzheimer disease led to examination of the dorsal raphe system and the locus coeruleus.

Tomlinson *et al* (1981) reported on sample counts of the pigmented cells of the locus coeruleus in 25 intellectually well preserved people and in 15 cases with pathological evidence for SDAT. This revealed an age-related decline in neurone population, with SDAT cases falling into two groups: about half the cases had slightly reduced counts within the lower range of those for age-matched controls (seven cases) while the remaining eight cases had severe depletion of neurones. Taken together, the SDAT cases had significantly lower counts than those in the controls, but the apparent existence within SDAT of two distinct sub groups was particularly interesting. The small number of cases examined did not allow this impression to be confirmed statistically, but later work confirmed these findings and suggested that marked reduction of cell counts in forebrain nuclei was typical of early onset and clinically more severe Type II cases of Alzheimer's disease (Rossor *et al*, 1984).

E. K. Perry and others (1984) examined cortical serotonin S2 receptor binding abnormalities in patients with Alzheimer's disease and confirmed a reduction in the number of binding sites for the serotonergic S2 receptor antagonist, ketanserin, in SDAT. S1 receptor binding sites were also found to be reduced to a smaller, but still significant degree.

## Discussion

The above account refers to the principal studies carried out by the team led by Sir Martin Roth between 1963 and 1977. After his appointment to the Chair of Psychiatry at the University of Cambridge, he swiftly established a team to continue the clinicopathological exploration of mental disorder in old age, and of dementia in particular. A special concern has been to refine further the clinical assessment of patients with dementia, and to improve instruments for the assessment of cognitive skills. However, details of these studies lie outside the brief of this communication.

It is probably too early to assess fully the significance of these studies. What they undoubtedly achieved was the demonstration that brain changes, readily detectable by neuropathological and neurochemical investigations, were of relevance for the development of certain psychiatric disorders in late life, and that careful evaluations of cases, augmented by comparatively simple tests of cognitive or daily living performance, could be related to the pathological and neurochemical data in a way that pointed to significant relationships between functional decline and brain dysfunction and/or pathology. This destroyed, once and for all, the notion that 'senile' decay of the brain, regarded as commonplace in the elderly, was of no significance in relation to the development of psychiatric disorder, and paved the way for more sophisticated studies. These have included: the development of more stringent clinical criteria including algorithms for the recognition of Alzheimer's disease; more elaborate and demanding tests of cognitive functioning in its various aspects; examination of a wide range of neurotransmitters; carefully controlled studies for evidence of reductions in neurone populations in various sites; ultramicroscopic studies of the neurofibrillary tangle and studies of the chemical and structural composition of the senile plaque. As well as stimulating scientific effort in laboratories throughout the Western world, Roth's painstaking work with elderly mentally ill people has certainly given impetus to the development of specialist clinical services for such patients and has raised the status of this new and rapidly growing sub-specialty of psychiatry.

## References

BLESSED, G., TOMLINSON, B. E. & ROTH, M. (1968) The association between quantitative measures of dementia and of senile change in the cerebral grey matter of elderly subjects. *British Journal of Psychiatry*, **114**, 797–811.

CORSELLIS, J. A. N. (1962) *Mental Illness and the Ageing Brain.* Oxford University Press.
HOPKINS, B. & ROTH, M. (1953) Psychological test performance in patients over 60. II. Paraphrenia, arteriosclerotic psychosis and acute confusion. *Journal of Mental Science*, **99**, 451–456.
PERRY, E. K., GIBSON, P. H., BLESSED, G., PERRY, R. H. & TOMLINSON, B. E. (1977) Neurotransmitter enzyme abnormalities in senile dementia. *Journal of the Neurological Sciences*, **34**, 247–265.
——, TOMLINSON, B. E., BLESSED, G., BERGMANN, K., GIBSON, P. H. & PERRY, R. H. (1978) Correlation of cholinergic abnormalities with senile plaques and mental test scores in senile dementia. *British Medical Journal*, **2**, (6150), 1457–1459.
—— & PERRY, R. H. (1980) The cholinergic system in Alzheimer's disease. In *Biochemistry of Dementia* (ed. P. J. Roberts). Chichester: John Wiley. 135–183.
——, ——, CANDY, J. M., FAIRBAIRN, A. F., BLESSED, G., DICK, D. J. & TOMLINSON, B. E. (1984) Cortical serotonin – S2 receptor binding abnormalities in patients with Alzheimer's disease: comparisons with Parkinson's disease. *Neuroscience Letters*, **51**, 353–357.
PERRY, R. H., CANDY, J. M., PERRY, E. K., IRVING, D., BLESSED, G., FAIRBAIRN, A. F. & TOMLINSON, B. E. (1982) Extensive loss of CAT activity is not reflected by neuronal loss in the Nucleus of Meynert in Alzheimer's Disease. *Neuroscience Letters*, **33**, 311–315.
RON, M. A., TOONE, B. K., GARRALDA, M. E. & LISHMAN, W. A. (1979) Diagnostic accuracy in presenile dementia. *British Journal of Psychiatry*, **134**, 161–168.
ROSSOR, M. N., IVERSEN, L. L., REYNOLDS, C. P., MOUNTJOY, C. Q. & ROTH, M. (1984) Neurochemical characteristics of early and late onset types of Alzheimer's disease. *British Medical Journal*, **288**, 961–964.
ROTH, M. & HOPKINS, B. (1953) Psychological test performance in patients over 60. I. Senile psychosis and the affective disorders of old age. *Journal of Mental Science*, **99**, 439–450.
—— (1955) The natural history of mental disorders arising in the senium. *Journal of Mental Science*, **101**, 281–301.
SHAPIRO, M. B., POST, F., LÖFVOING, B. & INGLIS, J. (1956) Memory function in psychiatric patients over 60; some methodological and diagnostic implications. *Journal of Mental Science*, **102**, 233–239.
SIMCHOVICZ, T. (1910) *Histologisches Studien über die Senile Demenz Arbeiten über die Grosshirnrinde.* (eds. Nissl & Alzheimer) Vol 4, 267.
TOMLINSON, B. E., IRVING, D. & BLESSED, G. (1981) Cell loss in the locus coeruleus in senile dementia of Alzheimer type. *Journal of Neurological Sciences*, **49**, 419–428.

# 34 Diagnosing dementia of the Alzheimer's type: the use of magnetic resonance imaging and single photon emission computed tomography

**HUGH C. HENDRIE** with Mary G. Austrom, Kathleen S. Hall, Martin R. Farlow and Henry N. Wellman

The application of the techniques of MRI and SPECT brain imaging to the study of dementing disorders is discussed. MRI performs functions similar to CT scanning in the differential diagnosis of dementia; that is, to rule out the presence of 'secondary' dementias due to brain structural disease. For this function, the superb anatomical detail and tissue differentiation available from MRI offers some advantages. The use of MR characteristics has so far been limited. Most promising is the ability of the weighted $T_2$ images to demonstrate small areas of infarction and patterns of high intensity which may indicate cerebro-vascular disease, although these patterns are also seen in the images of many apparently healthy elderly subjects. The ability of MRI to measure brain function depends on the future development of sodium and phosphorus imaging, blood flow measurements and spectroscopic techniques.

SPECT imaging represents a relatively less expensive and more easily accessible method of obtaining information about brain functioning in dementia than PET scanning. Alzheimer's patients have shown diverse patterns of reduced cortical and subcortical cerebral uptake which may be related to symptom clusters and which can be separated with some degree of reliability from the more focal changes which occur in multi-infarct dementia. The ability of SPECT imaging to detect the earliest brain changes in Alzheimer's disease remains questionable, but it is likely to prove a useful method to monitor alteration in brain functioning in the disease course and to assist in assessing treatment effectiveness. The development of specific radioactive neurotransmitter ligands in SPECT imaging is an exciting future prospect.

In 1975, when I assumed the chairmanship of the Department of Psychiatry at Indiana University School of Medicine, I was faced with a very momentous but pleasant task. Thanks to the efforts of my predecessor, Dr John Nurnberger, Sr, the Department of Psychiatry had been left an endowment fund to allow us to bring to Indianapolis every year a visiting professor; the post was to be named after the first professor of psychiatry and neurology at Indiana University, Dr Albert E. Sterne.

As this was to be the first occasion following the bequest, it was essential that we choose well to lay the foundation for the visiting professorship programme. We wanted to invite someone with a sufficient breadth of interest and knowledge to demonstrate to our somewhat sceptical academic community that psychiatry was able to produce outstanding academic physicians. We spent many hours deliberating, but really the choice quickly became clear. The most eminent practising psychiatrist in the opinion of all of us was Sir Martin Roth.

Sir Martin more than lived up to our expectations. He delighted and charmed our faculty, staff and students not only by his expected great erudition but also by his considerable clinical acumen and his exquisite sensitivity in conducting patient interviews.

The decision to whom to turn for advice when, in the early '80s, our School of Medicine decided to embark on clinical and research programmes in geriatric medicine and psychiatry was therefore easy. I understood that Sir Martin and his colleagues were preparing their new clinical schedule for diagnosing mental disorders in the elderly, the CAMDEX (Roth *et al*, 1986). In the summer of 1983 I spent a delightful three months at Cambridge with him and his colleagues, Chris Mountjoy, Liz Tym and Felicia Huppert, assisting them in their task.

The CAMDEX has been the clinical information basis for both our clinical and research work in geriatric psychiatry ever since. We have been able, with only a very few minor modifications in phraseology, to use the instrument with American patient populations with patient acceptance, and subscale scores for the various diagnostic groups similar to those attained at Cambridge. We have also been able to attain high degrees of reliability in training a number of physicians and non-physicians in its use (Hendrie *et al*, in press).

One of the continuing problems in clinical work with elderly patients remains the accurate diagnosis of the dementing disorders. The difficulties include the separation of dementia, particularly mild dementia, from non-dementing disorders which can affect intellectual function, and the distinction between Alzheimer's disease and the many other illnesses subsumed under the syndrome of dementia.

There have now been a few studies which have attempted to validate clinical diagnosis (Todorov *et al*, 1975; Sulkava *et al*, 1983; White & Heston, 1986) by subsequent post-mortem evaluation. All studies demonstrate the diagnostic difficulties but differ in their assessment of the extent of the problem. Rather encouragingly, it appears as if a more organised approach to data gathering and establishment of criteria such as those proposed by Roth *et al* provides better sensitivity and specificity for clinical diagnosis as determined by post-mortem evaluation (Sulkava *et al*, 1983). The possible development of new pharmacological methods of treating, at least symptomatically, Alzheimer's patients emphasises the increasing importance of accurate early diagnosis. One of the hopes for the future lies in the development of the new brain imaging techniques such as magnetic resonance imaging (MRI), cerebral scintigraphy using single photon emission tomography (SPECT), and positron emission tomography (PET), as well as the modern computer-assisted expansion of the old techniques of electro-encephalography.

In the course of our in-patient and out-patient clinical evaluation of psychogeriatric patients at Indiana University, we have been conducting ongoing studies using the techniques of MRI and SPECT in both patient populations and normal control subjects. For all these studies, the patients and control subjects are carefully evaluated independently by a psychiatrist (HCH) and a neurologist (MRF). Structured psychiatric (the CAMDEX) and neurological instruments are used. Laboratory testing including EEG and CT scans are performed.

Clinical diagnoses are made using primarily DSM–III criteria [for primary degenerative dementia (PDD), multi-infarct dementia (MID), major depressive disorder (MDD), etc.] although at times other sets of criteria are used, e.g. NINCDS for Alzheimer's disease (DAT) (McKhann *et al*, 1984), Roth's criteria, etc. The control subjects have to be healthy, with no evidence of dementia or other psychiatric or neurological disease and on no medication which could affect brain function. Findings from these studies will be discussed in this chapter, together with a review of MRI and SPECT studies on dementia.

## *Magnetic resonance imaging (MRI)*

The principles of MRI have been described well elsewhere (Pykett *et al*, 1982; DeMyer *et al*, 1985). MRI, derived as it is from information based upon chemical interactions within tissues, holds out the promise that analysis of MR characteristics will provide information about brain metabolism. Unfortunately, this promise has not yet been fulfilled and probably awaits the development of sodium and phosphorus imaging, blood flow measurements and the combination of imaging with spectroscopy (Steiner, 1986).

At the moment, however, clinically, MRI with its superb anatomical detail is used for diagnosing dementia in a manner similar to CT scanning, i.e. to rule out the presence of dementia secondary to brain structural disease (Bydder *et al*, 1982; Bydder *et al*, 1983). For this purpose, MRI holds some advantages over CT scanning as well as some disadvantages (Brant-Zawadzki *et al*, 1983). The advantages include

   (a)  better separation of grey from white matter because of MRI's high contrast resolution
   (b)  better imaging of posterior fossa masses
   (c)  a wider range of tissue characterisation and an ability to construct images in different planes
   (d)  safety (MRI does not use ionising radiation).

Some of the disadvantages of MRI compared with CT include the increased cost of MRI procedures and the relatively greater length which may be difficult for elderly and demented patients to tolerate. CT also delineates better brain calcification (Hendrie *et al*, 1985).

There have been some attempts to use MR parameters, e.g. $T_1$ values and $T_2$ values, to assist in the differential diagnostic process in dementia, particularly in separating Alzheimer's disease from multi-infarct dementia. Besson and his colleagues (1983, 1984 & 1985) have claimed to be able to distinguish groups of patients with senile dementia of the Alzheimer's type, multi-infarct dementia and healthy control subjects by means of a combination of $T_1$ and proton density measurements from varying parts of the brain, particularly from measurements of $T_1$ in white matter, even when lesions could not be detected visually on the images. There are, however, a number of difficulties in obtaining reliable $T_1$ values. These include partial volume artifact (the image slice may include more than one tissue, e.g. CSF underlying grey matter), imprecision in measurement techniques and the large normal variability in $T_1$ (and $T_2$) values in brain tissue which occurs not only between individuals but also within a given individual brain from slice to slice (DeMyer *et al*, in press). Rather than compare directly measurements derived from relaxation times from $T_1$ or other constructed images from brain areas, a few investigators have attempted to use the range of relaxation times (usually $T_1$ derived) associated with brain tissue or cerebro-spinal fluid to measure more accurately the presence of cerebral atrophy and ventricular dilatation. Condon *et al* (1986) reported on one such method to measure intracranial extraventricular and ventricular cerebro-spinal fluid volume with highly reproducible results. Using this method, they were able to distinguish ten normal subjects from four patients including one with Alzheimer's disease and one with normal pressure hydrocephalus.

In previous studies with schizophrenic patients and control subjects using a Teslacon 0.15 Tesla scanner where $T_1$ calculated images were obtained using a combined spin echo (SE)/inversion recovery (IR) pulse sequence (TE 30 msec., TR 1250 msec. and $T_1$ 400), we noted that the $T_1$ range for grey matter was approximately 400–600 msec., for white matter, 300–400 msec., and for cerebro-spinal fluid the range was 800–5000 msec. (DeMyer *et al*, in press). From a larger sample of MR imaged elderly subjects, we selected 11 PDD patients (seven males and four females, mean age 63 years, mean CAMCOG = 40) and ten control subjects (two males and eight females, mean age 69 years, mean CAMCOG = 93) based upon our ability to select from the slices available ones which were at closely comparable levels, i.e. the atrial region of the lateral ventricles. Applying our $T_1$ value limits to these slices, we estimated the amount of pixels corresponding to grey matter, white matter and CSF as demonstrated in Fig. 1 (Hendrie *et al*, 1987). Our results are shown in Table I.

There were highly significant differences between the patients with PDD and control subjects in amounts of cerebro-spinal fluid (PDD patients 3045 ± 766 pixels, control subjects 1267 ± 463 pixels $P < .0001$) and significant differences in the amount of white matter contained in the slice (PDD 4253 ± 1012 pixels, control subjects 5324 ± 1136 pixels $P = .034$). Differences in amount of grey matter did not reach significance (PDD patients 7969 ± 1213, control subjects 8838 ± 1065 n.s.). There were few correlations between brain tissue and CSF pixel counts and patient characteristics (see Table II).

The cerebro-spinal fluid measurements correlated significantly positively with age in both PDD patients and control subjects and significantly negatively with the CAMCOG memory subscale with control subjects but not with the PDD patients. The white matter measurements correlated significantly negatively with Blessed scores in the PDD patients and significantly positively with the Mini Mental State Examination scores in the control subjects but not the PDD patients. These correlations are all in the anticipated direction from previous studies using

TABLE I

*Mean and standard deviations of pixel counts of brain constituents between Alzheimer's patients and control subjects*

| Variables | Alzheimer's | Controls | $t$ | $P$ |
|---|---|---|---|---|
| CSF Pixels | 3045 ± 766 | 1267 ± 463 | 6.35 | .0001 |
| White matter Pixels | 4253 ± 1012 | 5324 ± 1136 | − 2.23 | .034 |
| Grey matter Pixels | 7969 ± 1213 | 8838 ± 1065 | − 1.70 | .098 |

(a)

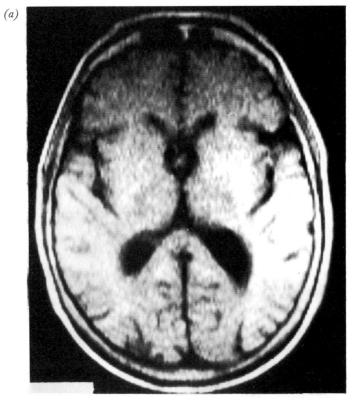

(b)

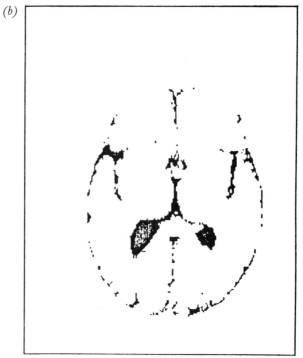

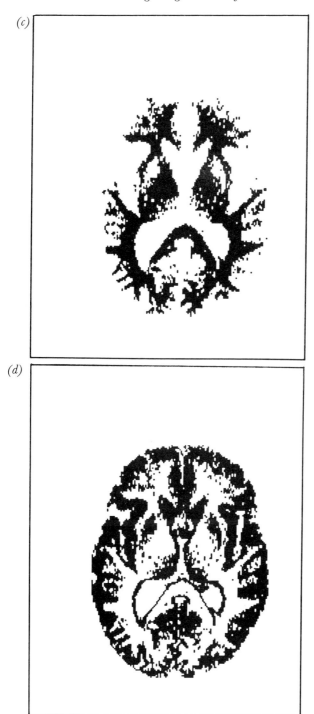

Fig. 1.(a) Original MRI transaxial slice (Spin Echo 30/250 sequence, not $OT_1$ image) at level of atrial region of lateral ventricle; (b) computer generated image using $OT_1$ range from 800–5000 msecs corresponding to CSF; (c) computer generated image using $OT_1$ range from 300–400 msecs corresponding to white matter; (d) computer generated image using $OT_1$ range from 400–600 msecs corresponding to grey matter.

Table II
*Significant correlations between atria pixel counts, age, behavioural and neuropsychological measurements of Alzheimer patients and control subjects*

|  | Age | Blessed | MMSE | CAMCOG memory subscale |
|---|---|---|---|---|
| *CSF* |  |  |  |  |
| Alzheimer patients | .58 |  |  |  |
| (n = 11) | P = .058 |  |  |  |
| Controls | .75 |  |  | – .67 |
| (n = 10) | P = .01 |  |  | P = .03 |
| *White matter* |  |  |  |  |
| Alzheimer patients |  | – .72 |  |  |
|  |  | P = .02 |  |  |
| Controls |  |  | .70 |  |
|  |  |  | P = .02 |  |
| *Grey matter* |  |  |  |  |
| Alzheimer patients |  |  |  |  |
| Controls | .74 |  |  |  |
|  | P = .01 |  |  |  |

CT scans (Brinkman *et al*, 1981; Gado *et al*, 1982; Creasey *et al*, 1986). The relationship of measurements of brain atrophy to cognitive scores in control subjects but not in Alzheimer's patients has been reported in at least one prior CT study (Jacoby & Levy, 1980). One correlation which was not expected was the significantly positive relationship between age and amounts of grey matter in control subjects. This last result probably points out the limitations of our method. In subsequent studies we are finding the greatest difficulty in defining reliable relaxation time limits using $T_1$ values for grey matter, probably because of the greater likelihood of partial voluming in these brain areas. Another problem, at least with the use of single slice comparisons, is the difficulty in positioning elderly patients to ensure that brain slices at comparable levels can be constructed, probably due to the prevalence of osteo-arthritic changes in the cervical spine in these populations. The wide variation that occurs in $T_1$ values from slice to slice within the same individual is also becoming more apparent as our studies proceed.

Considerable interest has been generated in observations documenting the presence of foci of increased $T_2$ signals particularly in the peri-ventricular region in MR imaging of elderly subjects (Bradley *et al*, 1984; Sze *et al*, 1985; Sarpel *et al*, 1987). These foci are sometimes associated with areas of hypodensity in the CT scan (Erkinjuntii *et al*, 1984) but frequently they are observed in the absence of any comparable CT changes (Awad *et al*, 1986). The cause and significance of these findings are not presently clear. It has been suggested that they represent evidence of subcortical arteriosclerotic encephalopathy akin to Binswanger's disease (Young *et al*, 1983) but these foci have been reported also in asymptomatic elderly subjects, as well as in patients with dementia and cerebro-vascular disease.

In a retrospective review of 151 patients over the age of 50 years who had been referred for MRI, Gerard & Weisberg (1986) concluded that the presence of a peri-ventricular high signal intensity pattern was associated with a history of cerebro-vascular risk factors (e.g. hypertension, cardio-vascular disease and diabetes and/or cerebro-vascular symptoms). Of patients with this history, 78% had peri-ventricular lesions compared with only 7.8% of patients who had no identified cerebro-vascular risk factors. Awad *et al* (1986) defined subcortical incidental lesions (ILs) as lesions of increased signal intensity $T_2$ weighted images, not visualised on CT scans and not explicable by the patient's clinical diagnosis or neurological examinations. They further graded the ILs on a four point scale depending upon their location, size and multiplicity. They then measured the incidence and severity of these ILs in 240 patients who had been referred for MR imaging. The incidence of the ILs was clearly related to age, being present in 22% of patients under the age of 40 and rising to 92% of patients 60 years or over. Brain ischaemia and hypertension in addition to age were identified as predictors of ILs in the elderly. Diabetes, coronary artery disease and sex were not significantly correlated. They concluded that the ILs may represent an index of chronic cerebro-vascular disease. In a further attempt to elucidate the pathological correlates of the increased $T_2$ signal areas, Awad and his colleagues (1986) conducted post-mortem *in vitro* proton MRIs on the brains of seven patients who died from non-neurological reasons and subsequently examined histopathologically these brain areas. The subcortical MRI lesions identified in this way were associated with areas of arteriosclerosis, dilated peri-vascular spaces and vascular ectasia.

In our first series of imaging studies using the 0.15 Tesla Magnet, a total of 17 subjects, seven patients with PDD and ten control subjects, had weighted $T_2$ images taken (Spin Echo TE 120 msecs., TR 2000 msecs.) in addition to the calculated $T_1$ images. Our radiologist semi-quantified the presence or absence of increased $T_2$ signals using a five point scale where "0" represented no evidence of increased signal and "4" extensive periventricular high intensity patterns. The results are shown in Table III.

While increased $T_2$ signals were a common finding in this population, their occurrence did not discriminate between the PDD patients and healthy control subjects. Three subjects had evidence of markedly increased $T_2$ patterns but two of these subjects were in our healthy control population. All three were in the oldest range of our population (75 years, 75 years and 78 years respectively).

We have now extended our imaging studies using an MR unit with a 1.5 Tesla super conductive magnet. Multi-slice $T_1$ as well as $T_2$ weighted images are being obtained (weighted $T_2$ sequence TR 2000 msecs. 30/90). So far we have imaged 21 carefully selected healthy elderly subjects 65 years or over. Increased $T_2$ signals were present in two-thirds (14 of 21) of these subjects. Again, this phenomenon appears to be age related. This sample will be enlarged and the subjects will be followed over time. If previous studies are correct, we would anticipate that the healthy subjects with evidence of extensive white matter lesions

TABLE III
*Presence of increased $T_2$ signals in weighted $T_2$ images in Alzheimer's patients and control subjects*

| *Radiologist's rating of severity of increased $T_2$ signal* | *0* | *1* | *2* | *3 & 4* |
|---|---|---|---|---|
| Alzheimer's patients ($n = 7$) | 2 (29%) | 3 (43%) | 1 (14%) | 1 (14%) |
| Control subjects ($n = 10$) | 2 (20%) | 4 (40%) | 2 (20%) | 2 (20%) |

$\chi^2 = 0.28$, N.S.

(a)

(b)

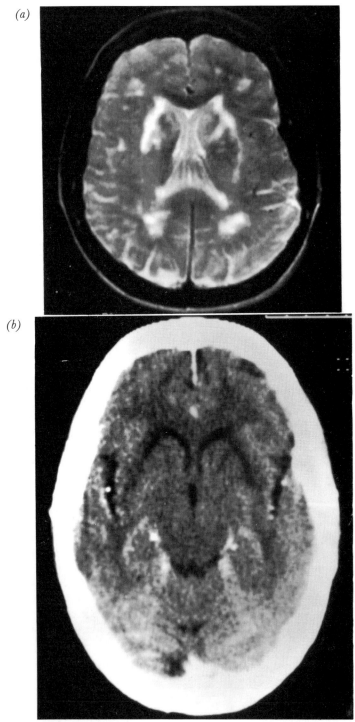

Fig. 2.(a) MR (weighted $T_2$) and (b) CT images on a 69 year old woman with a history of psychotic depression. Testing revealed mild cognitive deficit (MMSE – 24). MRI clearly shows multiple bilateral punctate and confluent white matter lesions both in periventricular area and scattered throughout image. CT image shows comparable areas of hypodensity but the lesions are not as obvious.

would be more likely to develop symptoms relating to cerebrovascular disease, including dementia.

Resolution of the nature of the white matter lesions would obviously be of great assistance in diagnosis and treatment. The patient whose MR images are shown in Fig. 2 was admitted to hospital with severe psychotic depression.

An MRI was performed as part of a workup for electro-convulsive therapy when she failed to respond to anti-depressant treatment and showed evidence of mild cognitive impairment (MMSE = 24, CAMCOG = 84). A subsequent SPECT evaluation showed increased hypoperfusion in the left temporal area. Despite this evidence of possible brain damage, a decision was made to proceed with ECT because of the severity of her depressive symptoms. She received four ECT and has so far demonstrated a considerable improvement in her depressive symptomatology, although after both her second and third treatments she did have a period of confusion lasting several hours. One week following her ECT she showed minimal improvement in her cognitive performance (MMSE = 25, CAMCOG = 88). The difficulty with distinguishing depression from dementia is of course well known. Follow-up studies of patients like this should help in the diagnostic process.

## Single photon emission computed tomography (SPECT)

The availability of single photon emitting radio labelled amines that cross the normal blood barrier has resurrected interest in cerebral scintigraphy as a potential diagnostic technique in dementia (English & Holman, 1987; Henkin, 1987). SPECT technology is quite new and rapidly developing. Until recently, the number of available pharmaceutical agents has been quite limited. They have included the iodine-123 ($^{123}$I)-labelled compounds N-isopropyl p-iodoamphetamine (IMP) (Johnson *et al*, 1985) and HHN-trimethyl-N- [2-hydroxy-3-methyl-5-iodobenzyl]-1, 3 propanediamine (HIPDM) (Kung *et al*, 1983). Technetium-99m labelled compounds which offer some advantages in expense, availability and physical characteristics to the radio-iodinated amines are now also available, e.g., $^{99m}$Tc-hexamethyl propylene amine oxime (HM-PAO) (Gemmell *et al*, 1987). Which agent or combination will ultimately prove to be the best for imaging Alzheimer's pathology is still uncertain. Integrated instrumentation systems for SPECT have been neglected by manufacturers compared with other imaging modalities, probably because of the relative paucity of radiopharmaceuticals. Imaging algorithms are inherently more difficult to develop with SPECT than with CT or MRI but newer methods of scatter correction and iterative or Monte Carlo reconstruction techniques promise to improve considerably the resolving power of the systems to approximate that of PET scanning.

One continuing problem with SPECT is the lack of ability to measure cerebral blood flow quantitatively. A number of semi-quantitative methods of measurement have been devised. These include estimating the cortical to cerebellar uptake ratio (Johnson *et al*, 1987) (the cerebellum seldom being abnormal in the dementias) or the cortical to hemispheric or whole slice uptake ratio (Bonte *et al*, 1986; Jagust *et al*, 1987). The reliability and validity of this approach, where comparisons can only be made within individual images to the more traditional pattern recognition approach of clinical radiology, is still open to question. Gemmell *et al* (1987), in their studies, have used a reliable rating system which involves the judgement of experienced observers.

The development of SPECT studies in the differential diagnosis of dementia has paralleled in many ways reports involving the use of PET (Friedland *et al*, 1983). The initial reports described a pattern of hypoperfusion in posterior parietal (and sometimes occipital) regions of the brain in patients with Alzheimer's disease (Gemmell *et al*, 1984; Sharp *et al*, 1986). This pattern could be distinguished reliably from the multiple randomly scattered focal areas of hypoperfusion found in patients with multi-infarct dementia and from normal patients. As more Alzheimer's patients were imaged, however, more diverse patterns of reduced cerebral uptake have been reported (DeRouesne *et al*, 1985; Hendrie *et al*, 1987). Hemispheric asymmetries were described as well as reduced cerebral uptake in brain regions other than the parietal lobes, e.g. the frontal lobes or subcortical areas (Gemmell *et al*, 1987). A few patients, particularly those with mild dementia, were reported to have normal images (Holman, 1986 and Hendrie *et al*, 1987). This pattern of diversity. found in SPECT images in Alzheimer's patients leads to potential diagnostic problems. Hemispheric asymmetries occurring in Alzheimer's patients might be mistaken for multiple infarct dementia (Cohen *et al*, 1986). The finding of at least a few mildly demented patients with normal images given present limitations of instrumentation may make SPECT less sensitive in detecting early Alzheimer's changes than PET where there is one report of PET changes preceding evidence of cognitive decline (Cutler *et al*, 1985).

The clinical significance of the SPECT image variability seen in DAT is not clear. It has been suggested that the different patterns of cerebral uptake are associated with different symptom clusters. Gemmell *et al* (1987) reported that Alzheimer's disease patients without bilateral temporo-parietal defects were less cognitively impaired than those patients who exhibited these defects. Holman (1986) describes one patient with aphasia who had a marked decrease in perfusion in the inferior temporal lobe of the dominant hemisphere, and another patient with visuo-spatial cognitive dysfunction who exhibited profound perfusion defects in the parieto-occipital cortex. DeRouesne (1987) has recently proposed three types of patients with Alzheimer's disease on the basis of SPECT imaging: Type I with bilateral decrease in occipito-parietal area whose predominant symptoms are partial amnesia and spatio-visual agnosia; Type II with asymmetrical temporo-parietal decrease with subcortical hypoperfusion who have, in addition to the symptoms of Type I, perseveration in image errors; and Type III with subcortical defects who have specific audio-verbal failure. Some studies have reported correlations of disease severity with degree of severity of hypoperfusion defect. Jagust *et al* (1987) reported a significant correlation between MMSE scores and temporo-parietal/whole slice perfusion ratio in nine patients with Alzheimer's disease and Holman & Johnson (1987) have reported a significant correlation between lowered mean parietal IMP activity ratios but not with other cortical areas and level of patient functioning and cognitive ability in 37 patients with probable Alzheimer's disease. There are few post-mortem studies available to check the validity of the SPECT findings. In one patient, the diagnosis of Alzheimer's disease was confirmed but the relative severity of the pathology in the posterior parietal lobe was not (Johnson *et al*, 1987).

TABLE IV
*Frequency distribution of SPECT images grouped according to patterns of reduced cerebral uptake*

| Diagnosis | n | Normal image | SPECT results Confined to one hemisphere | Bilateral | Multiple small areas |
|---|---|---|---|---|---|
| Healthy control subjects | 5 | 5 | | | |
| Major depressive disorder/cognitive impairment | 3 | 1 | 1 | 1 | |
| Multi-infarct dementia | 3 | | 1 | | 2 |
| Primary degenerative dementia | 21 | 3 | 7 | 9 | 2 |
| Dementia secondary to physical illness | 1 | 1 | | | |

So far SPECT imaging has been performed with agents that identify generalised perfusion and/or metabolic defects; it is likely that interest in the future as in PET scanning will focus on the use of specific receptor ligands (Holman, 1986). Already studies using [$^{123}$I]QNB, a muscarinic antagonist, in Alzheimer's patients have been reported (Holman *et al*, 1985).

In the SPECT imaging of our elderly subjects conducted at Indiana University, I-123 HIPDM is the agent used (Hendrie *et al*, 1987). Interpretations of cerebral uptake reported here represent the consensus opinion of physicians from the Division of Nuclear Medicine. So far we have imaged 33 subjects. The subjects consisted of 21 patients with primary degenerative dementia, three patients with multi-infarct dementia, three patients with major depressive disorder who exhibited some cognitive deficit, one patient with dementia secondary to physical illness and five healthy older control subjects. The resultant images have shown great diversity in patterns of cerebral uptake (see Table IV).

All control subjects had normal image interpretations, as did the patient with dementia secondary to physical illness. One patient with major depressive disorder (CAMCOG = 97) had a normal image, one depressed patient (CAMCOG = 84) had reduced cerebral uptake in the left hemisphere and one depressed patient (CAMCOG = 58) had reduced uptake bilaterally in the frontal areas. This apparent correlation between the extent of the area of reduced cerebral uptake and diminished cognitive performance was also suggested by the results of the imaging of patients with PDD. Nine of the 21 PDD patients had bilateral symmetrical areas of reduced cerebral uptake (mean CAMCOG = $43.1 \pm 27.7$, $n = 7$, two patients untestable). Seven patients had reduced uptake primarily confined to one hemisphere (mean CAMCOG = $54.1 \pm 17$). Three patients had normal images (mean CAMCOG = $67.7 \pm 4.9$) and two patients had multiple scattered areas of reduced cerebral uptake bilaterally (mean CAMCOG = $6 \pm 2.83$).

Diversity was also shown in the location of the cortical areas of reduced cerebral uptake in patients with a clinical diagnosis of PDD. In patients who showed either symmetrical or asymmetrical diffuse patterns of reduced cerebral uptake, four patients had predominantly reduced uptake in the fronto-parietal regions, four patients had reduced uptake in the parietal lobes, and four patients had reduced uptake in the occipital lobes in association with either temporal or parietal lobes. Our efforts to correlate symptom clusters with patterns of cerebral uptake will await the acquisition of larger numbers of patients and the application of semi-quantitative methods of analysing the SPECT images.

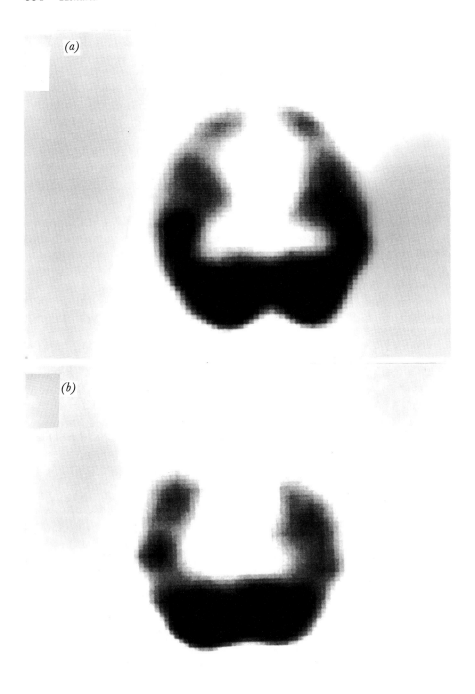

Fig. 3. Patient with normal cerebral uptake at time of first imaging (a) (CAMCOG = 70), now shows evidence of reduced cerebral uptake in bilateral frontal area after one year (b) (CAMCOG = 42).

So far we have been able to re-image five PDD patients after approximately one year. All patients showed a significant decline in cognitive function during this time. Several demonstrated changes in the SPECT imaging, others were unchanged. The patient whose SPECT imaging is illustrated in Fig. 3, at the time of the second reading showed evidence of bilateral frontal reduced uptake after having a previously normal pattern. During this time her CAMCOG had dropped from 70 to 42. The other PDD patient who presented first with a normal image now shows minimal areas of hypoperfusion in the left fronto-parietal areas (CAMCOG = 70 at the time of the first imaging, 47 at the time of the second imaging). One patient whose CAMCOG score declined from 69 to 23, had an identical pattern of reduced cerebral uptake in the left fronto-parietal region at both image times. Clearly more longitudinal studies are needed to understand the relationship between changes in SPECT patterns and disease progression.

# References

AWAD, I. A., SPETZLER, R. F., HODAK, J. A., AWAD, C. A. & CAREY, R. (1985) Incidental subcortical lesions identified on magnetic resonance imaging in the elderly. I Correlation with age and cerebro-vascular risk factors. *Stroke*, **17**, 1084–1089.

——, JOHNSON, P. C., SPETZLER, R. F. & HODAK, J. A. (1986) Incidental subcortical lesions identified on magnetic resonance imaging in the elderly. II Postmortem pathological correlations. *Stroke*, **17**, 1090–1097.

BESSON, J. A. O., CORRIGAN, F. M., FOREMAN, E. I., ASHCROFT, G. W., EASTWOOD, L. M. & SMITH, F. W. (1983) Differentiating senile dementia of Alzheimer's type and multi-infarct dementia by proton NMR imaging. *Lancet*, **ii**, 789.

——, ——, ——, EASTWOOD, L. M., SMITH, F. W. & ASHCROFT, G. W. (1985) Nuclear magnetic resonance (NMR) II imaging in dementia. *British Journal of Psychiatry*, **146**, 31–35.

——, ——, ——, —— & —— (1984) Proton NMR parameters and dementia. *Journal of Nuclear Medicine*, **8**, 94–99.

BONTE, F. J., ROSS, E. D., CHEHABI, H. H. & DEVOUS, SR, M. D. (1986) SPECT study of regional cerebral blood flow in Alzheimer's disease. *Journal of Computer Assisted Tomography*, **10**, 579–583.

BRADLEY, W. G., WALUCH, V., BRANT-ZAWADZKI, M., YADLEY, R. A. & WYCOFF, R. R. (1984) Patchy, periventricular white matter lesions in the elderly: A common observation during NMR imaging. *Noninvasive Medical Imaging*, **1**, 35–41.

BRANT-ZAWADZKI, M., DAVIS, P. L., CROOKS, L. E., MILLS, C. M., NORMAN, D., NEWTON, T. H., SHELDON, P. & KAUFMAN, L. (1983) NMR demonstration of cerebral abnormalities: Comparison with CT. *American Journal of Radiology*, **140**, 847–854.

BRINKMAN, S. D., SARWAR, M., LEVIN, H. S. & MORRIS, H. H. (1981) Quantitative indexes of computed tomography in dementia and normal imaging. *Radiology*, **138**, 89–92.

BYDDER, G. M., STEINER, R. E., YOUNG, I. R., HALL, A. S., THOMAS, D. J., MARSHALL, J., PALLIS, C. A. & LEGG, N. J. (1982) Clinical NMR imaging of the brain: 140 cases. *American Journal of Radiology*, **139**, 215–236.

——, ——, THOMAS, D. J., MARSHALL, J., GILDERDALE, D. J. & YOUNG, I. R. (1983) Nuclear magnetic resonance imaging of the posterior fossa: 500 cases. *Clinical Radiology*, **34**, 173–188.

COHEN, M. B., GRAHAM, S. L., LAKE, R., MELTER, J. E., FITTEN, J, KULKARNI, M. K., SERRIN, R., YAMADA, L., CHANG, C. C., WOODRUFF, N. & KLING, A. S. (1986) Diagnosis of Alzheimer's disease and multiple infarct dementia by tomographic imaging of iodine-123 IMP. *Journal of Nuclear Medicine*, **27**, 769–774.

CONDON, B., WYPER, D., GRANT, R., PATTERSON, J., HADLEY, D., TEASDALE, G. & ROWAN, J. (1986) Use of magnetic resonance imaging to measure intracranial cerebro-spinal fluid volume. *Lancet*, **i**, 1355–1357.

CREASEY, H., SCHWARTZ, M., FREDERICKSON, H., HAXBY, J. V. & RAPAPORT, S. I. (1986) Quantitative computed tomography in dementia of the Alzheimer's type. *Neurology*, **36**, 1563–1568.

CUTLER, N. R., HAXBY, J. V., DUARA, R., GRADY, C. L., MOORE, A. M., PAVISI, J. E., WHITE, J., HESTON, L., MARGOLIN, R. M. & RAPAPORT, S. I. (1985) Brain metabolism as measured with positron emission tomography: Serial assessment in a patient with familial Alzheimer's disease. *Neurology*, **35**, 1556–1561.

DeMyer, M. K., Hendrie, H. C., Gilmor, R. L. & DeMyer, W. E. (1985) Magnetic resonance imaging in psychiatry. *Psychiatric Annals*, **15**, 262–267.

——, Gilmore, R. L., Hendrie, H. C., DeMyer, W. E., Augustyn, G. T. & Jackson, R. K. (1988) MR Brain images in schizophrenics and normals: Influence of diagnosis and education. *Schizophrenia Bulletin*, **14**, 21–37.

DeRouesne, C., Rancurel, G., LePoncon Lafitte, M., Rapin, J. R. & Lassen, N. A. (1985) Variability of cerebral blood flow defects in Alzheimer's disease on [123]iodo-isopropyl-amphetamine and single photon emission tomography. *Lancet*, i, 1282.

—— (1987) Variability of cerebral blood flow defects. SPECT imaging in Alzheimer's disease (Abstract). *Third Congress of the International Psychogeriatric Association*, August, p. 131–132.

English, R. J. & Holman, B. L. (1987) Current status of cerebral perfusion radiopharmaceuticals. *Journal of Nuclear Medicine Technology*, **15**, 30–35.

Erkinjuntti, T., Sipponen, J. T., Iivanainen, M., Ketonen, L., Sulkava, R. & Sepponen, R. E. (1984) Cerebral NMR & CT imaging in dementia. *Journal of Computer Assisted Tomography*, **8**, 614–618.

Friedland, R. P., Budinger, T. F., Ganz, E., Yano, Y., Mathais, C. A., Koss, Q., Ober, B., Nussman, R. H. & Derenzo, S. E. (1983) Regional cerebral metabolic alterations in dementia of the Alzheimer's type: positron emission tomography with [ [18]F] fluorodeoxyglucose. *Journal of Computer Assisted Tomography*, **7**, 590–598.

Gado, M., Hughes, C. P., Danziger, W., Chi, D., Jost, R. G. & Berg, L. (1982) Volumetric measurements of the cerebro-spinal fluid spaces in demented patients & controls. *Radiology*, **144**, 535–538.

Gemmell, H. G., Sharp, P. F., Evans, N. T. S., Besson, J. A. O., Lyall, D. & Smith, F. W. (1984) Single photon emission tomography with [123]I-Isopropylamphetamine in Alzheimer's disease and multi-infarct dementia. *Lancet*, ii, 1348.

——, ——, Besson, J. A. O., Crawford, J. R., Ebmeier, K. P., Davidson, J. & Smith, F. W. (1987) Differential diagnosis in dementia using the cerebral blood flow agent [99m]Te HM-PAO: A SPECT study. *Journal of Computer Assisted Tomography*, **11**, 398–402.

Gerard, G. & Weisberg, L. A. (1986) MRI periventricular lesions in adults. *Neurology*, **36**, 998–1001.

Hendrie, H. C., Augustyn, G. T. & DeMyer, M. K. (1985) *Atlas of Brain Imaging in Masters in Psychiatry*. The Upjohn Company, Kalamazoo, Michigan, **5857**, Dec., 16–20.

——, Wellman, H. N., Hall, K. S., Farlow, M. R., Brittain, H. M. & DeMyer, M. K. (1987) Single photon emission tomography with Alzheimer's patients. *American Journal of Psychiatry*, **144**, 387.

——, Augustyn, G. T., Austrom, M. G., Farlow, M., Hall, K., Brittain, H. & DeMyer, M. (1987) Measurements of brain tissue and C.S.F. in Alzheimer's patients and control subjects using observed $T_1$ values from MRI. *Forty-Second Annual Convention & Scientific Program, Society of Biological Psychiatry Abstracts*, p. 387.

——, Hall, K. S., Brittain, H. M., Austrom, M. G., Farlow, M., Parker, J. & Kane, M. (1988) The CAMDEX: A standardised instrument for the diagnosis of mental disorders in the elderly: A replication with a U.S. sample. *Journal of the American Geriatric Society*, **36**, 402–408.

Henkin, R. E. (1987) SPECT and central nervous system studies. *Current Concepts in Diagnostic Nuclear Medicine*, **4**, 4–8.

Holman, B. L., Gibson, R. E., Hill, T. C., Eckelman, W. C., Albert, M., & Reba, R. C. (1985) Muscarinic acetylcholine receptors in Alzheimer's disease: In vivo imaging with iodine-123 labelled 3 quinuclidinyl-4-iodobenzilate and emission tomography. *Journal of the American Medical Association*, **254**, 3063–3066.

—— (1986) Perfusion & receptor SPECT in the dementias: George Taplin Memorial Lecture. *Journal of Nuclear Medicine*, **27**, 855–860.

—— & Johnson, K. A. (1987) SPECT in Alzheimer's disease. Abnormal IMP uptake reflects dementia severity (Abstract). *Third Congress of the International Psychogeriatric Association*, August, p. 125.

Jacoby, R. J. & Levy, R. (1980) Computerised tomography in the elderly with senile dementia: Diagnosis and functional impairment. *British Journal of Psychiatry*, **136**, 251–264.

Jagust, W. J., Budinger, T. F. & Reed, B. R. (1987) The diagnosis of dementia with single photon emission computed tomography. *Archives of Neurology*, **44**, 258–262.

Johnson, K. A., Mueller, S. T., Walshe, T. M., English, R. J., Holman, B. L. & Boston, M. A. (1985) Cerebral perfusion imaging in Alzheimer's disease with SPECT & I-123 IMP. *Neurology* (Suppl 1), **35**, 235.

——, ——, ——, —— & Holman, B. L. (1987) Cerebral perfusion imaging in Alzheimer's disease, use of single photon emission computed tomography and iofetamine hydrochloride I-123. *Archives of Neurology*, **44**, 165–168.

KUNG, H. F., TRAMPOSCH, K. M. & BLAU, M. (1983) A new brain perfusion imaging agent: (I-123)HIPDM: N,N,N¹-trimethyl-N¹-(2-hydroxy-3 methyl-5-iodobenzyl)-1; 3-propanediamine. *Journal of Nuclear Medicine*, **24**, 66–72.

McKHANN, G., DRACHMAN, D., FOLSTEIN, M., KATZMANN, R., PRICE, D. & STADLAN, E. M. (1984) Clinical diagnosis of Alzheimer's disease: Report of the NINCDS-ARDRA Work Group under the auspices of the Department of Health & Human Services Task Force on Alzheimer's Disease. *Neurology*, **34**, 939–944.

PYKETT, I. L., NEWHOUSE, J. H., BUONANNO, F. S., BRADY, T. J., GOLDMAN, M. R., KISTLER, J. P. & POHOST, G. M. (1982) Principles of nuclear magnetic resonance imaging. *Radiology*, **143**, 157–168.

ROTH, M., TYM, E., MOUNTJOY, C. Q., HUPPERT, F. A., HENDRIE, H. C., VERMA, S. & GODDARD, R. (1986) CAMDEX: A standardised instrument for the diagnosis of mental disorders in the elderly with special reference to the early detection of dementia. *British Journal of Psychiatry*, **149**, 698–709.

SARPEL, G., CHANDRY, F. & HINDO, W. (1987) Magnetic resonance imaging of periventricular hyperintensity in a Veterans Administration Hospital population. *Archives of Neurology*, **44**, 725–728.

SHARP, P., GEMMELL, H., CHERRYMAN, G., BESSON, J., CRAWFORD, J. & SMITH, F. (1986) The application of I-123 labelled isopropyl-amphetamine to the study of brain dementia. *Journal of Nuclear Medicine*, **27**, 761–768.

STEINER, R. E. (1986) Present and future clinical position of magnetic resonance imaging. *Magnetic Resonance in Medicine*, **3**, 473–490.

SULKAVA, R., HALTIA, M., PAETAU, A., WIKSTROM, J. & PALO, J. (1983) Accuracy of clinical diagnosis in primary degenerative dementia: Correlation with neuropathological findings. *Journal of Neurology, Neurosurgery & Psychiatry*, **46**, 9–13.

SZE, G., DeARMOND, S., BRANT-ZASADZKI, M. (1985) ''Abnormal'' MRI foci anterior to the frontal horns: pathological correlates of a ubiquitous finding. *American Journal of Neuroradiology*, **6**, 467–468.

TODOROV, A. B., GO, R. C., CONSTANTINIDIS, S. & ELSTON, R. C. (1975) Specificity of the clinical diagnosis of dementia. *Journal of the Neurological Sciences*, **26**, 81–98.

WHITE, J. A. & HESTON, J. L. (1986) The essential contribution of the autopsy in Alzheimer's disease and related disorders. *Pathologist*, **40**, 17–19.

YOUNG, I. R., RANDELL, C. P., KAPLAN, P. W., JAMES, A., BYDDER, G. M. & STEINER, R. E. (1983) (B) Nuclear magnetic resonance (NMR) imaging in white matter disease of the brain using spin-echo sequences. *Journal of Computer Assisted Tomography*, **7**, 290–294.

# 35 Histopathology of subtypes of Alzheimer's disease

## WILLIAM BONDAREFF*

Heterogeneity of neurobiological changes and clinical phenomena in Alzheimer's disease indicates the existence of two subtypes, which have been conveniently designated AD-1 and AD-2. These two subtypes are distinguishable on the basis of age, AD-2 being of earlier onset than AD-1. A greater deficit of neocortical transmitter substances, greater numbers of neocortical plaques and tangles, and a greater loss of locus coeruleus and nucleus basalis neurones characterise AD-2. It is unclear whether these two subtypes are categorically distinct. That they are distinguished by different degrees of age-related neuronal impairment suggests an aetiological distinction that remains to be proved.

That there might be two clinically distinct types of Alzheimer's disease (AD) became apparent when it was realised that senile dementia and the presenile dementia described by Alzheimer shared a common histopathology; namely, the presence of abundant plaques and tangles in cerebral cortex (Constantinidis, 1978). This set the stage for establishing a pragmatic definition of AD, which now is generally defined as a clinical picture meeting the DSM-III criteria of primary degenerative dementia (American Psychiatric Association, 1980) with a histopathological finding of abundant neuritic plaques and neurofibrillary tangles consistent with that described by Alzheimer (1907). The definition has been articulated with greater diagnostic utility by an *NINCDS-ADRDA* (National Institute of Neurological and Communicative Disorders and Stroke—The Alzheimer's Disease and Related Disorders Association) Work Group which set out criteria for the clinical diagnosis of 'probable AD', and enumerated clinical data which would make this diagnosis more or less likely (McKhann, G. *et al*, 1984). While the clinical criteria have been useful they clearly are not sufficiently specific to differentiate one type of dementia from all others, especially in the elderly. The histopathological criteria, on the contrary, do define a type of dementia. Whether the definition should be narrowed or broadened, however, is moot.

Tomlinson, Blessed & Roth (1970) examined the brains of 25 demented elderly patients and found an abundance of neurofibrillary tangles in neocortex in 20. Neuritic plaques were found in abundance in all these but one in which there were relatively few senile plaques and several minute infarcts in frontal grey matter.

*Supported in part by the Della Martin Foundation and the USC/St. Barnabas Alzheimer's Disease Diagnosis and Treatment Center.

In 28 non-demented elderly persons Tomlinson, Blessed & Roth (1968) found no neocortical neurofibrillary tangles in 25. In none of the three exceptions were neurofibrillary tangles abundant, and in only one were they generally distributed. Numbers of senile plaques were more variable, but the relationship between dementia and neocortical plaques and tangles in abundance was unquestionable. While, on the one hand, this relationship serves to establish a neuropathological diagnosis of Alzheimer's disease, it is apparent, on the other hand, that dementia in the presence of neocortical plaques or tangles in relatively smaller numbers does occur.

Terry *et al* (1987) have argued recently that AD in the elderly can exist even when tangles are not evident. They found demented elderly persons with plaques, but no neocortical tangles, who appeared clinically indistinguishable from those with abundant neocortical plaques and tangles. Terry *et al* (1987) considered these cases of dementia without neocortical neurofibrillary tangles as senile dementia of the Alzheimer type (i.e. AD). In doing so they assumed that the clinical characteristics of dementia in the elderly with plaques and tangles are similar to those unassociated with plaques and tangles, which seems unwarranted because the clinical characteristics of dementia have not been adequately correlated with histopathology. Clinical characteristics of specifically defined AD (histologically verified and meeting NICDS–ADRDA criteria for 'definite' AD) have also not been adequately correlated with histopathology. There is no known premorbid finding that is pathognomonic for AD. Until there is it would seem judicious to define AD conservatively as dementia in the presence of abundant neocortical plaques and tangles.

So defined, AD is a disease entity. It occurs typically in later years and is obviously an age-related disease, although its relationship with age is not adequately understood. Indeed, AD may be age-dependent in that its pathogenesis may directly involve ageing (Brody & Schneider, 1986). It is known, for example, that numbers of neurons in cerebral cortex (Brody, 1955), locus coeruleus (nLC) (Vijayashankar & Brody, 1979) and perhaps nucleus basalis (Chui *et al*, 1984), which decline normally during the course of ageing, decline to a much greater degree in AD (Terry *et al*, 1981; Mountjoy *et al*, 1983; Bondareff *et al*, 1982; Tomlinson, Irving & Blessed, 1981; Whitehouse *et al*, 1982; Davies & Maloney, 1976). The mechanism of this neuronal loss is not known, but in AD, and presumably in non-demented elderly persons as well, neuronal loss appears to be related to neurofibrillary degeneration (Sumpter *et al*, 1986). The processes of neuronal loss in AD in non-demented individuals certainly differ quantitatively; they may differ qualitatively also.

Neuronal loss is the end stage of progressive neuronal functional impairment leading to neuronal death. It is a directly measurable, unambiguous parameter of progressive neuronal impairment, certainly more reliably measured than are changes in the amounts of transmitter substances synthesised by individual neurons. While the latter are difficult to measure in humans, changes in the metabolic output of groups of neurons are, of course, more readily assessed. Changes, for example, in choline acetyltransferase (ChAT) activity have been compared by Rossor *et al* (1984) in patients younger and older than 79 years at the time of death, and appear to be age-related. Patients dying younger than 79 years showed a greater loss of ChAT activity in frontal, temporal, parietal, and occipital cortices, as well as in amygdala and hippocampus. Rossor *et al*

(1984) also found a greater loss of somatostatin in frontal and temporal cortices, and a greater loss of gamma-aminobutyric acid (GABA) in temporal cortex, amygdala and hippocampus in AD patients younger than 79 years of age at death. These younger patients were found to have also a greater loss of noradrenalin (NA) in cingulate cortex than did those older than 79 years.

The relationship between these data, age, and the virulence of AD was discussed by Roth (1986), who commented on the impossibility of bringing clinical phenomena into an unequivocal relationship with neurobiological changes. In part, this appears to have resulted from imprecision in the assessment of age of onset. The relationship between virulence and age, however, has also been suggested by numerous clinical (Bondareff, 1983; Mayeux, Stern & Spanton, 1985; Chui *et al*, 1985; Selzer & Sherwin, 1983; Roth, 1985), genetic (Heston, 1983; Heyman *et al*, 1983) and histological data (Hubbard & Anderson, 1985; Tagliavini & Pilleri, 1983; Mann, Yates & Marcyniuk, 1984). Age at death, which is reliably determined at the time biochemical and histological measurements are made, no longer predicts age of onset or duration of AD. Because the standard of contemporary medical practice is to control infection and maintain good physical health by active intervention, early onset cases are more likely to live longer and advanced age at death can as well be associated with an early as a late age of onset. Although more severe biochemical and histopathological impairment are more likely to be associated with AD of early onset (Table I), many cases with severe impairment are associated with older age at death. Because neuronal impairment of greater severity is more characteristic of younger AD patients than of older ones, greater mean neuronal losses are typically reported in younger patients. At the same time, individual older cases, characterised by extensive loss, are not unusual. For example, in the very elderly Rossor *et al* (1984) found numerous cases with severe loss of cortical ChAT activity. Iversen *et al* (1983) found severe loss of cortical dopamine-beta-hydroxylase activity and Bondareff *et al* (1982) found numerous cases characterised by extensive loss of nLC neurons. The murky relationship between age and neuronal impairment is likely, then, to blur any attempt to

TABLE I
*Biochemical and structural changes in early and late onset Alzheimer's disease*

| Variable | Non-demented elderly | Alzheimer's disease Late onset | Early onset | Reference |
|---|---|---|---|---|
| ChAT | ↓F | + + T | + + + FT | Rossor *et al* (1984) |
| NA | ? | | + + + FC | Rossor *et al* (1984) |
| GABA | ↓FT | | + + + FT | Rossor *et al* (1984) |
| 5-HT (S2 receptors) | ↓N | + + N | + + + N | Reynolds *et al* (1984) |
| Somatostatin | – N | + T | + + FT | Rossor *et al* (1984) |
| Plaques | ↑N | + + N | + + + N | Tomlinson, Blessed & Roth (1968, 1970) |
| Tangles | ↑H – N | + + HN | + + + HN | Tomlinson, Blessed & Roth (1968, 1970) |
| Neurones | F | – | + + FT | Terry *et al* (1981) Mountjoy *et al* (1983) |

Key: – change minimal or absent; + + moderate change, significantly greater than non-demented elderly; + + + severe change, significantly greater than non-demented elderly; F frontal cortex; T temporal cortex; C cingulate cortex; N neocortex, non-specific; H hippocampus.

TABLE II

*Clinical, neurochemical and histopathological characteristics (mean values with S.E.M. in parentheses) of two groups of AD patients: AD-1 (>65 nLC neurons) and AD-2 (<65 nLC neurons). Differences between means in the two groups were tested by Student's t-test for which t values, degrees of freedom (d.f.) and 2-tailed probabilities (P) are given (from Bondareff et al, 1987)*

|  | Number of nLC neurons | Age at death (years) | Duration (months) | ChAT[1] | NE[2] | SO[3] | P[4] | T[5] |
|---|---|---|---|---|---|---|---|---|
| AD-1 | >65 | 80.21 | 60 | 4.71 | 9.1 | 165.8 | 1.29 | 1.56 |
|  |  | (1.8) | (10.01) | (0.33) | (1.49) | (20.5) | (0.29) | (0.2) |
| AD-2 | <65 | 78.26 | 90 | 3.23 | 4.59 | 103.4 | 2.74 | 2.26 |
|  |  | (2.03) | (12.29) | (0.39) | (0.73) | (13.49) | (0.43) | (0.2) |
|  | $t$ = | − 1.83 | 1.94 | − 2.88 | − 2.72 | − 2.57 | 2.76 | 2.41 |
|  | $P$ = | 0.74 | 0.06 | 0.006 | 0.012 | 0.014 | 0.008 | 0.02 |
|  | d.f. | 44 | 39 | 44 | 26.11* | 37 | 44 | 44 |

*Separate variance estimate
1. ChAT = choline acetyltransferase (pmol/h/g protein): frontal cortex
2. NE = norepinephrine (ng/g tissue): cingulate cortex
3. SO = somatostatin (pmol/h/g protein): Brodmann area 21 temporal cortex
4. P = neuritic plaques/field: temporal cortex
5. T = neurofibrillary tangles/slide: cingulate cortex

segregate AD cases on the basis of age of death and perhaps on the basis of age of onset also, especially if the relationship between age and the biochemical or histological parameter being measured is not understood.

In a recent study of age and histologic heterogeneity in AD Bondareff *et al* (1987) found that histologically verified AD patients could be divided into two groups according to the number of noradrenergic neurons surviving in the nLC at the time of death. The distribution of neuronal counts in AD patients was distinctly different from that of non-demented patients of comparable age, which was continuous and roughly bell-shaped. There were some dips in the distribution of counts from AD patients, which suggested division into two subgroups, one with more than 65 neurons per representative section, the other with less than 65 neurons. This corresponded to two groups: one with a mean neuronal count of the entire nLC more than 5000 neurons; the other with a mean nLC count of less than 5000 neurons. These two subgroups were labelled, respectively, AD-1 and AD-2; in part as a matter of 'linguistic convenience', in part to suggest categorical distinction, the validity of which could be tested (cf. Jorm, 1985). Biochemical and histological parameters of neuronal function were found to be generally more impaired in AD-2 cases than they were in AD-1 cases (Table II). Neocortical ChAT activity, NA and somatostatin concentrations, neuritic plaque counts and neurofibrillary tangle counts were all more severely affected in AD-2 than in AD-1 cases, and in all cases the differences were statistically significant. AD-1 and AD-2 cases, however, did not differ significantly with regard to age at death, although AD-1 cases tended to be older than AD-2.

A series of discriminant function analyses was used to investigate further the relationship between age and neuronal impairment and criteria for the differentiation of AD cases into two subgroups (Bondareff *et al*, 1987). In an initial analysis the two groups were chosen on the basis of nLC neuronal counts and seven variables were submitted to analysis as possible discriminants (Table III). Only three variables were found to contribute significantly to the

TABLE III

*Discriminating variables and results of discriminant function analyses of two groups of AD patients defined by numbers of nLC neurons and age at death (from Bondareff et al, 1987)*

| Variables | Standard discriminant coefficients | |
|---|---|---|
| | Number of nLC neurons (>65 vs <65) | Age (>79 vs <79) |
| Age | NS | — |
| Number of nLC neurons | — | NS |
| ChAT (Area 24) | NS | 0.57 |
| Ne (Area 24) | 1.07 | − 0.65 |
| Tangles (Area 24) | 0.57 | 0.71 |
| ChAT (Area 21) | NS | NS |
| Tangles (Area 21) | NS | NS |
| Plaques (Area 21) | − 0.56 | 0.32 |
| Grouped cases | | |
| Correctly classified | 74.19% | 86.67% |

discrimination between the two groups into which 74.2% cases were correctly classified. Age of death made no contribution to the separation and, therefore, bore no relationship to the separation on the basis of neuronal counts. However, when the two groups were separated on the basis of age (those who died before 79 years of age and those who died later), 86.67% cases were correctly classified.

In these analyses, age at death proved superior to neuronal impairment (defined in terms of neuronal survival) in the definition of AD subtypes. As the greater part of the limited power of neuronal impairment to discriminate AD subtypes presumably derives from its correlation with age at death, it is reasonable to anticipate greater discrimination from age at onset or duration of disease. It is also reasonable to anticipate greater discrimination from a measure of neuronal impairment other than survival of nLC neurons. In this regard, it was noted that two histopathological indicators of increasing severity in AD ( numbers of cortical neuritic plaques and neurofibrillary tangles) emerged as variables with significant weights from each of the discriminant function analyses (Bondareff *et al*, 1987). In the discrimination of groups by nLC counts, neocortical tangle counts proved to have a high quantitative weight among the three significant discriminating variables (concentration of NA in cingulate cortex, neuritic plaque counts in the middle temporal gyrus, and neurofibrillary tangle counts in the anterior cingulate gyrus). Neurofibrillary tangles are also well-known to occur also in nLC (Ishii, 1966; Mann, Yates & Hawkes, 1983) but their possible contribution to neuronal death in nLC and to the differentiation of AD subtypes remains to be determined.

In a progressively degenerative neuronal disease such as AD, it seems reasonable to anticipate a period of functional neuronal impairment to precede neuronal death. While such functional impairment can sometimes be measured in individual neurons or even a small group of neurons (nucleus) in animals, in humans it is usually difficult to assess. Presumably, it precedes changes in neuronal counts, and in AD it can be assumed to change progressively through the course of the disease. As indicators of functional impairment in individual neurons, changes in nucleolar diameter (Mann *et al*, 1980), intensity of histofluorescence (Selemon & Sladek, 1986), the distribution of tyrosine hydroxylase activity demonstrated immunohistochemically (Nakashima & Ikuta, 1985) and neuronal size (Nakamura

& Vincent, 1986) have all been reported in the brains of AD patients. While unlikely, it is possible that changes in dendritic extent (Coleman & Flood, 1987), number of dendritic spines (Coleman & Flood, 1987) and number of synapses (Davies *et al*, 1987), also reported in the brains of AD patients, might serve as additional indicators of functional impairment in individual neurons. Data reported by Davies *et al* (1987), for example, showed reduced synaptic counts in biopsy specimens of younger AD patients (under 65 years of age) and suggested that synaptic loss probably occurs early in the disease. Most studies, however, have not attempted to relate morphometric changes in specific neurons with the functional capacities of those neurons, whether in terms of electrophysiological or metabolic output. Such studies, which usually depend upon the availability of biopsy specimens or tissue specimens obtained after very brief post-mortem delays, are very few.

The problem is more readily, although probably less reliably, dealt with indirectly by comparing neuronal loss in one part of the brain with amounts of substances synthesised by those neurons and delivered to a site distant from the cells of origin. Wilcock *et al* (1983), for example, found a more or less proportionate 49% loss of nucleus basalis neurons and a 70% loss of ChAT activity in the temporal cortex of AD patients. It is reasonable to assume that a large part, if not all, of the ChAT measured was synthesised by the surviving nucleus basalis neurons. A similarly greater loss of cortical ChAT activity, relative to neuronal loss in nucleus basalis (stated in terms of decreased neuronal density rather than numbers of neurons) was reported by Perry *et al* (1982).

Bondareff *et al* (unpublished data) compared neuronal loss in nLC with NA loss in the anterior cingulate gyrus. A disproportionately small loss of NA (2%) relative to neuronal loss in nLC (27%) was found, but only in AD cases more than 79 years of age. In AD patients less than 79 years of age, a 65% loss of anterior cingulate NA was found. It was associated with a more proportionate 48% loss of nLC neurons and suggests that 52% of the normal complement of nLC neurons was synthesising only 35% of the normal complement of anterior cingulate NA. These findings suggested that nLC neurons surviving in younger AD patients were functioning at only 67% of normal synthetic capacity. Surviving nLC neurons in older AD patients, contrarily, appeared to be functioning at 130% of normal capacity.

The effect of age of the synthetic capacity of the nLC, at least as it is known from studies with rodents (Ingvar *et al* , 1985), suggests that NA synthesis would decrease with advancing age. Because NA synthesis in nLC neurons appears to decrease with age in AD (Bondareff *et al*, unpublished data) a greater metabolic impairment in younger AD patients appears paradoxical. However, this finding as well as other data suggesting increased neuronal impairment in AD of early onset (for example, Rossor *et al* (1984)), might simply reflect the longer duration of disease in AD cases associated with earlier onset. In their study of 46 elderly AD patients, Bondareff *et al* (1987) found age of death tended to be less and the estimated duration of dementia tended to be greater in AD–2 patients, in whom the mean number of nLC neurons was less than in AD–1 patients. These findings might also be interpreted as indicating different histopathological lesions in AD of early and late onset, although this has not been shown to date. However, in a recent study of nLC in ten AD patients (Bondareff *et al*, unpublished data), neuronal counts tended to be less in AD patients younger than 79 years of age (at death) than in those more than 80 years. The difference between the two groups was not statistically significant ($t = 1.74$; $n = 10$; $P = 0.125$). There tended to be more neurofibrillary tangles in these younger AD patients but, again, the difference between them and older patients was not significant.

These same ten AD patients can also be grouped on the basis of the severity of neuronal impairment, the criterion used to define AD subtypes AD–1 and AD–2 (Bondareff *et al*, 1987). AD–1 and AD–2 are then characterised, respectively, as having more or less than 65 neurons in a representative transverse section of nLC (Bondareff & Mountjoy, 1986). The mean number of neurofibrillary tangles, associated with the greater loss of nLC neurons in AD–2 patients, was not significantly greater than that found in AD–1 patients. Although they tended to be greater in AD–2 patients, counts of neurofibrillary tangles, visualised with both polarising optics after Congo red staining and fluorescence optics after thioflavin-S staining, did not differ significantly in AD–1 and AD–2 patients.

These findings continue to support the existence of two AD subtypes, characterised by greater and lesser degrees of neuronal impairment. They also raise the possibility that neuronal loss in nLC might be unrelated to neurofibrillary degeneration, a possibility with precedence in AD. In this regard, axonal degeneration has been described in the optic nerves of AD patients. It was found to be associated with degenerative changes in retinal ganglion cells which did not include the presence of neurofibrillary tangles (Hinton *et al*, 1986). While they suggest that the existence of AD subtypes is unlikely to depend upon differences in the process of neurofibrillary degeneration, these findings do not provide a satisfactory explanation for the different degrees of neuronal loss in the two proposed AD–subtypes.

Although neuronal loss in nLC does not correlate with age at the time of death, it does appear to correlate with age of onset in that the degree of neuron loss in patients who became demented when less than 70 years old was significantly greater than that in patients who were older than 70 (Bondareff *et al*, unpublished data). That the duration of dementia was also significantly greater in these earlier onset cases, might suggest that the loss of neurons progresses relentlessly regardless of age of onset. Indeed, the loss of nLC neurons does appear to progress uniformly in AD, approximately 1000 neurons per year (Bondareff *et al*, unpublished data), unlike the less severe two-stage loss found in non-demented, elderly subjects (Vijayashankar & Brody, 1979). The occurrence of substantially greater neuronal loss in AD, especially in AD with onset before age 70 (Bondareff *et al*, 1982), and its association with greatly diminished neocortical stores of neurotransmitters, continues to suggest that the pathology underlying AD of younger onset (AD–2) may differ qualitatively as well as quantitatively from AD with onset after age 70.

As a disease that presents differently in younger and older persons, AD seems similar to diabetes mellitus. Heterogeneity of clinical signs and symptoms, while less well known in AD, is characteristic of both diseases. In both, heterogeneity depends upon age-related differences in cell pathology, involving primarily pancreatic beta cells in diabetes and neurons in AD. Very little is known about the genetic factors and mechanisms involved in the aetiologies of subtypes in both diseases and the effects of age are relatively unexplored. While insulin dependent (Type I) diabetes is more commonly of early onset, late onset Type I patients are well-recognised and appear to possess the same immunogenetic characteristics as those seen in more common early-onset insulin-dependent diabetes (Cudworth & Wolfe, 1987). Regardless of its age of onset, which is usually (but not always) before the age of 40, Type I diabetes is a clinical entity, biologically distinct from Type II.

While they are hardly analogous, AD and diabetes can be compared with regard to clinical heterogeneity and its biological underpinnings. The two AD subtypes defined in terms of age of onset appear, like the two subtypes of diabetes, to be structurally and biochemically distinct (Roth & Wischik, 1985). A cellular basis for the difference between the two AD subtypes is suggested by histopathological studies of nLC, the morphological and neurochemical characteristics of which made it a seemingly ideal model for the study of structure-function relationships in AD. This model is being used in an attempt to redefine the two age-related AD subtypes in terms of neuronal pathology. Although there can be little doubt that there are age-related differences between the two subtypes, it has not been proved that AD-1 and AD-2 are biologically distinct clinical entities. Severe structural and neurochemical changes are, indeed, associated frequently with the early onset AD-2 subtype and infrequently with the late onset AD-1, yet the genetic and pathophysiological mechanisms underlying these changes are not known. Until they are, differences in functional neuronal impairment remain an attractive but speculative basis for classifying AD subtypes.

# *References*

ALZHEIMER, A. (1907) Uber eine eigenartige Erkrankung der Hirnrinde. See Wilkens, R. H. & Brody, I. A. (1969) Alzheimer's disease. *Archives of Neurology*, **21**, 109–110.

AMERICAN PSYCHIATRIC ASSOCIATION (1980) Committee on Nomenclature and Statistics: *Diagnostic and Statistical Manual of Mental Disorders*, ed. 3. Washington, DC: American Psychiatric Association.

BONDAREFF, W. (1983) Age and Alzheimer's disease. *Lancet*, **i**, 1447.

—— (1987) Changes in the brain in aging and Alzheimer's disease assessed by neuronal counts. *Neurobiology of Aging*, **8**, 562–563.

—— & MOUNTJOY, C. Q. (1986) Number of neurons in nucleus locus ceruleus in demented and non-demented patients: Rapid estimation and correlated parameters. *Neurobiology of Aging*, **7**, 297–300.

——, —— & ROTH, M. (1982) Loss of neurons of origin of the adrenergic projection to cerebral cortex (nucleus locus ceruleus) in senile dementia. *Neurology*, **32**, 164–168.

——, ——, ——, ROSSOR, M. N., IVERSEN, L. L. & REYNOLDS, G. P. (1987) Age and histopathologic heterogeneity in Alzheimer's disease. Evidence for subtypes. *Archives of General Psychiatry*, **44**, 412–417.

BRODY, H. (1955) Organization of the cerebral cortex. *Journal of Comparative Neurology*, **102**, 511–556.

BRODY, J. A. & SCHNEIDER, E. L. (1986) Diseases and disorders of aging: an hypothesis. *Journal of Chronic Diseases*, **39**, 871–876.

CHUI, H. C., BONDAREFF, W., ZAROW, C. & SLAGER, U. (1984) Stability of neuronal number in the human nucleus basalis of Meynert with age. *Neurobiology of Aging*, **5**, 83–88.

——, TENG, E. L., HENDERSON, V. W. & MOY, A. C. (1985) Clinical subtypes of dementia of the Alzheimer type. *Neurology*, **35**, 1549–1550.

COLEMAN, P. D. & FLOOD, D. G. (1987) Neuron numbers and dendritic extent in normal aging and Alzheimer's disease. *Neurobiology of Aging*, **8**, 521–545.

CONSTANTINIDIS, J. (1978) Is Alzheimer's disease a major form of senile dementia? Clinical, anatomical, and genetic data. In *Alzheimer's Disease: Senile Dementia and Related Disorders* (eds. R. Katzman, R. D. Terry & K. L. Blick). New York: Raven Press, 15–25.

CUDWORTH, A. G. & WOLFE, E. (1987) Genetic basis of Type I (insulin-dependent) diabetes. In *Immunology of Clinical and Experimental Diabetes*, (ed. S. Gupta). New York: Plenum, 211–294.

DAVIES, C. A., MANN, D. M. A., SUMPTER, P. Q. & YATES, P. O. (1987) A quantitative morphometric analysis of the neuronal and synaptic content of the frontal and temporal cortex in patients with Alzheimer's disease. *Journal of the Neurological Sciences*, **78**, 151-164.

DAVIES, P. & MALONEY, A. F. (1976) Selective loss of central cholinergic neurons in Alzheimer's disease. *Lancet*, **i**, 1403.

HESTON, L. L. (1983) Dementia of the Alzheimer type: A perspective from family studies. In *Banbury Report 15: Biological Aspects of Alzheimer's Disease*, (ed. R. Katzman). New York: Cold Spring Harbor Laboratory, 183-192.

HEYMAN, A., WILKINSON, W. E., HURWITZ, B. J., SCHMECKEL, J., SIGMON, A. H., WEINBERG, T., HELMS, M. J. & SWIFT, M. (1983) Alzheimer's disease: genetic aspects and associated clinical disorders. *Annals of Neurology*, **14**, 507-515.

HINTON, D. R., SADUN, A. A., BLANKS, J. C. & MILLER, C. A. (1986) Optic-nerve degeneration in Alzheimer's disease. *New England Journal of Medicine*, **315**, 485-487.

HUBBARD, B. M. & ANDERSON, J. M. (1985) Age-related variations in the neuron content of the cerebral cortex in senile dementia of Alzheimer type. *Neuropathology and Applied Neurobiology*, **11**, 369-382.

INGVAR, M. C., MAEDER, P., SOKOLOFF, L. & SMITH, C. B. (1985) Effects of aging on local rates of cerebral protein synthesis in Sprague-Dawley rats. *Brain*, **108**, 155-170.

ISHII, T. (1966). Distribution of Alzheimer's neurofibrillary changes in the brain stem and hypothalamus of senile dementia. *Acta Neurologica*, **6**, 181-187.

IVERSEN, L. L., ROSSOR, M. N., REYNOLDS, G. P., HILLS, R., ROTH, M., MOUNTJOY, C. Q., FOOTE, S. L., MORRISON, J. H. & BLOOM, F. E. (1983) Loss of pigmented dopamine-hydroxylase positive cells from locus ceruleus in senile dementia of Alzheimer type. *Neuroscience Letters*, **39**, 95-100.

JORM, A. F. (1985) Subtypes of Alzheimer's dementia: a conceptual analysis and critical review. *Psychological Medicine*, **15**, 543-553.

MANN, D. M. A., LINCOLN, J., YATES, P. O., STAMP, J. E. & TOPER, S. (1980) Changes in the monoamine containing neurones of the human CNS in senile dementia. *British Journal of Psychiatry*, **136**, 533-541.

——, YATES, P. O. & HAWKES, J. (1983) The pathology of the human locus coeruleus. *Clinical Neuropathology*, **2**, 1-7.

——, —— & MARCYNIUK, B. (1984) Alzheimer's presenile dementia, senile dementia of Alzheimer type and Down's syndrome in middle age form an age-related continuum of pathological changes. *Neuropathology and Applied Neurobiology*, **10**, 185-207.

MAYEUX, R., STERN, Y. & SPANTON, S. (1985) Heterogeneity in dementia of the Alzheimer type: Evidence of subgroups. *Neurology*, **35**, 453-461.

MCKHANN, G., DRACHMAN, D., FOLSTEIN, M., KATZMAN, R., PRICE, D. & STADLAN, E. M. (1984) Clinical diagnosis of Alzheimer's disease: Report of the NINCDS-ADRDA Work Group under the auspices of Department of Health and Human Services Task Force on Alzheimer's Disease. *Neurology*, **34**, 939-944.

MOUNTJOY, C. Q., ROTH, M., EVANS, N. J. R. & EVANS, H. M. (1983) Cortical neuronal counts in normal elderly controls and demented patients. *Neurobiology of Aging*, **4**, 1-11.

NAKAMURA, S. & VINCENT, S. R. (1986) Somatostatin and neuropeptide Y-immunoreactive neurons in the neocortex in senile dementia of Alzheimer's type. *Brain Research*, **370**, 11-20.

NAKASHIMA, S. & IKUTA, F. (1985) Catecholamine neurons with Alzheimer's neurofibrillary changes and alteration of tyrosine hydroxylase. Immunohistochemical investigation of tyrosine hydroxylase. *Acta Neuropathologica*, **66**, 37-41.

PERRY, R. H., CANDY, J. M., PERRY, E. K., IRVING, D., BLESSED, G., FAIRBAIRN, A. F. & TOMLINSON, B. E. (1982) Extensive loss of choline acetyltransferase activity is not reflected by neuronal loss in the nucleus of Meynert in Alzheimer's disease. *Neuroscience Letters*, **33**, 311-315.

REYNOLDS, G. P., ARNOLD, L., ROSSOR, M. N., IVERSEN, L. L., MOUNTJOY, C. Q. & ROTH, M. (1984) Reduced binding of $^3$H-ketanserin to cortical 5HT-2 receptors in senile dementia of the Alzheimer type. *Neuroscience Letters*, **44**, 47-51.

ROSSOR, M. N., IVERSEN, L. L., REYNOLDS, G. P., MOUNTJOY, C. Q. & ROTH, M. (1984) Neurochemical characteristics of early- and late-onset types of Alzheimer's disease. *British Medical Journal*, **288**, 961-964.

ROTH, M. (1985) Evidence on the possible heterogeneity of Alzheimer's disease and its bearing on future inquiries into etiology and treatment. In *The Aging Process; Therapeutic Implications*, (eds. R. N. Butler & A. G. Bearn). New York: Raven Press, pp. 251-271.

—— (1986) The association of clinical and neurological findings and its bearing on the classification and aetiology of Alzheimer's disease. *British Medical Bulletin*, **42**, 42-50.

—— & WISCHIK, C. M. (1985) The heterogeneity of Alzheimer's disease and its implications for scientific investigations of the disorder. In *Recent Advances in Psychogeriatrics*, (ed. T. Arie). Edinburgh: Churchill Livingstone.

SELEMON, L. D. & SLADEK, J. R. (1986) Diencephalic catecholamine neurons (A-11, A-12, A-13, A-14) show divergent changes in the aged rat. *Journal of Comparative Neurology*, **254**, 113–124.

SELZER, B. & SHERWIN, I. (1983) A comparison of clinical features in early- and late-onset primary degenerative dementia. *Archives of Neurology*, **40**, 143–146.

SUMPTER, P. Q., MANN, D. M. A., DAVIES, C. A., YATES, P. O., SNOWDEN, J. S. & NEARY, D. (1986). An ultrastructural analysis of the effects of accumulation of neurofibrillary tangle in pyramidal neurons of the cerebral cortex in Alzheimer's disease. *Neuropathology and Applied Neurobiology*, **12**, 305–319.

TAGLIAVINI, F. & PILLERI, G. (1983) Neuronal counts in basal nucleus of Meynert in Alzheimer disease and in simple senile dementia. *Lancet*, **i**, 469–470.

TERRY, R. D., HANSEN, L. A., DeTERESA, R., DAVIES, P., TOBIAS, H. & KATZMAN, R. (1987) Senile dementia of the Alzheimer type without neocortical neurofibrillary tangles. *Journal of Neuropathology and Experimental Neurology*, **46**, 262–268.

——, PECK, A., DeTERESA, R., SCHECTER, R. & HOROUPIAN, D. S. (1981) Some morphometric aspects of the brain in senile dementia of the Alzheimer type. *Annals of Neurology*, **10**, 184–192.

TOMLINSON, B. E., BLESSED, G. & ROTH, M. (1968) Observations on the brains of non-demented old people. *Journal of the Neurological Sciences*, **7**, 331–356.

——, ——, —— (1970) Observations on the brains of demented old people. *Journal of the Neurological Sciences*, **11**, 205–242.

——, IRVING, D. & BLESSED, G. (1981) Cell loss in the locus ceruleus in senile dementia of Alzheimer type. *Journal of the Neurological Sciences*, **49**, 419–428.

VIJAYASHANKAR, N. & BRODY, H. (1979) A quantitative study of the pigmented neurons in the nucleus locus coeruleus and subcoeruleus in man as related to aging. *Journal of Neuropathology and Experimental Neurology*, **38**, 490–497.

WHITEHOUSE, P. J., STRUBLE, R. G., CLARK, A. W., COYLE, J. T. & DeLONG, M. R. (1982) Alzheimer's disease and senile dementia: loss of neurons in the basal forebrain. *Science*, **215**, 1237–1239.

WILCOCK, G. K., ESIRI, M. M., BOWEN, D. M. & SMITH, C. C. J. (1983) The nucleus basalis in Alzheimer's disease: Cell counts and cortical biochemistry. *Neuropathology and Applied Neurobiology*, **9**, 175–179.

# 36 Correlations between neuropathological and biochemical measures in dementia of Alzheimer type

## CHRISTOPHER MOUNTJOY

Sir Martin Roth's interest in the psychiatric disorders of old age in general, and dementia in particular, led to a series of publications, including his important paper on the natural history of mental illness in the elderly (Roth, 1955). From the very first he had an interest in the pathological changes found in the dementias, but his earliest efforts at Graylingwell Hospital in collaboration with Dr Harrison were brought to a close by Sir Martin's appointment to the chair of psychiatry at the University of Durham in 1956. Similar studies to those initiated at Graylingwell were set in progress at Newcastle in collaboration with Professor Sir Bernard Tomlinson and resulted in several publications, including those which related the clinical severity of dementia in life to the pathological changes found post mortem (Roth *et al*, 1967; Blessed *et al*, 1968). These studies showed that the number of senile plaques, counted in a reliable manner, correlated highly with measurements of the severity of dementia in life and indicated that plaques could no longer be considered as a mere epiphenomenon.

Sir Martin's work on dementia continued after his move to Cambridge, where he fostered a close collaboration with the MRC Neurochemical Pharmacology Unit (Director Dr L. L. Iversen). The biochemical deficits of Alzheimer's disease found elsewhere and in the Cambridge studies suggested that the relationship between these deficits and the classical pathological changes found in Alzheimer's disease should be examined in the hope that some clues might be found to the aetiology of dementia. The early investigations relied on simple statistical correlations which, of course, do not necessarily indicate a direct or causal relation. Some studies have depended on careful anatomical dissection and chemical measurement in the homogenate and others have used immunohisto-chemical techniques.

## Acetylcholine

The abnormality in the cholinergic system was first described in 1976 and was rapidly confirmed by two independent groups of workers (Bowen *et al*, 1976; Davies *et al*, 1976; Perry *et al*, 1977). It has proved to be a consistent finding in all subsequent studies.

348

## The basal nucleus

The cholinergic input to the cerebral cortex comes mainly from the substantia innominata (Emson & Lindvall, 1986). Evidence for the loss of neurons from the basal nucleus of Meynert was first described by Pilleri (1966) and has subsequently been confirmed by other workers. Loss of choline acetyl transferase (ChAT) activity has been shown in the substantia innominata (Rossor *et al*, 1982a).

Perry *et al* (1982), using an acetylcholinesterase stain, showed a 33% reduction in the neuron density in the basal nucleus in a group of 36 Alzheimer cases. This reduction is small compared with reports of reductions in choline acetyltransferase (ChAT) activity in the cortex of 75–90% and led the authors to suggest that the loss of cells in the basal nucleus was a secondary effect rather than a primary event. Pearson *et al* (1983) found no significant reduction in the number of cells stained for ChAT or acetyl choline esterase (AChE), though the size of the cells was reduced in the dements compared with the controls. Wilcock *et al* (1983) compared six patients with four normal subjects and showed a 50% reduction in basal nucleus count which was associated with a similar percentage reduction in the average ChAT activity. However, there were low and poor correlations between the neuron count in the nucleus basalis and the cortical ChAT activity.

## Plaques

Significant correlations ($r = -0.82$; $P<0.001$) between cortical plaque counts and ChAT activity were first reported by Perry *et al* (1978). AChE activity was significantly correlated with plaque counts but muscarinic cholinergic receptor binding was not. Perry *et al* (1980) showed that some plaques and tangles in the hippocampus of normal elderly people and patients suffering from Alzheimer's disease stained positively for AChE. The positive staining indicated that senile plaques in the hippocampus were at least partially derived from cholinergic fibres.

In a later paper Perry *et al* (1981a) demonstrated significant correlations between plaque counts and ChAT in non-demented and demented cases combined, and for Alzheimer cases alone in the temporal lobe ($r = -0.65$). By contrast Wilcock *et al* (1982), using an average plaque count for frontal and temporal lobes separately, were unable to show a significant correlation between the ChAT activity and plaque count in frontal ($r = -0.21$) or temporal ($r = -0.24$) lobes. Mountjoy *et al* (1984) found correlations between plaque counts that were of a similar order to those of Perry *et al* for the whole group of dements and controls in the nine areas studied ($r = -0.63$); however, in the demented group alone the correlations were lower and of the order of $r = -0.45$. Neary *et al* (1986) found significant correlations between ChAT activity and senile plaques ($r = -0.69$) but not acetyl choline synthesis in temporal lobe biopsy specimens taken for diagnostic purposes from patients with Alzheimer's disease.

## Neurofibrillary tangles

The tangle, which was first described by Alzheimer (1907a & b) and is the criterion for the pathological diagnosis of the disease when found in the neocortex, has been shown by Wilcock *et al* (1982) to be highly correlated with the severity of dementia and with ChAT activity. They found that a combined group of demented subjects and control subjects showed a statistically significant negative correlation between tangles and ChAT activity in the frontal lobe ($r = -0.3$) and temporal lobe ($r = -0.58$); when the demented group alone was examined a significant correlation was found only in the temporal lobe ($r = -0.43$). Mountjoy *et al* (1984) correlated ChAT activity in nine cortical areas with estimates of neurofibrillary change rated on a four point scale of severity. The correlations in the demented group alone were of the order of $r = -0.5$ and were significant only in the superior, middle and inferior frontal and middle temporal gyri. Correlations for the combined demented and control groups were of the order of $r = -0.8$ and were highly significant in all nine areas studied. Neary *et al* (1986) found the ChAT activity correlated significantly with neurofibrillary tangles in their biopsy samples but the order of correlation ($r = -0.55$) was lower than that found for plaques.

The correlation of tangles with other measures raises a particular problem of method. Neuronal counts and plaque counts show a continuum in the distribution between dements and controls but the tangles in the neocortex do not. In fact, the presence of tangles in the neocortex is regarded by many as the 'gold standard' for the pathological diagnosis of Alzheimer's disease. The consequence is that the two diagnostic categories provide two quite distinct clusters of tangle counts for control subjects and demented subjects. These two clusters can be joined by a straight line and therefore provide correlations of a high statistical significance.

## Cortical neurons

Attempts have been made to count cortical neurons by means of image analysing computers. The results of such studies have produced conflicting results. Early studies by Tomlinson & Henderson (1976) and by Terry *et al* (1977) failed to demonstrate significant loss of neurons in control subjects compared with Alzheimer subjects. Later studies (Terry *et al*, 1981; Mountjoy *et al*, 1983) showed a significant reduction in the number of large neurons in the frontal and temporal lobes in demented patients compared with control subjects. Correlations between counts of neurons made in this way with ChAT activity measured in the opposite hemisphere showed significant correlations in the total population, though not in the demented or control groups separately (Mountjoy *et al*, 1984). There are, however, results from a biopsy study which show that pyramidal cell loss in Layer III correlates as significantly with ChAT activity as do tangles and plaques (Neary *et al*, 1986).

## Noradrenaline

Abnormalities in noradrenaline activity have been found by a number of workers (Adolfsson *et al*, 1979; Perry *et al*, 1981(b); Rossor *et al*, 1984).

# Locus coeruleus

Counts of cells in the locus coeruleus, the nucleus which provides the bulk of the noradrenergic input to the cerebral cortex, have been shown to be reduced by 50–60% in SDAT (Bondareff *et al*, 1981; Tomlinson *et al*, 1981). In general, the greatest loss has been found in patients dying at a relatively young age (Bondareff *et al*, 1981; Mann *et al*, 1982) and this is in line with the finding of more severe pathological (Corsellis, 1962; Tomlinson & Corsellis, 1984) and biochemical (Bowen *et al*, 1979; Rossor *et al*, 1984) lesions in cases of early onset which has led to the suggestion that SDAT can be divided into two groups (Bondareff, 1983; Roth, 1985; Bondareff *et al*, 1987a). However, large reductions in cell counts in the locus coeruleus are not confined to the early onset group (Iversen *et al*, 1983). Perry *et al* (1981b) found no significant correlation between locus coeruleus counts and cortical dopamine-β-hydroxylase (DBH) activity in Brodmann areas 10 and 21, in either normal subjects or subjects with a diagnosis of SDAT. In contrast Iversen *et al* (1983) reported a 60% reduction in noradrenaline activity in Brodmann areas 21 and 38 which was comparable to the reduction found in locus coeruleus counts. ChAT activity was reduced only by 40% in this study and there was no change in the amount of dopamine in the cortex. Bondareff *et al* (1987b) found significant correlations between locus counts and noradrenaline activity in Brodmann area 24.

# Plaques and tangles

In the cortex Perry *et al* (1981a) found no significant correlations between plaque counts and DBH activity. Bondareff *et al* (1987b) found significant correlations between locus counts and plaque counts and neurofibrillary tangles.

# γ-Aminobutyric acid (GABA)

The activity of the GABAergic marker enzyme glutamic acid decarboxylase (GAD) is reduced in some areas of the post-mortem cerebral cortex and in the midbrain in cases of SDAT (Perry *et al*, 1977). However, this reduction is probably due to agonal effects because GAD activity is normal in biopsy material taken from the temporal lobe of SDAT subjects. GABA concentrations appear not to be affected by the agonal state and are significantly reduced in the temporal lobe in SDAT (Rossor *et al*, 1982b).

# Plaques

No significant correlations have been found between plaque counts and GAD activity (Perry *et al*, 1978) or GABA activity (Mountjoy *et al*, 1984).

# Tangles

A single correlation between tangle estimates and GABA activity was found in the superior temporal gyrus, only one of nine areas studied (Mountjoy *et al*, 1984).

## *Neurons*

Significant correlations were found between GABA activity and neuron counts in the inferior frontal and superior temporal gyri in a combined group of normal and demented subjects and the superior temporal gyrus in the demented group analysed separately but not elsewhere (Mountjoy *et al*, 1984). Perry *et al* (1984) studied the intralaminar patterns of GAD and GABA and found greater variation for GAD compared with GABA and found no change in pattern or amount of GABA in SDAT compared with control subjects.

## *5-Hydroxytryptamine*

Reductions in the 5-HT system have been reported by Adolfsson *et al* (1979) and by Benton *et al* (1982) in neocortical biopsy specimens. Subsequently Bowen *et al* (1983) showed a reduction in 5-HT1 receptors and Reynolds *et al* (1984) showed a significant reduction in ketanserin binding indicating a reduction in the 5-HT2 receptors. However, they were unable to show a significant reduction in 5-HT and 5-hydroxyindoleacetate (5-HIAA), although there was a trend for the levels in the demented subjects to be lower than in the control subjects. Mann & Yates (1983) showed a significant reduction in nucleolar volume and RNA content in the cells of both the medial and lateral dorsal tegmental nuclei, the cells of origin of some of the 5-HT input to the cortex. Direct correlations between cortical 5-HT and the nuclei were not reported. Palmer *et al* (1987) found no correlation between 5-HT activity and pyramidal neuronal counts or senile plaques. Neurofibrillary tangle counts were significantly correlated with concentrations of 5-HIAA.

## *Neuropeptides*

A number of neuropeptides have been studied in SDAT. Several of these including vasopressin, cholecystokinin and vasoactive intestinal peptide do not differ significantly from normal subjects (Rossor *et al*, 1980a,b ; Rossor *et al*, 1981; Perry *et al*, 1981(a)). Substance P is reduced by 30–50% in SDAT. Perry *et al* (1981a) showed a significant correlation between plaque counts and cholecystokinin and Substance P in a combined group of control and demented subjects, although not in demented subjects alone.

Somatostatin has been shown consistently to be reduced in SDAT (Rossor *et al*, 1980c; Davies *et al*, 1980; Ferrier *et al*, 1983). Although there is some disagreement about the areas affected there is agreement that there is a significant reduction in the temporal lobe of SDAT subjects. The distribution of somatostatin-like activity in the temporal cortex is reduced in the inner cortical layers (Perry *et al*, 1983).

Somatostatin has been demonstrated in the neuritic plaques (Morrison *et al*, 1985) and the somatostatin activity has been shown to correlate with plaque counts (Dawbarn *et al*, 1986). Struble *et al* (1987) used polyclonal antibodies directed against substance P, somatostatin, neurotensin, cholecystokinin, leucine enkephalin and vasoactive intestinal polypeptide to study the neurites of senile plaques and found that all the antibodies labelled neurites in some senile plaques. The transmitter specificities of the immunoreactive neurites tended to reflect the distribution of transmitter-associated fibres in normal tissues. This suggests that either there are a greater number of neurotransmitters involved in Alzheimer's disease than had been recognised in biochemical studies or that the plaque formation was non-specific and contained neurites that were from unaffected and affected neuronal systems.

## Conclusion

Significant correlations between pathological and biochemical measures are likely to be found whenever the measures are altered in SDAT, and both are related to measures of the clinical severity of the dementia. Correlations of this type have not helped in the understanding of the aetiology of the disease or diseases. In part this is due to the use of statistical methods rather than the use of immunohistochemical techniques which give precise information about type of neuron affected. Even these techniques give rise to uncertainty. It has now been shown that contributions from neurites of neurons of different neurotransmitter types make contributions to plaques in the appropriate areas of brain. In view of the different findings in biopsy and post-mortem material it is likely that advances will only be made by molecular biological studies of the abnormal proteins made in the failing neuron.

## References

ADOLFSSON, R., GOTTFRIES, C. G., ROOS, B. E. & WINBLAD, B. (1979) Changes in brain catecholamines in patients with dementia of Alzheimer's type. *British Journal of Psychiatry*, **135**, 216–223.

ALZHEIMER, A. (1907a) Ueber eine eigenartige Erkrankung der Hirnrinde. *Allgemeine Zeitschrift für Psychiatrie*, **64**, 146–148.

—— (1907b) Ueber eine eigenartige Erkrankung der Hirnrinde. *Zentralblatt für die gesamte Neurologie und Psychiatrie*, **18**, 177–179.

BENTON, J. S., BOWEN, D. M., ALLEN, S. J., HAAN, E. A., DAVISON, A. N., NEARY, D., MURPHY, R. P. & SNOWDEN, J. S. (1982) Alzheimer's disease as a disorder of the isodendritic core. *Lancet*, i, 456.

BLESSED, G., TOMLINSON, B. E. & ROTH, M. (1968) The association between quantitative measures of dementia and of senile change in the cerebral grey matter of elderly subjects. *British Journal of Psychiatry*, **114**, 797–811.

BONDAREFF, W., MOUNTJOY, C. Q. & ROTH, M. (1981) Selective loss of neurones of origin of adrenergic projection to cerebral cortex (nucleus locus coeruleus) in senile dementia. *Lancet*, i, 783–784.

—— (1983) Age and Alzheimer's disease. *Lancet*, i, 1447.

——, MOUNTJOY, C. Q., ROTH, M., ROSSOR, M. N., IVERSEN, L. L. & REYNOLDS, G. P. (1987a) Age and histopathological heterogeneity in Alzheimer's disease: evidence for subtypes. *Archives of General Psychiatry*, **44**, 412–417.

——, ——, ——, ——, ——, —— & HAUSER, D. L. (1987b) Neuronal degeneration in locus ceruleus and cortical correlates of Alzheimer disease. *Alzheimer Disease and Associated Disorders*, **1**, 256–262.

BOWEN, D. M., SMITH, C. B., WHITE, P. & DAVISON, A. N. (1976) Neurotransmitter-related enzymes and indices of hypoxia in senile dementia and other abiotrophies. *Brain*, **99**, 459–496.

——, WHITE, P., SPILLANE, J. A., GOODHARDT, M. J., CURZON, G., IWANGOFF, P., MEIER-RUGE, W. & DAVISON, A. N. (1979) Accelerated ageing or selective neuronal loss as an important cause of dementia. *Lancet*, i, 11–14.

——, ALLEN, S. J., BENTON, J. S., GOODHARDT, M. J., HAAN, E. A., PALMER, A. M., SIMS, N. R., SMITH, C. C. T., SPILLANE, J. A., ESIRI, M. M., NEARY, D., SNOWDEN, J. S., WILCOCK, G. K. & DAVISON, A. N. (1983) Biochemical assessment of serotonergic and cholinergic dysfunction and cerebral atrophy in Alzheimer's disease. *Journal of Biochemistry*, **41**, 266–272.

CORSELLIS, J. A. N. (1962) *Mental Illness and the Ageing Brain*. London: Oxford University Press.

DAVIES, P. & MALONEY, A. J. F. (1976) Selective loss of central cholinergic neurons in Alzheimer's disease. *Lancet*, **ii**, 1403.

DAVIES, P., KATZMAN, R. & TERRY, R. D. (1980) Reduced somatostatin-like immunoreactivity in cerebral cortex from cases of Alzheimer disease and Alzheimer senile dementia. *Nature*, **288**, 279–280.

DAWBARN, D., ROSSOR, M. N., MOUNTJOY, C. Q., ROTH, M. & EMSON, P. C. (1986) Decreased somatostatin immunoreactivity but not neuropeptide Y immunoreactivity in cortex in senile dementia of Alzheimer type. *Neuroscience Letters*, **70**, 154–159.

EMSON, P. C. & LINDVALL, O. (1986) Neuroanatomical aspects of neurotransmitters affected in Alzheimer's disease. *British Medical Bulletin*, **42**, 57–62.

FERRIER, I. N., CROSS, A. J., JOHNSON, J. A., CROW, T. J., CORSELLIS, J. A. N., LEE, Y. C., O'SHAUGHNESSY, D., ADRIAN, T. E., MCGREGOR, G. P., BARACESE-HAMILTON, A. J. & BLOOM, S. R. (1983) Neuropeptides in Alzheimer type dementia. *Journal of the Neurological Sciences*, **62**, 159–170.

IVERSEN, L. L., ROSSOR, M. N., REYNOLDS, G. P., HILLS, R., ROTH, M., MOUNTJOY, C. Q., FOOTE, S. L., MORRISON, J. H. & BLOOM, F. E. (1983) Loss of pigmented dopamine-β-hydroxylase positive cells from locus coeruleus in senile dementia of Alzheimer's type. *Neuroscience Letters*, **39**, 95–100.

MANN, D. M. A., YATES, P. O. & HAWKES, J. (1982) The noradrenergic system in Alzheimer and multi-infarct dementias. *Journal of Neurology, Neurosurgery and Psychiatry*, **45**, 113–119.

—— & —— (1983) Serotonin nerve cells in Alzheimer's disease. *Journal of Neurology, Neurosurgery and Psychiatry*, **46**, 96.

MORRISON, J. H., ROGERS, J., SCHERR, S., BENOIT, R. & BLOOM, F. E. (1985) Somatostatin immunoreactivity in neuritic plaques of Alzheimer's patients. *Nature*, **314**, 90–95.

MOUNTJOY, C. Q., ROTH, M., EVANS, N. J. R. & EVANS, H. M. (1983) Cortical neuronal counts in normal elderly controls and demented patients. *Neurobiology of Ageing*, **4**, 1–11.

——, ROSSOR, M. N., IVERSEN, L. L. & ROTH, M. (1984) Correlation of cortical cholinergic and GABA deficits with quantitative neuropathological findings in senile dementia. *Brain*, **107**, 507–518.

NEARY, D., SNOWDEN, J. S., MANN, D. M. A., BOWEN, D. M., SIMS, N. R., NORTHEN, B., YATES, P. O. & DAVISON, A. N. (1986) Alzheimer's disease: a correlative study. *Journal of Neurology, Neurosurgery and Psychiatry*, **49**, 229–237.

PALMER, A. M., FRANCIS, P. T., BENTON, J. S., SIMS, N. R., MANN, D. M. A., NEARY, D., SNOWDEN, J. S. & BOWEN, D. M. (1987) Presynaptic serotonergic dysfunction in patients with Alzheimer's disease. *Journal of Neurochemistry*. **48/1**, 8–15.

PEARSON, R. C. A., SOFRONIEW, M. V., CUELLO, A. C., POWELL, T. P., ECKENSTEIN, F., ESIRI, M. M. & WILCOCK, G. K. (1983) Persistence of cholinergic neurons in the basal nucleus in a brain with senile dementia of the Alzheimer's type demonstrated by immunohistochemical staining for choline acetyltransferase. *Brain Research*, **289**, 375–379.

PERRY, E. K., PERRY, R. H., BLESSED, G. & TOMLINSON, B. E. (1977) Neurotransmitter enzyme abnormalities in senile dementia—choline acetyltransferase and glutamic acid decarboxylase in necropsy brain tissue. *Journal of the Neurological Sciences*, **34**, 247–265.

——, TOMLINSON, B. E., BLESSED, G., BERGMANN, K., GIBSON, P. H. & PERRY, R. H. (1978) Correlation of cholinergic abnormalities with senile plaques and mental test scores in senile dementia. *British Medical Journal*, **ii**, 1457–1459.

——, BLESSED, G., TOMLINSON, B. E., PERRY, R. H., CROW, T. J., CROSS, A. J., DOCKRAY, G. J., DIMALINE, R. & ARREGUI, A. (1981a) Neurochemical activities in human temporal lobe related to aging and Alzheimer-type changes. *Neurobiology of Aging*, **2**, 251–256.

——, TOMLINSON, B. E., BLESSED, G., PERRY, R. H., CROSS, A. J. & CROW, T. J. (1981b) Neuropathological and biochemical observations on the noradrenergic system in Alzheimer's disease. *Journal of the Neurological Sciences*, **51**, 279–287.

——, ATACK, J. R., PERRY, R. H., HARDY, J. A., DODD, P. R., EDWARDSON, J. A., BLESSED, G. & FAIRBAIRN, A. F. (1984) Intralaminar neurochemical distributions in human midtemporal cortex: comparison between Alzheimer's disease and the normal. *Journal of Neurochemistry*, **42**, 1402–1410.

PERRY, R. H., BLESSED, G., PERRY, E. K. & TOMLINSON, B. E. (1980) Histochemical observations on cholinesterase activities in the brains of elderly normal and demented (Alzheimer-type) patients. *Age and Ageing*, **9**, 9–16.

——, CANDY, J. M., PERRY, E. K., IRVING, D., BLESSED, G., FAIRBAIRN, A. F. & TOMLINSON, B. E. (1982) Extensive loss of acetylcholinesterase activity is not reflected by neuronal loss in nucleus of Meynert in Alzheimer's disease. *Neuroscience Letters*, **33**, 311–315.

——, —— & —— (1983) Some observations and speculations concerning the cholinergic system and neuropeptides in Alzheimer's disease. In *Biological aspects of Alzheimer's disease. Banbury Report 15*, (eds. R. D. Terry & R. Katzman) 351–361.

PILLERI, G. (1966) Klüver-Bucy syndrome in man. A clinicopathological contribution to the function of the medial temporal lobe structures. *Psychiatria et Neurologia*, **152**, 65–103.

REYNOLDS, G. P., ARNOLD, L., ROSSOR, M. N., IVERSEN, L. L., MOUNTJOY, C. Q. & ROTH, M. (1984) Reduced binding of (3H) ketanserin to cortical 5-HT2 receptors in senile dementia of the Alzheimer type. *Neuroscience Letters*, **44**, 47–51.

ROSSOR, M. N., IVERSEN, L. L., MOUNTJOY, C. Q., ROTH, M., HAWTHORN, J., ANG, V. Y. & JENKINS, J. S. (1980a) Arginine vasopressin and choline acetyltransferase in brains of patients with Alzheimer type senile dementia. *Lancet*, **ii**, 1367–1368.

——, FAHRENKRUG, J., EMSON, P. C., MOUNTJOY, C. Q., IVERSEN, L. L. & ROTH, M. (1980b) Reduced cortical choline acetyltransferase activity in senile dementia of Alzheimer type is not accompanied by changes in vasoactive intestinal polypeptide. *Brain Research*, **201**, 249–253.

——, EMSON, P. C., MOUNTJOY, C. Q., ROTH, M. & IVERSEN, L. L. (1980c) Reduced amounts of immunoreactive somatostatin in the temporal cortex in senile dementia of Alzheimer type. *Neuroscience Letters*, **20**, 373–377.

——, REHFELD, J. F., EMSON, P. C., MOUNTJOY, C. Q., ROTH, M. & IVERSEN, L. L. (1981) Normal cortical concentration of cholecystokinin with reduced acetyltransferase activity in senile dementia of Alzheimer type. *Life Sciences*, **29**, 405–410.

——, SVENDSEN, C., HUNT, S. P., MOUNTJOY, C. Q., ROTH, M. & IVERSEN, L. L. (1982a) The substantia innominata in Alzheimer's disease: an histochemical and biochemical study of cholinergic marker enzymes. *Neuroscience letters*, **28**, 217–222.

——, GARRET, N. J., JOHNSON, A. L., MOUNTJOY, C. Q., ROTH, M. & IVERSEN, L. L. (1982b) A post-mortem study of the cholinergic and GABA systems in senile dementia. *Brain*, **105**, 313–330.

——, IVERSEN, L. L., REYNOLDS, G. P., MOUNTJOY, C. Q. & ROTH, M. (1984) Neurochemical characteristics of early and late onset types of Alzheimer's disease. *British Medical Journal*. **288**, 961–964.

ROTH, M. (1955) The natural history of mental disorder in old age. *Journal of Mental Science*, **101**, 281–301.

——, TOMLINSON, B. E. & BLESSED, G. (1967) The relationship between quantitative measures of dementia and of degenerative changes in the cerebral grey matter of elderly subjects. *Proceedings of the Royal Society of Medicine*, **60**, 254–259.

—— (1985) Evidence on possible heterogeneity of Alzheimer's disease and its bearing on aetiology and treatment. In *The Ageing Process: Therepeutic Implications* (eds. R. N. Butler & A. Bearn). New York: Raven.

STRUBLE, R. G., POWERS, R. E., CASANOVA, M. F., KITT, C. A., BROWN, E. C. & PRICE, D. L. (1987) Neuropeptidergic systems in plaques of Alzheimer's disease. *Journal of Neuropathology and Experimental Neurology*, **46**, 567–584.

TERRY, R. D., FITZGERALD, C., PECK, A., MILLNER, J. & FARMER, P. (1977) Cortical cell counts in senile dementia. *Journal of Neuropathology and Experimental Neurology*, **36**, 633.

——, PECK, A., DETERESA, R. & SCHECTER, R. (1981) Some morphometric aspects of the brain in senile dementia of the Alzheimer type. *Annals of Neurology*. **10**, 184–192.

TOMLINSON, B. E. & HENDERSON, G. (1976) Some quantitative cerebral findings in normal and demented old people. In *Neurobiology of Aging vol 3* (eds. R. D. Terry & S. Gershon). New York: Raven Press, p. 183–204.

——, IRVING, D. & BLESSED, G. (1981) Cell loss in the locus coeruleus in senile dementia of the Alzheimer type. *Journal of the Neurological Sciences*, **49**, 419–428.

—— & CORSELLIS, J. A. N. (1984) Ageing and the dementias. In *Greenfield's Neuropathology*, 4th edn. (eds. J. H. Adams, J. A. N. Corsellis & L. W. Duchen) London: Arnold, ch. 20, 951–1025.

WILCOCK, G. K., ESIRI, M. M., BOWEN, D. M. & SMITH, C. T. (1982) Correlation of cortical choline acetyltransferase activity with the severity of dementia and histological abnormalities. *Journal of the Neurological Sciences*, **57**, 407–417.

——, ——, —— & SMITH, C. C. T. (1983) The nucleus basalis in Alzheimer's disease cell counts and cortical biochemistry. *Neuropathology and Applied Neurobiology*, **9**, 175–179.

# 37 Neuronal lipopigment in relation to ageing, disease and chronic drug regimes

## JONATHAN H. DOWSON

In various neuronal groups the volume of neuronal lipopigment has been positively correlated with advancing age, Alzheimer dementia and the neuronal ceroidoses, while various changes in neuronal lipopigment have been reported in association with the chronic administration of dihydroergotoxine, ethanol, phenytoin, centrophenoxine, and chlorpromazine.

An increase in the volume of neuronal lipopigment may reflect a number of factors, including increased functional activity of the cell, impaired removal of pigment, the ageing process, anoxia, drug toxicity, or a degenerative disease. Chronic administration of agents which can be correlated with decreased neuronal lipopigment in animal models might protect neuronal function against certain adverse effects associated with lipopigment accumulation in normal ageing, anoxia or degenerative diseases. Long-term studies of the prophylactic use of such agents, or of drugs which neutralise free radicals, may be indicated in the healthy elderly and in early Alzheimer dementia. Other applications may include the protection of the brain and other organs against the effects of additional free radicals formed during periods of oxygen deprivation.

## Neuronal lipopigment

A tissue pigment has a naturally distinctive colour, and lipopigment consists of discrete or aggregated particles which appear yellow or brown in unstained tissue sections. Despite the large amounts of lipopigment which can be found in many cells, it has not attracted an equivalent degree of interest until the last decade, and it is an indication of Martin Roth's commitment to helping his colleagues and to obtaining the necessary funding for a wide range of research, that he encouraged my work in an area which was (and is!) a unique feature of a university department of psychiatry.

Lipopigment is present in many organs and cell types, and as it exhibits a striking yellow fluorescence in unstained tissue, fluorescence microscopy has proved useful for its identification and examination (Dowson & Harris, 1981). The gradual accumulation of neuronal lipopigment is one of the most consistent correlates of ageing in the mammalian nervous system and variations in lipopigment characteristics can be used to identify groups of neurones which share particular functions.

Lipopigment should be considered as an umbrella term for a variety of related pigments, and there are two main subcategories, *lipofuscin*, which accumulates during normal ageing, and *ceroid* which indicates a pathological process. However, each of these major subcategories is not homogeneous (Dowson, 1982a).

There is evidence that lipopigment contains protein and lipid debris derived from cell damage and from the normal processes of renewal of cellular constituents. It is believed that the reaction of unstable 'free radicals' with such constituents, in a process of lipid peroxidation, contributes to the formation of lipopigment (Halliwell & Gutteridge, 1984). Lipopigment is, therefore, usually considered as cellular rubbish, and it has been claimed that there may be a constant turnover of lipopigment, due to the extrusion of fragmented pigment particles or some constituents of lipopigment through the cell membrane (Glees & Spoerri, 1975). However, it is not certain that routine removal of intraneuronal lipopigment (or of certain constituents of lipopigment) takes place to a significant extent, and opinion also varies as to whether lipopigment is harmful. Although ageing is associated with a reduced number of neurones and structural changes with an impaired functional capacity of remaining neurones (Glick & Bondareff, 1979), there is no clear evidence that lipopigment accumulation is a causal factor (Mann *et al*, 1978). But possible factors include a toxic effect of the pigment or of other end products of lipid peroxidation (McBrian & Slater, 1982), the displacement of organelles, and the disruption of intracellular transport.

Any adverse effect of lipopigment may vary between different neuronal groups and interact with other factors; however, it seems clear that massive accumulation of intraneuronal lipopigment need not have a clinically significant effect as, for example, olivary neurones in elderly individuals with no known disease or neurological impairment are almost filled with lipopigment. Nevertheless, lipopigment accumulation may have subtle effects on cerebral function and make a significant contribution to the functional decline of ageing neurones.

## Correlates of changes in neuronal lipopigment

In addition to advancing age, the reported correlates of increased volume of neuronal lipopigment are Alzheimer dementia, the neuronal ceroidoses (ceroid-lipofuscinoses), the chronic administration of ethanol, phenytoin or dihydroergotoxine (Hydergine, Sandoz), and increased neuronal activity.

A decrease in the volume of intraneuronal lipopigment has been correlated with decreased neuronal activity or chronic administration of any of the following: centrophenoxine (meclofenoxate), chlorpromazine, vitamin E supplements (Rubra *et al*, 1975; Freund, 1979), acetylhomocysteine thiolactone (Totaro *et al*, 1985), or butylated hydroxytoluene (Constantinides *et al*, 1986). It has been suggested that chronic administration of antioxidants might have therapeutic applications in clinical practice, but on the basis of animal studies so far, a relatively large dose would probably be necessary to achieve even a modest suppression of lipopigment accumulation.

Of particular interest to psychiatrists is evidence which suggests that increased functional activity in neurones may be associated with increased lipopigment accumulation, and vice versa (Papafrangos & Lyman, 1982; Scholtz & Brown, 1978). Kerenyi *et al* (1968) subjected rats to a "repeated conflict of the feeding and defensive reflexes'' over a period of six months and it was claimed that this correlated with a marked increase in the volume of lipopigment in Purkinje cells. However, the lipopigment was only quantified by visual estimates. Basson *et al* (1982), in their study of the effects of a daily 'training programme' involving treadmill exercise on rats, for periods up to 17 months, claimed that brain lipopigment was increased, although this involved the analysis of tissue homogenates.

The correlates of changes in neuronal lipopigment which are of more immediate relevance to psychiatry are ageing, certain diseases and various drugs (including ethanol) which are relevant to clinical practice. These will now be considered in more detail, illustrated by data derived from fluorescence microscopy (Dowson & Harris, 1981; Dowson, 1982a).

## Neuronal lipopigment in relation to ageing and disease

### Neuronal lipopigment in ageing and Alzheimer dementia

The approximately linear rates of increase of neuronal lipopigment in ageing have been correlated with the rate of reduction of cytoplasmic RNA in certain neurones and it has been suggested that there is a threshold volume of lipopigment, above which further increases may be causally related to a more rapid rate of reduction of cytoplasmic RNA (Mann & Yates, 1974). However, another study has reported that the rate of decrease in cytoplasmic RNA, and also in nucleolar volume, is similar in Purkinje cells, neurones of the dentate nucleus and in pyramidal cells of the hippocampus, despite the different rates of lipopigment accumulation in these three cell populations (Mann *et al*, 1978).

It has been claimed that variations in the volume of neuronal lipopigment are correlated with the neuronal ceroidoses, progeria, Jakob-Creutzfeldt dementia, Huntington's chorea and Alzheimer dementia (Brizzee, 1975; Brizzee *et al*, 1975; West, 1979). Several studies have reported that Alzheimer dementia is associated with increased lipopigment in various populations of neurones (Kent, 1976; Malamud, 1972; Yamada, 1978), although it has also been claimed that there are no increases (Mann *et al*, 1977; Mann & Sinclair, 1978; Scholtz & Brown, 1978; Torack, 1978).

Dowson (1982b) reported measurements of the intensity of neuronal lipopigment fluorescence which were used to estimate the volume of neuronal lipopigment in a region of the parietal cortex and in the inferior olivary nucleus from post-mortem tissue affected by Alzheimer dementia and in control subjects. The results indicated a linear relationship between the accumulation of neuronal lipopigment and advancing age in both neuronal populations of the non-demented group and in the olivary neurones of the demented group. However, in the demented group, the estimated neuronal lipopigment volume in the parietal neurones was not significantly correlated with age, and the estimated neuronal lipopigment volume in the olivary neurones was significantly increased, when age had been taken into account.

This finding of increased lipopigment in the olivary neurones in Alzheimer dementia was consistent with a previous report of a greater reduction of cytoplasmic RNA and of nucleolar volume in olivary neurones in Alzheimer dementia, and it is possible that an increase in neuronal lipopigment has a secondary pathogenic effect on various neuronal populations in this disease.

### Neuronal lipopigment in the neuronal ceroidoses

The neuronal ceroidoses (ceroid-lipofuscinoses) are characterised by abnormally excessive amounts of neuronal lipopigment, although other types of cell are also affected (Zeman, 1976). The clinically heterogeneous ceroidoses are usually characterised by progressive blindness and neurological deficits, including dementia, and have been variously classified on the basis of age of onset, age at death, clinical presentation and pathological findings. Most occur in children but some present as a dementia in adult life when they are known as Kufs' disease, although the adult-onset cases show considerable variation (Badurska *et al*, 1981; Boehme *et al*, 1971; Chou & Thompson, 1970; Dom *et al*, 1979; Goebel *et al*, 1976, Kornfeld, 1972; Pallis *et al*, 1967; Zeman & Hoffman, 1962). Also, there are other rare disorders which can be associated with autofluorescent intraneuronal accumulations (Rapin *et al*, 1976; Suzuki *et al*, 1979; Lowden *et al*, 1981; Oldfors & Sourander, 1981).

The characteristics of the shape of the emission spectra of lipopigment fluorescence can be used to distinguish lipofuscin, which accumulates in non-diseased brains during ageing, from ceroid in the neuronal ceroidoses. Differences can be reliably quantified by calculating a ratio ('spectral ratio') between different points on the spectrum. Using this technique, the statistical significance of differences between the pigments in normal ageing, the ceroidoses and other disorders can be readily demonstrated.

Dowson (1983) reported characteristics of neuronal lipopigment fluorescence spectra from a case of adult-onset neuronal ceroidosis (Kufs' disease) in a patient who died from a seven-year dementia aged 41, and compared these with spectra from 14 brains which were unaffected by neurological disease. The results were also compared with emission spectra from childhood-onset ceroidoses (Batten's disease) and animal ceroidoses which had been previously reported (Dowson *et al*, 1982).

The emission spectra derived from abnormal lipopigment accumulations in cortex and cerebellum from the case of Kufs' disease could be distinguished from the spectra from lipofuscin in non-diseased brains, and from ceroid in the childhood-onset ceroidoses. The characteristics of an emission spectrum probably reflect the composition of the lipopigment, and spectral analysis may aid the identification of different pathogenic mechanisms which underlie the various types of neuronal ceroidosis. This technique has been used for the diagnosis of Kufs' disease in brain biopsies from dementias of uncertain aetiology.

## *Neuronal lipopigment in relation to chronic drug regimes*

The following psychotropic agents have been claimed to produce changes in neuronal lipopigment: dihydroergotoxine, centrophenoxine, chlorpromazine, phenytoin and ethanol. Chronic administration of agents which are correlated with decreased neuronal lipopigment might conceivably protect cerebral function against any adverse effects of lipopigment accumulation, while an increase in neuronal lipopigment may indicate increased functional activity of neurones or a toxic effect of a drug.

## Dihydroergotoxine

Dihydroergotoxine is the most extensively studied of all the drugs which have been used in attempts to alleviate chronic cognitive impairment in the elderly (Yesavage *et al*, 1979; McDonald, 1969) and many studies have reported significant improvements in various behavioural or psychological measures.

Huber *et al* (1986) have reported results after five years of a placebo-controlled long-term study to assess the preventative effects of dihydroergotoxine (4.5 mg daily) on several variables in healthy, elderly volunteers. Although statistical analysis of the data did not yield significant differences, the authors claimed that the pattern of several trends suggested that the drug regime did have a positive effect in maintaining physical and mental health.

There are a variety of reports of the pharmacological effects of dihydro-ergotoxine, including a claim that it can minimise the harmful effects of cerebral anoxia (Paoiorek & Wyllie, 1980). Dowson (1985) found that regular injections of dihydroergotoxine to rats over a period of 12 weeks was associated with a significant increase in mean area overlying neuronal lipopigment in a region of the hippocampus, which suggested that the drug regime was associated with an increase in neuronal lipopigment. Further studies on the effects of dihydroergotoxine on lipopigment may help to determine the effects of long-term administration at various dose levels on neuronal structures.

## Centrophenoxine

The clinical use of centrophenoxine has been advocated for various forms of dementia, cerebrovascular accidents and head injuries, although the clinical literature is sparse. One of the reported effects is to protect animals against the effects of cerebral anoxia or cyanide administration (Miyazaki *et al*, 1976). This suggests that centrophenoxine may be of value in some cases of cerebrovascular accident or arteriosclerotic dementia, in other pathological states in which there is reduced cerebral oxygenation, or in other conditions where there is tissue oxygen lack such as angina or intermittent claudication.

Many of the clinical studies of centrophenoxine were not controlled and involved diagnostically heterogeneous groups of elderly individuals. However, there have been four double-blind controlled studies. Oliver & Restell (1967) tested various cognitive functions in patients with evidence of memory impairment. No significant effect of centrophenoxine was detected, but this study did not investigate the process of learning new material. However, Gedye *et al* (1972) reported that administration of the drug to patients showing clinical evidence of a mild to moderate degree of either Alzheimer or arteriosclerotic dementia led to a statistically significant improvement in the performance of a task involving new learning. The third study, by Marcer & Hopkins (1977), examined the effects of centrophenoxine on memory for new information in normal elderly volunteers who were recruited from general practice, and there was a significant improvement in memory for new information.

The most recent study on the effects of centrophenoxine (Harris & Dowson, 1982, 1986) examined the effects of the drug, 600 mg twice daily for 12 weeks, on 20 residents in homes for the elderly who exhibited mild to moderate memory impairment which was probably due to senile dementia of the Alzheimer type. Although there was a trend towards improvement on word-learning performance, none of the cognitive tests showed statistically significant improvements with the drug. However, one subject showed a marked improvement in memory performance which coincided with centrophenoxine administration, and it may be that more individual case studies with a repeated cross-over design are indicated for this type of investigation.

Centrophenoxine is the p-chlorophenoxyacetic acid ester of dimethylamino-ethanol. In addition to its effect of reducing the adverse consequences of anoxia, many other effects have been reported, such as increased survival time in mice (Hochschild, 1973), an improved learning capacity in animals (Roy *et al*, 1983), increased RNA and protein synthesis in cultural human glial cells (Ludwig-Festl *et al*, 1983), neuronal electrolyte changes (Zs-Nagy *et al*, 1979), increased surface density of synapses in the rat cerebellum (Bertoni-Freddari *et al*, 1982) and increased nucleolar size in the aged rat brain. Several reports have claimed that centrophenoxine increases the activity of the pentose phosphate pathway and also increases the synthesis of phospholipid. Antioxidant enzymes oppose the harmful effects of oxidants, while the rate of lipopigment accumulation is thought to be related to the degree of peroxidative damage. Roy *et al* (1983) investigated the effects of centrophenoxine on the activity of antioxidant enzymes in the rat brain and the reported increases suggest that long-term prophylactic administration of centrophenoxine might have a role in preventing some of the adverse effects of ageing on neuronal structure and function.

Many studies have claimed that chronic administration of centrophenoxine leads to a reduction in the volume of neuronal lipopigment in many neuronal populations and that this is accompanied by ultrastructural changes and fragmentation of pigment aggregations. However, only five light-microscope studies which examined the effects of centrophenoxine on neuronal lipopigment have presented statistical analysis of data; three reported reduced neuronal lipopigment (Riga & Riga, 1974; Nandy 1978a,b) while two found no significant changes (Katz & Robison, 1983; Dowson 1985).

In conclusion, despite the many reported actions of centrophenoxine on the nervous system, there are no clear clinical indications for the use of this drug, and recent studies have not been able to confirm the many original claims that centrophenoxine can reduce neuronal lipopigment. Further research on the effects of this drug, including its effect on neuronal lipopigment, may help to indicate any potential clinical use. If further studies in animal models suggest that centrophenoxine can exert a prophylactic effect on the development of impaired neuronal function and structure due to normal ageing, then a long-term study in man would be indicated. Also, the reported dramatic ability of this drug to protect animals from the lethal effects of oxygen deprivation suggests that centrophenoxine may protect the brain, and other organs, from the destructive effects of those free radicals which are formed during periods of oxygen deprivation. In addition, compounds which appear to neutralise free radicals have been identified, and advances in this area could affect the viability of organs for transplantation surgery, and the management of cerebrovascular accidents and coronary thrombosis.

Other effects of centrophenoxine may have potential for therapeutic use; a recent uncontrolled study by Izumi *et al* (1986) claimed that centrophenoxine may be an effective treatment for tardive dyskinesia, and it was suggested that this may be related to an increase in cerebral cholinergic activity.

### Chlorpromazine

Samorajski & Rolsten (1976) administered chlorpromazine to mice and reported that lipopigment granules in certain neurones were markedly less numerous and more dispersed compared with control animals, although these observations were not backed up by a validated quantitative methodology. Also, there is a report by Ohtani & Kawashima (1983) which claimed that both chlorpromazine and centrophenoxine reduced the amount of intracellular pigment in cultural rat neurones, so that further histological studies of the effects of long-term chlorpromazine administration are indicated. If these findings are confirmed, it is possible that chronic neuroleptic administration may protect some neurones against certain adverse effects of ageing, although a decrease in neuronal lipopigment could be due to many factors.

### Phenytoin

Bernocchi *et al* (1983) claimed that daily administration of phenytoin to rats over eight months was associated with marked increases in the volume of lipopigment in Purkinje cell bodies. However, this was not confirmed in a recent study (Dowson & Wilton-Cox, 1988) although it was found that administration of phenytoin to rats was associated with an increased number of discrete lipopigment particles in Purkinje cells. As neuronal lipopigment accumulation in animal models may be an indication of the toxicity of anti-epileptic medication, further studies may help to determine the relative safety of various anticonvulsant regimes.

### Ethanol

Tavares & Paula-Barbosa (1983) administered a 20% aqueous ethanol solution to rats for periods of up to 18 months and claimed that Purkinje cell bodies contained considerably more lipopigment compared with control subjects, although this was not confirmed by Dowson & Wilton-Cox (1988). Also Borges *et al* (1986) reported that administration of a similar ethanol solution was associated with an increased lipopigment volume in hippocampal neurones after three months. Further studies in animal models may lead to an understanding of mechanisms responsible for the more subtle clinical features of alcohol abuse.

## Future studies

Future studies of neuronal lipopigment will contribute to the study of ageing, functional activity of neurones, pathogenic mechanisms and the effects of psychotropic drugs. They will also be concerned with the possible clinical applications of drugs which modify neuronal lipopigment, both in the treatment of degenerative disorders of the nervous system and in the possible reduction in some of the adverse effects of the normal ageing process. Such adverse effects might include an increased susceptibility to a variety of diseases, including neoplastic changes, atherosclerosis and dementia.

Of the various drugs which have been used clinically, and which have been examined in respect of their effect on lipopigment, centrophenoxine is of particular interest. However, conflicting results indicate the need for further investigations. If drug regimes can be identified which can consistently reduce neuronal lipopigment in animal models, these would be candidates for clinical trials in an increasingly elderly population, both in the healthy elderly and in early dementia.

The prophylactic effect of lipopigment-reducing regimes on normal elderly individuals could be examined in respect of the cognitive impairments which have been described in many elderly people without disease, although it should be noted that the effect of antioxidants may not significantly affect the maximum lifespan of a species (Pryor, 1982). However, adverse effects of the ageing process might be minimised, leading to an increase (of perhaps five years) in the mean lifespan, together with a reduced susceptibility to a variety of diseases and degenerative changes.

Although there is no evidence that any drug can modify the survival time of a patient with dementia, Halliwell & Gutteridge (1984) have pointed out that diseased tissue may undergo increased damage in a process which involves cytoxic end-products of lipid peroxidation, and increased lipopigment formation. Antioxidants, free-radical neutralisers, or drugs which reduce lipopigment accumulation, might have a beneficial effect in neuronal degeneration by preventing any such secondary damage, although the primary pathogenic mechanisms of the disease would not be halted.

However, this is likely to produce, at best, only modest clinical benefits, and investigating the effects of lipopigment-reducing drugs in normal ageing and anoxic conditions would seem to hold out more promise of real clinical benefit.

## Acknowledgement

The patient with Kufs' disease who was described was investigated at the University Department of Neurology, The Maudsley Hospital, London, under the care of Professor C. D. Marsden.

## References

BADURSKA, B., FIDZIANSKA, A. & JEDRZEJOWSKA, H. (1981) A dominant form of neuronal ceroid-lipofuscinosis. *Journal of Neurology*, **226**, 205–212.

BASSON, A. B. K., TERBLANCHE, S. E. & OELOFSEN, W. (1982) A comparative study of the effects of ageing and training on the levels of lipofuscin in various tissue of the rat. *Comparative Biochemical Physiology*, **71**, 369–374.

BERNOCCHI, G., BOTTIROLI, G., CAVANNA, O., ARRIGONI, E., SCELSI, R. & MANFREDI, L. (1983) Fluorescence histochemical patterns of Purkinje cell layer in rat cerebellum after long-term phenytoin administration. *Basic and Applied Histochemistry*, **27**, 45–53.

BERTONI-FREDDARI, C., GIULI, C. & PIERI, C. (1982) The effect of acute and chronic centrophenoxine treatment on the synaptic plasticity of old rats. *Archives of Gerontology and Geriatrics*, **1**, 363–373.

BOEHME, D. H., COTTELL, J. C., LEONBERG, S. C. & ZEMAN, W. (1971) A dominant form of neuronal ceroid-lipofuscinosis. *Brain*, **94**, 745–760.

BORGES, M. M., PAULA-BARBOSA, M. M. & VOLK, B. (1986) Chronic alcohol consumption induces lipofuscin deposition in the rat hippocampus. *Neurobiology of Aging*, **7**, 347–355.

BRIZZEE, K. R. (1975) Ageing changes in relation to diseases of the nervous system. In *Neurobiology of Ageing* (eds. J. M. Ordy & K. R. Brizzee). New York: Plenum Press.

——, KAACK, B. & KLARA, P. (1975) Lipofuscin: intra and extraneuronal accumulation and regional distribution. In *Neurobiology of Ageing* (eds. J. M. Ordy & K. R. Brizzee). New York: Plenum Press.

CHOU, S. M. & THOMPSON, H. G. (1970) Electron microscopy of storage cytosomes in Kufs' disease. *Archives of Neurology (Chicago)*, **23**, 489–501.

CONSTANTINIDES, P., HARKEY, M. & MCLAURY, D. (1986) Prevention of lipofuscin development in neurones by anti-oxidants. *Virchows Archives*, **409**, 583–593.

DOM, R., BRUCHER, J. M., CEUTERICK, C., CARTON, H. & MARTIN, J. J. (1979) Adult ceroid-lipofuscinosis (Kufs' disease) in two brothers. *Acta Neuropathologica*, **45**, 67–72.

DOWSON, J. H. (1982a) The evaluation of autofluorescence emission spectra derived from neuronal lipopigment. *Journal of Microscopy*, **128**, 261–270.

—— (1982b) Neuronal lipofuscin accumulation in ageing and Alzheimer dementia: a pathogenic mechanism? *British Journal of Psychiatry*, **140**, 142–148.

—— (1983) Autofluorescence emission spectra of neuronal lipopigment in a case of adult-onset ceroidosis (Kufs' disease). *Acta Neuropathologica*, **59**, 241–245.

—— (1985) Quantitative studies on the effects of ageing, meclofenoxate, and dihydroergotoxine on intraneuronal lipopigment accumulation in the rat. *Experimental Gerontology*, **20**, 333–340.

——, ARMSTRONG, D., KOPPANG, N., LAKE, B. D. & JOLLY, R. D. (1982) Autofluorescence emission spectra of neuronal lipopigment in animal and human ceroidoses (ceroid-lipofuscinoses). *Acta Neuropathologica*, **58**, 152–156.

—— & HARRIS, S. J. (1981) Quantitative studies of the autofluorescence derived from neuronal lipofuscin. *Journal of Microscopy*, **123**, 249–258.

—— & WILTON-COX, H. (1988) The effect of drugs on neuronal lipopigment. In *Lipofuscin-1987: State of the Art* (ed. I. Zs-Nagy). Amsterdam: Elsevier.

EARNEST, M. P., HEATON, R. K., WILKINSON, W. S. & MANKE, W. F. (1979). Cortical atrophy, ventricular enlargement and intellectual impairment in the aged. *Neurology*, **29**, 1138–1143.

FREUND, G. (1979) The effects of chronic alcohol and vitamin E consumption on ageing pigments and learning performance in mice. *Life Science*, **24**, 145–152.

GEDYE, J. L., EXTON-SMITH, A. N. & WEDGEWOOD, J. (1972) A method for measuring mental performance in the elderly and its use in a pilot clinical trial of meclofenoxate in organic dementia. *Age and Ageing*, **1**, 74–80.

GLEES, P. & SPOERRI, P. E. (1975) Centrophenoxin-induced dissolution and removal of lipofuscin. An electron microscopic study. *Arzneimittel-Forschung*, **25**, 3–9.

GLICK, R. & BONDAREFF, W. (1979) Loss of synapses in the cerebellar cortex of the senescent rat. *Journal of Gerontology*, **24**, 818–822.

GOEBEL, H. H., PILZ, H. & GULLOTTA, F. (1976) The protracted form of juvenile neuronal ceroid-lipofuscinosis. *Acta Neuropathologica*, **36**, 393–396.

HALLIWELL, B. & GUTTERIDGE, J. M. C. (1984) Lipid peroxidation, oxygen radicals, cell damage, and antioxidant therapy. *Lancet*, **i**, 1396–1397.

HARRIS, S. J. & DOWSON, J. H. (1982) Recall of a 10-word list in the assessment of dementia in the elderly. *British Journal of Psychiatry*, **141**, 524–527.

—— & —— (1986) The effects of meclofenoxate on cognitive performance in elderly individuals with memory impairment: a placebo-controlled study. *International Journal of Geriatric Psychiatry*, **1**, 93–98.

HOCHSCHILD, R. (1973) Effect of dimethylaminoethyl p-chlorophenoxyacetate on the life span of male Swiss Webster albino mice. *Experimental Gerontology*, **8**, 177–183.

HUBER, F., KOBERLE, S., PRESTELE, H. & SPIEGEL, R. (1986) Effects of long-term ergoloid mesylates (Hydergine) administration in healthy pensioners: 5 year results. *Current Medical Research and Opinion*, **10**, 256–279.

Izumi, K., Tominaga, H., Koja, T., Nomoto, M., Shimizu, T., Sonoda, H., Imamura, K., Igata, A. & Fukuda, T. (1986) Meclofenoxate therapy in tardive dyskinesia: a preliminary report. *Biological Psychiatry*, **21**, 151–160.

Katz, M. L. & Robison, W. G. (1983) Lipofuscin response to the "aging-reversal" drug centrophenoxine in rat retinal pigment epithelium and frontal cortex. *Journal of Gerontology*, **38**, 525–531.

——, ——, Herrmann, R. K., Groome, A. B. & Bieri, J. G. (1984) Lipofuscin accumulation resulting from senescence and vitamin E deficiency: spectral properties and tissue distribution. *Mechanisms of Ageing and Development*, **25**, 149–159.

Kent, S. (1976) Solving the riddle of lipofuscin origin may uncover clues to the ageing process. *Geriatrics*, **31**, 128–137.

Kerenyi, T., Haranghy, L. & Huttner, I. (1968) Investigations on experimentally produced age-pigment in the nervous system. *Experimental Gerontology*, **3**, 155–158.

Kornfeld, M. (1972) Generalized lipofuscinosis (generalized Kufs' disease). *Journal of Neuropathology and Experimental Neurology*, **3**, 608–682.

Lowden, J. A., Callahan, J. W., Gravel, R. A., Skomorowski, M. A., Becker, C. & Groves, J. (1981) Type 2 $GM_1$ gangliosidosis with long survival and neuronal ceroid lipofuscinosis. *Neurology (NY)*, **31**, 719–724.

Ludwig-Festl, M., Grater, B. & Bayreuther, K. (1983) Meclofenoxate-induced increase in cell metabolic activities in normal diploid human glia cells in a stationary cell culture system. *Arzneimittel-Forschung*, **33**, 495–501.

Malamud, N. (1972) Neuropathology of organic brain syndromes associated with ageing. *Advances in Behavioural Biology*, **3**, 63–88.

Mann, D. M. A. & Sinclair, K. G. A. (1978) The quantitative assessment of lipofuscin pigment, cytoplasmic RNA and nucleolar volume in senile dementia. *Neuropathology and Applied Neurobiology*, **4**, 129–135.

—— & Yates, P. O. (1974) Lipoprotein pigments—their relationship to ageing in the human nervous system. *Brain*, **97**, 481–488.

——, —— & Barton, C. M. (1977) Cytophotometric mapping of neuronal changes in senile dementia. *Journal of Neurology, Neurosurgery and Psychiatry*, **40**, 299–302.

——, —— & Stamp, J. E. (1978) The relationship between lipofuscin pigment and ageing in the human nervous system. *Journal of the Neurological Sciences*, **37**, 83–93.

Marcer, D. & Hopkins, S. M. (1977) The differential effects of meclofenoxate on memory loss in the elderly. *Age and Ageing*, **6**, 123–131.

McBrien, D. C. H. & Slater, T. F. (eds.) (1982) *Free Radicals, Lipid Peroxidation and Cancer*. London: Academic Press.

McDonald, C. (1969) Clinical heterogeneity in senile dementia. *British Journal of Psychiatry*, **115**, 267–271.

Miyazaki, H., Nambu, K. & Hashimoto, M. (1976) Antianoxic effect of meclofenoxate related to its disposition. *Chemical and Pharmacological Bulletin*, **24**, 822–825.

Nandy, K. (1978a) Lipofuscinogenesis in mice early treated with centrophenoxine. *Mechanisms in Ageing and Development*, **8**, 131–138.

—— (1978b) Centrophenoxine: effects on ageing mammalian brain. *Journal of the American Geriatrics Society*, **26**, 74–81.

Ohtani, R. & Kawashima, S. (1983) Reduction of lipofuscin by centrophenoxine and chlorpromazine in the neurones of rat cerebral hemisphere in primary culture. *Experimental Gerontology*, **18**, 105–112.

Oldfors, A. & Sourander, P. (1981) Storage of lipofuscin in neurones in mucopolysaccharidoses. *Acta Neuropathologica*, **54**, 287–292.

Oliver, J. E. & Restell, M. (1967) Serial testing in assessing the effect of meclofenoxate on patients with memory defects. *British Journal of Psychiatry*, **113**, 219–222.

Pallis, C. A., Duckett, S. & Pearce, A. G. E. (1967) Diffuse lipofuscinosis of the central nervous system. *Neurology (NY)*, **17**, 381–395.

Paoiorek, P. M. & Wyllie, M. G. (1980) The effects of drugs on cerebral cortex ATP levels in normal and hypoxic rats. *British Journal of Pharmacology*, **70**, 92–93.

Papafrangos, E. S. & Lyman, C. P. (1982) Lipofuscin accumulation and hibernation in the Turkish hamster, Mesocricetus trandti. *Journal of Gerontology*, **37**, 417–421.

Pryor, W. A. (1982) Free radical biology: xenobiotics, cancer and aging. *Annals of the New York Academy of Sciences*, **393**, 1–22.

Rapin, I., Suzuki, K. & Valsarnis, M. P. (1976) Adult (chronic) $GM_2$ gangliosidosis. *Archives of Neurology*, **33**, 120–130.

Riga, S. & Riga, D. (1974) Effects of centrophenoxine on the lipofuscin pigments in the nervous system of old rats. *Brain Research*, **72**, 265–275.

ROY, D., PATHAK, D. N. & SINGH, R. (1983) Effects of centrophenoxine on the antioxidative enzymes in various regions of the aging rat brain. *Experimental Gerontology*, **18**, 185–197.

RUBRA, D. N., DICKERSON, J. W. T. & WALKER, R. (1975) The effect of some antioxidants on lipofuscin accumulation in rat brain. *Proceedings of the Nutrition Society*, **34**, 122.

SAMORAJSKI, T. & ROLSTEN, C. (1976) Chlorpromazine and ageing in the brain. *Experimental Gerontology*, **11**, 141–147.

SCHOLTZ, C. L. & BROWN, A. (1978) Lipofuscin and transynaptic degeneration. *Virchows Archives*, **281**, 35–40.

SUZUKI, Y., FURUKAWA, T., HOOGEUBEN, A., VERHEIJEN, F. & GALJAARD, H. (1979) Adult type GM$_1$ gangliosidosis: a complementation study on somatic hybrids. *Brain Development*, **1**, 83–86.

TAVARES, M. A. & PAULA-BARBOSA, M. M. (1983) Lipofuscin granules in Purkinje cells after long-term alcohol consumption. *Alcoholism: Clinical and Experimental Research*, **7**, 302–306.

TORACK, R. M. (1978) In *The Pathologic Physiology of Dementia*. Berlin: Springer.

TOTARO, E. A., PISANTI, F. A., CONTINILLO, A. & LIBERATORI, E. (1985) Morphological evaluation of the lipofuscinolytic effect of acetylhomocysteine thiolactone. *Archives of Gerontology and Geriatrics*, **4**, 67–72.

WEST, C. D. (1979) A quantitative study of lipofuscin accumulation with age in normals and individuals with Down's syndrome, phenylketonuria, progeria and transneuronal atrophy. *Journal of Comparative Neurology*, **186**, 109–116.

YAMADA, M. (1978) On the distribution of senile changes in the spinal cord. *Folio psychiatrica et neurologica Japonica*, **32**, 249–251.

YESAVAGE, J. A., TINKLENBERG, J. R., HOLLISTER, L. E. & BERGER, P. A. (1979) Vasodilators in senile dementias. *Archives of General Psychiatry*, **36**, 220–232.

ZEMAN, W. (1976) The neuronal ceroid-lipofuscinoses. In *Progress in Neuropathology, Vol. III* (ed. H. H. Zimmerman). New York, San Francisco, London: Grune & Stratton.

—— & HOFFMAN, J. (1962) Juvenile and late forms of amaurotic idiocy in one family. *Journal of Neurology, Neurosurgery and Psychiatry*, **25**, 352–362.

ZS-NAGY, I., PIERI, C. & DEL MORO, M.. (1979) Effects of centrophenoxine on the monovalent electrolyte contents of the large brain cortical cells of old rats. *Gerontology*, **25**, 94–102.

# V. Schizophrenia: Organic aspects and problems of drug treatment

# 38 The EEG in schizophrenia: the first 50 years

## A. ARTHUR SUGERMAN

The EEG in schizophrenia has been investigated ever since Hans Berger first recorded cerebral potentials. As in so many other areas of schizophrenia research, the study of the EEG has been confounded by the problem of heterogeneity of diagnosis. Another major obstacle to research has been the pervasive presence of artefact. The use of quantitative methods of EEG analysis has produced considerably more information but has not eradicated these difficulties. Reduced amplitude variability, a consistent finding in many studies, may indicate a form of hyperarousal or the schizophrenic patient's lack of reactivity to changing environmental stimuli.

## *The search for specific EEG abnormalities*

Since the first use of electroencephalography in man many attempts have been made to show differences among the EEGs of schizophrenic patients, other psychiatric patients and normal subjects.

Many studies have claimed that schizophrenic patients have more EEG abnormalities than normal subjects; others have pointed to quantitative variations in normal activity, and more recently to differences in lateralisation of EEG activity. Evaluation of early studies is made difficult by problems common to all research in schizophrenia, specifically the heterogeneity of the disorder with an absence of reliable diagnostic criteria in early studies; the many artefacts to which EEGs of schizophrenic patients are especially subject—muscle artefacts due to tension, eye blinks, eyelid tremors and perspiration; the difficulty of controlling for age, institutionalisation, cooperativeness and the perhaps long-lived effects of somatic treatment such as ECT, insulin therapy and, in the last 30 years, neuroleptic therapy and its neurological effects. More specific to EEG research are the relatively primitive nature of the technology in the early studies and the subjective nature of clinical EEG interpretation. The following selective review surveys representative studies in order to indicate the nature of research during the past 50 years.

### (a) Visual inspection

The earliest researchers attempted to relate psychopathology to the obvious features of the clinical EEG; the alpha, beta, delta and theta activities, as well as to any abnormal, especially paroxysmal, activity. Berger, the originator of the EEG, suspected (1937) that high frequency (40–90 Hz) beta waves were implicated in schizophrenia and other disorders, while Lemere (1936, 1938) believed that an absent or weak alpha rhythm was more frequent in apathetic schizophrenic subjects. Other authors also implicated increased fast activity and decreased alpha activity in schizophrenia. Pauline Davis (1940) claimed that "choppy activity" (disorganised low voltage fast activity) was common in schizophrenic patients and she suggested it was an indication of overstimulation or irritation of the cortex due to unsynchronised activity at lower levels. Newman (1938) & Newman & Lawrence (1952) found an increased number of abnormalities, with fast activity as the predominant index of abnormality. He found this in 17% of chronic schizophrenic in-patients and 21% of those with psychopathic states, but in only 6% of depressive and psychoneurotic patients. Finley & Campbell (1941) compared the records of 500 'unselected' schizophrenic patients with those of 215 healthy (non-patient) controls. They found 28% abnormal and 34% borderline records in the patient group compared with 7% abnormal and 22% borderline records in the control group. Abnormal records included those with high frequency activity of 25 $\mu$V or more, whether or not superimposed upon slow activity, as well as records with short runs of slow activity, and records which showed increased amplitude and slowing on hyperventilation.

Ninety-eight of Finley & Campbell's schizophrenic subjects were placed in a catatonic-hebephrenic group and this group showed more abnormalities than other groups including dementia simplex and paranoid schizophrenia. It is noteworthy that this group included cases with an affective admixture as well as "any acute psychoses of uncertain prognosis with considerable emotional tension", which they refer to as schizophrenic "turmoil". Finley & Campbell refer briefly to a comparison they made among EEGs of schizophrenic, manic–depressive and epileptic patients, finding fewer manic subjects in the borderline groups and more in the abnormal group; as might be expected, the epileptic group showed the greatest proportion of abnormal records.

A large controlled survey of EEG in schizophrenic patients and normal subjects was reported by Colony & Willis (1956). One thousand schizophrenic patients admitted to an Oakland, California, naval hospital were compared with 474 non-psychotic control patients without discernible neurological disorder. The control patients showed EEG abnormalities in 8.3% and the schizophrenic patients in 5.0%. A small group of 18 patients with asocial, amoral or aggressive personality disorders in the control group had an incidence of 27.7% abnormal tracings; all had paroxysmal 4–6 Hz activity, generally fronto-temporal. Without this group the remaining controls had a 7.5% incidence of abnormal records.

In comparing the findings of Colony & Willis with those of Finley & Campbell, it appears that abnormalities were at least five times as frequent in Finley & Campbell's patient group; the control groups did not show such a major disparity. Some of the possible reasons for such a great difference are evident in differences in methodology. It is difficult to compare the patient populations since we are given no information about such basic data as age, sex, length of illness, medication or other somatic treatment in Finley & Campbell's group. The Colony & Willis group were all male, aged 17 to 35, mean 20.4 years. The major difference is in how records were judged to be abnormal; Colony & Willis did not consider any fast activity to be abnormal; "grades of abnormality were recorded as mild, moderate or severe corresponding to the degree of slowing and the increase in amplitude". Their reason for neglecting fast activity, which, as noted earlier was considered important by Berger, Davis and others, was that they considered low-voltage fast activity to be "influenced by the emotional state of the individual rather than a static condition", and in their examination of EEGs in schizophrenia they were searching for *organic* rather than *psychogenic* indicators of abnormality.

A subject of interest for nearly 50 years is the resemblance between schizophrenia and epilepsy, especially psychomotor, temporal lobe or complex partial epilepsy. The earliest report of similarities between cortical dysrhythmias in schizophrenia and psychomotor epilepsy was that of Gibbs, Gibbs & Lennox (1938). Many others since then have described "epileptic" discharges, "paroxysmal" discharges and "epileptic-like" potentials in schizophrenic patients. Hill (1963) reported on a group of 80 schizophrenic subjects (how these were selected is not mentioned), of whom 33 had abnormal EEGs, but more of the younger acute subjects (47%) than of the older chronic subjects (25%) were abnormal. Of 28 recent (acute) schizophrenic patients with abnormal EEGs, 10 had mild 'non-specific' abnormalities (non-paroxysmal, non-focal theta rhythm) while nine had generalised non-paroxysmal dysrhythmia of fast and slow activity, and in a further nine paroxysmal grouped slow and fast activity with low voltage spikes occurred. The latter nine showed findings "indistinguishable from those seen in many epileptics". Hill found a definite association in this group with catatonic illness and with histories of convulsions in the patients themselves and their families. Of the other nine patients with generalised non-paroxysmal dysrhythmia of fast and slow activity, six had had convulsions during insulin coma therapy. Although Hill suggests that they may have been carriers of 'hereditary' cerebral dysrhythmia, one wonders whether their EEG abnormalities may not have been a result of their therapy.

Catatonia is frequently mentioned in the older studies, although it is rarely seen nowadays and when seen appears to be more often part of an affective disorder rather than schizophrenia (Barnes *et al*, 1986; Abrams & Taylor, 1976). Gjessing's periodic catatonia has been reported by Bonkalo *et al* (1955) to show reduced alpha incidence and amplitude and increased frequency in the catatonic phases, and by Gjessing *et al* (1967) to show decreased alpha amplitude and increased frequency in the same phases.

What is missing in most of the older studies of the EEG in schizophrenia is any attempt to reduce the large variance by cutting the group of schizophrenic subjects (or schizophrenias) into any more homogeneous subgroups than the classical catatonic, paranoid or simple symptomatic groups. Little attention was given to differences in age at time of recording, age of onset of illness, duration of illness, acute versus insidious onset and premorbid personality, although Langfeldt (1937) had already made the distinction between true schizophrenia and schizophreniform states, and Wittman (1941) and Phillips (1953) had separated process and reactive schizophrenia, and good—and poor—premorbid schizophrenia, and shown the differences in outcome associated with premorbid personality and acute versus insidious onset.

However, some investigators (e.g. Igert & Lairy, 1962) have noted that differences in outcome are associated with different EEG appearances.

Commonly records which were characterised as normal were associated with a poor outcome, showing a more severe and prolonged course, while those with distinct focal or paroxysmal abnormalities had a better prognosis. Small & Small (1965) studied 88 acutely ill, schizophrenic patients, all recent urgent admissions to a city psychiatric hospital, selected to participate in a study of phenothiazine treatment. A variety of symptoms were listed which would qualify the patients for admission to the study. These included thinking and speech disorder, catatonic motor behaviour, paranoid ideation and behaviour as well as others, so it is likely that many patients would not fit DSM–III or research diagnostic criteria. Waking records were classified as normal if they showed a background of alpha and /or low voltage fast activity (not more than 25 $\mu$V) without focal or paroxysmal features. Abnormal records were either records with diffuse non-paroxysmal background irregularities with fast frequencies of more than 25 $\mu$V and/or diffuse slowing without other manifestations, or records with distinct paroxysmal features (abrupt alterations of voltage exceeding 50% of the resting background amplitude) and/or focal abnormalities with or without background changes.

Available clinical data were compared for the normal and two abnormal groups. Fifty-two patients had normal records (59%) while 17 or 19% had diffuse background abnormalities and 19 or 22% had distinct focal and/or paroxysmal features. Diagnostically, 10 of 12 catatonic patients had normal records while 10 of 15 acute schizophrenic patients had normal records. There were evident medication effects; 13 of 15 patients who had no medication had normal records while 13 of 27 patients given parenteral sodium amytal for sedation had abnormal records, with 11 showing diffuse background abnormalities.

At follow-up six months later, although statistically significant differences were not found, patients with normal or diffusely abnormal records tended to have longer hospital stays; and slightly more returned to hospital or transferred elsewhere for long-term care, while those patients with focal or paroxysmal abnormalities tended to have fewer hospital stays and be more asymptomatic. It should be noted that patients with normal records were found to have a significantly earlier onset of illness and more previous psychiatric hospital admissions. Small & Small concluded that a clinically normal EEG was correlated with a more severe form of illness and that the more striking the EEG abnormalities, the milder the course and outlook of the disorder appeared to be.

This result and others previously cited might suggest that schizophrenia diagnosed by strict criteria (to exclude organic, affective, schizophreniform and other short-lasting psychotic states) might show few abnormalities. One major study addressed this point directly. Small *et al* (1984) reviewed the clinical and EEG records of 759 patients seen from 1965 to 1972 and bearing DSM–I or DSM–II diagnoses of schizophrenia. Analysis of the EEGs of the total group supported previous findings showing a high incidence of EEG abnormalities and lower mean alpha frequency. Furthermore, EEG abnormalities predicted a better outcome while 'hypernormal' records were associated with a poor outcome. All the patients were rediagnosed according to strict Feighner *et al* (1972) criteria. One-third of the schizophrenic patients were rediagnosed as having affective, organic or other disorders. The presence of EEG abnormalities predicted diagnostic change and a relatively favourable outcome. However, 38% of the reclassified (Feighner) schizophrenic patients still had abnormal records, compared with 48% to 54% in other diagnostic categories. The standards of normality and abnormality were those of Kellaway (1979). One finding tending to confirm that a normal EEG in schizophrenia is a bad omen is that, of the 343 patients remaining in the schizophrenic category, 11% of those with normal EEGs versus 3% with EEG abnormalities were transferred to long-stay institutions. On the other hand, although EEG abnormalities were most prevalent in patients reclassified into organic, neurotic and personality disorder categories, those patients so reassigned had a better outcome if the EEG was normal. A tentative conclusion may be that an abnormal EEG in an apparently schizophrenic patient may indicate a good prognosis only if the correct diagnosis proves to be another illness; however, a normal EEG carries a poor prognosis only in strictly diagnosed schizophrenic patients.

## (b) Electronic methods of EEG analysis

*Frequency analysis*
Quantitative analysis of the EEG by means of a Fourier analyser developed by Grass was used by Gibbs as early as 1939. He reported that schizophrenic patients had less alpha and more fast activity than normal subjects; however, Gibbs & Gibbs (1963) later concluded that these findings resulted from more muscle artefacts in the patient records. The Walter-type analogue frequency analyser displays integrated voltage in a selected series of frequency bands. Kennard & Schwartzman (1957) used a Walter-type analyser and an array of electrodes over the head. They compared EEGs of patients and control subjects and also looked at changes after treatment. They found alpha activity less sharply defined in patients, with a greater frequency spread within the alpha range, and more activity outside of this range. There also appeared to be less synchrony between the two hemispheres in the patient group. They noted that more deviant EEG measurements were associated with acute and severe onset of illness and a greater degree of dissociation from the environment, so their results may reflect mainly acute disturbance.

Itil, Saletu & Davis (1972) also used a Walter-type analyser to compare right occipital EEG in 10 chronic schizophrenic patients and 100 age (and sex) matched controls. They found that their schizophrenic patients had significantly higher power (voltage) in high frequency bands (24, 27, 30 and 33 Hz), with significantly lower voltage in fast alpha frequencies (11, 12 and 12 Hz) and slow beta bands (15 Hz), and higher voltage in low frequencies (3, 4, 5 and 6.5 Hz). The same investigators reported a similar study two years later (1974) using digital computer analysis and had similar findings; the schizophrenic patients showed more slow and fast and less alpha activity.

Stevens & Livermore (1982) derived power spectra from EEGs of schizophrenic patients recorded by telemetry during free behaviour on psychiatric wards. In comparison with normal control subjects the schizophrenic patients showed more delta and theta activity and less alpha activity, as previously reported by others. Patients showed more delta and theta activity over the right temporal lobe than the left during all abnormal events except auditory hallucinations, during which left central–parietal delta predominated. The authors did not find evidence for a specific left temporal abnormality in schizophrenia as proposed by Flor-Henry (1976) and Shaw *et al* (1979). It must be noted that in subsequent correspondence Flor-Henry (1983) disputed this, finding ample evidence for left hemisphere involvement in the report of Stevens & Livermore (1982); and Stevens (1983) replied to Flor-Henry stating "our interpretation of the data did not allow us to specify which was the abnormal hemisphere for the few statistically significant changes emerging from our extensive studies of scalp EEG in schizophrenic patients".

Stevens & Livermore (1982) found ramp spectra, characterised by a smooth decline in power from lowest to highest frequencies in 45 of 120 patient spectra (9/18 patients) and in no normal control subjects. Ramp spectra had been previously found in conjunction with subcortical spike activity of epilepsy. As they can also emerge from eye and body movement the authors note that they may be interpreted as consistent with, not diagnostic of, remote spike or slow activity only when movement is meticulously excluded. They conclude that their findings are consistent with Pauline Davis's early (1940) report of EEGs in catatonic schizophrenia resembling those of convulsive disorder, suggesting inappropriate focal cortical arousal, episodic remote spike or slow activity and slower frequencies in the EEGs of many schizophrenic patients.

With the development of computer-based EEG analysis many channels can be analysed at the same time and statistical data can be presented without significant delay. Brain maps can be shown on the computer monitor which reveal patterns of activity in individuals, or differences between individuals and group means which cannot be recognised by the naked eye.

As Small (1983) points out, these methods, while more sensitive, are extremely vulnerable to artefact contamination and distortion. Multi-channel recordings, with numerous scalp and extracranial electrodes, must be used. She notes that certain types of artefact, such as muscle tension, eye movement, and restlessness, may be more typical of schizophrenic patients, while comparison groups might have such different sources of potential distortion as drowsiness and boredom.

A recent study by Karson *et al* (1987) illustrates this point. They cite a number of studies in which the results of power spectral analysis are presented in topographic maps showing bilateral slowing in the frontal regions of patients with schizophrenia (e.g. Morihisa *et al* 1983; Morstyn *et al*, 1983; Guenther *et al*, 1986). Karson *et al* used superorbital and lateral canthus electrodes to detect eye movements and deleted EEG epochs during eye movements in 15 medication-free patients with schizophrenia and in 13 normal control subjects. Power spectral analysis of the 28 channel EEG showed a diffuse mild increase in delta activity in the patients compared with the control subjects but no tendency for frontal localisation of this slow activity. There were no differences between patients and control subjects in other frequency bands. Their findings emphasise the importance of excluding artefact when computing EEG maps, and this requires that specific channels be dedicated to the measurement of horizontal eye movements.

*Amplitude analysis*

In amplitude analysis of the EEG as originally performed by Drohocki (1948) and applied to schizophrenia by Goldstein *et al* (1963) frequency is ignored, and measurements are made on cumulative amplitudes regardless of the frequency band to which they belong. The integrator is set to deliver a pulse whenever a certain cumulative voltage level is reached. The number of pulses recorded continuously expresses the integrated amplitude of the EEG channel analysed. The mean integrated amplitude per unit time and its standard deviation are easily calculated. The standard deviation as a percentage of the mean, or coefficient of variation, has been used as a measure of the variability of the EEG. Goldstein *et al* (1965) reported data obtained from 101 chronic male schizophrenic patients and 104 non-patient control subjects. All recordings were obtained with subjects supine, eyes closed, and the only lead analysed was left occipital with reference to both ears. Although no difference was found in amplitude levels between patients and normal subjects, the coefficient of variation in patient groups was about half of that in normal controls, with means of 7.39% in catatonic, 9.18% in chronic undifferentiated, 9.98% in paranoid and 10.02% in hebephrenic patients compared with 17.52% and 19.62% in two groups of male control subjects and 17.42% in a group of female control subjects. The patients are described as having been selected according to strict criteria (DSM-I), absence of neurological abnormalities and little or no response to somatic therapies. They were stated to be a representative sample of male chronic 'process' schizophrenic patients. Age range was 17 to 49; 57 patients had had both electroconvulsive therapy and insulin coma therapy, averaging about 55 ECT and 40 ICT; 33 had only ECT (average about 40) and two only ICT. None had received medication for at least one month before the recordings. The authors do not break down their results by previous somatic treatments. In similar patients in the same facility, Sugerman *et al* (1964) showed that the CV varied over the course of one year's treatment with psychotropic drugs and these variations occurred *pari passu* with changes in mental disorganisation. Goldstein *et al* (1963, 1965) suggested that the relative invariability of the EEG in these patients is a manifestation of hyperactivation, hyperarousal or "information input overload". The variability is subject to change under the influence of drugs with decrease being produced by stimulants and increase by sedatives and neuroleptics.

The hypovariability of the EEG has probably been the most reliable of all EEG findings in schizophrenia; according to Etevenon *et al* (1982) 30 publications from many different laboratories had confirmed this finding by 1982. Etevenon *et al* went further by analysing frequency as well as amplitude parameters on four EEG channels recorded simultaneously. Using five frequency bands (delta, theta, alpha, beta 1 and beta 2) and amplitude values for each frequency band and the raw EEG signal for each channel, they carried out quadratic discrimination analysis which was sufficient to classify three groups of schizophrenic subjects (residual, paranoid and 'other', using Feighner and DSM-III criteria) and two groups of normals (high alpha and low alpha EEGs). Only 10 parameters were enough for 99% correct recognition; of course this important study needs cross-replication in other patients.

Müller *et al* (1986) have also carried out interesting studies of amplitude variability in chronic schizophrenic patients and normal subjects. They examined 23 frequency bands from 5.2 to 14 Hz. They found EEG amplitude variability was significantly lower for the schizophrenics in ten posterior areas with eyes closed, resting, when alpha and theta functions were considered jointly. For alpha alone this was true for seven areas and for theta alone for four. They also found more slow (theta) activity in frontal areas, although they eliminated artefacts by hand before computer analysis. They found the amplitude variability (posterior) and theta activity (anterior) to correlate with ratings of psychopathology in the expected direction. They report that the variability is increased by unstructured perception, probably as an expression of readiness or search for structures in the input, and that it shows persistent topographic patterns over time in individuals. They theorise that it is "one of several spontaneous oscillatory functions which are diminished in chronic psychosis, perhaps as a consequence of prefrontal malfunction". They believe their results suggest a diminished guiding function by the anterior cortex and a diminished readiness for perception of exogenous structured information in chronic psychosis. Shagass (1976) stated that the amplitude variability results in male chronic schizophrenic patients appear to show hyperarousal in schizophrenic patients compared with normal subjects, but as Lifshitz & Gradijian (1972) found that the greater variability in control subjects was due to more variability in the slow bands, the differences between control subjects and patients might reflect no more than greater tendency for a state shift into drowsiness in the normal subjects. In later reports Shagass and his colleagues (1982, 1984) not only replicated the reduced variability of amplitude in overt schizophrenics, "consistent with a higher than normal level of 'resting' activation", but showed that EEGs of patients with personality disorders suggested lower than normal levels of activation. Further analysis used amplitude, frequency and wave symmetry measures to make useful discriminations between neurotic and personality disordered patients on the one hand and psychotic patients (overtly and latently schizophrenic and manic) on the other; major depressive patients from latent schizophrenic and manic patients, and non-patients from schizophrenic subjects, depressive or manic patients. If these results are confirmed by replication it would appear that a combination of amplitude and frequency variables would be most useful in discrimination of normal, non-psychotic and psychotic individuals. However, it must be emphasised that at the present time there is no characteristic EEG pattern, or frequency or amplitude derived variable, or discriminant function, which has been shown to be diagnostic of schizophrenia.

*Laterality and coherence studies*

Many investigators have studied a variety of EEG parameters to compare left and right sided brain functioning. The methods of frequency and amplitude analysis described above, as well as derived functions such as coherence (which gives a measure of the amount of power in common between two signals from different areas for each frequency, and thus measures the degree of similarity of the signals) and ratios of left/right coherences, to assess relative organisation or disorganisation of function in both sides of the brain, and complex multivariate statistical procedures, applied to all these variables, have resulted in many contradictory findings. It is often hypothesised that the cognitive deficits of schizophrenia are associated with dominant (usually left) hemisphere impairment, while the affective disorders are localised on the nondominant (usually right) side. Serafetinides (1984) reported that even among schizophrenic patients the use of power spectral density analysis could differentiate between patients with 'left' hemisphere symptoms (e.g. thought disorder) who had large amplitude high frequency activity in the left fronto-temporal area and patients with 'right' hemisphere symptoms (e.g. anxiety) who had bilateral activity of this type. Like many other studies in this area, the findings are in great need of replication.

Merrin *et al* (1986) list previous studies by others which show relatively higher left-sided alpha power in schizophrenics than in normals, especially posteriorly; higher right-sided alpha; relative normalisation of anomalous alpha asymmetry by neuroleptic medication; differences in alpha asymmetry between paranoid and hebephrenic schizophrenics; and no differences in alpha asymmetry from controls. They point out that the studies show differences in sample selection, recording techniques, data analysis, medication, and artefact detection and removal. They also pay little attention to the possible effects of differences in ongoing mental state between schizophrenic and normal subjects. Their own study looked at lateral asymmetry of EEG spectra in 10 predominantly unmedicated schizophrenic in-patients and nine normal control subjects performing monitored cognitive tasks during bilateral recording of EEG from parietal and temporal sites. They compared left and right power in five frequency bands between groups, with separate analyses for linked ears and vertex reference. They found that group differences were revealed only with the linked ears reference, showing the previously underappreciated effect of recording montage on spectral values. The schizophrenic group showed relatively less alpha power over the right hemisphere than controls during all conditions, particularly in the parietal leads. After treatment with neuroleptics a subsample of patients were retested and showed a significant shift in alpha, and to a lesser extent theta, towards the control values.

In the amplitude variability domain, Rochford *et al* (1976) studied right/left ratios of variances of the distribution of amplitudes in patients with depression, schizophrenia and personality disorders, finding that in depressive patients the ratio was close to 3.0, with variability much higher on the right; the schizophrenic group of patients showed a ratio of 0.48, with variability on the right about half that on the left, and the other group had a ratio of 0.95. Recordings were made from left and right occipital and temporal leads with vertex reference. The authors found that some patients showed the abnormality to a greater extent temporally and others occipitally, and selected the most deviant value. Etevenon *et al* (1979) confirmed Rochford *et al*'s finding in hebephrenic patients with regard to parieto-occipital derivations but found an opposite ratio for the same patients in more central (rolando-parietal) areas.

Ford *et al* (1986) studied coherence and power variables in attempts to discriminate between four patient groups (those suffering from paranoid schizophrenia; dysthymia; major affective disorders and receiving tricyclics, neuroleptics, or no medication; and geriatric patients). They found that coherence measures, usually in the alpha band, were more sensitive than power measures in differentiating the various groups. Coherence was greatest in the paranoid group, decreased with age and neuroleptic medication and increased with tricyclic antidepressants. Group differences were interpreted in accordance with an arousal model for coherence.

Flor-Henry *et al* (1982) used power spectral analysis and coherence measures to compare depressive psychotic, manic, schizophrenic and normal control subjects, all unmedicated and right-handed. They interpreted their results as suggesting a perturbation of right hemisphere systems in depression, a more profound such disturbance in mania, and left parietal and interhemispheric disorganisation in schizophrenia. Flor-Henry & Koles (1984) reported on a larger series containing the patients of the earlier study. The data now suggested increasing disorganisation of the right hemisphere (least in depression, intermediate in mania and maximal in schizophrenia) together with left hemisphere disorganisation in both mania and schizophrenia, again maximal in schizophrenia.

Although Flor-Henry and his colleagues used complex methods of analysis, they did not edit their EEGs for muscle artefacts. They recognise that this led to increasing myogenic contribution in the faster frequencies, and as there was a trend to increasing left hemisphere energy both parietally and temporally, least in normal subjects, and most in schizophrenic subjects, with increasing frequency, this was interpreted as either left hemisphere activation or asymmetrical activation of temporalis musculature due to increased activation of the motor nucleus of the right trigeminal nerve.

## Conclusion

The best established finding in the early years of EEG in schizophrenia was that these patients have a higher incidence of abnormalities in their records, but as schizophrenia is diagnosed more narrowly, excluding schizo-affectives, schizophreniform disorders, temporal lobe epilepsy and other 'organic' conditions, drug, ECT and insulin effects, fast activity due to muscle artefact (the 'myogenic contribution' mentioned above), and slow activity due to eye movements, the remaining records appear to be at least as normal as those of normal control subjects. They may in fact show very regular, very invariable activity, which is only statistically abnormal, but this may indicate defective homeostasis with sustained hyperactivation (Goldstein & Sugerman, 1969; Flekkøy, 1975) or some associated overactivity of dopaminergic or other catecholamine systems (see discussion in Small, 1983).

Alternatively, the schizophrenic subject's low variability, especially of occipital alpha, with eyes closed, may reflect a lack of attention to outer influences, or a preoccupation with inner fantasy; perhaps Müller *et al*'s diminished readiness to perceive outside structure.

The results of power spectrum and period analysis suggest a greater spread of alpha frequencies, reduced alpha activity and a lower average alpha frequency; also more lower and higher (delta, theta, beta) frequency activity. Laterality and coherence studies are suggestive of left hemisphere disorganisation but a great deal needs to be done with regard to standardisation of research methodology before consistent results can be obtained in this very complex field. The next 50 years may provide enough time for this.

## References

ABRAMS, R. & TAYLOR, M. A. (1976) Catatonia: a prospective study. *Archives of General Psychiatry*, **33**, 579–581.
BARNES, M. P., SAUNDERS, M., WALLS, T. J., SAUNDERS, I. & KIRK, C. A. (1986) The syndrome of Karl Ludwig Kahlbaum. *Journal of Neurology, Neurosurgery & Psychiatry*, **49**, 991–996.

BERGER, H. (1937) On the electroencephalogram of man. Thirteenth report. (Published in *Archiv für Psychiatrie und Nervenkrankheiten*, **106**, 557–584.) In *Hans Berger on the electroencephalograph of man* (ed. P. Gloor) *Electroencephalography and Clinical Neurophysiology*, Suppl. No. 28, 291–297, 1969.

BONKALO, A., LOVETT-DOUST, J. & STOKES, A. M. (1955) Physiological concomitants of the phasic disturbances seen in periodic catatonia. *American Journal of Psychiatry*, **112**, 114–122.

COLONY, H. S. & WILLIS, S. E. (1956) Electroencephalographic studies of 1,000 schizophrenic patients. *American Journal of Psychiatry*, **113**, 163–169.

DAVIS, P. (1940) Evaluation of the electroencephalograms of schizophrenic patients. *American Journal of Psychiatry*, **96**, 851–860.

DROHOCKI, A. (1948) L'intégrateur de l'électroproduction cérébrale pour l'électroencéphalographie quantitative. *Revue Neurologique,* **80**, 619–624.

ETEVENON, P., PIDOUX, B., RIOUX, P., PERON-MAGNON, P., VERDEAUX, G. & DENIKER, P. (1979) Intra- and interhemispheric EEG differences quantified by spectral analysis. *Acta Psychiatrica Scandinavica*, **60**, 57–68.

——, ——, PERON-MAGNON, P., RIOUX, P., VERDEAUX, G. & DENIKER, P. (1982) Computerized EEG in schizophrenia and pharmacopsychiatry. In *Kyoto Symposia (EEG Supplement No 36).* (eds P. A. Buser, W. A. Cobb & T. Okuma). Amsterdam: Elsevier.

FEIGHNER, J. P., ROBINS, E., GUZE, S. B., WOODRUFF, R. A., WINOKUR, G. & MUNOZ, R. (1972) Diagnostic criteria for use in psychiatric research. *Archives of General Psychiatry*, **26**, 57–63.

FINLEY, K. H. & CAMPBELL, C. M. (1941) Electroencephalography in schizophrenia. *American Journal of Psychiatry*, **98**, 374–381.

FLEKKØY, K. (1975) Psychophysiological and neurophysiological aspects of schizophrenia. *Acta Psychiatrica Scandinavica*, **51**, 234–248.

FLOR-HENRY, P. (1976) Lateralized temporal-limbic dysfunction and psychopathology. In *Origins and Evolution of Language and Speech* (eds. S. R. Harnad, J. D. Steklis & J. Lancaster) *Annals of New York Academy of Science*, **280**, 777–797.

—— (1983) Telemetered EEG in schizophrenia. *Journal of Neurology, Neurosurgery and Psychiatry*, **46**, 287.

——, KOLES, Z. J. & TUCKER, D. M. (1982) Studies in EEG power and coherence (8–13 Hz) in depression, mania and schizophrenia compared to controls. *Advances in Biological Psychiatry*, **9**, 1–7.

—— & —— (1984) Statistical quantitative EEG studies of depression, mania, schizophrenia and normals. *Biological Psychiatry*, **19**, 257–279.

FORD, M. R., GOETHE, J. W. & DEKKER, D. K. (1986) EEG coherence and power in the discrimination of psychiatric disorders and medication effects. *Biological Psychiatry*, **21**, 1175–1188.

GIBBS, F. A. (1939) Cortical frequency spectra of schizophrenic, epileptic and normal individuals. *Transactions of American Neurological Association*, **65**, 141–144.

—— & GIBBS, E. L. (1963) The mitten pattern. An electroencephalographic abnormality correlating with psychosis. *Journal of Neuropsychiatry*, **5**, 6–13.

——, —— & LENNOX, W. G. (1938) The likeness of cortical dysrhythmias of schizophrenia and psychomotor epilepsy. *American Journal of Psychiatry*, **95**, 255–269.

GJESSING, L. R., HARDING, G. F. A., JENNER, F. A. & JOHANNESEN, N. B. (1967) The EEG in three cases of periodic catatonia. *British Journal of Psychiatry*, **113**, 1271–1282.

GOLDSTEIN, L., MURPHREE, H. B., SUGERMAN, A. A., PFEIFFER, C. C. & JENNEY, E. H. (1963) Quantitative electroencephalographic analysis of naturally occurring (schizophrenic) and drug-induced psychotic states in human males. *Clinical Pharmacology & Therapeutics*, **4**, 10–21.

——, SUGERMAN, A. A., STOLBERG, H., MURPHREE, H. B. & PFEIFFER, C. C. (1965) Electrocerebral activity in schizophrenic and non-psychotic subjects: quantitative EEG amplitude analysis. *Electroencephalography and Clinical Neurophysiology*, **9**, 350–364.

—— & —— (1969) EEG correlates of psychopathology. In *Neurobiological Aspects of Psychopathology* (eds. J. Zubin & C. Shagass). New York: Grune & Stratton.

GUENTHER, W., BREITLING, D., BANQUET, J. P., MARCIE, P. & RONDOT, P. (1986) EEG mapping of left hemisphere dysfunction during motor performance in schizophrenia. *Biological Psychiatry*, **21**, 249–262.

HILL, D. (1963) The EEG in psychiatry. In *Electroencephalography* (eds. J. D. N. Hill & G. Parr). New York: Macmillan.

IGERT, C. & LAIRY, G. C. (1962) Intérêt pronostique de L'EEG au cours de l'évolution des schizophrènes. *Electroencephalography & Clinical Neurophysiology*, **14**, 183–190.

ITIL, T. M., SALETU, B. & DAVIS, S. (1972) EEG findings in chronic schizophrenics based on digital computer period analysis and analog power spectra. *Biological Psychiatry*, **5**, 1–13.

——, —— & ALLEN, M. (1974) Stability studies in schizophrenics and normals using computer-analyzed EEG. *Biological Psychiatry*, **8**, 321–335.

KARSON, C. N., COPPOLA, R., MORIHISA, J. M. & WEINBERGER, D. R. (1987) Computer electroencephalographic activity mapping in schizophrenia. *Archives of General Psychiatry*, **44**, 514–517.

KELLAWAY, P. (1979) An orderly approach to visual analysis: the parameters of the normal EEG in adults and children. In *Current Practice of Clinical Electroencephalography* (eds. D. W. Klass & D. D. Daly). New York: Raven Press.

KENNARD, M. A. & SCHWARTZMAN, A. F. (1957) A longitudinal study of electroencephalographic frequency patterns in mental hospital patients and normal controls. *Electroencephalography and Clinical Neurophysiology*, **9**, 263–274.

LANGFELDT, G. (1937) Prognosis in schizophrenia and factors influencing the course of the disease. *Acta Psychiatrica Neurologica Scandinavica*, **13**, 1–228.

LEMERE, F. (1936) The significance of individual differences in the Berger rhythm. *Brain*, **59**, 366–375.

—— (1938) Effects on electroencephalogram of various agents used in treating schizophrenia. *Journal of Neurophysiology*, **1**, 590–595.

LIFSHITZ, K. & GRADIJIAN, J. (1972) Relationships between measures of the coefficient of variation of the mean absolute EEG voltage and spectral intensities in schizophrenic and control subjects. *Biological Psychiatry*, **5**, 149–163.

MERRIN, E. L., FEIN, G., FLOYD, T. C. & YINGLING, C. D. (1986) EEG asymmetry in schizophrenic patients before and during neuroleptic treatment. *Biological Psychiatry*, **21**, 455–464.

MORIHISA, J. M., DUFFY, F. H. & WYATT, R. J. (1983) Brain electrical activity mapping (BEAM) in schizophrenic patients. *Archives of General Psychiatry*, **40**, 719–728.

MORSTYN, R., DUFFY, F. H., MCCARLEY, R. W. (1983) Altered topography of EEG spectral content in schizophrenia. *Electroencephalography & Clinical Neurophysiology*, **56**, 263–271.

MULLER, H. F., ACHIM, A., LAUR, A. & BUCHBINDER, A. (1986) Topography and possible physiological significance of EEG amplitude variability in psychosis. *Acta Psychiatrica Scandinavica*, **73**, 665–675.

NEWMAN, H. W. (1938) Electroencephalography. *American Journal of Medical Science*, **196**, 882–887.

NEWMAN, H. W. & LAWRENCE, R. (1952) The electroencephalogram in functional psychiatric disorders. *Stanford Medical Bulletin*, **10**, 76–77.

PHILLIPS, L. (1953) Case history data and prognosis in schizophrenia. *Journal of Nervous and Mental Disease*, **117**, 515–525.

ROCHFORD, J. M., SWARTZBURG, M., CHOWDHREY, S. M. & GOLDSTEIN, L. (1976) Some quantitative EEG correlates of psychopathology. *Research Communications in Psychology, Psychiatry and Behavior*, **1**, 211–226.

SERAFETINIDES, E. A. (1984) EEG lateral asymmetries in psychiatric disorders. *Biological Psychiatry*, **19**, 237–246.

SHAGASS, C. (1976) An electrophysiological view of schizophrenia. *Biological Psychiatry*, **11**, 3–30.

——, ROEMER, R. A. & STRAUMANIS, J. J. (1982) Relationships between psychiatric diagnosis and some quantitative EEG variables. *Archives of General Psychiatry*, **39**, 1423–1435.

——, ——, —— & JOSIASSEN, R. C. (1984) Psychiatric diagnostic discriminations with combinations of quantitative EEG variables. *British Journal of Psychiatry*, **114**, 581–592.

SHAW, J. C., BROOKS, S., COULTER, N. & O'CONNOR, K. P. (1979) A comparison for schizophrenic and neurotic patients using EEG power and coherence spectra. In *Hemisphere Asymmetries of Function in Psychopathology* (eds. J. H. Gruzelier & P. Flor-Henry). Amsterdam: Elsevier/North Holland.

SMALL, J. G. (1983) EEG in schizophrenia. In *EEG and Evoked Potentials in Psychiatry and Behavioral Neurology* (eds. J. R. Hughes & W. P. Wilson). London: Butterworths.

—— & SMALL, I. F. (1965) Re-evaluation of clinical EEG findings in schizophrenia. *Diseases of the Nervous System*, **26**, 345–349.

——, MILSTEIN, V., SHARPLEY, P. H., KLAPPER, M. & SMALL, I. F. (1984) Electro—encephalographic findings in relation to diagnostic constructs in psychiatry. *Biological Psychiatry*, **19**, 471–487.

STEVENS, J. R. & LIVERMORE, A. (1982) Telemetered EEG in schizophrenia: spectral analysis during abnormal behaviour episodes. *Journal of Neurology, Neurosurgery and Psychiatry*, **45**, 385–395.

—— (1983) Telemetered EEG in schizophrenia [reply to Flor-Henry]. *Journal of Neurology, Neurosurgery and Psychiatry*, **46**, 287–288.

SUGERMAN, A. A., GOLDSTEIN, L., MURPHREE, H. B., PFEIFFER, C. C. & JENNEY, E. H. (1964) EEG and behavioral changes in schizophrenia. *Archives of General Psychiatry*, **10**, 340–344.

WITTMAN, P. (1941) Scale for measuring prognosis in schizophrenia. *Elgin Papers*, **4**, 20–33.

# 39 Clear consciousness and the diagnosis of schizophrenia: An irreconcilable problem?

**MALCOLM P. I. WELLER**

Most diagnostic schemes take pains to differentiate schizophrenia, a 'functional' illness, from toxic confusional psychosis. Attempts are made to exclude organic conditions by stipulating that the hallucinations, delusions and thought disorder of schizophrenia must occur in clear consciousness. Since we do not know the aetiology of schizophrenia it seems inappropriate to exclude cases where we believe that there is an organic explanation.

---

Despite the diagnostic requirements that clouded consciousness is incompatible with a diagnosis of schizophrenia, there are many examples of such schizophrenic psychoses which appear to fit the criteria for clouding of consciousness specified by Engel & Romano (1959), Slater & Roth (1969) and Lipowsky (1980, see appendix). This is hardly surprising having regard to the growing evidence for organic disturbances in schizophrenia, but constitutes a diagnostic impropriety that seems inescapable.

## *The organic–functional dichotomy*

In order to distinguish schizophrenic phenomena from delirium, twilight states and intoxication, Schneider (1957) asserts that if a first rank symptom occurs "*in a non-organic psychosis* then we call that psychosis schizophrenia" (author's italics). He lists a number of somatic factors which lead to clouded consciousness, such as an acute response to intoxications, GPI and other infections and internal disorders (p 2). The Registrar-General's (1968) *Glossary of Mental Disorders* specifies the need for clear consciousness in the assessment of those symptoms which form the basis for a diagnosis of schizophrenia. One of the intentions for invoking the term 'clear consciousness' is to distinguish schizophrenia from delirium, toxic psychosis and abnormal states of consciousness, such as hypnogogic and hypnopompic experiences, but it begs important questions. Aetiological theories of schizophrenia include: auto-intoxication, biochemical abnormalities, synaptic receptor abnormalities, traumatic brain damage, epilepsy, epileptic kindling and viral infections. If an organic explanation, such as one of the above, is confirmed, at least for some patients, is it likely that consciousness is indeed clear? Is it not equally plausible that the psychotic experiences are manifestations of disordered brain mechanisms, postulated by Kraepelin (1920) as the source of the disorder, and that some disturbance of consciousness is an inevitable and central component of the experiences?

Roth & McClelland (1979), in accord with Ferraro (1943), considered schizophrenia to be a phenomenological rather than a neurological entity, and repudiated Schneider's view that "the presence of a coarse brain disease excludes all other kinds of diagnosis"; they take the contrary view that, "As its (schizophrenia's) aetiological basis, the hereditary factors apart, is not understood, it is illogical and circular to exclude cases with associated organic lesions from the outset".

The problem may be more deeply ingrained than appears at first sight. Roth & McClelland implied that there is a substantial group of schizophrenic patients who are excluded from their discussion because they display organic phenomena. It is the burden of this paper to stress that organic psychological phenomena are common in schizophrenic patients, an observation that is reinforced by evidence of brain lesions or malfunction, but that either this knowledge is suppressed to accommodate the requirement that consciousness should be clear in the definition of the disorder, or the clinical examination is insufficiently searching to reveal the clouding which is identified in the research literature.

The situation is inconsistent and relaxation of the exclusion of clouded consciousness is explicitly countenanced in the case of acute schizophrenic episodes, which are described in the ninth edition of the *International Classification of Diseases* as often being characterised by "a dream-like state with slight clouding". (There is a further problem here in the implicit assumption that we can prospectively differentiate between acute and chronic conditions on the basis of the history and phenomenology.)

## *The problems of detection of clouded consciousness*

The vigour with which we pursue investigations depends on our preconceptions. Leff (1977) has pointed out that in documenting a psychiatric interview, the importance attached to the phenomena is largely determined by the psychiatrist's theoretical frame of reference. When we are alert to the presence of a physical illness, as in a fever, it is not difficult to detect clouding of consciousness and natural to attribute the clouding to the illness. On the other hand, in the case of an occult physical illness accompanied by slight clouding, we may fail to detect the clouding for want of repeated, careful observations. Even if detected the cause of the clouding may remain obscure. "In investigating the possible cause of the delirious state, it must be remembered that when associated with an acute infection, such as pneumonia, the condition may not start until the convalescent stage, perhaps one or two weeks after the febrile illness has subsided. Careful history-taking is therefore essential if some specific cause is not to be over-looked". (Slater & Roth, 1969, p. 602.)

Is such a cause being overlooked when Kraepelin (1920) asserts (p. 19), "Delirious states may appear under extremely varied conditions, not only as a result of toxic substances or infection, as in fever of brain injury, but also in epilepsy, general paresis, manic depressive insanity, dementia praecox, . . .".

This association between delirium and psychosis is implied in the description of acute schizophrenic episodes in the ninth edition of the *International Classification of Diseases*, already discussed, as often being characterised by "a dream-like state with slight clouding of consciousness and perplexity".

## Similarities between delirium and the cognitive impairments of schizophrenia

Two statements describing clouded consciousness taken from Slater & Roth (1969) demonstrate the close similarity between this state and schizophrenia.

> "Conceptual thinking (in clouded consciousness) breaks down and becomes cluttered with incoherent and fragmentary matter, often visualised and taking on an hallucinatory or delusional quality. Even the self and the environment are incompletely differentiated". (p. 347)

> "An increase in suspiciousness, and the occurrence of delusional ideas is a feature of importance. These experiences may occur with suddenness and conviction, *in a form indistinguishable from the primary delusional experience*, in states of clouding so mild as to be unrecognisable as such". (p. 348) (my italics).

Kraepelin (1919) stated that, "[dementia praecox] patients complain frequently of passing dullness of consciousness which should probably be regarded as a condition of very slight stupor." (p. 17). Romano & Engel (1944) considered the corollary, "essentially, delirium is a psychotic syndrome in which the basic psychologic symptom is a disturbance in the level of consciousness . . .". As Lipowski (1980) points out in his monograph on delirium, it may be doubtful whether a patient is suffering from delirium "rather than from one of the functional psychoses . . . Acute schizophrenia, schizophreniform, or atypical psychosis is particularly likely to give rise to diagnostic difficulties" (p. 210).

In Table I defining characteristics of clouding of consciousness, as described by Slater & Roth (1969), are contrasted with statements in the literature on schizophrenia to illustrate how commonly clouding occurs, despite the fact that clouding of consciousness is an exclusion criterion for diagnosis (Registrar-General, 1968).

## Nocturnal deterioration

In addition to these features, and in accord with Lipowski (1980), Slater & Roth mention fluctuations in the intensity of clouding of consciousness, with a tendency for it to become much more prominent at night. In order to differentiate 'true' schizophrenic phenomena from hypnogogic and hypnopompic experiences little regard is paid to experiences which occur in bed at night. Nevertheless, patients frequently report such experiences, particularly haptic ones of being touched or given electric shocks, and others describe an intensification of daytime auditory hallucinations. These features are so commonly encountered in clinical practice that it is difficult to find them specifically mentioned in contemporary accounts, but in the words of one early author describing a schizophrenic patient,

TABLE I

| States of clouded consciousness (Slater & Roth, 1969) | Quotations from the literature on schizophrenia |
| --- | --- |
| "The patient has difficulty in maintaining attention." | "It is our contention that many of the behavioural deficits seen in the schizophrenic can be accounted for by a primary attentional disorder." (Kornetsky & Orzack, 1978) |
| "He tends to be easily distracted." | "Thinking becomes distracted by external events. It also becomes distracted by irrelevant personal thoughts and emotions which may even become mixed up with the problem." (Payne, 1964) |
| "He cannot dismiss from his mind the irrelevant sensory experience or the irrelevant idea." | "Schizophrenics have difficulty in maintaining a perceptual set and in concentrating on part of the perceptual field to the exclusion of other parts . . . these patients are less capable of shutting off information which is irrelevant to the task in hand." (Weckowicz & Witney, 1960) |
| "Perception is affected so that sense data are misjudged" | "In early phases of their illness, schizophrenic patients, together with difficulty in thinking, such as an inability to concentrate and to control their thoughts, may experience perceptual difficulty and may even complain of an impairment of vision." (Weckowicz, 1960) |
| | ". . . distance constancy is poorer in schizophrenics than in non-schizophrenics and also . . . related to the poorer size constancy found in these patients . . . The lack of depth and 'flatness' of the visual world of schizophrenics has theoretical implications for the phenomenology of schizophrenia. Together with impaired form constancy it can change, foreshorten and distort the appearance of the perceived objects. Perhaps this change in depth perception would account for the complaint of some schizophrenics that things look different, unfamiliar and strange . . ." (Weckowicz, Sommer & Hall, 1958) |
| "Illusions, especially visual illusions . . . are very much more likely to arise than in the normal state . . ." | "Schizophrenics are more susceptible to the Muller-Lyer illusion than non-schizophrenics." (Weckowicz & Witney, 1960) |
| "There are corresponding difficulties in comprehension shown at first only at the highest and most abstract level." | "Some investigators [Cameron (1939), Vigotsky (1934), Kasanin *et al* (1944)] have, on the basis of cognitive testing, concluded that the schizophrenic is unable to form the abstractions necessary for normal thinking in much the same manner in which the patient with organic brain defect is unable to deal with abstractions." (Freeman, Cameron & McGhie, 1958) |
| "Called on to respond to a complex situation, the patient is likely to be slow." | "Although complete diagnostic specificity is lacking, there seems to be a remarkable correlation between . . . reaction time phenomena and those behaviours that lead diagnosticians at many different times and places to a diagnosis of schizophrenia." (Zahn, 1977) |
| ". . . and to show some perseveration in thought and speech" | "The tendency toward stereotyping, combined with a lack of purposeful goal in their thinking, leads on the one hand to 'Klebendenken' (adhesive, sticky type of thinking), to a kind of *perseveration*, and on the other hand to a general impoverishment of thought." (Bleuler, 1911, p. 27) |
| | "We frequently observe written verbigeration in random repetition of words and sentences, and particularly of single letter and punctuation marks, either in a characteristic pattern or mixed with crosses, circles, triangles and other figures. For many years a hebephrenic always wrote the same row of numbers whose zeros were always continued to the end of each line." (Bleuler, 1911, p. 159) |

Table I (continued)

| | |
|---|---|
| "Judgements also will be less balanced and less adequate" | ". . . the weakening of judgement . . . would have to be reckoned among the fundamental disorders of dementia praecox." (Kraepelin, 1919, p. 248) |
| "Gestalts are not sharply circumscribed and finely differentiated; figure-background differentiation is blurred, and is much less open to goal directed action." | "Selective perception becomes impossible so that instead of dealing with the essence of the problem irrelevant aspects are perceived and thought about . . ." (Payne, 1964) |
| "The difficulties in attention, comprehension etc., can be described as difficulties in raising the figure from the background, in maintaining it against disturbing forces arising from the background and in manipulating it." | "these irrelevant associations to which the normal is also subject but to a much lesser degree would appear to arise from three sources: chance distractors from the environment; irrelevancies from the stimulus situation; and irrelevancies from past experience . . . the mere presence of these irrelevant factors . . . seems to lead the schizophrenic to give them focal rather than ground significance, signal rather than noise import" (Shakow, 1962). |

"he continued, however, to suffer much from noise in his ears, hearing voices, etc., especially at night" (Rorie, 1862–63). The abnormal nighttime experiences occurring without any such daytime experiences probably represent an incipient phase when psychotic phenomena, like epileptic and delirious phenomena, are highlighted.

## Memory

Memory disturbance is stressed by Slater & Roth (1969) as an indication of clouded consciousness. Subcortical neurones in the hippocampus and caudate nucleus compare stimuli and respond to novelty, and are therefore part of the mechanism of memory (see Luria, 1973 and Buchwald & Humphrey, 1973 for reviews, including the important Russian literature) and structural abnormalities have been found in the hippocampi and caudate nuclei of schizophrenic patients (Davison & Bagley, 1969; Roberts *et al*, 1984; Roberts, 1988).

Memory disturbances are common in schizophrenia, including delusional memories. The imagined events are often intensely significant and the false memory may become the basis of paranoid misinterpretation.

Dodge (1924), in an interesting article entitled 'Problems of human variability', wrote: "Variations are not artifacts to be statistically lumped and treated as though they were errors of measurement, but they represent features which might well be quite as significant as the conscious aim of measurement in which they occurred". The variability of the schizophrenic patient's performance on test procedures is notorious and any group of schizophrenic patients seemingly inevitably vary more than non-psychiatric control subjects. I believe one would expect just such variability in a brain-damaged group. In the World Health Organization's international pilot study of schizophrenia, the test–retest reliability had a mean intra-class correlation coefficient of only 0.49 (Hays, 1967). Since the patients were describing the same illness episode to trained observers, who used the same structured interview with which the inter-observer reliability averaged 0.83, the memory and reporting of the illness episode must have varied over the few days between the two interviews.

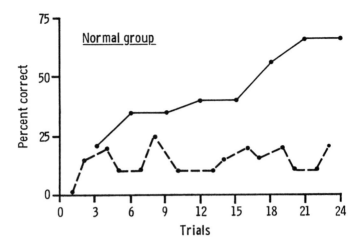

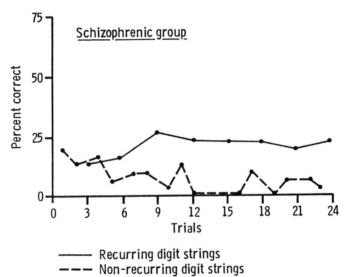

Fig. 1. *Comparison of performances of control subjects and schizophrenic patients on the Hebb recurring-digits test*

This well authenticated example of recent memory disturbance cannot be easily disregarded.

There is no evidence of a temporal gradient to memories in schizophrenia, such as occurs in non-psychiatric patients, whereby the more recent memories are stronger than the more distant (Calev *et al*, 1987) and unmedicated, as well as medicated, schizophrenic patients rapidly forget verbal material (Calev *et al*, 1987).

A defect of cumulative memory in schizophrenia has been demonstrated experimentally (Kugler & Weller, 1983). In this study a chain of digits, exceeding the subject's memory capacity, was repeated seven times alternatively with two novel chains. Control subjects, matched for initial digit span, improved their performance steadily and significantly on the repeated chain, while schizophrenic patients did not (Fig. 1). This pattern of results is consonant with left hippocampal damage (Corsi, 1967), the deficits being proportional to the extent of the hippocampal damage.

## Orientation

Memory defects may account for some of the temporal disorientation in schizophrenia. Stevens *et al* (1978), supplementing the work of Crow & Mitchell (1975), found that 25% of 357 patients with a consistent case-note diagnosis of schizophrenia underestimated their age by more than five years; 11% underestimated their age by a mean of 28.9 years. The phenomenon was associated with early onset and a poor prognosis. Six further studies were reviewed with similar findings; Crow & Stevens (1978) went on to demonstrate what they believed was a "continuum of increasing temporal disorientation" which was associated with age disorientation.

The phenomenon of 'double orientation', admittedly of person rather than of place, is considered characteristic of schizophrenia and actually facilitated by clear consciousness (Slater & Roth, 1969, p. 276), although these authors also stated that a "co-existence of two or more totally incompatible orientations" is a feature of clouding of consciousness (Slater & Roth, 1969, p. 602). One patient treated by the author thought it was afternoon although he agreed that the clock told the right time (11 a. m.) and that he had not yet had his lunch (he has subsequently remained unwell for six years).

## Perception

Many perceptual abnormalities have been described in schizophrenic patients, including phoneme recognition (Caudrey & Kirk, 1979), auditory acuity with normal otology and tympanography (Burtt & Weller, 1984), stereognosis under bimanual conditions (Beaumont & Dimond, 1973; Green, 1978) and unimanually (Weller & Kugler, 1979) and size and distance constancy (Weckowicz, 1957; Weckowicz, Sommer & Hall, 1958).

## Schizophrenic symptoms as a product of brain malfunction and the probability of altered consciousness

We must be sensitive to even slight indications of perceptual and cognitive impairment such as disorientation, since gross insults to the brain may result in only subtle changes, requiring careful testing and evaluation. Indubitable and substantial changes occur in cerebral function in advanced hydrocephalus, sub-total hemispherectomy and callosectomy yet such conditions betray nothing more than subtle changes in perception and cognition, advanced hydrocephalus being compatible with high intelligence (Lewin, 1981), and do not produce any obvious changes in consciousness. From the examples just cited, one may conclude that gross changes in cerebral functioning will not necessarily lead to obvious changes in the level of consciousness, and if there *is* evidence of clouding of consciousness it therefore probably implies marked alterations in brain functioning.

## Subcortical abnormalities

Malfunctions of subcortical structures, particularly the basal ganglia and mid-brain, are particularly liable to cause disturbances of consciousness (Reichardt, 1929; Jefferson, 1944; Penfield & Jasper, 1947; Cairns, 1952) and there is a concept of subcortical dementia (see Foster, 1986). So-called schizophreniform psychoses have been associated with many different disease processes affecting the basal ganglia (see Davison & Bagley, 1969), including post-encephalitic psychosis (Fairweather, 1947), hepatolenticular degeneration (Beard, 1959), Huntington's chorea (Heathfield, 1967) and calcification of the basal ganglia (Kasanin & Crank, 1935; see Cummings *et al*, 1983), which may include the striopallidodentate system (Lowenthal & Bruyn, 1968) and the cerebellum (Kalamboukis & Molling, 1962).

Cerebellar dysfunction, disorders of equilibrium, staggering, adiadochokinesia, and tremor had been noted in schizophrenic patients before the introduction of phenothiazines (Dufour, cited by Kraepelin, 1919, p. 79) and tapping speed is slow in schizophrenia (Weller *et al*, 1988). The anterior cerebellar vermis has been found to be atrophic in some schizophrenic patients on CAT scans (Weinberger *et al*, 1979, 1981; Reider *et al*, 1981). The frequency is variable but reached 40% (34 out of 85 patients) in one study (Heath, Franklin & Shraberg, 1979). Recent animal experiments have shown that this structure is essential for long-term habituation (Leaton & Supple, 1986). Although this recent finding was unknown to the anatomical workers, in accord with the general theme adopted here Heath, Franklin & Shraberg were clearly impressed by the brain pathology in a population allegedly suffering from a functional psychiatric disorder and entitled their paper 'Gross pathology of the cerebellum in patients diagnosed and treated as functional psychiatric disorders'.

Corpus callosal degeneration with demyelination and subsequent cavitation, and destruction of central axis cylinders in the Marchiafava–Bignami syndrome is associated with psychosis (Marchiafava, 1932–33; Ironside, Bosenquet & McMenemy, 1961; Victor & Adams, 1961). The syndrome usually occurs in alcoholics, but can occur with accompanying psychosis without alcohol consumption (Nielsen, 1958). Anatomical evidence of abnormalities of the corpus callosum have been alleged in some schizophrenic patients (Bigelow, Nasrallah & Rauscher, 1983) and defects of stereognosis have been shown, suggestive of defects of corpus callosal function (Beaumont & Dimond, 1973; Green, Glass & O'Callaghan, 1979; Weller & Kugler, 1979).

Abnormalities of limbic neurones have been found in young schizophrenic patients whose brains were examined post mortem (Averback, 1981a and b). The youth of the patients made it unlikely that these abnormalities represented senile degenerative changes. More recently an abnormal cellular architecture has been found in the alpha and pre-beta layers of the parahippocampal/entorhinal cortex (Roberts, 1988).

Neurotransmitter and neuromodulator differences have been found in limbic structures of schizophrenic brains examined at post-mortem. An abnormal asymmetry of dopamine has been found in the amygdalae of post-mortem schizophrenic brains (Reynolds, 1983) (although this may also occur in depression; see Weller, 1986b), and peptide abnormalities have been found in the hippocampus and amygdala (Roberts *et al*, 1984).

The abnormalities of oculo-motor control (Holzman, Proctor & Hughes, 1973; Latham *et al*, 1981) are further examples of subcortical malfunction.

## Electrophysiological abnormalities

Consonant with the pathological findings, several neurophysiological abnormalities have been found in schizophrenic subjects which are interpreted as indicative of limbic malfunction. These include orienting response abnormalities (Gruzelier & Venables, 1972; Gruzelier *et al*, 1981), which are particularly evident in those patients who respond poorly to treatment (Frith *et al*, 1978; Zahn *et al*, 1981) and illustrate a fundamental defect in the attentive mechanisms.

Using indwelling electrodes, abnormal discharges have been recorded from the septal nuclei in schizophrenic patients, and the onset and offset of these correlated with psychotic experiences and behaviour (Heath, 1966). Such discharges could also be induced by low frequency stimulation of the hippocampus at 3–6 Hz, the same frequencies that showed excessive synchronous activity from temporal EEG derivations (Weller & Montagu, 1979). When the recording abnormality appeared, the patients showed what Heath (1966) described as "classical psychotic symptoms", and in an interesting aside, he remarks, "after recovering from the effects of stimulation, (the patients) described the experience as dream-like".

## Electroencephalographic findings

Lipowski (1980, p. 41, see Appendix) influenced by the findings of Engel & Romano (1959), points out that in delirium slow waves are more prominent in the electroencephalogram. Statistical analysis of the EEG recordings from schizophrenic subjects has shown an excess of slow wave activity (Coger, Dymond & Serafetinides, 1979; Weller & Montagu, 1979; Fenton *et al*, 1980) and an increase in the degree of synchrony between certain brain regions (Flor-Henry & Yeudall, 1979; Weller & Montagu, 1979). Bilateral spikes and waves and paroxysmal slow wave activity have been described in non-epileptic schizophrenic patients (Hill & Parr, 1963). Non-specific EEG abnormalities are detected in many psychiatric conditions, but, since they occur in a proportion of non-psychiatric patients, they do not have diagnostic implications. Nevertheless, the frequency of such abnormalities is greater among abnormal personalities (Schwade & Geiger, 1956; Hill, 1963) and borderline psychotic conditions are probably more frequent in this group (Hoch & Polatin, 1949).

## Cerebral insufficiency

Engel & Romano (1959) consider that delirium is "a syndrome of cerebral insufficiency", which takes its origin from changes in the functional metabolism of cerebral neurones. "As with the more familiar concepts of organ insufficiency, this refers to what evolves when the function of the organ as a whole is interfered with, for whatever reason". The metabolic rate and blood flow are lower in the frontal area in schizophrenia in all but one study, when there was a generalised reduction in metabolic activity (see Buchsbaum & Ingvar, 1982, for experiments and review; DeLisi *et al*, 1985; Weinberger, Berman & Zec, 1986).

## Conclusion

Differences between psychotic states and clouded consciousness are clearly difficult to demonstrate. This conclusion corresponds to Kraepelin's (1920, p. 19) position: "There is a strong argument for classifying delirium as one of those forms of psychiatric disorder which are based on primarily mental reactions. It takes the place of orderly, clear, conscious thought, as soon as consciousness becomes clouded under the influence of any morbid process. It is not surprising that the particular form which delirium takes may be partly determined by the nature of the morbid process in question, as well as by the patient's own previous history."

From the many examples that have been cited, it is difficult to escape the conclusion that at least subtle examples of clouded consciousness can be detected in many schizophrenic patients. This would accord with organic explanations for at least a sub-group of patients, and reinforces the arguments of Ferraro (1943) and Roth & McClelland (1979), who challenge Schneider's (1957) view that "the presence of coarse brain disease excludes all other kind of diagnosis". There is no unequivocal diagnostic test of schizophrenia analogous to diagnostic tests in physical medicine. In the end one is reliant on the presenting phenomena, the previous history and clinical judgement. The desirability of excluding cases where there is a presumed organic aetiology inevitably results in an idiopathic group, in which the hope of finding a specific locus, or loci, of lesions causing the symptoms is diminished. It also creates a further group for whom there is no suitable diagnostic category. In any event, organic features are so readily demonstrated in so many patients diagnosed as schizophrenic that attempts to exclude organic cases, and to sieve out a 'functional' disorder, are doomed to failure from the outset. The conviction of Kraepelin that organic explanations for dementia praecox would ultimately be demonstrated is vindicated by the phenomenological features of clouded consciousness which are so obviously apparent in so many patients allegedly suffering from schizophrenia—despite the fact that none of them is schizophrenic if the diagnostic requirement of clear consciousness is rigorously enforced.

## Acknowledgements

I thank the Wellcome Trust, the North East Thames Regional Health Authority, and the National Schizophrenia Fellowship for grants for the experimental work discussed in this paper, Dr K. Davison for helpful comments, and Friern Hospital and the Royal Society of Medicine for library assistance. An earlier formulation of the problem was first expressed in 'Some problems in the diagnosis of schizophrenia and the problems of clear consciousness' in *Aspects of Consciousness*, vol. 4 (ed. R. Stevens, Academic Press, 1984).

# References

AVERBACK, P. (1981a) Lesions of the nucleus ansae peduncularis in neuropsychiatric disease. *Archives of Neurology*, **38**, 230–235.
—— (1981b) Structural lesions of the brain in young schizophrenics. *Canadian Journal of Neurological Science*, **8**, 73–76.
BEARD, A. E. (1959) The association of hepato-lenticular degeneration with schizophrenia. *Acta Psychiatrica et Neurologica Scandinavica*, **34**, 411–428.
BEAUMONT, J. G. & DIMOND, S. J. (1973) Brain disconnection and schizophrenia. *British Journal of Psychiatry*, **123**, 661–662.
BIGELOW, L. B., NASRALLAH, H. M. A. & RAUSCHER, P. R. (1983) Corpus callosum thickness in chronic schizophrenia. *British Journal of Psychiatry*, **142**, 284–287.
BLEULER, E. (1911) *Dementia praecox or The Group of Schizophrenias*. Translated 1950, J. Zinkin and N. C. D. Lewis. New York: International Universities Press.
BUCHSBAUM, M. S. & INGVAR, D. H. (1982) New visions in the schizophrenic brain: regional differences in electrophysiology, blood flow and cerebral glucose use. In *Schizophrenia as a brain disease* (eds F. A. Henn & H. A. Nasrallah). New York and Oxford: Oxford University Press.
BUCHWALD, J. S. & HUMPHREY, G. L. (1973) An analysis of habituation in the specific sensory systems. In *Progress in Physiological Psychology* vol. 5 (eds E. Stellar & J. M. Sprague). New York and London: Academic Press. pp. 1–76.
BURTT, C. & WELLER, M. P. I. (1984) Diminished auditory acuity in schizophrenia. *Journal of Physiology*, **351**, 20.
CAIRNS, H. (1952) Disturbances of consciousness with lesions of the brain-stem and diencephalon. Victor Horsley Memorial Lecture, December 8, 1949. *Brain*, **75**, 8–146.
CALEV, A., BERLIN, H. & LERE, B. (1987) Remote and recent memory in long-hospitalized chronic schizophrenics. *Biological Psychiatry*, **22**, 79–85.
CAUDREY, D. J. & KIRK, K. (1979) *The perception of speech in schizophrenia and affective disorder*. In *Hemisphere Asymmetries of Function and Psychopathology* (eds J. Gruzelier & P. Flor-Henry). North Holland: Elsevier. pp. 581–601.
COGER, R. W., DYMOND, A. M. & SERAFETINIDES, E. A. (1979) Electroencephalographic similarities between chronic alcoholics and chronic, non-paranoid schizophrenics. *Archives of General Psychiatry*, **36**, 91–94.
CORSI, P. M. (1967) Unpublished MA thesis, McGill University, Montreal; reported in Milner, B. (1971) Interhemispheric differences in localisation of psychological processes in man. *British Medical Bulletin*, **27**, 272–277.
CROW, T. J. & MITCHELL, W. S. (1975) Subjective age in chronic schizophrenia: evidence for a sub-group of patients with defective learning capacity. *British Journal of Psychiatry*, **126**, 360–363.
—— & STEVENS, M. (1978) Age distortion in chronic schizophrenia: the nature of the cognitive defect. *British Journal of Psychiatry*, **133**, 137–142.
CUMMINGS, J. L., GOSENFELD, L. F., HOULIHAN, J. P. & McCAFFREY, T. (1983) Neuropsychiatric disturbances associated with idiopathic calcification of the basal ganglia. *Biological Psychiatry*, **18**, 591–601.
DAVISON, K. & BAGLEY, C. (1969) Schizophrenia-like psychoses associated with organic disorders of the CNS: A review of the literature. In *Current Problems in Neuropsychiatry* (ed. R. N. Herrington). British Journal of Psychiatry Special Publication No. 4, p. 113. Ashford, Kent: Headley Bros.
DeLISI, L. E., BUCHSBAUM, M. S., HOLCOMB, H. H., DOWLING-ZIMMERMAN, S., PICKAR, D. *et al* (1985) Clinical correlates of decreased antero-posterior metabolic gradients in positron emission tomography (PET) of schizophrenic patients. *American Journal of Psychiatry*, **142**, 78–81.
DODGE, R. (1924) Human variability. *Science*, **59**, 263.
ENGEL, G. L. & ROMANO, J. (1944) Delirium II Reversibility of the electroencephalogram with experimental procedures. *AMA Archives of Neurology and Psychiatry*, **51**, 378–392.
—— & —— (1959) Delirium, a syndrome of cerebral insufficiency. *Journal of Chronic Diseases*, **9**, 260–277.

FAIRWEATHER, D. S. (1947) Psychiatric aspects of the post encephalitis syndrome. *Journal of Mental Science*, **93**, 201-254.

FENTON, G. W., FENWICK, P. B. C., DOLLIMORE, J., DUNN, T. L. & HIRSCH, S. R. (1980) EEG spectral analysis in schizophrenia. *British Journal of Psychiatry*, **136**, 445-455.

FERRARO, A. (1934) Histopathological findings in two cases clinically diagnosed dementia praecox. *American Journal of Psychiatry*, **90**, 883-903.

—— (1943) Pathological changes in the brain of a case clinically diagnosed dementia praecox. *Journal of Neuropathology and Experimental Neurology*, **2**, 84-94.

FLOR-HENRY, P. & YEUDALL, L. T. (1979) Neuropsychological investigation of schizophrenia and manic-depressive psychoses. In *Hemisphere Asymmetries of Function in Psychopathology* (eds. J. Gruzelier & P. Flor-Henry). North Holland: Elsevier. pp. 341-362.

FOSTER, J. B. (1986) Subcortical dementia. Leader, *British Medical Journal*, **292**, 1035-6.

FREEMAN, T., CAMERON, J. L. & MCGHIE, A. (1958) *Chronic Schizophrenia*. London: Tavistock Publications.

FRITH, C. D., STEVENS, M., JOHNSTONE, E. C. & CROW, T. J. (1978) Skin conductance responsivity during acute episodes of schizophrenia as a predictor of symptomatic improvement. *Psychological Medicine*, **9**, 101-106.

GREEN, P. (1978) Interhemispheric transfer in schizophrenia: recent developments. *Behavioural Psychotherapy*, **6**, 105-110.

——, GLASS, A. & O'CALLAGHAN, M. A. J. (1979) Some implications of abnormal hemisphere interaction in schizophrenia. In *Hemisphere Asymmetries of Function and Psychopathology*. (eds. J. H. Gruzelier & P. Flor-Henry) Amsterdam: Elsevier/North Holland Biochemical Press. pp. 431-448.

GRUZELIER, J. H. & VENABLES, P. H. (1972) Skin conductance orienting activity in a heterogenous sample of schizophrenics: possible evidence of limbic dysfunction. *Journal of Nervous and Mental Disease*, **155**, 277-287.

——, CONNOLLY, J., EVES, F., HIRSCH, S. R., WELLER, M. P. I. & YORKSTON, M. (1981) Effects of propranolol and phenothiazines on electrodermal orienting and habituation in schizophrenia. *Psychological Medicine*, **11**, 93-188.

HAYS, W. L. (1967) *Statistics for Psychologists*. New York: Brooks-Cole.

HEATH, R. G. (1966) Schizophrenia: biochemical and physiologic aberrations. *International Journal of Neuropsychiatry*, **2**, 597-610.

——, FRANKLIN, D. E. & SHRABERG, D. (1979) Gross pathology of the cerebellum in patients diagnosed and treated as functional psychiatric disorders. *Journal of Nervous and Mental Disease*, **167**, 585-592.

HEATHFIELD, K. W. G. (1967) Huntington's chorea. Investigations into the prevalence of this disease in the area covered by the North East Metropolitan Regional Hospital Board. *Brain*, **90**, 203-232.

HILL, D. (1963) The EEG in psychiatry. In *Electroencephalography* (eds. D. Hill & G. Parr). London: Macdonald. p. 368.

—— & PARR, G. (1963) *Electroencephalography*, 2nd edn. A symposium of various aspects. London: Macdonald.

HOCH, P. & POLATIN, P. (1949) Pseudoneurotic forms of schizophrenia. *Psychiatric Quarterly*, **23**, 248-276.

HOLZMAN, P. S., PROCTOR, L. R. & HUGHES, D. W. (1973) Eye tracking patterns in schizophrenia. *Science*, **181**, 179-181.

INGVAR, D. H. & FRANZEN, G. (1974) Abnormalities of cerebral blood flow distribution in patients with chronic schizophrenia. *Acta Psychiatrica Scandinavica*, **50**, 425-462.

IRONSIDE, R., BOSANQUET, G. D. & MCMENEMY, W. H. (1961) Central demyelination of the corpus callosum. (Marchiafava-Bignami disease). *Brain*, **84**, 212-230.

JEFFERSON, G. (1944) The nature of concussion. *British Medical Journal*, i, 1-5.

KALAMBOUKIS, Z. & MOLLING, P. (1962) Symmetrical calcification of the brain: predominance in the basal ganglia and cerebellum. *Journal of Neuropathology and Experimental Neurology*, **21**, 364-371.

KASANIN, J. & CRANK, R. P. (1935) A case of extensive calcification of the brain. *Archives of Neurology and Psychiatry*, **34**, 164-178.

KORNETSKY, C. & ORZACK, M. H. (1978) Physiological and behavioural correlates of attention dysfunction in schizophrenic patients. *Journal of Psychiatric Research*, **14**, 69-79.

KRAEPELIN, E. (1919) *Dementia Praecox* (trans. M. Barclay; ed. G. M. Robertson). Edinburgh: E. and S. Livingstone.

—— (1920) Patterns of mental disorder. In *Themes and Variations in European Psychiatry* reprinted 1974 (eds. M. Shepherd & S. Hirsch). Bristol: Wright & Sons.

KUGLER, B. T. & WELLER, M. P. I. (1983) Memory impairment in schizophrenia: Hebb's recurring digits. In *Laterality and Psychopathology* (eds. P. Flor-Henry & J. Gruzelier). North Holland: Elsevier. pp. 493–495.

LATHAM, C., HOLTZMAN, P. S., MANSCHRECK, T. C. & TOLE, J. (1981) Optokinetic nystagmus and pursuit eye movements in schizophrenia. *Archives of General Psychiatry*, **38**, 997–1003.

LEATON, R. N. & SUPPLE, JR, W. F. (1986) Cerebellar vermis: essential for long-term habituation of the acoustic startle response. *Science*, **232**, 513–515.

LEFF, J. (1977) International variations in the diagnosis of psychiatric illness. *British Journal of Psychiatry*, **131**, 329–338.

LEWIN, R. (1981) Is your brain really necessary? *Science*, **210**, 1232–1234.

LIPOWSKI, Z. J. (1980) *Delirium: Acute Brain Failure in Man.* Illinois: Charles C. Thomas.

LOWENTHAL, A. & BRUYN, G. W. (1968) Calcification of the strio-pallido-dentate system. In *Handbook of Clinical Neurology, Diseases of the Basal Ganglia*, (eds. P. J. Vinken & G. W. Bruyn) **6**, 703–725.

LURIA, A. R. (1973) *The Working Brain: An Introduction to Neuropsychology*, (trans. B. Haigh) Harmondsworth, Middlesex: Penguin.

MARCHIAFAVA, E. (1932–33) The degeneration of the brain in chronic alcoholism. *Proceedings of the Royal Society of Medicine*, **26**, 1151–1158.

NIELSEN, J. M. (1958) Cerebral localization and the psychoses. *Research Publications. Association for Research in Nervous and Mental Disease*, Baltimore, **36**, 467–477.

PAYNE, R. W., CAIRD, W. K. & LAVERTY, S. G. (1964) Overinclusive thinking and delusions in schizophrenic patients. *Journal of Abnormal Social Psychology*, **68**, 562–566.

PENFIELD, W. & JASPER, H. H. (1947) Highest level seizures. *Association for Research In Nervous and Mental Disease, Proceedings*, **24**, 252–271. Baltimore: Williams & Wilkins.

REGISTRAR-GENERAL (1968) *A Glossary of Mental Disorders.* London: HMSO.

REICHARDT, M. (1929) Brain and psyche (trans. F. I. Wertham) *Journal of Nervous and Mental Disease*, **70**, 390–396.

REIDER, R. O., MANN, L. S., WEINBERGER, D. R., VAN KAMMEN, D. P. & POST, R. M. (1981) CAT-scans in patients with schizophrenia, schizo-affective disorder and affective disorder, presented at APA Annual Meeting New Orleans, cited Weinberger, D. R. & Wyatt, R. J. Chapter 8 In *Schizophrenia as a Brain Disease* (eds F. A. Henn & H. A. Nasrallah). New York and Oxford: Oxford University Press, 1982.

REYNOLDS, G. P. (1988) Lateral asymmetries in neurochemical measurements in human brains. Paper read at Schizophrenia Group Meeting, 20 April 1983. Wellcome Trust, London. (In press, *Nature*).

ROBERTS, G. W., FERRIER, N., LEE, Y., CROW, T. J., JOHNSTONE, E. C., OWENS, D. G. C., BACARESE-HAMILTON, A. J., McGREGOR, G., O'SHAUGHNESSEY, D., POLAK, J. M. & BLOOM, S. R. (1984) Peptides, the limbic lobe and schizophrenia. *Brain Research*, **288**, 199–211.

—— (1988) Brain development and CCK systems in schizophrenia: a working hypothesis. In *Advances in Biological Psychiatry* (eds. M. P. I. Weller, John Libby, London [in press] ).

ROMANO, J. & ENGEL, G. L. (1944) Physiologic and psychologic considerations of delirium. *Medical Clinics of North America*, **28**, 629–638.

RORIE, J. (1862–63) The treatment of hallucinations by electrization. *Journal of Mental Science*, **8**, 363–365.

ROTH, M. & McCLELLAND, H. (1979) The relationship of 'nuclear' and 'atypical' psychoses. *Psychiatrica Clinica*, **12**, 23–54.

RUSSELL, W. (1934) The after-effects of head injury. *Medical Journal*, **41**, 129–141. Extracts in *The Traumatic Amnesias.* London, Glasgow, New York: Oxford University Press (1971).

SCHNEIDER, K. (1957) Primary and secondary symptoms in schizophrenia. Reprinted 1974 in *Themes and Variations in European Psychiatry.* (eds M. Shepherd & S. Hirsch). Bristol: Wright.

SCHWADE, E. D. & GEIGER, S. G. (1965) Abnormal electroencephalographic findings in severe behaviour disorders. *Diseases of the Nervous System*, **17**, 307–317.

SHAKOW, D. (1962) Segmental set: a theory of the formal psychological deficit in schizophrenia. *Archives of General Psychiatry*, **6**, 1–11.

SLATER, E. & ROTH, M. (1969) *Clinical Psychiatry.* 3rd edition. London: Baillière, Tindall & Cassell.

STEVENS, M., CROW, T. J., BOWMAN, M. & COLES, E. C. (1978) Age disorientation in chronic schizophrenia: a constant prevalence of 25% in a mental hospital population? *British Journal of Psychiatry*, **133**, 130–136.

—— (1982) Neurology and neuropathology of schizophrenia. Chap. 7 pp. 112–147. In *Schizophrenia as a Brain Disease.* (eds F. A. Henn & H. A. Nasrallah). New York and Oxford: Oxford University Press.

SYMONDS, C. P. & RUSSELL, W. R. (1943) Accidental head injuries: prognosis in severe patients. *Lancet*, **i**, 7–10.

THOMPSON, R. F. (1987) The cerebellum and memory storage. *Science*, **238**, 1729–1730.

VICTOR, M. & ADAMS, R. D. (1961) On the etiology of the alcoholic neurologic diseases with special reference to the role of nutrition. *American Journal of Clinical Nutrition*, **9**, 379–397.

WECKOWICZ, T. E. (1957) Size constancy in schizophrenic patients. *Journal of Mental Science*, **103**, 432–486.

——, SOMMER, R. & HALL, R. (1958) Distance constancy in schizophrenic patients. *Journal of Mental Science*, **104**, 1174–1182.

—— (1960) Perception of hidden figures by schizophrenic patients. *Archives of General Psychiatry*, **2**, 521–527.

—— & WITNEY, G. (1960) The Muller-Lyer illusion in schizophrenic patients. *Journal of Mental Science*, **106**, 1002–1009.

WEINBERGER, D. R., TORREY, E. F. & WYATT, R. J. (1979) Cerebellar atrophy in chronic schizophrenia. *Lancet*, **i**, 718–719.

——, DeLISI, L. E., NEOPHYTIDES, A. N. & WYATT, R. J. (1981) Familial aspects of CT abnormalities in chronic schizophrenic patients. *Psychiatric Research*, **4**, 65–71.

——, BERMAN, K. F. & ZEC, R. F. (1986) Physiologic dysfunction of dorsolateral prefrontal cortex in schizophrenia. *Archives of General Psychiatry*, **43**, 114–124.

WELLER, M. P. I. & MONTAGU, J. D. (1979) Electroencephalographic coherence in schizophrenia; a preliminary study. In *Hemisphere Asymmetries of Function in Psychopathology* (eds. J. Gruzelier & P. Flor-Henry). North Holland: Elsevier. pp. 285–292.

—— & KUGLER, B. T. (1979) Tactile discrimination in schizophrenic and affective psychoses. In *Hemisphere Asymmetries of Function in Psychopathology* (eds. J. Gruzelier & P. Flor-Henry). North Holland: Elsevier. pp. 463–474.

—— (1986a) Cognitive and sensory defects in schizophrenia. In *The Long-term Management of Patients Suffering from Schizophrenia* (eds R. R. R. Tilleard-Cole & M. Lader). London and Geneva: Franklyn Scientific.

—— (1986b) Report of the 3rd Biannual International Workshop on Schizophrenia 1985, Schladming. *Bulletin of the Royal College of Psychiatrists*, **10**, 277.

——, KIDD, J., CALEV, A., CHAZEN, S., NIGAL, D. & LERER, B. (1988) Laterality in schizophrenia measured by tapping speed. Presented at Biannual Workshop on Schizophrenia, Badgastein, Jan., abstract in press, *International Journal of Schizophrenia*.

WHITTY, C. W. M. & ZANGWILL, O. L. (1966) Traumatic amnesia. In *Amnesia* (eds. C. W. M. Whitty & O. L. Zangwill). London: Butterworths. pp. 92–108.

ZAHN, T. P. (1977) Comments on reaction time and attention in schizophrenia. *Schizophrenia Bulletin*, **3**, 452–456.

—— *et al* (1981) cited Zahn, T. P., Rapoport, J. L. and Thompson, C. L. (1981) Autonomic effects of dextroamphetamine in normal men: implications for hyperactivity and schizophrenia. *Psychiatric Research*, **4**, 39–47.

# *Appendix*

Lipowski (1980, p. 41) gives a comprehensive list of what he terms essential characteristics of delirium: "an organic brain syndrome of acute onset and transient duration, characterized by global impairment, and due to widespread disturbance of cerebral metabolism. The term encompasses 'acute confusional states' and 'simple confusion' of other authors, provided that they use these terms to designate organic mental disorders" (pp. 38–39).

(1) Impaired awareness of self and surroundings and their relationships.
(2) Impairment of memory.
(3) Disturbance of attention.
(4) Impairment of directed thinking.
(5) Diminished perceptual discrimination with a tendency to illusions and hallucinations.
(6) Impairment of spatiotemporal orientation.
(7) Increased or decreased alertness.
(8) Sleep disturbance, usually drowsiness during the day, or insomnia at night, or both.
(9) Relatively rapid fluctuations in awareness and severity of symptoms (2) through (7) during daytime and tendency to their exacerbation at night or in the dark.
(10) Acute onset and relatively short duration.
(11) Laboratory evidence of cerebral dysfunction, especially diffuse changes of background activity in the electroencephalogram.

# 40 Organic cerebral concomitants of schizophrenia: Association greater than chance?

## KENNETH DAVISON

A variety of organic CNS disorders is found in a minority of sufferers from schizophrenia, or a clinically similar psychosis. Evidence is evaluated to determine the frequency of this concurrence and whether or not it exceeds chance expectation. In some conditions the verdict is not proven, but in many others the association appears to be more than fortuitous.

## Definitions

The frequency of occurrence of schizophrenia in association with various organic cerebral disorders will be compared with the frequency of schizophrenia in the general population using standard epidemiological terms.

*Incidence* is the number of *new* cases developing per unit of population during a stated period. In several studies the annual incidence of schizophrenia is quoted as 0.01% to 0.05% (Dunham, 1965). *Prevalence* is the number of cases per unit of population present at some specific point in time (point prevalence) or over some period of time (period prevalence), often one year or a lifetime. It reflects not only incidence but also duration. The point prevalence of schizophrenia in various parts of the world lies between 0.1% and 0.6%, although an unusually high prevalence of over 1% is reported from parts of Sweden and Ireland (Torrey, 1987). Point prevalence of DSM-III schizophrenia in a US community is reported as 0.46% for active cases and 0.64% for active and remitted cases combined (Von Korff *et al*, 1985) and lifetime prevalence for DSM-III schizophrenia and schizophreniform disorder as 1.1-2% (Robins *et al*, 1984). *Morbidity risk* is the expectation of a person developing a condition between specified ages. For schizophrenia the maximum risk is concentrated between age 15 and 40 years. The morbidity risk in the general population is 0.8% to age 40 years and 1% to age 55 years (Slater & Cowie, 1971).

## Organic CNS disorders and schizophrenia

The association of schizophrenia (or a schizophrenia-like psychosis) with organic brain disorder (and also extra-cerebral somatic disease, toxins and drugs) is

TABLE I

*Organic disorders discovered in 462 patients with a first episode of schizophrenia, 268 of whom fulfilled PSE diagnostic criteria (Johnstone et al, 1986)*

| Diagnosis | N |
|---|---|
| Alcohol abuse | 3 |
| Syphilis | 3 |
| Drug abuse | 2 |
| Sarcoidosis | 2 |
| Auto-immune disease | 1 |
| Bronchial carcinoma | 1 |
| Cerebral cysticercosis | 1 |
| Hypothyroidism, overtreated | 1 |
| Head injury/hemiparesis | 1 |

not easily quantified. Population studies are rare and hospital-based studies are biased by selection for the presence of psychiatric disorder.

Apart from the continuing problem of the definition of schizophrenia, diagnostic systems often obscure the association, as the identification of an organic disorder often results in the diagnosis of schizophrenia being changed. Fifty years ago Mapother commented on psychoses occurring after head injury: ''The term 'schizophrenia' is withheld from traumatic cases to which it would be applied if a history of injury were absent. There is naturally little schizophrenia as a sequel of head injury if they are diagnosed as 'insanity with gross brain lesion' '' (Mapother, 1937). Today it could well be organic delusional disorder (DSM–III, 1980).

One survey of 318 consecutive admissions with a clinical diagnosis of schizophrenia found 25(7.9%) with an antecedent organic cerebral disorder and an autopsy study of 200 schizophrenic patients yielded 22 (11%) with structural brain disease thought to be causally related. Schizophrenia-like psychoses associated with organic brain disease account for 1.25% to 3% of all admissions to psychiatric hospitals and constituted 17% of all psychiatric in-patients with chronic brain disorder in the Australian State of Victoria (Davison, 1983).

In a recent study of first episodes of schizophrenia, 462 patients referred with a clinical diagnosis of schizophrenia included 15 (3.25%) in whom the psychosis was thought to be organically determined (Johnstone *et al*, 1986, 1987). Only 268 fulfilled Present State Examination (PSE) diagnostic criteria for schizophrenia (Wing *et al*, 1974), thus raising the proportion of organic cases to 5.6%. Only seven (2.8%) had intrinsic brain disease but the method of collection excluded obvious cases of organic disorder. The full list of diagnoses is shown in Table 1.

CT scans of chronic schizophrenic patients often detect unsuspected organic brain disease. For example, one study of 136 patients yielded 12 cases of which 10 (7.4%) were regarded as of possible aetiological relevance (Owens *et al*, 1980). The diagnoses in this study are listed in Table II.

From a review of 10 years admissions to a London neuropsychiatric hospital, the author calculated that patients with organic brain disease developed a schizophrenia-like psychosis at least twice as often, and very probably a good deal more, than expected on a chance association hypothesis (Davison, 1966).

Organic brain disease is of particular significance at the extremes of age. Childhood schizophrenia is often associated with a history of peri-natal injury

TABLE II
*Clinically undiagnosed organic brain disease revealed by CT scan*
*in 136 patients with chronic schizophrenia (Owens et al, 1980)*

| Diagnosis | N |
|---|---|
| Cerebral infarction | 7 |
| Porencephalic cyst | 1 |
| Meningioma | 1 |
| Subdural haematoma | 2 |
| Pineal cyst | 1 |

or anoxia or concurrent organic disease. Thus one series of 100 children with a diagnosis of schizophrenia contained 12 with epilepsy, one with congenital hemiplegia, two with cerebral lipoidosis (unsuspected in life) and two with other forms of brain damage (17% in all) (Creak, 1963). A series of 63 patients with 'infantile psychosis' included 18 (28%) with definite and 16 (25%) with possible brain damage (Rutter & Lockyer, 1967). Likewise, groups of patients with an onset of schizophrenia after age 60 years yield prevalence rates for organic brain disorder of 5% to 17% initially with an additional 8% to 18% appearing later (Davison, 1983). A recent 10-year follow-up of 42 cases of non-affective paranoid-hallucinatory psychosis occurring after age 60, diagnosed as late paraphrenia, found that five (11.9%) were symptomatic of organic disease on first referral and a further 13 (31%) became demented within three years. The organic group showed an excess of visual hallucinations but was otherwise clinically indistinguishable from the other cases at presentation (Holden, 1987).

A significant minority of patients with a clinical diagnosis of schizophrenia or psychoses usually included in the schizophrenia category, therefore, also manifests some form of organic cerebral disorder.

Some specific brain disorders will now be considered in detail.

## Epilepsy

An association between epilepsy and schizophrenia has long been suspected, even though convulsion therapy was introduced on the basis of the entirely opposite premise. It is the persistent inter-ictal psychosis of epilepsy that is the most schizophrenia-like.

A review of early literature quotes the prevalence of schizophrenia in epileptic patients as 0.2% to 0.8%, and the prevalence of epilepsy in schizophrenia patients as 0.06% to 19.5% (Davison & Bagley, 1969). Confounding variables were so great, however, as to render these figures virtually meaningless. Slater *et al* (1963) attempted to avoid some of the pitfalls by calculating the expected number of random combination cases in the general population from the product of the individual expectations of developing epilepsy and schizophrenia independently ($0.005 \times 0.008 = 0.00004$ or 40 per million over the entire risk period). Making the assumption that epilepsy would precede psychosis in 75% of cases, they calculated that in a population of 10 million, as in the London area, there would be 148 chance association cases and three to five new cases would appear each year. Allowing for selective referral, they still regarded the collection of 69 such cases at two hospitals as greater than chance expectation.

This conclusion has been challenged on the grounds that the patients were drawn from the population of two prestigious London hospitals, both containing neuropsychiatric units and without defined catchment areas. According to this argument, selective referral would therefore be likely to occur and might well account for the facility with which cases were acquired. At that time in the UK, however, most patients with epilepsy and psychosis were located in the long-stay wards of large psychiatric hospitals.

This controversy has recently been brought up-to-date by McKenna *et al* (1985). From recent community surveys they arrive at an estimate of the point prevalence of 'psychosis' in epileptic subjects as 7%. They point out, however, that this does not necessarily reflect a statistical association as the prevalence of psychosis, which here includes major depression as well as schizophrenia-like states, in the general population is difficult to ascertain as it varies according to definition. Nevertheless it is unlikely to be as high as 7% (Myers *et al*, 1984).

McKenna *et al* examine the prevalence of epilepsy in psychosis and rely heavily on the study of Betts (1981), who screened every patient in two long-stay psychiatric hospitals and found the point prevalence of epilepsy in patients with functional psychosis, mainly paranoid or schizophreniform, to be "somewhat greater than 2.1%". As the point prevalence of epilepsy in the general population is 0.3% to 0.5%, this result is a four to seven-fold over-representation of epilepsy in psychosis. This, of course, rests on the assumption that the epilepsy played no part in the patient's admission to, or retention in, hospital.

After considering all the evidence, McKenna *et al* conclude that the risk of developing a psychosis is 6 to 12 times greater in epileptic patients.

## Association with temporal lobe epilepsy (TLE)

Discussion of this topic is bedevilled by varying definitions of TLE, from clinical presentations, such as psychomotor attacks, to EEG or radiological evidence of structural lesions in the temporal lobes. As the clinical manifestations of TLE are protean, the objective technical criteria are preferable.

Several studies have found the proportion of TLE cases in series of epileptic inter-ictal schizophrenia-like psychosis to be about 80%. This leads to the assumption of a specific association of these psychoses with TLE, a view that has been criticised by several workers, notably Janice Stevens (1966) who comments: "The assumed relationship between psychomotor epilepsy (sic) and psychosis can be explained by the coincident statistical rise in incidence of both disorders with increasing age." More recently, in response to a phenomenological study of epileptic psychosis (Perez *et al*, 1985), she has conceded an association between TLE and a psychosis with Schneider's first rank symptoms (nuclear syndrome on the PSE), although forbearing to label it schizophrenia-like (Stevens, 1985). Her claim that TLE accounts for 55% to 80% of all epileptics (Stevens, 1985) is not supported by several large-scale surveys that found proportions of 27% to 43% (Zielinsky, 1982).

Several studies have found a disparity in the rate of psychotic development between TLE and idiopathic epilepsy, TLE being greater by a factor of 2 to 12 (McKenna *et al*, 1985). The important prospective study of Lindsay *et al* (1979) of 100 children with TLE followed for 13 years demonstrated the occurrence of a schizophreniform psychosis in nine of the 87 survivors (10.4%), some 20 times the expected incidence.

There is evidence, not entirely undisputed, of an association between schizophreniform psychoses and left-sided TL lesions. Perez *et al* (1985) pooled data from 180 patients in ten reports and produced proportions of left-sided foci 62.2%, right-sided foci 15% and bilateral foci 22.7%, although comparative data for non-psychotic TLE patients were not provided.

The preponderant association of discrete TL pathology with these psychoses suggests that the development of the latter is related, not to the occurrence of seizures, but to the presence of an underlying cerebral lesion of which both the seizures and the psychosis are manifestations. This hypothesis reconciles the conflicting views of the relationship between epilepsy and schizophrenia as either one of biological affinity or antagonism. The antagonism hypothesis was derived from observations of the beneficial effects of spontaneous seizures in some schizophrenic patients that led to the introduction of convulsive therapy, subsequently electro-convulsive therapy (ECT). There can, therefore, be said to be an affinity between the psychosis and the underlying brain lesion, but antagonism between the psychosis and the actual seizures. Such a hypothesis also predicts the association of schizophrenia-like psychoses with other brain lesions, with or without associated epilepsy.

The alternative hypothesis is that of kindling, a model of epilepsy in which recurrent sub-convulsive electrical stimulation of certain brain areas results in a lowering of an animal's seizure threshold to a point where generalised convulsions occur in response to stimuli that were previously ineffective. In the limbic system this process is accompanied by behavioural abnormalities and neurotransmitter changes suggesting that temporal lobe sub-ictal electrical activity might underlie the development of epileptic psychoses in man (McKenna *et al*, 1985).

These hypotheses are not necessarily mutually exclusive.

## Cerebral trauma

The notion of 'insanity' as a sequel to brain injury came to prominence towards the end of the last century and many of the reported cases are recognisably schizophreniform. Arguments about the severity of brain injury and latent interval before onset of psychosis to be regarded as of aetiological significance can be avoided by following an unselected series of brain-injured patients over a long period and comparing the observed incidence of schizophrenia with that expected from a purely chance association.

In several such reports, covering some 15,000 patients followed for up to 20 years, the observed incidence of schizophrenia is two to three times the expected incidence (Davison & Bagley, 1969). In one series of 415 brain-injured war veterans, it is possible to calculate from the age-structure that the number of expected cases of schizophrenia is two whereas the actual number observed was 11 (Hillbom, 1960). Of 3552 brain-injured war veterans followed for 22 to 26 years, schizophrenic psychoses developed in 2.1%, paranoid psychoses in 2% and 'epileptic psychoses' in 1.3% (Achté *et al*, 1969). In 291 survivors of severe peacetime head injuries who had been unconscious for at least a week and followed for ten to 24 years, psychoses designated schizophreniform developed in 2.4% (Lewin *et al*, 1979). There is, therefore, reasonably strong evidence that the occurrence of schizophrenia-like psychoses after brain trauma exceeds chance expectation.

## Cerebral tumour

Autopsy studies of psychiatric hospital patients usually yield a prevalence of cerebral tumours much in excess of the general prevalence of cerebral tumours at autopsy of 1% to 1.5% (Russell & Rubenstein, 1963). A review of nine mental hospital studies between 1909 and 1949 found prevalence rates of 1.7% to 11.2%, of which 31% to 72% were undiagnosed in life (Davison & Bagley, 1969). Despite the advent of modern investigative techniques, frequencies of up to 5.5% are still found (Cole, 1978).

Autopsy studies of long-term hospitalised schizophrenic patients yield prevalence rates for cerebral tumour similar to those at autopsy on unselected groups. For example, 1275 cases yielded 16 patients with primary lesions and four with metastatic brain tumours (1.6% in all), only four of which were diagnosed in life (Hussar, 1966). However, these populations are selected for chronicity and maintenance of a schizophrenic clinical picture. The discovery of a cerebral tumour is itself likely to change the psychiatric diagnosis, and in other patients an initial schizophrenic picture progresses to a chronic brain syndrome with similar result. Such cases appear in the overall hospital statistics but not in the schizophrenic group. Others might be transferred out of the mental hospital altogether. Autopsy statistics, therefore, do not accurately reflect the extent of any association between cerebral tumour and schizophrenia.

Of cases diagnosed in life, two patients with a paranoid psychosis and two with hebephrenic schizophrenia were found in 34 cases of cerebral tumour with a psychiatric presentation (Remington & Rubert, 1962) and two schizophrenic reactions occurred in 33 mental hospital patients with cerebral tumours (Selecki, 1965). Routine skull radiography of 1200 schizophrenic in-patients revealed 17 unsuspected tumours (1.4%) (Kraft *et al*, 1965), more than the prevalence of cerebral tumours of all kinds in the general population of 0.05% (Brewis *et al*, 1966).

The prevalence of schizophrenia in eight published cerebral tumour series, totalling over 3000 patients, varied from 0 to 3.5% with a mean and standard error of 1.2 ± 0.2% (Davison, 1983). This is somewhat greater than the prevalence of schizophrenia in the general population of up to 0.6%. Since the life expectancy of cerebral tumour patients is usually severely curtailed and the constraints on diagnosis already discussed apply, the association of cerebral tumour with schizophrenia probably significantly exceeds chance expectation.

## Cerebral infections

Although 'schizophrenia' has been reported to develop during or after various viral and bacterial encephalitides (Davison, 1983), its occurrence appears to be sporadic. Certain specific infections do, however, have a more frequent association with schizophrenia-like psychoses.

## Encephalitis lethargica

After the great epidemics of the 1920s, schizophrenia was a common sequel to encephalitis lethargica, often associated with narcolepsy or Parkinsonism. A paranoid-hallucinatory psychosis is estimated to have developed in 15% to 30% of post-encephalitic patients, and in one series of 113 patients 16% developed psychoses "resembling manic–depressive insanity or dementia praecox". Psychoses indistinguishable from paraphrenia or dementia praecox accounted for 10% of all post-encephalitic patients admitted to one mental hospital (Davison & Bagley, 1969).

Analysis of 40 such cases conforming to ICD-8 diagnostic criteria for schizophrenia revealed that the psychosis developed at a mean interval of five years after the encephalitic episode and Parkinsonism was associated in 50%. Only one patient had a previously schizoid personality and two had a family history of schizophrenia (Davison & Bagley, 1969).

## Cerebral syphilis

Tertiary syphilis of the brain producing general paresis is another variety of encephalitis in which a schizophreniform presentation has long been recognised. In one large series of 3889 cases of general paresis, admittedly selected for a psychiatric presentation, schizophrenia developed in 19%, compared with dementia in 34%, mania in 23.8% and depression in 9.6% (Cheney, 1935). Other surveys yield prevalences of schizophrenia of 3.5% to 20% (Davison, 1983).

Even allowing for possible selection bias, these figures exceed chance expectation and most observers accept an aetiological connection between the cerebral lesion and the psychosis.

## Rheumatic (Sydenham's) chorea

Sydenham's chorea is produced by an allergic cerebral vasculitis rather than an infection, but since it is often termed rheumatic encephalitis it can be included here.

Sydenham's chorea is now comparatively rare but in the days when it was a common disorder its association with various psychiatric disorders was recognised and is implicit in the term "chorea insaniens" (Hammes, 1922). These disorders included "complex hallucinatory psychoses in a setting of clear consciousness in which the symptomatic resemblance to schizophrenia is often striking" (Shaskan, 1938). Such psychoses occurred concurrently with the chorea in 2.3% to 7.5% of cases (Kleist, 1907; Hammes, 1922), whereas others were a late sequel to the choreic episode (Keeler & Bender, 1952).

A significant excess of chronic insidious schizophrenia developed subsequently in 891 males who had suffered from chorea or acute rheumatism before age 18 years, compared with a matched group with orthopaedic disabilities (Wertheimer, 1963). Of 20 children with chorea followed for five years, three developed schizophrenia and one developed a "psychosis associated with psychopathic personality" (Keeler & Bender, 1952). A review of Maudsley Hospital, London in-patients in the 1930s found that a previous history of chorea was twice as common in schizophrenic as in manic–depressive patients (Guttman, 1936).

A related claim was that of Bruetsch who found rheumatic cerebral vasculitis in the brains of 5% to 9% of schizophrenic patients coming to autopsy. The introduction of non-psychotic controls, however, nullified the significance of these observations (Davison & Bagley, 1969).

## Basal ganglia disorders

The occurrence of Parkinsonism in some 50% of post-encephalitic psychoses has already been noted. Schizophrenia has occurred in association with other basal ganglia degenerations including torsion spasm, Wilson's disease and Huntington's chorea. Similar psychoses occur in association with familial basal ganglia calcification, including six cases in four generations of one family (Francis, 1979). Of all recorded patients with idiopathic basal ganglia calcification, 50% are reported to have developed a schizophrenia-like psychosis (Cummings *et al*, 1983) and this lesion has been found unexpectedly at autopsy in schizophrenic patients (Davison & Bagley, 1969).

### Paralysis agitans

In contrast to post-encephalitic Parkinsonism, there are relatively few reports of schizophrenia associated with paralysis agitans (idiopathic Parkinsonism). One series of 282 patients contained six (2.1%) with schizophrenic symptoms and in ten years' admissions to a mental hospital, eight of 36 patients with paralysis agitans displayed schizophrenic reactions that were not drug-induced (Davison, 1983).

### Huntington's chorea (HC)

Psychoses diagnosed as schizophrenia and paranoid-hallucinatory psychoses resembling paranoid schizophrenia occur quite often in patients with HC. Prevalence rates in various series are listed in Table III (Davison, 1983) and considerably exceed chance expectation. Three of these reports are population surveys and therefore unselected for psychiatric disorder (Bolt, 1970; Heathfield, 1967; Oliver, 1970). Some authors do not distinguish between diagnoses of schizophrenia and paranoid psychosis.

TABLE III
*Prevalence of schizophrenia and paranoid psychosis in HC (Davison, 1983)*

| Number of cases of HC | Schizophrenia ($\% \pm$ SE) | Paranoid psychosis ($\% \pm$ SE) |
|---|---|---|
| 461 | $5.0 \pm 1.0$ | — |
| 1200 | $1.7 \pm 0.4$ | $4.0 \pm 0.6$ |
| 102 | $6.9 \pm 2.5$ | — |
| 199 | $19.6 \pm 2.8$ | |
| 71 | $14.1 \pm 4.1$ | $15.5 \pm 4.3$ |
| 43 | $2.3 \pm 2.3$ | $7.0 \pm 3.9$ |
| 334* | $2.4 \pm 0.8$ | $15.0 \pm 1.9$ |
| 100* | $12.0 \pm 3.2$ | — |
| 81* | $11.0 \pm 3.5$ | — |

* = population survey

Schizophrenia is a common initial diagnosis and said to be the most frequent persisting misdiagnosis. A recent Norwegian review (Saugstad & Ødegard, 1986) comments: "In several cases this diagnosis [of schizophrenia] was preserved during as many as three or four readmissions. The disease [HC] should be considered in the differential diagnosis of schizophrenia."

Streletzki (1961) recognised an early-onset psychosis indistinguishable from "endogenous schizophrenia" and a late-onset paranoid-hallucinatory psychosis often on a background of early dementia "reminiscent of general paresis". Panse (1942) also remarked on the close resemblance to schizophrenia, but only one of his 23 cases had a family history of schizophrenia which, in his view, excluded the possibility of the genetic combination postulated by others.

**Hepato-lenticular degeneration (Wilson's disease)**

Wilson's disease, a rare recessive genetic disorder, is characterised by the deposition of copper in the liver and basal ganglia, leading sometimes to liver failure but more often to the development of an extra-pyramidal syndrome and progressive intellectual impairment in early adult life. Its estimated prevalence is 0.00003% (Scheinberg & Sternlieb, 1985).

The 520 case reports of Wilson's disease in the literature up to 1959 include eight definite (1.5%) and 11 doubtful (2.1%) associated schizophrenic psychoses (Davison, 1983), significantly greater than the general population prevalence for schizophrenia of 0.1% to 0.6%, even before allowance is made for the curtailed life-span of Wilson's disease sufferers. In a recent review of 646 cases published since 1959 (Dening, 1985), 14 (2.1%) were psychotic (unspecified) and an additional three to eight (0.5% to 1.2%) exhibited psychoses described as schizophrenia-like. It is of some interest that two of the 14 patients (cases 2 & 3) in Wilson's original series presented with schizophrenic symptomatology (Wilson, 1912).

A recent report of the response of a schizophreniform psychosis associated with Wilson's disease to a critical dose of penicillamine (Modai et al, 1985) supports an aetiological relationship of the psychosis to the Wilson's disease.

## Demyelinating diseases

Sporadic reports of schizophrenia-like psychoses associated with multiple sclerosis (MS) have appeared for the past century. Analysis of 39 such case reports that fulfilled ICD-8 diagnostic criteria for schizophrenia revealed a mean age of onset of MS of 30 years and of the psychosis, 33 years. In 36% psychosis and neurologic signs appeared contemporaneously and in a further 25% the psychosis appeared within two years before or after the first neurological signs (Davison, 1983).

The prevalence of MS in mental hospital populations varies from 0.05% to 0.65%, compared with the prevalence of MS in the general population of 0.05%. Neither the incidence nor prevalence of schizophrenia in MS has been definitely shown to exceed chance expectation but the clustering of psychosis onset around the time of MS onset suggests that the two disorders are not independent (Davison & Bagley, 1969).

Similar psychoses occur in association with other demyelinating conditions such as diffuse sclerosis (Schilder's disease), diffuse encephalo-myelitis (Davison & Bagley, 1969), the rare adult form of metachromatic leukodystrophy (Finelli, 1985; Manowitz *et al*, 1978) and the even rarer adreno-myelo-neuropathy (James *et al*, 1984; Luauté, 1985). However, the reports are too few to draw any statistical conclusion.

## Narcolepsy

The association of a schizophrenia-like psychosis with narcolepsy has been recognised for over 100 years and several examples were reported before the introduction of amphetamine therapy in 1935. Although the possibility of psychostimulant intoxication cannot always be excluded, there are at least 20 published cases in which amphetamines played no part (Davison & Bagley, 1969). A follow-up study of 75 cases of primary narcolepsy over 30 years yielded nine who developed a "schizophrenic reaction" unrelated to the consumption of amphetamines (Sours, 1963), an incidence (12%) in excess of chance expectation.

## Cerebral vascular disease

Although paranoid-hallucinatory psychoses are reported as developing soon after sub-arachnoid haemorrhage, cerebral fat embolism and bilateral carotid artery occlusion, the prevalence of cerebro-vascular disease in middle-aged schizophrenic subjects does not appear to exceed that of the general population (Davison & Bagley, 1969). It is not, however, in long-standing psychoses with onset in early life but rather in late-onset psychoses that any significant association is likely to be found. Thus one series of 93 elderly paraphrenic patients included seven (7.5%) with signs of cerebro-vascular disease. In 99 patients with onset of schizophrenia over age 60 years, 5% showed focal cerebral abnormalities initially and a further 9% later, mainly of vascular origin, and two of 50 similar patients (4%) developed their psychoses soon after cerebro-vascular accidents. Of 90 patients with paranoid psychoses developing after age 50 years observed for five to ten years, 14 (15.6%) developed vascular dementia (Davison, 1983).

These figures suggest that vascular brain disease is significantly associated with the paraphrenic syndrome, and it is probably the major contributor to the organic component of this syndrome to which reference has previously been made.

## Other cerebral disorders

Psychoses occur in association with many other cerebral disorders, including degenerative ataxias, motor neurone disease and the early stages of various dementing processes (Davison & Bagley, 1969). Reports, however, are not sufficiently numerous or systematic to allow any valid conclusion about degree of association.

# Genetic disorders

In an important recent review of the literature on the association of genetic disorders with schizophrenia, Propping (1983) lists those genetic disorders in which an increased risk of developing a schizophrenia-like psychosis is established or very probable, or possible (Table IV). It will be seen that many of these conditions are associated with brain dysfunction, either primarily or secondary to metabolic defects.

TABLE IV
*Genetic disorders with an increased risk of developing a schizophrenia-like psychosis (Propping, 1983)*

| Established or very probable | Possible |
|---|---|
| Klinefelter karyotype (XXY) | Turner(45,XO) or Noonan syndrome |
| XXX karyotype | XYY karyotype |
| 18q or r(18) constitution | Erythropoietic protoporphyria |
| Huntington's chorea | Niemann-Pick's disease, late type |
| Acute intermittent porphyria | Gaucher's disease, late type |
| Porphyria variegata | Fabry disease |
| Metachromatic leukodystrophy adult type | Amaurotic idiocy, late type |
| Familial basal ganglia calcification | Congenital adrenal hyperplasia |
| | Homocystinuria |
| | Wilson's disease |
| | Haemochromatosis |
| | Icthyosis vulgaris |
| | Laurence–Moon–Biedl syndrome |
| | Glucose-6-PD-deficiency |
| | Phenylketonuria |
| | Albinism |
| | Kartagener's syndrome |
| | Ataxia, dominant type |
| | Hyperasparaginaemia |

An example is Klinefelter's syndrome in which the sex chromosome constitution is XXY. A review of 48 studies involving 411 cases found 179 (43.5%) with a psychiatric disorder, including 26 (6.3%) with schizophrenia and 29 (7.1%) with ''psychoses of uncertain type with paranoid delusions'' (Nielsen, 1969).

# Somatic and toxic disorders

Schizophrenia-like psychoses also occur in association with various somatic diseases and drug intoxications (Davison, 1976, 1987; Cummings, 1986) but these are beyond the scope of this article.

# Significance of the 'organic schizophrenias'

Statistical association does not necessarily imply causation but the author has previously marshalled evidence in support of a causal link between the brain disorder and the psychosis in most cases (Davison & Bagley, 1969). This raises some interesting questions:

(a)  *Are organically determined schizophrenia-like psychoses clinically distinguishable from spontaneously occurring schizophrenia?*
     Several studies have found that these organic psychoses fulfil operational diagnostic criteria for schizophrenia (Davison, 1983). For example, a recent review of 55 epileptic patients with various psychiatric disorders attending the author's clinic revealed 22 who fulfilled Research Diagnostic Criteria (Spitzer *et al*, 1975) for schizophrenia and five for schizo-affective disorder (Oyebode & Davison, unpublished data).

(b)  *Do these organic psychoses develop* de novo *or are they precipitated in predisposed subjects?*
     The evidence concerning personality predispostion is largely impressionistic but tends to support the former view (Davison & Bagley, 1969). As for genetic predisposition, several studies have found an absence of family loading for schizophrenia in the organic cases (Davison, 1983).

(c)  *Is any particular brain locus preferentially affected?*
     There is weighty evidence pointing to the temporo-limbic system (Torrey & Peterson, 1974) and sub-cortical brain areas (Cummings, 1986; Davison & Bagley, 1969) as the commonest sites for the lesions associated with schizophrenia-like psychoses.

(d)  *What are the implications for the concept of schizophrenia?*
     The occurence of psychoses resembling schizophrenia, yet apparently organically determined, supports the syndromic, as opposed to the disease entity, concept of schizophrenia. Should such psychoses, then, be labelled schizophrenic if they satisfy phenomenological criteria? DSM–III (1980) classifies them separately as ''organic delusional disorder''. Does this illuminate or obfuscate our understanding of schizophrenia? I much prefer the dual aetiological-descriptive classification long advocated by Essen-Möller (1961, 1982).

## Conclusion

A substantial minority of patients with a clinical diagnosis of schizophrenia has an associated organic cerebral disorder of possible aetiological significance and, conversely, sufferers from organic brain disorders show a significantly increased risk of developing a psychosis indistinguishable from schizophrenia.

Study of the 'organic schizophrenias' should surely teach us something about the cerebral dysfunction underlying the idiopathic variety.

## Acknowledgement

It is a great pleasure to acknowledge the advice and encouragement of Professor Sir Martin Roth in the formulation of these ideas over many years. I am indebted to him for a thorough training in clinical psychiatry, insight into the significance of organic factors and an example of intellectual rigour to emulate.

# References

ACHTÉ, K. A., HILLBOM, E. & AALBERG, V. (1969) Psychoses following war brain injuries. *Acta Psychiatrica Scandinavica*, **45**, 1–18.

AMERICAN PSYCHIATRIC ASSOCIATION (1980) *Diagnostic and Statistical Manual of Mental Disorders* (3rd edn) (DSM–III). Washington, DC: APA.

BETTS, T. A. (1981) Epilepsy and the mental hospital. In *Epilepsy and Psychiatry* (eds. E. H. Reynolds & M. R. Trimble). New York: Raven Press.

BOLT, J. M. W. (1970) Huntington's chorea in the West of Scotland. *British Journal of Psychiatry*, **116**, 259–270.

BREWIS, M., POSKANZER, D. C., ROLLAND, C. & MILLER, H. (1966) Neurological disease in an English city. *Acta Neurologica Scandinavica*, Supplement 24.

CHENEY, C. O. (1935) Clinical data on general paresis. *Psychiatric Quarterly*, **9**, 467–485.

COLE, G. (1978) Intracranial space-occupying masses in mental hospital patients: necropsy study. *Journal of Neurology, Neurosurgery & Psychiatry*, **41**, 730–736.

CREAK, M. (1963) Childhood psychosis. A review of 100 cases. *British Journal of Psychiatry*, **109**, 84–89.

CUMMINGS, J. L., GOSENFELD, L. F., HOULIHAN, J. P. & McCAFFREY, T. (1983) Neuropsychiatric manifestations of idiopathic calcification of the basal ganglia: case report and review. *Biological Psychiatry*, **18**, 591–601.

—— (1985) Organic delusions: phenomenology, anatomical correlations and review. *British Journal of Psychiatry*, **146**, 184–197.

—— (1986) Organic psychoses: delusional disorders and secondary mania. *Psychiatric Clinics of North America*, **9**, 293–311.

DAVISON, K. (1966) Schizophrenia-like psychoses associated with organic brain disease. Preliminary observations on 50 patients. *Newcastle Medical Journal*, **29**, 67–73.

—— & BAGLEY, C. R. (1969) Schizophrenia-like psychoses associated with organic disorders of the CNS: a review of the literature. In *Current Problems in Neuropsychiatry* (ed. R. N. Herrington). *British Journal of Psychiatry* Special Publication No. 4, pp. 113–184. Ashford: Headley Bros.

—— (1976) Drug-induced psychoses and their relationship to schizophrenia. In *Schizophrenia Today* (eds. D. Kemali, G. Bartholini & D. Richter) pp. 105–133. Oxford & New York: Pergamon.

—— (1983) Schizophrenia-like psychoses associated with organic cerebral disorders: a review. *Psychiatric Developments*, **1**, 1–34.

—— (1987) Organic and toxic concomitants of schizophrenia. In *Biological Perspectives of Schizophrenia* (eds. H. Helmchen & F. Henn). Dahlem Konferenzen. Chichester: John Wiley.

DENING, T. R. (1985) Psychiatric aspects of Wilson's disease. *British Journal of Psychiatry*, **147**, 677–682.

DUNHAM, H. W. (1965) *Community and Schizophrenia: An Epidemiological Analysis*. Detroit: Wayne State University.

ESSEN-MÖLLER, E. (1961) On classification of mental disorders. *Acta Psychiatrica Scandinavica*, **37**, 119–126.

—— (1982) Gutenberg and the ICD-9 of mental disorders. *British Journal of Psychiatry*, **140**, 529–531.

FINELLI, P. F. (1985) Metachromatic leukodystrophy manifesting as a schizophrenic disorder: computed tomographic correlation. *Annals of Neurology*, **18**, 94–95.

FRANCIS, A. F. (1979) Familial basal ganglia calcification and schizophreniform psychosis. *British Journal of Psychiatry*, **135**, 360–362.

GUTTMAN, E. (1936) On some constitutional aspects of chorea and on its sequelae. *Journal of Neuropathology and Psychopathology*, **17**, 16–26.

HAMMES, E. M. (1922) Psychoses associated with Sydenham's chorea. *Journal of the American Medical Association*, **79**, 804–807.

HEATHFIELD, K. W. G. (1967) Huntington's chorea. Investigation into the prevalence of this disease in the area covered by the North-East Metropolitan Regional Hospital Board. *Brain*, **90**, 203–232.

HOLDEN, N. L. (1987) Late paraphrenia or the paraphrenias? A descriptive study with a 10-year follow-up. *British Journal of Psychiatry*, **150**, 635–639.

HILLBOM, E. (1960) After effects of brain injuries. *Acta Psychiatrica Scandinavica*, Supplement 142.

HUSSAR, A. E. (1966) Gross anatomic lesions of the brain in 1275 autopsies of long-term hospitalised schizophrenic patients. *Diseases of the Nervous System*, **27**, 743–747.

JAMES, A. C. D., KAPLAN, P., LEES, A. & BRADLEY, J. T. (1984) Schizophreniform psychosis and adreno-myelo-neuropathy. *Journal of the Royal Society of Medicine*, **77**, 882–884.

JOHNSTONE, E. C., CROW, T. J., JOHNSON, A. L. & MACMILLAN, J. F. (1986) The Northwick Park study of first episodes of schizophrenia. *British Journal of Psychiatry*, **148**, 115–120.

——, MacMillan, J. F. & Crow, T. J. (1987) The occurrence of organic disease of possible or probable aetiological significance in a population of 268 cases of first episode schizophrenia. *Psychological Medicine*, **17**, 371–379.

Keeler, W. R. & Bender, L. (1952) A follow-up study of children with behaviour disorder and Sydenham's chorea. *American Journal of Psychiatry*, **109**, 421–428.

Kleist, K. (1907) Über die psychischen Störungen bei der Chorea minor. *Allgemeine Zeitschrift für Psychiatrie*, **64**, 769–855.

Kraft, E., Schillinger, A., Finby, N. & Halperin, M. (1965) Routine skull radiography in a neuropsychiatric hospital. *American Journal of Psychiatry*, **121**, 1011–1012.

Lewin, W., Marshall, T. F. de C. & Roberts, A. H. (1979) Long-term outcome after severe head injury. *British Medical Journal*, **ii**, 1533–1539.

Lindsay, J., Ounsted, C. & Richards, P. (1979) Long-term outcome in children with temporal lobe seizures. III. Psychiatric aspects in childhood and adult life. *Developmental Medicine & Childhood Neurology*, **21**, 630–636.

Luauté, J. P. (1985) Schizophreniform psychosis and adreno-myelo-neuropathy (AMN). *Journal of the Royal Society of Medicine*, **78**, 512–513.

Manowitz, P., Kling, A. & Kohn, H. (1978) Clinical course of adult metachromatic leukodystrophy presenting as schizophrenia. A report of two living cases in siblings. *Journal of Nervous and Mental Disease*, **166**, 500–506.

Mapother, E. (1937) Mental symptoms associated with head injury. *British Medical Journal*, **ii**, 1055–1073.

McKenna, P. J., Kane, J. M. & Parrish, K. (1985) Psychotic syndromes in epilepsy. *American Journal of Psychiatry*, **142**, 895–904.

Modai, I., Karp, L., Liberman, U. A. & Munitz, H. (1985) Penicillamine therapy for schizophreniform psychosis in Wilson's disease. *Journal of Nervous and Mental Disease*, **173**, 698–701.

Myers, J. K., Weissman, M. M., Tischler, T. L., Holzer, C. E., Leaf, P. J., Orvaschel, H., Anthony, J. C., Boyd, J. H., Burke, J. D., Kramer, M. & Stoltzmann, R. (1984) Six-month prevalence of psychiatric disorders in three communities. *Archives of General Psychiatry*, **41**, 959–967.

Nielsen, J. (1969) Klinefelter's syndrome and the XYY syndrome. *Acta Psychiatrica Scandinavica*, **45**, Supplement 209.

Oliver, J. E. (1970) Huntington's chorea in Northamptonshire. *British Journal of Psychiatry*, **116**, 241–253.

Owens, D. G. C., Johnstone, E. C., Bydder, G. M. & Kreel, L. (1980) Unsuspected organic disease in chronic schizophrenia demonstrated by computed tomography. *Journal of Neurology, Neurosurgery & Psychiatry*, **43**, 1065–1069.

Panse, F. (1942) *Die Erbchorea*. Leipzig.

Perez, M. M., Trimble, M. R., Murray, N. M. F. & Reider, I. (1985) Epileptic psychosis: an evaluation of PSE profiles. *British Journal of Psychiatry*, **146**, 155–163.

Propping, P. (1983) Genetic disorders presenting as "schizophrenia". Karl Bonhoeffer's early view of the psychoses in the light of medical genetics. *Human Genetics*, **65**, 1–10.

Remington, F. B. & Rubert, S. L. (1962) Why patients with brain tumors come to a psychiatric hospital. *American Journal of Psychiatry*, **119**, 256–263.

Robins, L. N., Helzer, J. E., Weissman, M. M., Orvaschel, H., Gruenberg, E., Burke, J. D. & Regier, D. A. (1984) Lifetime prevalence of specific psychiatric disorders in three sites. *Archives of General Psychiatry*, **41**, 949–958.

Russell, D. S. & Rubinstein, L. J. (1963) *Pathology of Tumours of the Nervous System* (2nd edn). London: Arnold.

Rutter, M. & Lockyer, L. (1967) A five to fifteen year follow-up study of infantile psychosis. I. Description of sample. *British Journal of Psychiatry*, **113**, 1169–1182.

Saugstad, L. & Ødegård, Ø. (1986) Huntington's chorea in Norway. *Psychological Medicine*, **16**, 39–48.

Scheinberg, I. H. & Sternlieb, I. (1985) *Wilson's Disease*. (Major Problems in Internal Medicine, vol 23). Philadelphia: W. B. Saunders.

Selecki, B. R. (1965) Intracranial space-occupying lesions among patients admitted to mental hospitals. *Medical Journal of Australia*, **1**, 383–390.

Shaskan, D. (1938) Mental changes in chorea minor (Sydenham's). *American Journal of Psychiatry*, **95**, 193–202.

Slater, E., Beard, A. W. & Glithero, E. (1963) The schizophrenia-like psychoses of epilepsy. *British Journal of Psychiatry*, **109**, 95–150.

—— & Cowie, V. (1971) *The Genetics of Mental Disorders*. London: Oxford University Press.

SOURS, J. A. (1963) Narcolepsy and other disturbances in the sleep-waking rhythm: a study of 115 cases with review of the literature. *Journal of Nervous and Mental Disease*, **137**, 525–542.

SPITZER, R., ENDICOTT, J. & ROBINS, E. (1975) *Research Diagnostic Criteria*. New York: New York State Psychiatric Institute.

STEVENS, J. R. (1966) Psychiatric implications of psychomotor epilepsy. *Archives of General Psychiatry*, **14**, 461–471.

—— (1985) Epilepsy and psychosis. *British Journal of Psychiatry*, **146**, 321–322.

STRELETZKI, F. (1961) Psychosen im Verlauf der Huntingtonscher Chorea unter besonderer Berücksichtigung der Wahnbildungen. *Archive für Psychiatrie und Nervenkrankheiten*, **202**, 202–214.

TORREY, E. F. & PETERSON, M. R. (1974) Schizophrenia and the limbic system. *Lancet*, ii, 942–946.

—— (1987) Prevalence studies in schizophrenia. *British Journal of Psychiatry*, **150**, 598–608.

VON KORFF, M. V., NESTADT, G., ROMANOSKI, A., ANTHONY, J., EATON, W., MERCHANT, A., CHAHAL, R., KRAMER, M., FOLSTEIN, M. & GRUENBERG, E. (1985) Prevalence of treated and untreated DSM–III schizophrenia. Results of a two-stage community survey. *Journal of Nervous and Mental Disease*, **173**, 577–581.

WERTHEIMER, N. M. (1963) A psychiatric follow-up of children with rheumatic fever and other chronic diseases. *Journal of Chronic Diseases*, **16**, 223–237.

WILSON, S. A. K. (1912) Progressive lenticular degeneration: a familial nervous disease associated with cirrhosis of the liver. *Brain*, **34**, 295–309.

WING, J. K., COOPER, J. E. & SARTORIUS, N. (1974) *The Description and Classification of Psychiatric Symptoms: An Instruction Manual for the PSE and Catego Systems*. Cambridge: Cambridge University Press.

ZIELINSKY, J. J. (1982) Epidemiology. In *A Textbook of Epilepsy* (eds. J. Laidlaw & A. Richens). Edinburgh: Churchill Livingstone.

# 41 Tardive dyskinesia: The natural history and outcome

## HAMISH McCLELLAND and ALAN KERR

The study of the natural history of mental disorder has a hallowed tradition extending back to classical times. In our work with Martin Roth in earlier years the importance of course and outcome, and the identification of factors of predictive importance, were important lessons. Determination of the mortality, and whether there is an altered risk, of the patients under scrutiny also forms an important component.

The ideal objective is a methodological design in which a large sample of patients is studied in the context of a prospective follow-up, with detailed assessments made both at initial presentation and at the time of follow-up, by independent observers of proven reliability and free from bias and preconception. Such investigations were more practicable 20 years ago when there was greater availability of manpower, more generous funding, absence of a need to fulfil educational requirements and easier access to computing and statistical facilities. To mount a sizeable prospective study nowadays is a formidable undertaking and this is a pity as longitudinal studies have never been over-worked and have been confined to comparatively few groups of illnesses. What Aubrey Lewis said 50 years ago remains true, ''It will be a pity if other quests kept us from making sure of all the plain clinical things that have yet to be seen and studied'' (Lewis, 1936). From the investigator's point of view such projects have the agreeable features that they always produce a result, and one which should be publishable.

The interest of one of us (H.A.McC) in the problem of tardive dyskinesia began 25 years ago when the disorder had only recently been identified (Schonecker, 1957). Interest at that time focused on problems of identification, assessment and prevalence and subsequently on risk and predisposing factors. About one-fifth of chronic psychotic patients are estimated to be affected by dyskinesia, with some in-patient populations having a reported prevalence rate of up to 50%; Jeste & Wyatt (1981) have argued convincingly that there has been a true increase in prevalence rates in recent years.

While tardive dyskinesia as a clinical syndrome is linked to the administration of neuroleptics, persistent minor facial movements can occur spontaneously in the elderly and have been reported as occurring in psychotic patients independent of medication (Owens et al, 1982). However, precise and agreed diagnostic criteria for the condition are essential for satisfactory communication and meaningful research and there is as yet no general agreement, particularly in relation to the minor forms of abnormal movements. It seems likely that the writings of

410

Kraepelin and Bleuler refer to such disorders rather than the more complex and distinctive movements of tardive dyskinesia. It is generally agreed that tardive dyskinesia occurs with more or less equal frequency in all forms of neuroleptic-treated functional psychosis.

Although it is generally accepted that neuroleptic medication plays a causal role in the development of tardive dyskinesia, there have been difficulties in firmly establishing this aetiology due to the paucity of prospective studies. A good deal of the evidence has been based on a clinical observation of psychotic patients receiving such drugs, the development of movements in non-schizophrenic neuroleptic-treated patients, the absence of dyskinesia on long-stay wards in countries such as Turkey where neuroleptics have not been used (Crane, 1968) and a few prospective studies (Kane *et al*, 1985). Only a few cross-sectional studies examining retrospective data have found an aetiological role for neuroleptics (Tarsey & Baldessarini, 1984).

In the past decade attention has been focused on subtle cognitive changes in chronic schizophrenia. Recent work has shown that schizophrenic patients with tardive dyskinesia are more likely to have cognitive impairment than those without dyskinesia (Famuyiwa *et al*, 1979; Waddington *et al*, 1987). However, while cognitive impairment is increasingly believed to be a clinical manifestation of chronic schizophrenia, the possibility that neuroleptics may in part be responsible has hitherto not been systematically evaluated.

In our own follow-up study, prospective and over a 16-year period, we examined the course and outcome of a large group of mental hospital patients suffering from movement disorders. Prospective studies such as this and that by Kane *et al* (1985) have the advantage of being able to disentangle risk factors and specifically the aetiological contributions of neuroleptics in relation to outcome. Cross-sectional studies have to depend on retrospective scanning of unsystematically recorded pharmacological data and uncertainty about when the dyskinesia began so that the duration and dosage of medication prior to the onset is difficult to determine and therefore the causal role of medication cannot be clarified with confidence. The mortality rate and factors related to death were determined and the relationship between psychiatric diagnosis, age, sex, neuroleptic prescribing and other variables in predisposing to subsequent dyskinesia in the survivors was examined. Interest in the organic basis of schizophrenia, particularly among the more chronic forms, encouraged us to take an interest in possible cognitive impairment and cerebral pathology. Awareness of the medico-legal implications of drug-induced disorders gives a heightened if unwelcome contemporary addition to a natural scientific interest in this subject.

The large prevalence survey carried out in Newcastle in 1965 on facial dyskinesia (Brandon *et al*, 1971) served as the starting point for our follow-up enquiries which were completed in 1981. In 1965, all 910 patients in the Newcastle mental hospital (St Nicholas) who had been resident for over three months were examined for the presence of facial dyskinesia which was found in 15% of the men and 30% of the women. (Facial dyskinesia is the commonest manifestation of tardive dyskinesia, being present in over 80% of cases—Jeste & Wyatt, 1982). Increasing age was found to be the most significant factor in determining the risk of developing dyskinesia. Neuroleptics were significantly associated with facial dyskinesia in patients aged over 50. However, 25% of the patients with facial dyskinesia had never been exposed to neuroleptics and such patients spanned all age groups.

Two previous studies on *mortality* had produced conflicting results. Mehta *et al* (1978) followed up 35 patients with dyskinesia, and 35 patients without, for five years and found reduced survival time in the dyskinetic group while Kucharski *et al* (1979) followed up 377 patients for 18 months but found no association between dyskinesia and early death. In our follow-up we were able to trace the outcome in terms of death or age at survival for 408 (84%) of the 484 females originally examined (McClelland *et al*, 1986) of whom 249 and 159 suffered from functional and organic disorders respectively. While no reduced life expectancy for patients with primary organic disorder who had facial dyskinesia was found, the patients with functional disorders who had moderate and severe dyskinesia had significantly reduced survival time. However, those patients with mild dyskinesia, sometimes described as low-grade oral movements, did not die prematurely. As minor dyskinesia is more common in older patients, this suggests that it may represent a normal ageing process unconnected with psychiatric disorder or neuroleptic prescribing.

A recent investigation by Youssef & Waddington (1987) of 101 schizophrenic in-patients has confirmed that only more prominent dyskinesia is associated with increased mortality. Our study gave no firm reason for the reduced life expectancy, although a significant association was found between the number of infections in the 12 months before death and the presence of dyskinesia. Interestingly, Youssef & Waddington found that their surviving dyskinetic patients, compared with those without dyskinesia, were more likely to have repeated respiratory tract infections and to suffer from more cardiovascular disorders. They found that smoking was equal in their dyskinetic and non-dyskinetic groups but those with involuntary movements who died were more likely to be smokers than those who died without involuntary movements. Furthermore, dyskinetic patients were more likely to die of a vascular problem. The authors suggested that patients with dyskinesia were more vulnerable to the effects of smoking.

At follow-up we found, of the original 484 women, 356 had died, 14 could not be traced, four had moved away and one refused to be interviewed; 77 were still in hospital and 32 living in the community, making a total of 109 patients available for study.

Details of neuroleptic medication taken at five-year intervals during the total follow-up period in terms of graded chlopromazine equivalents were calculated. Other types of psychotropic medication (antiparkinsonian drugs, benzodiazepines, antidepressants) were graded. Details regarding length of psychiatric illness and physical treatment (ECT, insulin coma, psychosurgery) were also determined. The AIMS (Abnormal Involuntary Movements Scale) was used to rate dyskinesia. A simple parkinsonian rating scale was used with single items (rigidity, loss of arm swing, tremor) and an overall score. The mental state (cognitive) examination was tested using patients' subjective age against chronological age (Crow & Stevens, 1978), the Face/Hand test (Irving *et al*, 1970) and the Newcastle Dementia Scale (Blessed *et al*, 1968). Brain scan (CT) studies were carried out on a sub-group of 25 patients in 1985.

# The findings

The 109 survivors had an overall dyskinesia prevalence of 17.4% in 1965 which had risen to 43.1% in 1981. The prevalence of dyskinesia increased with age as has been found in other studies (Table I).

The overall dyskinesia severity among the patients had also increased during the follow-up period. In 1965 there were six cases of moderate but no severe dyskinesia and in 1981 fourteen moderate and two severe cases.

Psychiatric diagnoses were based on DSM–III criteria. Table II gives details in relation to dyskinesia status. The five patients with organic brain syndrome were excluded from subsequent analysis. The 104 patients with functional diagnoses were divided into four groups:

  (a)  Dyskinesia positive in 1965 to negative in 1981. Six patients—four with moderate and two mild dyskinesia. Only three of the six had stopped neuroleptics by 1981.

  (b)  Dyskinesia positive in 1965 and 1981. Eight cases—six with mild dyskinesia in 1965 of whom three remained mild and three increased to moderate. Of the two who were moderate in 1965 one remained unchanged and one improved to mild. No case who had dyskinesia in 1965 deteriorated to the severe grade by 1981.

  (c)  Dyskinesia free in 1965 and 1981; 52 patients.

  (d)  Dyskinesia negative in 1965 and dyskinesia positive in 1981; 38 patients, of whom 25 developed mild, 11 moderate and two severe dyskinesia.

Eight patients, all long-term in-patients, had never received any neuroleptics. Each was dyskinesia free in 1965; seven remained so in 1981 while one patient developed mild dyskinesia.

As the mortality study had shown that patients with mild dyskinesia may represent a non-pathological variant, analyses were performed first with all

TABLE I

*Facial dyskinesia in 109 survivors in 1965 and 1981 (Figures in brackets are percentages of total)*

| Age 1981 | Total | Dyskinesia + 1965 | Dyskinesia + 1981 |
|---|---|---|---|
| 50 years | 17 | 1 (5.5) | 2 (11.8) |
| 51–60 | 21 | 1 (4.8) | 9 (42.9) |
| 61–70 | 27 | 4 (14.8) | 9 (33.3) |
| Over 70 | 44 | 13 (29.6) | 27 (61.4) |
| | 109 | 19 (17.4) | 47 (43.1) |

TABLE II

*Psychiatric diagnosis and dyskinesia status (1981)*

| Diagnosis | Total number | No dyskinesia | Number with dyskinesia | | | % with dyskinesia |
|---|---|---|---|---|---|---|
| | | | Mild | Moderate | Severe | |
| Schizophrenia | 62 | 35 | 15 | 10 | 2 | (43.5) |
| Schizo-Affective | 15 | 7 | 5 | 3 | 0 | (53.3) |
| Manic Depressive | 17 | 8 | 8 | 1 | 0 | (52.9) |
| Other | 10 | 8 | 1 | 1 | 0 | (20) |
| Organic Brain Syndrome | 5 | 4 | 1 | 0 | 0 | (20) |
| | 109 | 62 | 30 | 15 | 2 | |

TABLE III
*Treatment items and dyskinesia development*

| Treatment item | Dyskinesia defined as mild, moderate, severe | | Dyskinesia defined as moderate and severe only | |
| --- | --- | --- | --- | --- |
| | Dyskinesia neg. 1965 and 1981 (n = 52) Dyskinesia neg. 1965 and pos. 1981 (n = 38) | | Dyskinesia neg. 1965 and 1981 (n = 82) Dyskinesia neg. 1965 and pos. 1981 (n = 16) | |
| Psychosurgery | NS | | NS | |
| ECT | NS | | NS | |
| Neuroleptics 1975–1981 | NS | | NS | |
| Duration (short) of neuroleptics to 1965 | NS | | * | |
| Duration (long) of neuroleptics to 1981 | * | | * | |
| Increasing amounts of neuroleptics to 1981 | $P = 0.09$ | | ** | |
| Overall amounts of neuroleptics to 1981 | ** | | ** | |
| Total antidepressants | NS | | NS | |
| Total benzodiazepines | NS | | NS | |
| Total lithium | NS | | NS | |
| Total amount of antiparkinsonian drugs | * | | $P = 0.06$ | |

\*$P < 0.05$  1-sided alternative hypothesis        $P$-values between 0.05 and 0.1 are given (1-sided alternative)
\*\*$P < 0.01$  1-sided alternative hypothesis
Psychiatric diagnosis has been allowed for. A linear allowance has been made for age.

gradings of dyskinesia (mild, moderate and severe) and secondly with moderate and severe dyskinesia only. Of the treatment items shown in Table III, "overall amount of neuroleptics", "longer duration of neuroleptics to 1981", and "increasing amounts of neuroleptics" were significantly associated with the development of dyskinesia between 1965 and 1981. "Short duration of neuroleptic prescribing (prior to 1965)" was significantly but negatively correlated when dyskinesia was restricted to moderate and severe grades. Other drugs (anti-depressants, benzodiazepines and lithium) and physical treatments were not associated with dyskinesia development. It will be seen that restricting dyskinesia to moderate and severe grades only had the effect of increasing the significance of certain neuroleptic items.

The use of antiparkinsonian medication was significantly associated with dyskinesia development (moderate and severe grades only) and these drugs may have masked the role of parkinsonism. Parkinsonism itself is not significantly associated with dyskinesia development, though in the under-fifty age group there was a non-significant trend. Dyskinesia was only slightly less frequent in schizophrenic patients than in the other major functional psychoses (Table I).

Patients who developed dyskinesia during the follow-up period, in contrast to those who remained dyskinesia-free, scored significantly worse on the dementia scale and the subjective age test. Only one treatment item, "being on neuroleptics 1975–1981", was significantly associated with increased dementia score. Analyses with interactional items which took into account diagnosis, duration of illness and neuroleptic prescribing showed that, for schizophrenic patients, the dementia score increased with the length of the illness but not for non-schizophrenic patients. Poor subjective age performance was also significantly linked to the duration of illness in the schizophrenic patients.

*Brain scan studies* were carried out on 25 of the patients. Seventeen suffered from schizophrenia, three manic–depressive disorder, four schizo-affective psychosis and one from an "other" functional disorder. Only two of these 25 patients were graded as "dubious or minimal" dyskinesia in 1965 and the remainder were dyskinesia negative. By 1981 12 had developed facial dyskinesia (eight mild and four moderate).

There was no significant association between dyskinesia development and Ventricle Brain Ratio (VBR) in the group as a whole. However, of the 14 patients under 65 years, there were three cases of facial dyskinesia and these were significantly associated with increased ventricle size. Age, as expected, was very significantly associated with increased ventricle size. "Overall amount of neuroleptics" was highly significantly associated with high brain scan scores even when allowing for the contribution of diagnosis and length of illness. "Longer duration of neuroleptics to 1981" was also significantly related. Thus, there was clear evidence of an association between increased ventricle size and neuroleptic medication. Analyses of dementia and subjective age scores also (allowing for age) showed a significant association between subjective age score results and ventricular enlargement.

## Comment

A major problem in defining control groups for dyskinesia is that, in populations taken into a study at any defined point, an unknown number of patients, though initially dyskinesia negative, will in time develop dyskinesia. The Newcastle study, prospective and with a 16-year follow-up period, and with neuroleptic data extending up to ten years before 1965, will have as valid a dyskinesia-resistant population as it is practicable to collect.

Recent work suggests that the outlook for tardive dyskinesia is not as serious as was once thought (Casey, 1985). The American Task Force (1980) reviewing dyskinesia studies estimated that 22% of patients went into remission when neuroleptics were discontinued and, even when continued, stability of dyskinesia severity or a degree of spontaneous improvement in up to 50% of cases studied takes place (Klawans *et al*, 1984; Casey *et al*, 1986; Seeman, 1981; Robinson & McCreadie, 1986). In our group of 14 functional patients who had dyskinesia in 1965, six became dyskinesia-free and only three had stopped neuroleptics. Of the eight who remain dyskinesia-positive, none had progressed to a severe grade by 1981. In contrast, only two patients had developed severe dyskinesia at follow-up and both had been dyskinesia-free in 1965. Both these patients were in their late 60s in 1965, both had had schizophrenic illnesses for many years prior to 1965 and neither had received neuroleptics until the early 1970s. This emphasises the vulnerability of the elderly to the comparatively rapid onset of such movements after neuroleptic prescribing is initiated (Toenniessen *et al*, 1985).

Patients who developed dyskinesia by 1981, compared with the control group, had taken significantly larger and increasing amounts of neuroleptics, and were still receiving neuroleptics in 1981. That long duration of neuroleptic prescribing prior to 1965 was negatively correlated with the development of moderate or severe dyskinesia suggests that there are patients with a high constitutional resistance and, further, that for most patients dyskinesia starts within a comparatively short time of starting neuroleptics. Crane & Smeets (1974) found no simple relationship between tardive dyskinesia and the length of neuroleptic intake. In their study tardive dyskinesia was commoner in patients receiving neuroleptics for six to eight years than those who had received shorter or longer courses. Kane and his colleagues (1985) found that their younger patients showed a steady annual incidence of 3–4%, implying a linear relationship, while Toenniessen and colleagues (1985) claimed that older patients showed no significant difference in tardive dyskinesia over a duration of treatment range of 5–25 years.

The role of antiparkinsonian drugs has been a matter of dispute. Some investigators argue that such medication has a direct aetiological role in dyskinesia while others suggest, and our findings support, that parkinsonism occurs in a vulnerable brain predisposed to dyskinesia (Kane *et al*, 1986; Chouinard *et al*, 1986).

Dyskinesia development in the younger patients (under 65) was significantly associated with ventricle enlargement. Waddington (1987) reviewed 11 CT studies of patients with and without dyskinesia. Three showed no abnormality of the VB ratio but four studies showed ventricular abnormality in all dyskinetic patients. The other four studies did not evaluate VB ratio: they examined and found caudate or cerebral atrophy.

The patients who developed dyskinesia between 1965 and 1981 were more likely to have had poorer scores on the subjective age test and dementia rating scale than the persistently dyskinesia-free population. This would fit a commonsense view that dyskinesia is an indicator of brain damage which is also reflected in cognitive impairment. But the issue of cognitive impairment is a complex one. It is now generally accepted that schizophrenia is an organic brain disorder and Waddington (1987), reviewing studies in the past decade, has shown that cognitive dysfunction and the defect state (negative symptoms) are present to a greater extent in schizophrenic patients who have involuntary movements than those that do not. A prospective study by Struve & Wilner (1983) showed that the patients with tardive dyskinesia had greater cognitive dysfunction and they found that the cognitive dysfunction predated the development of tardive dyskinesia.

The possibility that neuroleptics themselves can bring about, or increase, cognitive impairment as well as causing dyskinesia has to be considered. Our findings showed that, when diagnosis and neuroleptic prescribing were allowed for, the schizophrenic patients showed a significant correlation between the duration of illness and increased cognitive impairment suggesting an intrinsic deterioration during the course of their illness. But when the matter was examined further in the group of patients who had CT scans, analyses showed that (even when allowing for age) psychiatric diagnosis, length of illness and a possible differential effect of neuroleptics on the psychiatric diagnosis, "overall amount" and "longer duration of neuroleptics to 1981" were still significantly associated with increased ventricle size.

These results do not therefore necessarily incriminate neuroleptics as an aetiological factor, as the patients with ventricle enlargement could have been more psychiatrically ill over the decades and therefore required more neuroleptics. However, this seems less likely as schizophrenics with negative symptoms (now assumed to be the more brain-damaged) receive less neuroleptic medication than those with positive symptoms (Opler *et al*, 1984). Our results support the findings of Famuyiwa and his colleagues (1979) who found a significant correlation between dyskinesia, cognitive impairment and abnormal brain scans;

these authors suggested, though could not confirm from their own data, an aetiological role for neuroleptics. However, a large brain scan study (Owens, 1985) of 110 patients with and without dyskinesia showed no significant relationship between VBR and past neuroleptic exposure. But this latter study did show a significant correlation between the severer forms of dyskinesia and ventricular enlargement.

## Concluding remarks

Our findings indicate that patients with functional psychosis who manifest dyskinesia have a shortened life expectancy and greater cognitive impairment. They are a biologically disadvantaged group.

However, our long-term follow-up confirms other findings of the past decade that the abnormal movements themselves do not inexorably progress. Nearly half of the patients with dyskinesia in 1965 had lost their movements by 1981. The only patients who developed severe movements by 1981 were the two women who were free of dyskinesia in 1965 but later commenced neuroleptics in their old age.

Cognitive impairment was associated with dyskinesia, ventricle enlargement and longer duration of illness in schizophrenia. There was only a weak association between cognitive impairment and neuroleptic prescribing. The significant association between ventricle enlargement and neuroleptics may be causal, though an alternative explanation is that the patients were more ill for sustained periods with probable intrinsic deficits and therefore received more enthusiastic treatment.

The modern view (Waddington, 1987) is that patients with schizophrenia have intrinsic organic deficits which may lead to spontaneous dyskinesia with neuroleptics bringing out or exacerbating dyskinesia. The basic deficits also seem associated with minimal cognitive impairment and one can postulate that treatment factors such as neuroleptics can increase such impairment. In our follow-up study the link between neuroleptic prescribing, dyskinesia development and ventricle enlargement is strong; the link between dyskinesia and cognitive impairment is also strong. However, we could not firmly establish an association between neuroleptics and cognitive impairment, though neuroleptics were significantly associated with increased ventricle size. We consider it is a matter of urgency that further studies should examine the possible role of neuroleptics in causing, or exacerbating, more generalised brain damage.

In the meantime, clinicians should carefully tailor the amount of neuroleptic prescribing to what is needed by the patient rather than by the standard dosages which may be unnecessarily high. Recent work has explored the benefits of low-dosage neuroleptic therapy (Manchanda & Hirsch, 1986; Marder *et al*, 1987). Low dosage not only entails a lower risk of tardive dyskinesia and associated movement disorders but may also have implications for less cognitive impairment and less behavioural abnormality. The need for new antipsychotic drugs with different modes of action is great, not only to reduce the increasing list of side-effects attributed to neuroleptics but to provide more effective treatment.

## Acknowledgement

We thank Andrew Metcalfe, Department of Mathematics, University of Newcastle-upon-Tyne, for statistical help.

## References

BARNES, T. R. E. & BRAUDE, W. M. (1985) Akathisia variants and tardive dyskinesia. *Archives of General Psychiatry*, **42**, 874–878.

BLESSED, G., TOMLINSON, B. E. & ROTH, M. (1968) The association between quantitative measures of dementia and senile change in the cerebral grey matter of elderly subjects. *British Journal of Psychiatry*, **114**, 797–811.

BRANDON, S., McCLELLAND, H. A. & PROTHEROE, C. (1971) A study of facial dyskinesia in a mental hospital population. *British Journal of Psychiatry*, **181**, 171–184.

CASEY, D. E. (1985) Tardive dyskinesia: reversible and irreversible. In *Dyskinesia—Research and treatment* (eds. D. E. Casey, T. N. Chase, A. V. Christensen & J. Gerlach). Berlin: Springer-Verlag (pp. 88–96).

——, POVISEN, U. J., MEIDAHL, B. M. & GERLACH, J. (1986) Neuroleptic-induced tardive dyskinesia and parkinsonism changes during several changes of treatment. *Psychopharmacology Bulletin*, **22**, 250–253.

CHOUINARD, G., ANNABLE, L., MERCIER, P. & ROSS-CHOUINARD, A. (1986) A five-year follow-up study of tardive dyskinesia. *Psychopharmacology Bulletin*, **22**, 259–263.

CRANE, G. E. (1968) Dyskinesia and neuroleptics. *Archives of General Psychiatry*, **19**, 700–703.

—— & SMEETS, R. A. (1974) Tardive dyskinesia and drug therapy in geriatric patients. *Archives of General Psychiatry*, **30**, 341–343.

CROW, T. J. & STEVENS, M. (1978) Age disorientation in chronic schizophrenia: the nature of the cognitive deficit. *British Journal of Psychiatry*, **133**, 137–142.

FAMUYIWA, O. O., ECCLESTON, D., DONALDSON, A. A. & GARSIDE, R. F. (1979) Tardive dyskinesia and dementia. *British Journal of Psychiatry*, **135**, 500–504.

GARDOS, G. & COLE, J. O. (1980) Problems in the assessment of tardive dyskinesia. In *Tardive Dyskinesia: Research and Treatment* (eds. W. E. Fann, R. C. Smith, J. M. Davis & F. E. Domino). New York: Spectrum Publications.

IRVING, G., ROBINSON, R. A. & McADAM, W. (1970) The validity of some cognitive tests in the diagnosis of dementia. *British Journal of Psychiatry*, **117**, 149–156.

JESTE, D. V. & WYATT, R. J. (1981) The changing epidemiology of tardive dyskinesia. *American Journal of Psychiatry*, **138**, 297–309.

—— & —— (1982) *Understanding and Treating Tardive Dyskinesia*. New York and London: The Guilford Press.

KANE, J. M., WOEVNER, M., BORENSTEIN, M., WEGNER, J. & LIEBERMAN, J. (1986) Integrating incidence and prevalence of tardive dyskinesia. *Psychopharmacology Bulletin*, **22**, 254–258.

——, —— & LIEBERMANN, J. (1985) Tardive dyskinesia: prevalence, incidence and risk factors. In *Dyskinesia: Research and Treatment* (eds D. E. Casey, T. N. Chase, A. V. Christensen & J. Gerlach). Berlin: Springer-Verlag. (pp. 72–78).

—— & SMITH, J. M. (1982) Tardive dyskinesia: prevalence and risk factors 1959–1979. *Archives of General Psychiatry*, **39**, 473–481.

——, WOEVNER, M., WEINHOLD, P., WEGNER, J., KINON, B. & BORENSTEIN, M. (1984) *Psychopharmacology Bulletin*, **20**, 387–389.

KLAWANS, H. L., TANNER, C. M. & BARR, A. (1984) The reversibility of permanent tardive dyskinesia. *Clinical Neuropharmacology*, **7**, 153–159.

KUCHARSKI, L. T., SMITH, J. M. & DUNN, D. D. (1979) Mortality and tardive dyskinesia. *American Journal of Psychiatry*, **168**, 215.

LEWIS, A. J. (1936) Melancholia: a prognostic study. *Journal of Mental Science*, **82**, 488–588.

MANCHANDA, R. & HIRSCH, S. R. (1986) Low dose maintenance medication for schizophrenia. *British Medical Journal*, **293**, 515–516.

MARDER, R. S., VAN PUTTEN, T., MINTZ, J., LEBELL, M., McKENZIE, J. & MAY, P. R. A. (1987) Low—and conventional—dose maintenance therapy with fluphenazine decanoate. *Archives of General Psychiatry*, **44**, 518–521.

McCLELLAND, H. A., DUTTA, D., METCALF, A. & KERR, T. A. (1986) Mortality and facial dyskinesia. *British Journal of Psychiatry*, **148**, 310–316.

MEHTA, D., MALLYE, A. & VOLARKA, J. (1978) Mortality of patients with tardive dyskinesia. *American Journal of Psychiatry*, **135**, 371-372.

NATIONAL INSTITUTE OF MENTAL HEALTH (1976) Abnormal Involuntary Movement Scale. In *ECDEU Assessment Manual* (ed. W. Guy). Rockville: US Department of Health, Education and Welfare.

OPLER, L. A., KAY, S. R., ROSADO, V. & LINDENMAYER, J. P. (1984) Positive and negative syndromes in schizophrenic inpatients. *Journal of Nervous and Mental Disease*, **172**, 317-325.

OWENS, D. G. C. & JOHNSTONE, E. C. (1982) Spontaneous involuntary disorders of movement. *Archives of General Psychiatry*, **39**, 452-461.

—— (1985) Involuntary disorders of movement in chronic schizophrenia—the role of the illness and its treatment. In *Dyskinesia: Research of Treatment* (eds. D. E. Casey, T. N. Chase, A. V. Christensen & J. Gerlach). Berlin: Springer-Verlag, (79-87).

ROBINSON, A. D. T. & MCCREADIE R. G. (1986) The Nithsdale Schizophrenia Survey v. follow-up of tardive dyskinesia after 31/2 years. *British Journal of Psychiatry*, **149**, 621-623.

SCHONECKER, M. (1957) Ein eigentumliches Syndrom im oralen Bereich bei Megaphen Applikation. *Nervenarzt*, **28**, 35.

SCHOOLER, N. R. & KANE, J. M. (1982) Research diagnoses for tardive dyskinesia. *Archives of General Psychiatry*, **39**, 486-487.

SEEMAN, M. V. (1981) Tardive dyskinesia: two year recovery. *Comprehensive Psychiatry*, **22**, 189-192.

SIGWALD, J., BOUTTIER, D., RAYMONDEAUD, C. *et al* (1959) Quatre cas de dyskinesie facio-bucco-lingui-masticatrice à evolution prolongée secondaire à un traitment par les neuroleptiques. *Revue Neurologique*, **100**, 751-755.

STAHL, S. M. (1986) Natural history studies assist the pursuit of preventive therapies. *Psychological Medicine*, **16**, 491-494.

STRUVE, F. A. & WILLNER, A. E. (1983) Cognitive dysfunction and tardive dyskinesia. *British Journal of Psychiatry*, **143**, 597-600.

TARSEY, D. & BALDESSARINI, R. J. (1984) Tardive dyskinesia. *Annual Review of Medicine*, **35**, 605-623.

TASK FORCE ON LATE NEUROLOGICAL EFFECTS OF ANTIPSYCHOTIC DRUGS (1980) Tardive dyskinesia. *American Journal of Psychiatry*, **137**, 1163-1172.

TOENNIESSEN, L. M., CASEY, D. E. & MCFARLAND, B. H. (1985) Tardive dyskinesia in the aged. *Archives of General Psychiatry*, **42**, 278-284.

WADDINGTON, J. L. (1987) Tardive dyskinesia in schizophrenia and other disorders: associations with ageing, cognitive dysfunction and structural brain pathology in relation to neuroleptic exposure. *Human Psychopharmacology*, **2**, 11-22.

——, YOUSSEF, H. A., DOLPHIN, C. & KINSELLA, A. (1987) Cognitive dysfunction, negative symptoms and tardive dyskinesia in schizophrenia. *Archives of General Psychiatry*, **44**, 907-912.

—— & —— (1986) Late onset involuntary movements in chronic schizophrenia. *British Journal of Psychiatry*, **149**, 616-620.

WILSON, I. C., GARBUTT, J. C., LANIER, C. F., MOYLAN, J., NELSON, W. & PRANGE, A. J. (1983) Is there a tardive dysmentia? *Schizophrenia Bulletin*, **9**, 187-192.

YOUSSEF, H. A. & WADDINGTON, J. L. (1987) Morbidity and mortality in tardive dyskinesia. *Acta Psychiatrica Scandinavica*, **75**, 74-77.

# 42  An investigation to determine the clinical characteristics of acute akathisia

## WALTER M. BRAUDE

This study was completed in collaboration with Dr Thomas R. E. Barnes, in the University Department of Psychiatry, Cambridge, between 1980 and 1983. It was supervised by Professor Sir Martin Roth, to whom I personally owe a great debt of gratitude and who was a source of wisdom and inspiration both through the study and in my formative years as a psychiatric trainee. I have written this selected account of the study so as to represent most accurately Sir Martin's impression on my endeavours. I have thus highlighted the form and detail of the enquiry with particular reference to the methodology, as much as its clinical utility, as my tribute. This study was published in more complete form in the *British Journal of Psychiatry* (Braude *et al*, 1983). It has also formed part of my MD thesis.

## Background to the study

Akathisia is a syndrome of motor restlessness associated with the administration of antipsychotic drugs. Despite its being a common and distressing condition in clinical practice, phenomenological descriptions at the time of the study were noted for their inconsistency and a generally accepted clinical definition had hitherto not been established. This may explain the variability of reported prevalence and treatment response of the condition. The lack of precise diagnostic criteria may be related to the composite nature of the syndrome, which comprises both a subjective sense of restlessness and observable motor signs. Clinicians have differed in their opinion regarding the relative importance of these two aspects of the condition and confusion has also arisen in distinguishing it clinically from psychotic illness.

The main aims of this study were firstly to identify the characteristic phenomena of the syndrome in acute psychiatric in-patients receiving antipsychotic medication and, secondly, to study the clinical behaviour of the condition during these patients' hospital stay.

## Method

Over a six-month period, consecutive admissions were monitored throughout their hospital stay. All patients who required antipsychotic medication following admission during this period were considered suitable for the study and 104

TABLE I

*Incidence of items derived from 'restlessness' questionnaire and examination schedule in 'akathisia' and 'illness-related movement' groups*

| | 'Akathisia' group | | | | Illness-related movement group |
|---|---|---|---|---|---|
| | Mild ($n = 8$) n(%) | Moderate ($n = 13$) n(%) | Severe ($n = 6$) n(%) | Total ($n = 27$) n(%) | ($n = 35$) n(%) |
| *Symptoms (Patient report)* | | | | | |
| Limb sensations | 6(75%) | 6(46%) | 3(50%) | 15(56%) | 7(20%) |
| Inner restlessness | 7(88%) | 9(69%) | 6(100%) | 22(81%) | 23(66%) |
| Inability to remain still | 7(88%) | 12(92%) | 6(100%) | 25(93%) | 11(31%) |
| Inability to keep legs still | 7(88%) | 13(100%) | 6(100%) | 26(96%) | 7(20%) |
| Symptoms worse while standing | 2(25%) | 9(69%) | 5(83%) | 16(59%) | — |
| Associated moderate/severe distress | 2(25%) | 9(69%) | 5(83%) | 16(59%) | — |
| *Signs* | | | | | |
| (i) Sitting | | | | | |
| Semipurposeful feet movements for more than half the time | 2(25%) | 3(23%) | 5(83%) | 10(37%) | 4(11%) |
| Shifting position in chair | 1(13%) | 5(38%) | 5(83%) | 11(41%) | 1(3%) |
| Inability to remain seated | 0 | 1(8%) | 4(67%) | 5(19%) | 3(9%) |
| Semipurposeful hand/arm movements for more than half the time | 2(25%) | 3(23%) | 1(17%) | 6(22%) | 18(51%) |
| Purposeless normal hand/arm movements | 2(25%) | 2(15%) | 1(17%) | 5(19%) | 10(29%) |
| (ii) Standing | | | | | |
| Rocking from foot to foot etc. (more than half the time) | 0 | 9(69%) | 6(100%) | 15(56%) | 0 |
| Other normal purposeless foot movements | 1(13%) | 7(54%) | 2(33%) | 10(37%) | 1(3%) |
| Inability to remain standing | 1(13%) | 2(15%) | 5(83%) | 8(30%) | 1(3%) |
| (iii) Lying | | | | | |
| Coarse tremor | 0 | 8(62%) | 6(100%) | 14(52%) | 1(3%) |
| Myoclonic jerks of the feet | 0 | 11(85%) | 5(83%) | 16(59%) | 0 |
| Semipurposeful feet movements | 0 | 4(31%) | 5(83%) | 9(33%) | 2(6%) |
| Shifting position of legs | 0 | 4(31%) | 5(83%) | 9(33%) | 5(14%) |
| Trunk movements | 0 | 0 | 2(33%) | 2(7%) | 2(6%) |
| Inability to remain lying | 0 | 0 | 2(33%) | 2(7%) | 0 |

patients were initially assessed. The investigation was intended as a 'naturalistic' study, all patients at risk of developing akathisia by virtue of their receiving antipsychotic drug treatment being monitored throughout their hospital admission. The assessment procedure included demographic and clinical data and the Brief Psychiatric Rating Scale (Overall & Gorham, 1962). Parkinsonism (Simpson & Angus, 1970) and tardive dyskinesia (Barnes & Trauer, 1982) were assessed independently. In addition to the use of the specific rating scales, a structured interview and standardised examination were included, which had been designed to identify subjective symptoms of restlessness and determine the presence of motor restlessness and other purposeless movements. The interview began with open questions such as whether the medication was suiting the patient or whether the patient had been aware of any adverse effects over the previous week. Subsequently, specific enquiry was made regarding particular symptoms, as listed in Table I, derived from a wide variety of clinical descriptions of akathisia in the literature (Hodge, 1959; Sigwald & Raymondeaud, 1968; Sigwald &

Solgnac, 1968; Raskin, 1972; Van Putten, 1975; Marsden *et al*, 1975). The examination was conducted with the patient sitting, standing and lying. The site and type of movements were recorded and rated according to severity. The criterion of severity was the proportion of time that movement was present during the observation period. Abnormal movements were classified according to the definitions proposed by the Research Group on Extrapyramidal Disorders of the World Federation of Neurology (1981).

Before beginning the study, both investigators saw a number of patients using the questionnaire and standard examination, and satisfactory agreement on procedure was reached. On completion of the data collection, both investigators reviewed all the data directly referrable to akathisia. A global clinical assessment of each case was made. A joint decision was reached regarding the presence or absence of akathisia and, if present, a grading of mild, moderate or severe was agreed upon.

## Data analysis

The main aim of the study was to identify the constituent signs and symptoms of the akathisia syndrome. A multivariate statistical method was considered an appropriate technique for objective classification in such a context, where a large number of clinical phenomena are involved and the weight to be attached to the different features in diagnosis is uncertain (Garside & Roth, 1978). In this study the technique was to be used to indicate whether, in our patient sample, certain of the patient variables recorded tended to occur together, i.e. would emerge as correlated items in distinct clusters of symptoms. However, should symptom groupings emerge from such a procedure, it must then be established whether one or more of these groupings allows a more precise delineation of akathisia as a clinical entity. The statistical method chosen was a principal components analysis. For each patient only one set of ratings from a single assessment was included in this multivariate analysis. In each case the set of ratings used was from the occasion on which the maximum number of items were scored on the questionnaire and examination schedule.

# Results

## Principal components analysis

Eighteen items (listed in Table IIa), derived only from the 'restlessness' questionnaire and examination schedule, were subjected to a principal components analysis. Oblique rotation revealed four components which jointly accounted for 68% of the total variance; Component 1 accounted for 44%, Component 2 for 11%, Component 3 for 8% and Component 4 for 5%. Table IIa indicates the loadings of the individual items on each of the four components. Item loadings indicating a major contribution to a component are marked with an asterisk.

The main items making a positive contribution to Component I were a complaint of an inability to keep the legs still, semipurposeful leg and foot movements while sitting, shifting body weight from foot to foot and

TABLE IIa

*Component loadings on 18 items derived from 'restlessness' questionnaire and examination schedule*

| | | Components | | | |
|---|---|---|---|---|---|
| | | 1 | 2 | 3 | 4 |
| | *Questionnaire items* | | | | |
| | Limb sensations | .27 | − .17 | .36* | − .39* |
| | Inner restlessness | − .08 | .12 | .79* | − .14 |
| | Inability to remain still | .22 | .03 | .51* | − .54* |
| | Inability to keep legs still | .67* | .02 | .06 | − .48* |
| | *Examination items* | | | | |
| (i) | Sitting | | | | |
| | Semipurposeful or purposeless normal leg/feet movements | .71* | − .04 | .27 | .09 |
| | Shifting body position in chair | .15 | .30* | .10 | − .46* |
| | Inability to remain seated | .20 | .49* | .11 | .09 |
| | Semipurposeful hand/arm movements | − .07 | .03 | .57* | .09 |
| | Purposeless, normal hand/arm movements | .13 | .02 | .31* | .36* |
| (ii) | *Standing* | | | | |
| | Shifting weight from foot to foot and/or 'walking on the spot' | .67* | .22 | − .06 | − .31* |
| | Other purposeless foot movements (normal) | .63* | .04 | .07 | .19 |
| | Inability to remain standing on one spot (walked or paced) | .19 | .44* | .11 | − .11 |
| (iii) | Lying | | | | |
| | Coarse tremor of legs/feet | .77* | .03 | − .07 | − .17 |
| | Myoclonic jerks of the feet | .83* | .06 | − .13 | − .12 |
| | Semipurposeful or purposeless leg/feet movements | .74* | .12 | − .09 | .09 |
| | Shifting position of legs | .33* | .50* | .10 | .03 |
| | Shifting position of trunk/buttocks | − .09 | .85* | − .05 | − .02 |
| | Inability to remain lying down | − .07 | .99* | .00 | .03 |

TABLE IIb

*Component inter-correlations*

| | 1 | 2 | 3 | 4 |
|---|---|---|---|---|
| 1 | | | | |
| 2 | 0.44 | | | |
| 3 | 0.38 | 0.19 | | |
| 4 | − 0.26 | − 0.09 | − 0.05 | |
| | 1 | 2 | 3 | 4 |

*Components*

'walking-on-the-spot', and other purposeless leg and foot movements (e.g. lateral kicking movements) while standing. A few of these items, such as rocking from foot to foot while standing, have been specifically mentioned in some previous descriptions of the akathisia syndrome (Raskin, 1972; Marsden *et al*, 1975). In addition, several items, apparent on lying, made a significant positive contribution: coarse tremor and myoclonic jerks of the feet, and semipurposeful/purposeless movements and shifting of the legs. The 'myoclonus' appeared as intermittent, jerky activity in the feet, consistent with Halliday's (1967) description of extrapyramidal myoclonus i.e. "broken-up beats of extrapyramidal tremor".

Component 2 was notable for small positive loadings for many of the items which made a major contribution to Component 1 (see Table IIa). This implied an affinity between Components 1 and 2 which was reflected in a 0.44 correlation between them. In addition, the following items made a marked positive contribution to Component 2: shifting body position while seated; the inability to remain sitting down, the inability to remain standing on one spot; shifting the position of legs while lying; shifting the trunk while lying and the inability to remain lying down. All of these items represent gross body movements. Overall, Component 2 appeared to correspond to a severity variant of Component 1.

Component 3 received major positive contributions from three of the four questionnaire items; the item with the highest loading being a patient report of 'inner restlessness'. Also, semipurposeful and purposeless hand and arm movements while seated had high positive loadings. This component was interpreted as representing non-specific emotional unease with associated fidgety movements of the upper limbs.

Component 4 was characterised by strong negative loadings for many of the items making a positive contribution to Component 1. This was reflected in a $-0.26$ correlation between these two components (see Table IIb).

## Classification of patients

Component scores were calculated for each patient. These scores were then simplified, being expressed in terms of a simple 0–3 grading, which was based on the distribution of scores in the patient sample for each component. Cases were then grouped together according to the similarity of their component score profiles. By this method two main patient groupings emerged. Table III lists the group of patients characterised by relatively high Components 1 and 2 scores and negative Component 4 scores. Based on the item loadings for these components, this group of patients appeared to manifest a specific syndrome of motor restlessness, particularly referrable to the legs and feet. The phenomena present were considered to be consistent with a clarification and refinement of the akathisia syndrome. This hypothesis is tested below.

A second main patient grouping was apparent. This group of patients was characterised by relatively high Components 3 and 4 scores and negative Components 1 and 2 scores. The component scores in this group would appear to correspond to the non-specific movements observed in psychiatric illness with respect to emotional disturbance. Although diagnostically heterogeneous, this group contained a significant excess of depressive patients ($x^2 = 4.74$, d.f. = 1, $P < 0.05$). Clinically, the movements present in this group were manifestations of agitated depression, psychotic excitement and overactivity, stereotypies and mannerisms, and catatonic posturing.

## Clinical validation of the putative 'akathisia' group

In order to support the contention that the specific features of motor restlessness present in the putative 'akathisia' group derived from principal components analysis (see Table III) represented a more precise delineation of akathisia, it was necessary to demonstrate that the syndrome identified in these patients conformed to the more established clinical and pharmacological characteristics of the akathisia syndrome.

TABLE III
*Component scores of 27 patients assigned to 'akathisia' group*

| Patient number | Component scores 1 | 2 | 3 | 4 | Akathisia Grading | Clinical diagnosis |
|---|---|---|---|---|---|---|
| 19 | 1.7 | 0.1 | 0.7 | − 2.2 | | Schizophrenia |
| 21 | 2.4 | 0.9 | 0.3 | − 1.9 | | Manic–depressive disorder |
| 26 | 2.1 | 7.1 | 0.7 | 1.1 | severe | Schizo-affective psychosis |
| 77 | 3.0 | 6.5 | 1.5 | 0.5 | | Manic–depressive disorder |
| 91 | 1.5 | 0.2 | 1.0 | − 2.4 | | Schizophrenia |
| 95 | 1.7 | 0.3 | 0.8 | − 1.2 | | Schizophrenia |
| 5 | 2.4 | − 0.2 | 0.5 | − 1.0 | | Manic–depressive disorder |
| 15 | 2.0 | 0.0 | − 0.4 | − 2.0 | | Schizophrenia |
| 18 | 2.1 | − 0.1 | − 0.7 | − 0.4 | | Schizophrenia |
| 28 | 2.1 | 0.3 | − 0.5 | − 0.4 | | Schizophrenia |
| 31 | 1.4 | 0.1 | − 0.2 | − 0.6 | | Manic–depressive disorder |
| 38 | 1.2 | − 0.1 | 0.9 | − 1.1 | | Manic–depressive disorder |
| 42 | 2.2 | − 0.1 | 0.1 | − 0.2 | moderate | Manic–depressive disorder |
| 50 | 0.1 | 0.1 | − 0.1 | − 1.9 | | Schizophrenia |
| 58 | 2.5 | 0.4 | 2.1 | 0.7 | | Neurotic depression |
| 64 | 1.8 | 0.1 | − 1.1 | − 0.8 | | Schizophrenia |
| 66 | 1.5 | 0.5 | 0.2 | − 0.1 | | Manic–depressive disorder |
| 71 | 1.7 | − 1.0 | 1.7 | 0.1 | | Schizophrenia |
| 101 | 0.9 | 0.1 | 1.2 | − 1.0 | | Manic–depressive disorder |
| 8 | 0.1 | − 0.1 | 0.9 | − 0.2 | | Schizophrenia |
| 46 | − 0.2 | − 0.4 | 0.1 | − 1.5 | | Schizophrenia |
| 63 | 0.4 | 0.3 | − 0.4 | − 0.7 | | Schizophrenia |
| 92 | 0.1 | − 0.2 | 0.7 | − 1.8 | mild | Endogenous depression |
| 93 | 0.1 | − 0.2 | 0.2 | 0.5 | | Schizophrenia |
| 97 | 0.4 | − 0.3 | 1.4 | − 1.2 | | Schizophrenia |
| 99 | 0.1 | − 0.1 | 0.6 | − 0.4 | | Manic–depressive disorder |
| 104 | 0.3 | − 0.5 | 1.5 | − 0.9 | | Schizophrenia |

## 1. *Clinical diagnosis*

As previously mentioned, global clinical assessment of each case was carried out following the completion of data collection. A diagnosis of akathisia was made in 28 out of the 104 patients. Subsequently, all cases were classified into groups according to their component score profiles, as described above. All 27 of the cases allocated to the group listed in Table III had received a clinical diagnosis of akathisia. Thus, only one patient (number 94), with a tentative clinical diagnosis of akathisia, was not classified within this putative 'akathisia' group.

## 2. *Incidence*

Twenty-seven out of the 104 patients in our sample were included in the putative 'akathisia' group. However, when 'akathisia' incidence was calculated, one patient (number 28) in this group had to be excluded as his signs and symptoms of motor restlessness had been present prior to admission. Thus, the incidence figure in our sample was 25% which is in accord with a reported incidence of akathisia in the literature of approximately 20% (Ayd, 1961; Marsden *et al*, 1975).

### 3. *Antipsychotic drug treatment*

The first ten days of drug treatment was found to be the period of maximum drug dose increase for all patients in the study. Within this period the maximum antipsychotic drug dose was identified for the 26 cases of acute akathisia in this group listed in Table III. In 22 (85%) of these patients, signs and symptoms appeared within seven days after reaching this maximum dose. Three of these patients developed akathisia within 12 hours of the administration of their first antipsychotic drug dose. In all 26 cases the condition developed within 14 days after the first administration of their maximum drug dose.

In order to compare the groups derived from the principal components analysis in terms of antipsychotic drug treatment, an index of dose change over the first ten days of treatment was calculated. As the patients had received a variety of antipsychotic drugs, all drug doses in this period (including the dose each patient was receiving immediately prior to hospital admission) were converted into chlorpromazine equivalents per day (Davis, 1974; Wyatt & Togrow, 1976;

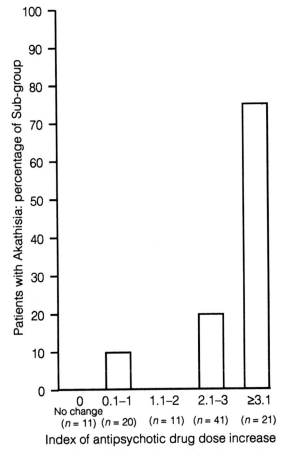

Fig. 1. *Proportion of patients with 'akathisia' according to index of antipsychotic drug dose increase,* $log \left( \frac{CPZ\ max + 1}{CPZ\ min + 1} \right).$

Ezrin-Waters *et al*, 1981). The index of dose change was expressed as a logarithmic ratio, log $[(CPZ \max + 1)/(CPZ \min + 1)]$, where 'CPZ max' and 'CPZ min' were the maximum and minimum antipsychotic drug doses administered during this period in chlorpromazine equivalents, respectively. In no case did this index represent a decrease in medication. Fig. 1 reveals that all patients in the putative 'akathisia' group had experienced an increase in antipsychotic drug dosage during the first ten days of drug treatment. Furthermore, the proportion of 'akathisia' patients increases sharply at log ratio levels greater than 3:1; a figure indicative of a large increase in dosage. For example, an increase in drug dose from 0–1000 chlorpromazine equivalents per day would give a log ratio of 3:0.

These results show that for patients in the putative 'akathisia' group, the specific signs and symptoms of motor restlessness developed rapidly following a relatively large initial increase in drug dosage. This is entirely in accord with descriptions of akathisia as an acute, dose-related, antipsychotic drug side-effect (Ayd, 1961; Marsden *et al*, 1975). In addition, akathisia usually improves following drug reduction or withdrawal (Hodge, 1959; Raskin, 1972; Van Putten, 1974). Only ten patients in the 'akathisia' group had a significant reduction in antipsychotic drug dosage (decreased by at least one-third of their maximum) early enough for the subsequent effects to be assessed during their hospital stay. Relief of akathisia signs and symptoms occurred in eight of these cases within seven days, and in the remaining two cases within three weeks of this dose reduction.

In summary, the 'akathisia' group listed in Table III was found to conform closely to generally accepted clinical and pharmacological criteria for a diagnosis of akathisia.

## Results and conclusions

### Phenomenological characteristics

The patients in the akathisia group were further subdivided into severity gradings of mild, moderate and severe akathisia, based on their component score profiles and the clinical global ratings (see Table III).

Table III lists the items from the restlessness questionnaire and examination and gives their incidence within the akathisia and illness-related movement groups. This information is also provided for the three gradings of severity within the akathisia group. This allows us to identify and delineate the clinical features of akathisia and its grades of severity. The results of this investigation allow us to describe 'mild', 'moderate' and 'severe' akathisia in terms of their characteristic signs and symptoms.

Mild akathisia presents, principally, as the subjective symptoms of the condition, with very few observable signs. Van Putten (1975) and Gagrat *et al* (1978) have referred to feelings of unease, and in particular 'inner restlessness', as being typical of mild akathisia. But, our results showed 'inner restlessness' to be a common, non-specific symptom, occurring in nearly half of the total sample. In addition, it has been suggested that mild akathisia is not only difficult to diagnose but also difficult to differentiate from generalised anxiety

(Raskin, 1972; Van Putten, 1975, 1978). However, we found complaints specifically referable to the legs discriminated most effectively between mild akathisia, and restlessness due to underlying psychiatric illness. These complaints were, typically, abnormal leg sensations, such as 'drawing' or 'pulling' feelings, and the experience of being unable to keep the legs still. Abnormal sensations in the legs in association with akathisia have been previously described (Sigwald & Solgnac, 1968; Sigwald & Raymondeaud, 1968; Marsden *et al*, 1975).

Patients with moderate akathisia expressed the same complaints as the mild group, but, in addition, characteristic observable features were noted. These patients would typically rock from foot to foot or 'walk-on-the-spot' while standing, for most of the time they were being observed. In addition, these patients exhibited both coarse tremor and myoclonic jerks in their feet. Myoclonic jerks in the legs have been described in association with the restless legs syndrome, a condition phenomenologically similar to akathisia (Behrman, 1958; Boghen & Peyronnard, 1976; Hussey, 1976). Myoclonus has also been reported as accompanying acute dystonias (Marsden *et al*, 1975) and tardive dyskinesia (Degwitz & Wentzel, 1967; Marsden *et al*, 1975), a syndrome that may include signs and symptoms of akathisia (Ayd, 1961; Brandon *et al*, 1971; Kennedy *et al*, 1971; Simpson, 1977; Forrest & Fahn, 1979).

In a further investigation tremographic techniques were employed to characterise this motor activity (Braude *et al*, 1984). This controlled investigation indicated that akathisia patients were characterised by the presence of large amplitude, low frequency (less than four Hz) rhythmic foot movements. Changes in the severity of akathisia at follow-up were reflected in changes in the amplitude and frequency of this dyskinesia.

Patients suffering from severe akathisia manifested features of moderate akathisia, but also exhibited difficulty in maintaining their position. For example, when seated they would stand up from the chair, when standing they would begin to walk or pace, or, when lying would feel compelled to leave the couch to take a few steps. These features are consistent with the descriptions of 'tasikinesia', which has been regarded as indicative of severe akathisia (Delay & Deniker, 1968; Raskin, 1972; Sovner & DiMascio, 1978). Most cases with moderate or severe akathisia were markedly distressed by their symptoms (see Table I). Although 'akathisia' literally means 'inability to remain seated', most of these patients described the condition as being worse when they were required to stand still (see Table I), for example, when queuing for their meals or medication, on the ward.

The group of patients with movements related to their underlying psychiatric illness was characterised by a significantly higher number of cases with a diagnosis of depressive illness, and also had a significant excess of semipurposeful hand and arm movements. This would suggest that much of the movement recorded in this group represented the typical hand wringing and fidgety movements of agitated depressive patients. Other movements scored in this group were related to psychotic excitement and overactivity, stereotypies and mannerisms, and catatonia.

### Drug treatment and relationship to parkinsonism

In all ten akathisia patients whose antipsychotic medication was significantly reduced, the condition improved. However, this was the only pharmacological manipulation which proved to be invariably beneficial. Four patients with akathisia received a benzodiazepine drug but this was not helpful, despite previous encouraging reports (Donlon, 1973; Gagrat *et al*, 1978; Director & Muniz, 1982).

Twenty patients with akathisia were treated with anticholinergic agents. Only six (30%) showed a clinically significant improvement. These six responders were characterised by concomitant severe parkinsonism according to the Simpson & Angus rating scale (1970) which showed a parallel response to these agents. Thus, in these cases, akathisia appeared to behave as a parkinsonism symptom. In common with most of the cases of akathisia identified, the remaining 14 patients who received anticholinergic drugs had only relatively mild parkinsonism. In these 14 cases akathisia did not respond to these agents and their parkinsonism either failed to improve or, in a few cases, became worse. These results suggest that there may be two distinct types of early-onset akathisia, one related to severe parkinsonism and one not, possibly reflecting different pathophysiological mechanisms. This may help to explain the variable response of akathisia to anticholinergic treatment (Marsden *et al*, 1975; Sovner & DiMascio, 1978).

**Pathophysiological implications**

The presentation of the six patients with akathisia and severe parkinsonism, where both conditions responded to anticholinergic medication, is compatible with an overwhelming blockade of post-synaptic dopamine receptors in the nigrostriatal system by antipsychotic drugs. However, an alternative explanation of pathophysiology may be required for the majority of akathisia patients in this study, as they had only mild parkinsonism and those who received anticholinergic medications were without benefit. Akathisia in such cases may either be related to antagonism of a group of dopamine receptors within the nigrostriatal system distinct from those whose blockade results in parkinsonism, or produced by dopamine receptor blockade in a separate dopaminergic system.

With regard to the latter proposal, animal experiments have suggested that the mesocortical dopamine system may exert an inhibitory role on locomotor behaviour (Iversen, 1971; Tassin *et al*, 1978; Koob *et al*, 1981). Lesions of the pre-frontal cortex have been found to lead to increased activity in the subcortical dopamine systems, with an associated increase in locomotor activity (Carter & Pycock, 1980; Pycock *et al*, 1980a, b).

Marsden & Jenner (1980) have hypothesised that the equivalent result in man, following meso-cortical dopamine receptor blockade by antipsychotic drugs, may be the psychological and motor manifestations of akathisia. Such an explanation of the pathophysiological mechanism of akathisia appears relatively plausible at present, although recent animal work identifying dopamine receptors in the spinal cord which can modulate motor output (Carp & Anderson, 1982) raises the possibility that antipsychotic drug activity at dopamine receptors in the spinal cord might also be relevant.

## References

AYD, F. J. (1961) A survey of drug-induced extrapyramidal reactions. *Journal of the American Medical Association*, **175**, 1054–1060.

BARNES, T. R. E. & TRAUER, T. (1982) Reliability and validity of a tardive dyskinesia videotape rating technique. *British Journal of Psychiatry*, **140**, 508–515.

BEHRMAN, S. (1958) Disturbed relaxation of limbs. *British Medical Journal*, i, 1454–1457.

BOGHEN, D. & PEYRONNARD, J. M. (1976) Myoclonus in familial restless legs syndrome. *Archives of Neurology*, **33**, 368–370.

BRANDON, S., MCCLELLAND, H. A. & PROTHEROE, C. (1971) A study of facial dyskinesia in a mental hospital population. *British Journal of Psychiatry*, **118**, 171–184.

BRAUDE, W. M., BARNES, T. R. E. & GORE, S. M. (1983) Clinical characteristics of akathisia. A systematic investigation of acute psychiatric inpatient admissions. *British Journal of Psychiatry*, **143**, 139–150.

——, CHARLES, I. P. & BARNES, T. R. E. (1984) Coarse, jerky foot tremor: Tremographic investigation of an objective sign of acute akathisia. *Psychopharmacology*, **82**, 95–101.

CARP, J. S. & ANDERSON, R. J. (1982) Dopamine receptor-mediated depression of spinal monosynaptic transmission. *Brain Research*, **242**, 247–254.

CARTER, C. J. & PYCOCK, C. J. (1980) Behavioural and biochemical effects of dopamine and noradrenaline depletion within the medial prefrontal cortex of the rat. *Brain Research*, **192**, 163–176.

DAVIS, J. M. (1974) Dose equivalence of the antipsychotic drugs. *Journal of Psychiatric Research*, **11**, 65–69.

DEGKWITZ, R. & WENZEL, W. (1967) Persistent extrapyramidal side-effects after long-term application of neuroleptics. In *Neuropsychopharmacology* (eds. H. Brill, J. O. Cole, H. Hippius & P. B. Bradley), pp. 608–618. Excerpta Medica International Congress Series 129. Amsterdam, Excerpta Medica Foundation.

DELAY, J. & DENIKER, P. (1968) Drug-induced extrapyramidal syndromes. In *Handbook of Clinical Neurology* (eds. P. J. Vinken & G. W. Bruyn), pp. 248–266, Vol. 6. Amsterdam: North Holland.

DIRECTOR, K. L. & MUNIZ, C. E. (1982) Diazepam in the treatment of extrapyramidal symptoms: A case report. *Journal of Clinical Psychiatry*, **43**, 160–161.

DONLON, P. T. (1973) The therapeutic use of diazepam for akathisia. *Psychosomatics*, **14**, 222–225.

EZRIN-WATERS, C., SEEMAN, M. V. & SEEMAN, P. (1981) Tardive dyskinesia in schizophrenic outpatients: prevalence and significant variables. *Journal of Clinical Psychiatry*, **42**, 16–22.

FORREST, D. V. & FAHN, S. (1979) Tardive dysphrenia and subjective akathisia. *Journal of Clinical Psychiatry*, **40**, 206.

GAGRAT, D., HAMILTON, J. & BELMAKER, R. H. (1978) Intravenous diazepam in the treatment of neuroleptic-induced acute dystonia and akathisia. *American Journal of Psychiatry*, **135**, 1232–1233.

GARSIDE, R. F. & ROTH, M. (1978) Multivariate statistical methods and problems of classification in psychiatry. *British Journal of Psychiatry*, **133**, 53–67.

HALLIDAY, A. M. (1967) The clinical incidence of myoclonus. In *Modern Trends in Neurology 4* (ed. D. Williams), pp. 69–105. London: Butterworths.

HODGE, J. R. (1959) Akathisia: the syndrome of motor restlessness. *American Journal of Psychiatry*, **116**, 337–338.

HUSSEY, H. H. (1976) Restless legs syndrome. *Journal of American Medical Association*, **235**, 2224.

IVERSEN, S. D. (1971) The effect of surgical lesions to frontal cortex and substantia nigra on amphetamine responses in rats. *Brain Research*, **31**, 295–311.

KENNEDY, P. F., HERSHON, H. I. & MCGUIRE, R. J. (1971) Extrapyramidal disorders after prolonged phenothiazine therapy. *British Journal of Psychiatry*, **118**, 509–518.

KOOB, G. F., STINUS, L. & LE MOAL, M. (1981) Hyperactivity and hypoactivity produced by lesions to the mesolimbic dopamine system. *Behavioural Brain Research*, **3**, 341–359.

MARSDEN, C. D. & JENNER, P. (1980) The pathophysiology of extrapyramidal side-effects of neuroleptic drugs. *Psychological Medicine*, **10**, 55–72.

——, TARSY, D. & BALDESSARINI, R. J. (1975) Spontaneous and drug-induced movement disorders in psychotic patients. In *Psychiatric Aspects of Neurological Disease* (eds. D. F. Benson & D. Blumer), pp. 219–265. New York: Grune & Stratton.

OVERALL, J. E. & GORHAM, D. R. (1962) The brief psychiatric rating scale. *Psychological Reports*, **10**, 799–812.

PYCOCK, C. J., KERWIN, R. W. & CARTER, C. J. (1980a) Effect of lesion of cortical dopamine terminals on subcortical dopamine receptors in rats. *Nature*, **286**, 74–77.

——, CARTER, C. J. & KERWIN, R. W. (1980b) Effect of 6-hydroxydopamine lesions of the medial prefrontal cortex on neurotransmitter system in subcortical sites in the rat. *Journal of Neurochemistry*, **34**, 91–99.

RASKIN, D. E. (1972) Akathisia: a side-effect to be remembered. *American Journal of Psychiatry*, **129**, 345–347.

RESEARCH GROUP ON EXTRAPYRAMIDAL DISORDERS OF THE WORLD FEDERATION OF NEUROLOGY (1981) Classification of extrapyramidal disorders: proposal for an international classification and glossary of terms. *Journal of the Neurological Sciences*, **51**, 311–327.

SIGWALD, J. & RAYMONDEAUD, C. I. (1968) Les réactions désagréables ou douloureuses de la maladie de Parkinson et de la thérapeutique neuroleptique (paresthésies impatiences, crampes, akathisie). Leur amélioration par l'alimémazine. *Semaine des Hôpitaux de Paris*, **4**, 2897–2899.

—— & SOLGNAC, J. (1968) Manifestations douloureuses de la maladie de Parkinson et paresthéses provoquées par les neuroleptiques. *Semaine des Hôpitaux de Paris*, **36**, 2222–2225.

SIMPSON, G. M. (1977) Neurotoxicology of major tranquillisers. In *Neurotoxicology* (eds. L. Roizin, H. Shiraki & N. Grcević), Vol. 1, pp. 1–7. New York: Raven Press.

—— & ANGUS, J. W. S. (1970) A rating scale for extrapyramidal side-effects. *Acta Psychiatrica Scandinavica*, **212**, 11–19.

SOVNER, R. & DiMASCIO, A. (1978) Extrapyramidal syndromes and other neurological side-effects of psychotropic drugs. In *Psychopharmacology: A Generation of Progress* (eds. M. A. Lipton, A. DiMascio & K. F. Killam), pp. 1021–1032. New York: Raven Press.

TASSIN, J-P., STINUS, L., SIMON, H., BLANC, G., THIERRY, A-M., LE MOAL, M., CARDO, B. & GLOWINSKI, J. (1978) Relationship between the locomotor hyperactivity induced by A10 lesions and the destruction of the frontocortical dopaminergic innervation in the rat. *Brain Research*, **141**, 267–281.

VAN PUTTEN, T. (1974) Why do schizophrenic patients refuse to take their drugs? *Archives of General Psychiatry*, **31**, 67–72.

—— (1975) The many faces of akathisia. *Comprehensive Psychiatry*, **16**, 43–47.

—— (1978) Drug refusal in schizophrenia: causes and prescribing hints. *Hospital and Community Psychiatry*, **29**, 110–112.

WYATT, R. J. & TOGROW, J. S. (1976) A comparison of equivalent clinical potencies of neuroleptics as used to treat schizophrenia and affective disorders. *Journal of Psychiatric Research*, **13**, 91–98.

# 43  A study of drug-induced akathisia in schizophrenic out-patients

**THOMAS R. E. BARNES**

The work discussed here was carried out by Walter Braude and myself during the last two years of my five year appointment in the Department of Psychiatry in Cambridge under Professor Sir Martin Roth. Throughout this research work, Sir Martin provided encouragement and support and made some invaluable suggestions. He had the rare ability of being able to maintain the issue under scrutiny in sharp focus while viewing it from a number of perspectives and within a number of contexts. His comments were drawn from an extraordinary depth and breadth of academic knowledge and clinical understanding, and to appreciate their relevance and importance could take more than a few moments' reflection and some conceptual reorganisation.

## Introduction

Acute akathisia develops soon after starting or increasing antipsychotic drugs or other dopamine antagonist such as reserpine or metoclopramide, and seems to be dose dependent (Braude *et al*, 1983; Ayd, 1961). The onset may be very rapid in some cases, sometimes within an hour or so of pre-operative treatment with droperidol and metoclopramide (Barnes *et al*, 1982).

Our initial study of acute akathisia, reported by Braude in the previous chapter, found that acute akathisia developed in approximately 25% of acute psychiatric admissions in patients receiving antipsychotic drugs. Although akathisia is usually thought of as an early-onset phenomenon it can be a persistent problem, often following a fluctuating course over many years, and even continuing after drug withdrawal (Weiner & Luby, 1983).

The first of the two main problems envisaged in this investigation of chronic akathisia was the absence of established diagnostic criteria for akathisia. This has been reflected in the wide range of prevalence figures reported in the literature, inconsistent findings in treatment studies and diagnostic confusion in clinical practice with failure to distinguish between akathisia and agitation related to psychiatric illness. Secondly, there was the associated difficulty of discriminating between the variety of abnormal movements observed in chronic schizophrenic patients. These include the restless movements of akathisia, and the abnormal movements of tardive dystonia, tardive dyskinesia, tics, stereotypies, mannerisms, and restlessness related to psychotic agitation. The distinction between tardive dyskinesia and chronic akathisia is complicated by the common coexistence of the two conditions in the same individuals (Barnes *et al*, 1983). Descriptions of tardive dyskinesia have consistently mentioned motor restlessness, and subjective distress has been found to correlate better with trunk and limb movements than with oro-facial movement (Rosen *et al*, 1982).

## Aims and methods

The aims of this study (Barnes & Braude, 1985) were to examine the nature and prevalence of drug-induced akathisia in a population of out-patients with established schizophrenia who were receiving long-term antipsychotic drugs. The principal strategy was the application of diagnostic criteria for acute akathisia which we derived from our previous work (Braude *et al*, 1983). All patients attending either of two out-patient 'depot neuroleptic' clinics over a period of three months were screened, and 82 patients out of the total of 89 fulfilled DSM–III criteria for schizophrenia. Mental state was assessed using the Manchester Scale (Krawiecka *et al*, 1977), the Extrapyramidal Side Effects scale of Simpson & Angus (1970) was used to evaluate parkinsonism, and tardive dyskinesia was rated according to the scale of Barnes & Trauer (1982).

A second patient sample was studied as a control group for the effects of the interview and examination procedure in the context of an out-patient clinic. Fifty-four consecutive attenders at a surgical out-patient clinic were assessed for movement disorders in the same manner as the psychiatric patients. None of these control subjects had a psychiatric history and none had received or were taking any psychotropic drugs except for three individuals taking small doses of benzodiazepines.

The first diagnostic criterion for akathisia was a subjective complaint of restlessness, particularly referable to the legs. This would be reported as a desire to move the legs to gain relief or the awareness of an inability to keep the legs still, usually against a background of non-specific feelings of inner tension which are less specific to the condition. The second criterion was the observation of characteristic patterns of restless movements during a standard examination procedure. Most characteristically, patients with akathisia rock from foot to foot and also 'walk on the spot' while standing. If such movements were present for more than half the time the patient would fulfil this criterion. If such movements were present for less than half of the time they were being observed then the patient needed to display the fidgety leg movements, shuffling or tramping their feet, or swinging one leg while sitting or an inability to stand without walking or pacing, or fidgety leg movements while lying.

## Results and discussion

Twenty-nine (35%) of the schizophrenic patients fulfilled both criteria for akathisia. None of the surgical out-patients satisfied either criterion, although eight reported abnormal, uncomfortable sensations in the lower limbs. These sensations were experienced only at rest, either sitting in the evening or lying in bed at night, and were accompanied by a need to move the legs to gain respite.

In all cases these episodes occurred only sporadically and were consistent with the spontaneous condition of restless legs or Ekbom's syndrome (Ekbom, 1960; Gibb & Lees, 1986), a syndrome resembling akathisia. This presents as an aching discomfort in the legs at rest, associated with restlessness of the legs and the irresistable urge to move. Walking usually affords some relief. The syndrome occurs in approximately 5% of healthy people with an increased frequency in late pregnancy and in several specific disorders including iron deficiency anaemia.

The findings suggested several variants of the acute akathisia picture in this population (Barnes & Braude, 1985). Ten patients fulfilled the objective criterion of observable restless movements but not the subjective criterion for akathisia. That is, they manifested obvious, complex, repetitive movements resembling those seen in acute akathisia. These movements were of a volitional rather than choreic nature and appeared as motor restlessness. However, these patients did not report a sense of inner restlessness or a compulsion to move. This syndrome was called pseudoakathisia, a term previously used by Munetz & Cornes (1982). The main feature was rocking from foot to foot while standing. It is uncertain whether this should be considered as merely a stereotypy resembling akathisia, or an end-stage akathisia in which the subjective component had faded. While the natural history of akathisia remains obscure, this study provided limited evidence that the feelings of restlessness and associated distress may become less intense with time, and this small group of patients with pseudoakathisia were relatively old within this population, with a mean age of 51 years. However, the failure to obtain a report of feelings of restlessness in these patients with pseudoakathisia may also reflect the presence of negative schizophrenic features, specifically poverty of speech and flattening of affect, which were very common in this group.

Twenty-nine patients fulfilled both diagnostic criteria. Six of these cases were classified as suffering from acute akathisia, in that the onset of the condition had occurred within the previous six months, coincident with an increase in drug dose. The clinical picture was the same as that observed in the earlier study of acute akathisia in psychiatric in-patients.

After exclusion of the cases of acute akathisia, there remained 23 patients who qualified for a diagnosis of akathisia but whose signs and symptoms had not developed in association with a recent increase in drug dose. These cases were referred to as having chronic akathisia, but this could be sub-classified further, principally on the basis of the relationship with changes in drug dose. In 12 cases the chronic akathisia appeared to represent a continuation of the acute form of the condition. Although the symptoms had been present for periods ranging from seven months to seven years, these patients were able to date the onset of their symptoms precisely enough for examination of their medical records to reveal that there had been marked increase in drug dosage at that time. These patients were considered to manifest an 'acute persistent' variant of akathisia.

Of the remaining 11 patients with chronic akathisia, two reported that they had first become aware of their symptoms in the preceding month, a period during which their antipsychotic medication had been progressively reduced. An additional three patients reported that they were only aware of symptoms within the week before their regular depot injection, the time when drug plasma levels reach their minimum. The akathisia in these cases had emerged during long-term antipsychotic drug treatment and appeared to be related to drug withdrawal.

This syndrome was referred to as tardive akathisia. This condition has been previously identified in the literature (Fahn, 1983; Braude & Barnes, 1983; Jeste & Wyatt, 1982). It is associated with oro-facial dyskinesia, and is reported to share the pharmacological characteristics of tardive dyskinesia on the basis that it is exacerbated or provoked by drug reduction or withdrawal and improves at least temporarily when the dose is increased.

Whether these akathisia variants represent stages in the progression of the condition is unclear. The mixed picture of chronic akathisia could represent a transitional stage in the natural history of the condition, while the presence of motor signs without a subjective sense of restlessness would be the final stage of the evolution. We found that certain subjective symptoms of akathisia, specifically limb paraethesiae and distress related to restlessness, were less common in the chronic akathisia group than in those patients suffering from acute akathisia. Nevertheless, the main finding of this study was that the restless movements that characterise akathisia commonly co-existed with signs of tardive dyskinesia. Overall, oro-facial dyskinesia was present in 16 (41%) of the 39 patients with motor manifestations of akathisia compared with only five (12%) of the 43 patients without evidence of akathisia. Oro-facial dyskinesia was limited to the patients with the more chronic forms of akathisia. Further, 30 (77%) of the 39 patients with signs of akathisia displayed choreo-athetoid limb dyskinesia compared with only four (9%) of the 43 patients without akathisia. One interpretation of these findings would be that the more chronic forms of akathisia are part of the tardive dyskinesia syndrome. This close association between symptoms of akathisia and tardive dyskinesia has also been found in a similar study by Gibb & Lees (1986), who further concluded that approximately 50% of chronic psychiatric patients had some signs and symptoms of akathisia.

## The akathisia syndrome

Our approach to the diagnosis of akathisia in this study was to set up operational criteria related to both subjective and objective features. Patients were classified according to whether they exhibited subjective features, objective features or both, and we then attempted to clarify the nature of the subtypes in terms of their relationship to other movement disorder and the natural history of schizophrenia in these cases. This approach raises problems with individuals who fulfil only one of the two criteria. The presence of a subjective report of restlessness without observable restless movements may be found in mild akathisia (Braude *et al*, 1983), so called 'subjective akathisia' (Van Putten & Marder, 1986). In practice it may be difficult to differentiate between this condition and subtle presentations of anxiety or emotional unease in psychiatric patients. Further, the presence of objective features only, so-called pseudoakathisia, may not represent a variant of akathisia, as already discussed, but rather a stereotypy closely resembling the movements of akathisia, or as suggested by Stahl (1985) and Munetz (1986), a variant of tardive dyskinesia. In the latter case, non-dyskinetic movements are being included within the tardive dyskinesia syndrome which traditionally comprises choreiform oro-facial trunk and limb movements.

Problems also arise when attempting to delimit these akathisia variants from other movement disorders, particularly tardive dyskinesia. Our approach to discriminating between these two movement disorders has been to attempt a qualitative assessment. Thus, movements that are choreiform or choreo-athetoid in nature are considered part of tardive dyskinesia while akathisia is characterised by restless movements that are not abnormal in the sense that they can be mimicked and are not dyskinetic in character; that is, they do not appear to be choreic, dystonic, tic-like etc. This distinction is crucial to the interpretation of the results of our study, but clinically the differentiation may be difficult. Munetz (1986) assumes that the movements of akathisia are a consequence of internal restlessness, and takes the subjective report of restlessness as a defining characteristic. That is, if the patient is restless, and therefore moving, this represents akathisia while if a patient is moving, and therefore restless, this is tardive dyskinesia. Such a distinction rests heavily upon a clear subjective report which may be difficult to obtain in chronic psychiatric patients.

Thus, there is a major methodological problem facing researchers in this area. The descriptive categories of dyskinesia, such as choreiform and dystonic, may be useful, as may distinction into purposeful or purposeless or voluntary and involuntary, but none of these analyses guarantees differentiation between akathisia and tardive dyskinesia, or even drug-related and illness-related motor abnormalities seen in drug-treated schizophrenic patients. Such patients may well manifest movements inherent to their illness.

The problems of classification and interpretation of movement disorder within schizophrenia pre-date the introduction of antipsychotic drugs. Before such medication was available, various motor disorders were described in psychiatric patients, particularly those with catatonic and other types of schizophrenia (Marsden *et al*, 1975). In addition to disturbances of voluntary motor activity, classified as stereotypies and mannerisms, perseverative movements, tics, grimaces and general clumsiness and lack of coordination, abnormal involuntary movements (dyskinesia) such as choreiform and oro-facial dyskinesia were also clearly described (Kraepelin, 1919; Farran-Ridge, 1926; Jones & Hunter, 1969). Such movements were interpreted by Kraepelin (1919) and Bleuler (1950) as being essentially a manifestation of the disturbances of thought, emotion and will that characterise schizophrenia (Barnes & Liddle, 1985).

Rogers (1985) argues convincingly that the vocabulary used to describe abnormal movements will reflect the conceptual view of the phenomena. His study provided detailed description of motor disorder in 100 patients with severe psychiatric illness and eschews any interpretation of movement referring to neurological or psychiatric diagnosis. However, concepts such as tone, posture, purposefulness and judgement as to whether the movements are abnormal, still underlie the descriptions in his report. Such an approach does not lend itself easily to attempts to measure change in the severity of movement over time, which may be necessary in the context of a treatment trial or a follow-up assessment, and some categorisation of the movements observed is necessary. However, as already mentioned, a spectrum of motor disturbance is seen in chronic psychotic patients. The various dyskinesias, and the myriad disorders of posture, tone, gait, speech, and purposive movement that are found are not readily reduced to items suitable for a rating scale. The Abnormal Involuntary Movement Scale (AIMS), the most popular instrument for rating tardive dyskinesia, is a checklist for abnormal movements at various body sites which refers only to broad descriptions of movement rather than the nature and quality of the movement. Thus, the scale may have limitations in terms of its ability to distinguish between the various motor syndromes, or to provide scores that reflect the severity of these syndromes.

The validity of the variants of akathisia identified in the study discussed here remains to be established, but the findings should allow working hypotheses to be generated regarding the natural history of the condition and the relationship between akathisia and both tardive dyskinesia and schizophrenia. Undoubtedly, further research in this area would be enhanced by a consensus between clinicians on the definition and appropriate use of terms employed to describe movement disorder in patients with established schizophrenia.

# References

AYD, F. J. (1961) A survey of drug-induced extrapyramidal reactions. *Journal of the American Medical Association*, **175**, 1054–1060.

BARNES, T. R. E. & LIDDLE, P. F. (1985) Tardive dyskinesia. Implications for schizophrenia? In *Schizophrenia: New Pharmacological and Clinical Developments* (eds. A. A. Schiff, Sir Martin Roth & H. L. Freeman). London, Royal Society of Medicine Services.

——, BRAUDE, W. M. & HILL, D. J. (1982) Acute akathisia after oral droperidol and metoclopramide preoperative medication. *Lancet*, ii, 48–49.

—— & TRAUER, T. (1982) Reliability and validity of a tardive dyskinesia videotape rating technique. *British Journal of Psychiatry*, **140**, 508–515.

——, KIDGER, T. & GORE, S. M. (1983) Tardive dyskinesia: a 3-year follow-up study. *Psychological Medicine*, **13**, 71–81.

—— & BRAUDE, W. M. (1985) Akathisia variants and tardive dyskinesia. *Archives of General Psychiatry*, **42**, 874–878.

BLEULER, E. (1950) *Dementia Praecox or the Group of Schizophrenias*. Translated by J. Zinkin. New York: International Universities Press.

BRAUDE, W. M., BARNES, T. R. E. & GORE, S. M. (1983) Clinical characteristics of akathisia: a systematic investigation of acute psychiatric inpatient admissions. *British Journal of Psychiatry*, **143**, 139–150.

—— & —— (1983) Late-onset akathisia—an indicant of covert dyskinesia: two case reports. *American Journal of Psychiatry*, **140**, 611–612.

EKBOM, K. A. (1960) Restless legs syndrome. *Neurology*, **10**, 868–873.

FAHN, S. (1983) Long-term treatment of tardive dyskinesia with presynaptically acting dopamine-depleting agents. In *Advances in Neurology, Volume 37: Experimental Therapeutics of Movement Disorders* (eds S. Fahn, D. B. Calne & I. Shoulson). New York: Raven Press.

FARREN-RIDGE, C. (1926) Some symptoms referable to the basal ganglia occurring in dementia praecox and epidemic encephalitis. *Journal of Mental Science*, **72**, 513–523.

GIBB, W. R. G. & LEES, A. (1986) The clinical phenomenon of akathisia. *Journal of Neurology, Neurosurgery and Psychiatry*, **49**, 861–866.

—— & LEES, A. J. (1986) The restless legs syndrome. *Postgraduate Medical Journal*, **62**, 329–333.

JESTE, D. & WYATT, R. J. (1982) *Understanding and Treating Tardive Dyskinesia*. New York: Guildford.

JONES, M. & HUNTER, R. (1969) Abnormal movements in patients with chronic psychiatric illness. In *Psychotropic Drugs and Dysfunction of the Basal Ganglia* (eds G. E. Crane & R. Gardner). Washington: US Public Health Service.

KRAEPELIN, E. P. (1919) *Dementia Praecox and Paraphrenia* (ed. G. M. Robertson), Translated by R. M. Barclay. Edinburgh: Livingstone.

KRAWIECKA, M., GOLDBERG, D. & VAUGHN, M. (1977) A standardised psychiatric assessment scale for rating chronic psychotic patients. *Acta Psychiatrica Scandinavica*, **55**, 299–308.

MARSDEN, C. D., TARSY, D. & BALDESSARINI, R. J. (1975) Spontaneous and drug-induced movement disorders in psychotic patients. In *Psychiatric Aspects of Neurological Disease* (eds D. F. Benson & D. Blumer). New York: Grune and Stratton.

MUNETZ, M. R. (1986) Akathisia variants and tardive dyskinesia (letter). *Archives of General Psychiatry*, **43**, 1015.

—— & CORNES, C. L. (1982) Akathisia, pseudoakathisia and tardive dyskinesia: clinical examples. *Comprehensive Psychiatry*, **23**, 345–352.

ROGERS, D. (1985) The motor disorders of severe psychiatric illness: a conflict of paradigms. *British Journal of Psychiatry*, **147**, 221-232.

ROSEN, A. M., MUKHERJEE, S., OLARTE, S., VARIA, V. & CARDENAS, C. (1982) Perception of tardive dyskinesia in outpatients receiving maintenance neuroleptics. *American Journal of Psychiatry*, **139**, 372-373.

SIMPSON, G. M. & ANGUS, J. W. S. (1970) A rating scale for extrapyramidal side-effects. *Acta Psychiatrica Scandinavica*, **212** (suppl. 44), 11-19.

STAHL, S. M. (1985) Akathisia and tardive dyskinesia: changing concepts. *Archives of General Psychiatry*, **42**, 874-878.

VAN PUTTEN, T. & MARDER, S. R. (1986) Toward a more reliable diagnosis of akathisia (letter). *Archives of General Psychiatry*, **43**, 1016.

WEINER, W. J. & LUBY, E. D. (1983) Persistent akathisia following neuroleptic withdrawal. *Annals of Neurology*, **13**, 466-467.

# VI. Aspects of ethology

# 44 Psychopathology of emotions in view of neuroethology

## DETLEV PLOOG

Feelings, emotions and affects are products of evolution and based upon the evolution of the central nervous system in vertebrates. While human emotions as subjective experience can only be expressed by language, expressions of emotions can be performed and perceived without the faculty of language. An ethological approach to the study of the expression of emotions is presented which permits a comparison of man and animal in regard to expressive behaviour and its underlying causes. Facial expressions, chosen as the chief paradigm, are innate behaviour patterns which in the course of human ontogeny are subject to volitional control. The hierarchically organised cerebral system which mediates facial (and similarly vocal) expressions is delineated, and clinical examples underpin the conclusion that under pathological conditions volitional and emotional facial expressions (as well as vocal expressions) can be disconnected from emotional experience. On these neuroethological grounds, facial expressions in the course of depressive disorders are studied which reflect the individually differing changes of the physical condition. It is assumed that these expressions of emotion are linked to certain brain processes. It will be up to explanatory psychopathology to assign the spectrum of affective disorders to system-related more specific regional brain functions.

## In quest of causal connections in psychopathology

When theorising on the development of mental disorders, psychiatrists ought to consider heterogeneous sources of different origin. On the one hand, there are the patients with their life histories and personal experiences, their individual personalities and social environments, all of which may contribute to the understanding of the given mental or affective or behavioural disorder. On the other hand, there is an ever-increasing body of facts that lead us to search for the underlying physical causes of mental, emotional or behavioural disorders common to the human race. Almost 75 years ago, it was Karl Jaspers who wrote in the preface of his *General Psychopathology*: "My efforts have been directed towards sorting these approaches out, separating them clearly and at the same time demonstrating the many-sided nature of our science". The distinction between the psychology of meaningful connections ('understanding') and the causal connections of psychic life ('explaining') came into the minds

441

of psychopathologists. Nowadays it still seems appropriate to remind the psychiatric community that Jaspers' approach was methodological and anything but dogmatic. We must admit that we are still far away from bringing these two inconsistent approaches together, and we still keep asking how they are intertwined, interdependent or related to each other. Since we cannot assume that the mind/body problem can be 'solved' like a mathematical equation, which then would resolve the inconsistency of the two approaches, are we perhaps asking the wrong questions? Should we instead look for theories in biology which offer explanations for the behaviour of living organisms without the need of understanding their inner lives, i.e. their subjective feelings, as many as there may exist?

It is the theory of ethology, which is based on the theory of natural evolution, that I proposed on several occasions (e.g. 1964, 1976, 1980) would be helpful in advancing the theoretical framework in psychopathology and psychiatry. Kraepelin was the first who approached psychopathology in an evolutionary context:

> "The phylogenetic development of the human personality was an infinitely slow evolutionary process, with progress being made in innumerable minute, barely perceptible steps; some steps backward probably also occurred; byroads were taken and then abandoned. By its very nature the final outcome of this endless and complex evolutionary process contains signs and vestiges of widely differing phases of phylogeny, though the vast majority of mechanisms that were developed along the way and then superseded have probably been completely lost. If therefore we attempt today to establish the relationship between the manifestation of mental illness and the individual stages in the evolution of personality, we lack almost all of the prerequisites. If in our attempts we are to do more than merely grope our way, it will be necessary to search everywhere for the roots of the manifestations of our inner lives—in the minds of children, of primitive men, of animals. Furthermore, it will be necessary to establish to what degree lost emotions of the individual and of the phylogenetic past are reborn in illness. The prospects opened up by such an approach appear to be encouraging ones in spite of the meagerness of our present knowledge; the new insights gained might perhaps contribute to making somewhat easier our impossibly difficult central task, a clinical understanding of the different forms of [mental] illness." (Kraepelin, 1920)

Ethology, the comparative biology of behaviour, permits a comparison of man and animal in regard to behaviour and its underlying causes. It is an approach that is common in medicine, where we look for commonalities and differences in animals and man, say, in the immune system, the organs of the body, and the brains. But it is still uncommon in psychiatry, where mental phenomena and behaviour are the objective of our studies.

This behavioural theory is based on the theory of evolution, according to which man ranks highest in the primate species. His unique species-specific characteristics may be easier to explain by considering their phylogenetic development and taking into account that they are the result of an evolutionary process of the primates over millions of years. The ethological theory does not suffice, however, for understanding man completely. The behavioural analysis connected with it, in particular, does not yield direct access to introspective experience. That can be achieved only by speech and language.

Allowing for this significant restriction, we can conclude that common to both man and monkey are certain characteristics which play a central role in psychology and psychopathology: their behavioural development is strongly dependent on their environment; they are highly socialised creatures, expressing emotions and affects. Their behaviour is co-determined by their life history and modifiable by learning. Belonging to the anthropoid suborder of the primate species, man and monkey also have much in common, physiologically and morphologically, on the biochemical and molecular level and their sensory and motor systems. Furthermore, we may assume that their feelings, emotions, or affects—these terms are used here synonymously as defined by Gruhle (1948)—are similar and are mediated via homologous brain structures. It seems that not only ethology should be based on the theory of evolution of the nervous system, but explanatory psychopathology as well. I shall therefore also discuss the evolutionary aspects of emotions and their expression within the framework of neuroethology. Neuroethology is concerned with the analysis of the neural substrates and mechanisms that underlie species-typical behaviour (Ploog, 1987). In view of this young branch of behavioural physiology, the cerebral substrates of emotional expressions will be examined.

## Emotions as compared to sensations

My comments will be concerned with the question of what emotions are and how they are registered by the individual. It is a very old question but for some reason has played only a minor role in psychopathology. Up to the age of romanticism, feelings were considered to be of a secondary nature, dependent on perception, recognition, thinking. More attention is given now to affectivity in the pathogenesis of mental disorders; this does not mean, however, that in psychopathology the chapter entitled 'From mental to affective disorders' has been completed. Still, based on the observations of experts as well as the patients themselves, we now try to measure metrically conditions, moods, feelings, emotions and affects—these terms are listed in the order of duration of the emotional occurrence— and include them in our diagnoses. When taking a closer look, however, it becomes apparent that all these diagnostic means are based on language. Language, it is presumed, adequately describes the emotional occurrence. A clinician, however, relying on direct observation, will intuitively register the patient's facial, verbal and other motor patterns—the so-called psychomotility. Based on these observations, he will define the emotion and describe the individual as being cheerful, sad, desperate, indifferent, etc. In other words, language turns objective observations of expressed emotions into assessments of subjective feelings.

Only man can speak about his emotional experiences, and in every language there are words for describing them. Nevertheless, he has no way of knowing whether his individual experience of joy, sadness, or despair is equal to that of his fellow man. Emotions are innate and cannot be learned from a model. In this regard, they are similar to sensations. Although, unlike emotions, sensations can be measured by psychophysical rules, it is impossible to say whether the taste or pain sensations of one person are equal to those of another.

The qualities of sensations are innate, as in the case of emotions, and there are words in all languages for describing them. But, contrary to emotions, a sensation is linked to an object—something that can be seen, heard, felt or tasted. The specific object connected with the specific sensation must be learned; it must be learned that the white cube tastes sweet. Boiling water, an initially unknown neutral stimulus, can elicit the innate sensation of pain. The fact that the relationship between the perceived stimulus and the elicited sensation is invariant makes sensations equivalent to reflexes. The counterparts of sensations are the emotions. Their qualities are also innate and can neither be learned nor copied. The releasers of emotions, however, like the stimuli of sensations, may be learned through experience. But, as is characteristic of motivated behaviour, the relationship between releasers and emotional response is not invariant but fluctuating, depending on the internal state of the organism. Take hunger as an example.

It is my contention that emotions are the subjective equivalent of certain innate behaviour patterns which will be discussed in the following section. Most of man's goal-oriented actions are extremely variable and have been learned, but the ensuing emotions are remarkably universal and cannot be copied from a pattern. And just as emotional experiences are universal, so are emotional expressions. This is probably what Darwin meant when he wrote that certain actions "are the direct result of the constitution of the nervous system, and have been from the first independent of the will and, to a large extent, of habit" (Darwin, 1872, p. 66). More than 100 years have passed since then. The physiology of emotions is still in a state of flux; current theories on emotion were supplied by psychologists, and a theory on the psychopathology of emotions is still lacking.

## *The expression of emotion as a social signal*

According to ethology, facial expressions of animal and man are social signals belonging to the fixed action patterns defined by Lorenz (1937; 1965). Each facial expression corresponds to a mood, a sensation, an emotion. Like all socio-communicative signals, a facial expression exercises a dual function: it expresses an emotion and transmits a message to the recipient of the signal.

In man, contrary to animal, the innate behaviour patterns are subjected to volitional control in the course of ontogeny. Depending on the cultural and social level, the child and the juvenile learn when, where and to whom such signals are sent; the forms of expression become more complex and distinctive. The face expresses not only the affect, but also volitionally controlled representations and messages co-determined by social rules, e.g., the noncommittal party smile. It is difficult for the observer to separate the volitionally controlled patterns from the innate ones. And since understanding the socio-communicative signals is also based on innate perception mechanisms, the recipient of a message can be misled by volitionally controlled signals.

The smiles displayed in Fig. 1 were shown to 50 test persons who were to describe them by using the words listed (upper row) for the emotions of surprise (SUR), contempt (CON), fear (FEA), anger (ANG), joy (JOY), disgust (DIS), and sadness (SAD), and indicate the intensity of the emotion on a 5-step scale. On another 5-step scale (lower row) the test persons were to indicate whether

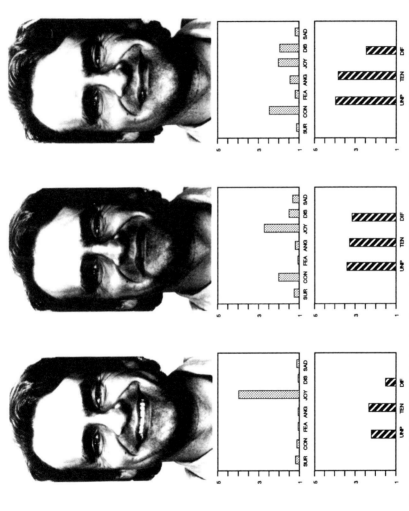

Fig. 1. *Variations of smiling, assessed by 50 subjects viewing the photographs. SUR—surprise; CON—contempt; FEA—fear; ANG—anger; JOY—joy; DIS—disgust; SAD—sadness; UNP—unpleasant; TEN—tensed; DIF—difficult to evaluate*

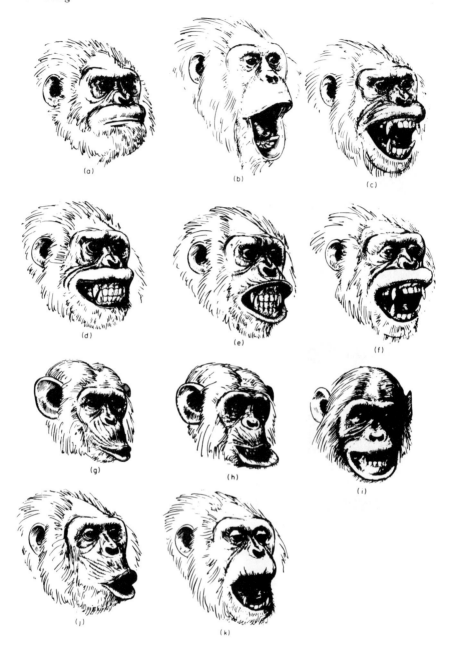

*Fig. 2. Some facial expressions of chimpanzees. (a) "Glare"; anger, type 1. (b) "Waa bark"; anger, type 2. (c) "Scream calls"; fear-anger. (d) "Silent bared-teeth"; "type 1, horizontal bared-teeth"; submission. (e) "Silent bared-teeth"; "type 2, vertical bared-teeth"; fear-affection (?). (f) "Silent bared-teeth"; "type 3, open-mouth bared-teeth"; affection. (g) "Pout face"; desiring-frustration (?). (h) "Whimper face"; frustration-sadness (?), type 1, or type 1–2 transition (infant). (i) "Cry face"; frustration-sadness, type 2 (infant). (j) "Hoot face"; excitement-affection (?). (k) "Play face"; playfulness.*

*Note—these drawings are presented for illustrative purposes only. They are diagrammatic and do not claim to precisely depict actual expressions of emotion. They are drawn after photographs and descriptions from van Hooff (1971); and van Lawick-Goodall (1968a, b). All expressions were drawn from the same angle in order to facilitate comparisons (Chevalier-Skolnikoff, 1973)*

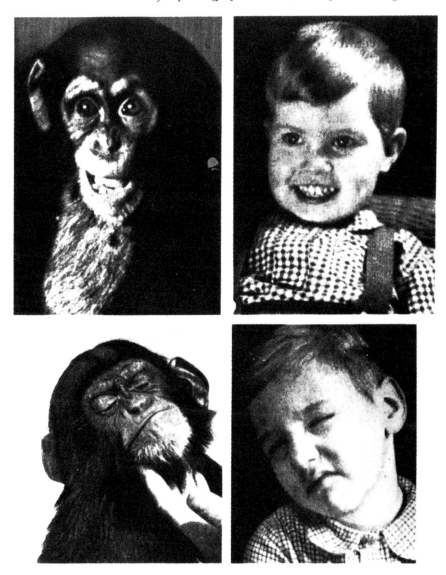

*Fig. 3. Homologous facial expressions in a boy and a young chimpanzee: curious smiling (above); displeasure (below) (Ploog, 1964)*

they found the faces unpleasant (UNP), tense (TEN) or difficult (DIF) to rate. The picture on the left impressed the test persons as being joyful, pleasant, relaxed, and easy to describe. In the centre picture, they still registered joy but mixed with contempt and disgust. They found the face unpleasant, tense, difficult to describe. The smile in the picture on the right was found to express contempt, joy, disgust; the face was found to be unpleasant, tense and difficult to rate.

The facial expressions of monkeys can also be classified according to signal effect and intensity of emotion. Similar to the observations by Lorenz (dogs),

Schenkel (wolves) and Leyhausen (cats), the facial expressions of macaques can be classified according to the degree of their attack or flight motivation. Intermediate forms between these two extremes are overlappings of both motivational states in various intensities (Chevalier-Skolnikoff, 1973).

In higher primates, the facial expressions become more complex and distinctive. Shown in Fig. 2 are several facial expressions of chimpanzees. When studying these facial expressions, it becomes obvious that the distance between man and subhuman primates has become smaller. Definition of a really homologous expression requires thorough familiarity not only with the facial expression but also with the situation in which it occurs. Sometimes the similarity appears to be obvious (Fig. 3).

To recapitulate, facial expressions belong to the class of social signals used in species-specific communication. These signals exercise a dual function: they express the sender's emotion and transmit a message to the recipient. With higher mammals, emotional expressions become more distinctive and, consequently, the signal effect more differentiated. This is an indication of an increase of discrete emotions in the evolutionary history of mammals. In order for emotions to become more distinct, specific peripheral structures capable of conveying the expressive variety need to be developed. Social signals, and this includes facial signals, are innate instinctive behaviour patterns and as such differ from other, primarily learned behaviour patterns. Ethological studies have shown that these innate behaviour patterns, in the course of human ontogeny, have come under volitional control (Ploog, 1977).

## About the cerebral organisation of facial movements

Based on the concept outlined above, it may be assumed that, together with the evolutionary development of the sender equipment—in our case man's developed facial musculature—the cerebral development of the structures required to put the equipment into a working condition continued. The more complex and differentiated the cerebral structures responsible for this behaviour are, the more complex and differentiated are the facial expressions as well as the corresponding emotions. I cannot describe the cerebral organisation of the facial musculature in detail here. All I want to do is give an outline of the cerebral representation of facial movements in relation to volitionally controlled as well as emotional (uncontrolled) facial expressions.

We are all familiar with the homunculus representation of the body in the sensory motor cortex. The cortical representation of the facial musculature in man is much more extensive than that of other parts of the body. From neurophysiological, neuropsychological, and clinico-neurological findings we conclude that the motor cortex in the precentral gyrus is directly involved in the voluntary control of the facial musculature but not so where facial expressions are concerned. The first neuron runs within the pyramidal tract from Area 4 to the facial nucleus directly, on the one hand, with the synapses in the facial nucleus, on the other hand, indirectly via interneurons in the reticular formation of the brain stem (Fig. 4). All of the direct fibres innervating the lower half of the face, i.e., nose, mouth, and chin, ascend from the contralateral cortex, while of the direct fibres ending in that part of the facial nucleus representing the

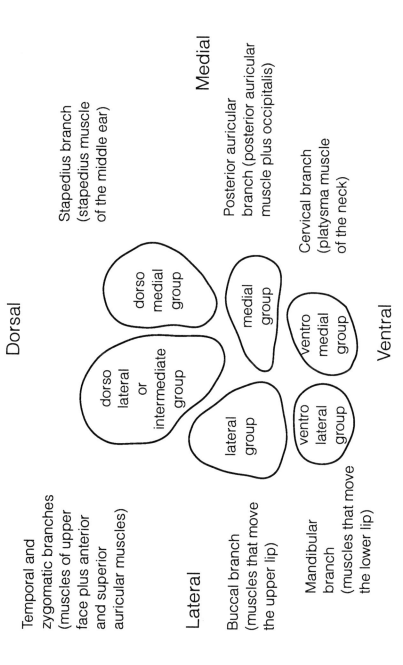

Fig. 4. *The facial nerve nucleus. (A schematic composite drawing based on drawings by Courville, 1966b.) The peripheral branches of the facial nerve that map to each grouping of cell bodies within the nucleus are indicated (after Rinn, 1984)*

orbicularis-oculi region, only 75% come from the contralateral cortex; the remaining 25% come from the ipsilateral cortex. As regards the upper third of the face, i.e., the glabella region, eyebrow and forehead musculature, half of the fibres rise from the ipsilateral, half of them from the contralateral cortex. This topographical difference in the projections to the facial nucleus is the reason for the fact that a lesion of the first neuron does not cause a paresis of the forehead musculature. That contralaterally innervated muscles show a greater independence than bilaterally innervated ones is of consequence for mimic behaviour. Contralaterally innervated muscles are also subjected to a more differentiated voluntary control. That is why all people can make unilateral lip and mouth movements but find it difficult to make unilateral voluntary movements in the eye region—and almost impossible in the forehead region—without accompanying movements on the other side. Learned movements requiring skill, such as lip and mouth movements during speech, are only possible by contralaterally innervated muscles. Finally, the contralaterally innervated muscles have a much larger cortical representation than the bilaterally innervated muscles, especially where the upper and lower face is involved; homunculus has a small forehead and a huge mouth. Another type of dichotomy results from the indirect connections via the reticular formation and other extrapyramidal structures. They transmit impulses bilaterally into the left as well as right facial nucleus. More connections, however, go to that part of the facial nucleus representing the upper face than to that representing the lower face. Furthermore, there are direct connections from the contralateral nucleus ruber (Tr. rubrofacialis) to that part of the facial nucleus representing the upper face, while such fibres are absent from the lower face. Roughly speaking, the lower face receives mainly pyramidal innervation, the upper face predominantly extrapyramidal innervation. The pyramidal motor control, especially the contralateral one, serves voluntary control, while the extrapyramidal motor control seems to have greater importance for nonvoluntary emotional motor behaviour (Courville, 1966; Rinn, 1984).

The clinician knows, of course, how to distinguish neuro-anatomically volitional from emotional facial expressions and uses this information for diagnostic purposes. A patient with a lesioned pyramidal tract, for example, cannot move the paralysed corner of his mouth on command but he may show a bilaterally symmetric smile. On the other hand, patients with lesions of the basal ganglia and persons suffering from Parkinson's disease can move their facial muscles when asked to do so, but eventually they become unable to express emotions spontaneously, while still being capable—at least for a while—of going through emotions. And then there are patients with lesions at various subcortical brain sites who laugh and cry pathologically without having the corresponding emotions. In other words, they can feel anger or pain and still utter a stereotyped laughter (Poeck, 1969).

Based on these examples, we may draw the conclusion that under pathological conditions volitional and emotional facial expressions can be dissociatively disconnected from emotional experience so that either the innate pattern is performed but no emotion experienced, or the emotion is experienced but cannot be expressed. This fact seems to support the assumption of emotions being subjective correlates of innate behaviour. Without these dissociation examples one could still argue that emotions are conditional (learned) responses to motor behaviour or, vice versa, motor behaviour a conditional response to emotions. This does not mean, of course, that emotions cannot be conditioned. It merely means that there are unconditioned emotions as there are unconditioned fixed action patterns, such as facial expressions. The disconnection of facial expressions from emotional experiences leads to the question where, in the brain stem, the innate behaviour patterns are integrated and where they are executed. Although the integration level has not been precisely described so far neurophysiologically, there is sufficient information concerning its location. In behavioural pathology, observations of infants with anencephalic malformations have shown that even those born with only an intact midbrain can still exhibit expressions of crying and laughing. Also, according to investigations in comparative anatomy, it may be assumed that on this level the motor organisation of facial expressions is closely connected to that of the voice topographically and functionally.

As far as the voice is concerned—the most refined instrument for emotional expressions (Ploog, 1986)—there is evidence that all direct and indirect references participating in phonation converge in the periaqueductal grey-parabrachial area at the dorsal midbrain-pons transition, with the limbic pathways contributing significantly to this pool. If this emotional phonation centre is destroyed, mutism results. When stimulated electrically, coordinated natural vocalisations are emitted from this area; caudal stimulation will yield only fragmentary calls (Jürgens, 1979; Ploog, 1981; Jürgens & Ploog, 1985). This corresponds to the fractioned movements of the facial musculature when stimulated (supranuclear). From these findings we may assume that the integration centre of facial expressions, where the situation-specific and disposition-dependent behaviour patterns are combined and released, is also located in this area, probably just above the integrative phonation centre in the mesencephalic tegmentum.

I think that here is the border between the neurologically observable disturbance of an affective expression and the affective disorder. Quite frequently a patient with Parkinson's disease is, at its beginning, considered endogenously depressive before a diagnosis has been made, although he does not have to be depressive even at an advanced stage of the disorder. It will be up to explanatory psychopathology to study the cerebro-structural aspects of affective disorders and provide, together with an anatomy of emotions, a physiology of emotions. By way of the various disorder patterns we will gain access to the brain structures which produce, control and express emotions. In psychiatry, we use psychopharmacy in dealing with this complex system of which we know so little.

## *The facial expression in the course of a depressive disorder*

Each clinician will give the facial expressions of a depressive patient much attention: it will help him in making a diagnosis or registering changes in the patient's condition. Still, there are only a few investigations which dealt with the problem of exactly which facial expressions the clinician selects for his purposes and, more important, which he can perceive at all. It is his hope that a thorough study of the patient's facial expressions will yield information the patient cannot disclose.

Heimann & Spoerri (1957) were the first to approach this problem in their paper on the disintegration of facial expressions in schizophrenic subjects,

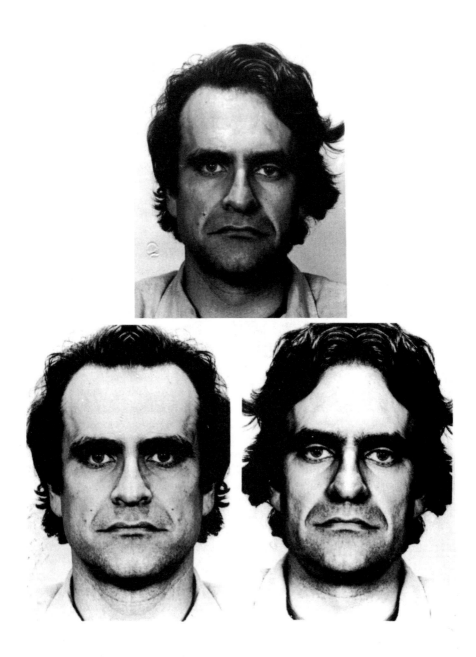

Fig. 5. *Hemispheric dominance for the expression of the face. Above—normal face; right—the left half of the face is duplicated; left—the right half of the face is duplicated.*

an approach Heimann later adapted to psychopharmacological purposes. At the Max Planck Institute of Psychiatry in Munich we have been concerned for some time with nonverbal communication (Ploog, 1964, 1980) and, more recently, with the facial expressions of depressive patients in the course of their illness (Ellgring, 1981, 1984; Ellgring & Ploog, 1985). While vocal behaviour can be recorded on tape and sonographically analysed, the analysis of facial expressions has to overcome other, more complicated, methodical difficulties.

Time, for instance, is of the essence. Some fleeting expressions, such as the eyebrow flash described by Eibl-Eibesfeldt (1979, 1984), last only for 100–200 ms; still they are perceived—if only subconsciously—by the observer. Other affect expressions last from several seconds—a baby's sleepy smile—to several minutes when expressing rage or fear (Ploog, 1964). It is important to register the lasting expression of an emotion, among others, because it modulates all other expressive behaviour or inhibits certain groups of facial signals, such as expressions of happiness or sadness. In this connection, reference is made to Veraguth's fold, the classic example of the lasting expression of depression. It occurs under bilateral moderate tension of the M. frontalis medialis and the M. corrugator glabellae. Here is where the lasting expression of depression, which corresponds to an equivalent central process, can be localised. In this connection, it is interesting to note the EMG investigations revealed an increased activity of the M. corrugator in depressive patients (Greden *et al*, 1985).

Also, it is noteworthy that the right half of the face differs from the left half in expressing emotions. In the centre of Fig. 5 the normal face is shown, on the right a double of the left side, on the left a double of the right side. Obviously, the left side of the face is more expressive, which is the case with all right-handers. Neuropsychologists have come to assume that the right hemisphere has a dominating effect on the expression of emotions (Bear, 1983). Of course, there is also the opinion that the left hemisphere has an impeding effect. The result remains the same: on the left side of the face of a right-hander the facial expression is stronger.

Confronted with these methodical difficulties, we selected the Facial Action Coding System (FACS) introduced by the Swedish anatomist Hjortsjoe (1970) and developed by Ekman & Friesen (1978) for our analyses of facial expressions. Displayed in Fig. 6 are three examples of combining three so-called action units of the forehead. Action units 1, 2, and 4 in the upper row are combined in the lower row. With the aid of this coding system, it is possible, in a step-by-step analysis of a video tape, also to code the sequential occurrence of all facial expressions for subsequent quantitative analysis (Ekman, 1979).

In a depression study conducted by Ellgring (1984), video recordings were made of 20 patients with endogenous depression, 16 patients with neurotic depression—classified according to Martin Roth's classification of affective disorders (1978) as well as DSM–III and ICD–9 and nine control persons while subjected to standardised interviews and talking freely, and their facial expressions analysed by FACS. The results were impressive in many respects: the facial activity changed quantitatively in the course of the depression; the qualitative and quantitative changes differed in endogenous and neurotic patients; the type of the change was person-specific.

In 75% of the endogenous patients (E), as compared to 31% of the neurotic patients (N), a reduction of the general facial activity was observed when the

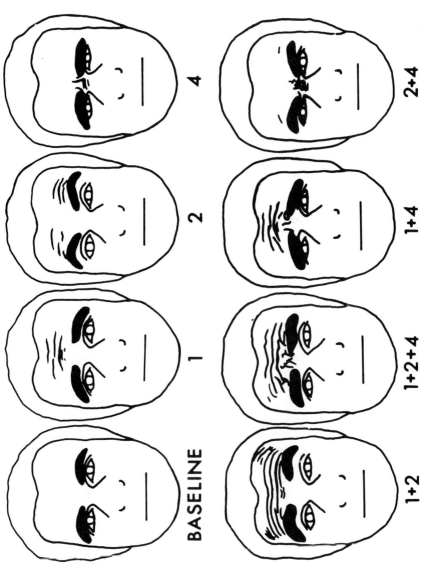

*Fig. 6. Facial Coding System (FACS) for facial expressions. Action Units for the brow/forehead 1, 2 and 4, and combinations of them (after Ekman, 1979)*

patients felt bad (self-rating scale). When comparing E and N patients over a period of three months, the tendency was quite different: in E patients, reduced facial expressions decreased from 75% to 43% to 25%, while in N patients it increased from 31% to 63%. In other words, the amount of facial activity increased in E patients as the illness improved, and it decreased in N patients. These observations may be explained as follows: N patients express the degree of their suffering by their facial expressions; when they feel bad, they display more of it, when they feel better, fewer. In contrast, E patients express the degree of their suffering by reducing their facial expressions which increase when they feel better.

As may be expected, the production of smiles is strongly reduced in E and N patients; even when the patient's condition improves he does not smile as often as a control person. In the majority of cases, however, smiles were shown more often when the physical condition improved. The ratings registered for E patients in bad condition were considerably lower than those of N patients. However, in comparison with the general expressive activity, for smiles no contrasting tendency has been recorded for the two patient groups.

With the aid of a cluster method, it was possible to show the individual specificity of facial patterns in depression and in the course of improvement. Configuratively similar patterns, obtained in 120 interviews, were classified according to the relative frequency with which specific facial units were displayed by a person. Typical for the depression-specific patterns was a dominance of the facial expressions of annoyance, fear and tension, while those of sadness were rarely shown.

Other studies of the nonverbal behaviour of depressive and healthy persons, in particular glances of the eye, eye contact, gestures and content-independent verbal activity in the course of a depression, support the findings with respect to facial expressions: only a small person-specific part of the nonverbal repertoire is subject to change.

In summary, it can be said that depressive patients display a variety of facial and other nonverbal expressions which reflect the individually differing changes of the physical condition. Reductions of the nonverbal repertoire differ individually and change in accordance with the improvement of the physical condition. Only in a few cases, all registered nonverbal characteristics are involved; usually only two or three of them change in the course of the depression. According to the individual pattern developed, only part of the behavioural repertoire is subject to change. The clinician seems to sort out this part intuitively and makes diagnostic use of it.

Another, quite significant, sign in affective disorders should be mentioned here briefly, and that is the change in the prosody of the voice in the course of depression. We know much more about the neuroanatomy and neurophysiology of vocal behaviour than that of facial expressions, of its many roots in the limbic system and brain stem sites which are also essential for facial expressions (Jürgens & Ploog, 1985; Jürgens, 1986). Consequently, we should be able to define the brain system, perhaps even the specific brain sites responsible for disturbances of vocal behaviour, i.e. prosodic defects of speech in depressive patients. There is evidence that the anterior cingulate cortex is involved (Jürgens & von Cramon, 1982).

In view of all these complexities and individual particularities, it seems amazing how successful clinicians can be in dealing with the facial, vocal, and other nonverbal indications of depressive behaviour intuitively without having to analyse individual patterns of expression. After inspection of our video material, Pattay (1982) and Avarello (1983) proved that only by evaluating the answers to two standard questions or the information obtained from viewing a video film of 10 seconds, which showed the behaviour of the interviewee as well as the interviewer, conclusions may be drawn as to the condition of the patient. Other studies indicate that an experienced clinician only needs a few behavioural spot checks and comparative data to be able to register changes in the depression of a patient.

It seems doubtful, however, whether the judgement of the clinician as to the degree and course of the affective disorder suffices for diagnosing the complex expression patterns of disturbed emotionality so as to utilise them in his treatment. On account of the analysis of nonverbal behaviour and the brain structures involved, it is assumed that these expression patterns are linked to certain system-related regional brain processes. This assumption is supported by the findings of EMG investigations conducted by Greden *et al* (1984, 1985) and Schwartz *et al* (1976) and their predictions as to the effect of psychopharmacy. I believe that future causality-directed psychopathology, in particular where affectivity is concerned, will have to deal with system-related regional processes, and not so much with global changes (e.g. changes of transmitter balances in endogenous psychoses). Although the delineation of the regional processes responsible for affective disorders will rather be achieved by future brain mapping methods than by application of the time-consuming analysis of nonverbal behaviour, it may possibly lead to a finer graduation of the spectrum of depressive disorders for which Martin Roth (1977; 1978) has laid the foundation. In any event, the neuro-ethological approach to the study of emotions and their disturbances will increase our knowledge of the cerebral organisation of expressive behaviour and the influences exercised by internal (neuronal and humoral) and external (social) processes.

## Conclusions

Ethologically, feelings, emotions and affects are evolutionary products, having developed in the course of natural history from a primitive to a highly complex form. Neuroethologically, the cerebral structures responsible for emotions went through the same evolutionary process (Ploog, 1986). While human emotions as subjective experience can be expressed only by language, comparative ethology has shown that the expression of emotions has an evolutionary history. Darwin realised that facial expressions are the result of cerebral processes from the first independence of the will and habit. The emotional expression—focusing here on facial expressions—has a dual function: it expresses an emotion and serves as a social signal to the conspecific. Social signals, on the other hand, are the basic elements of communication and govern life in the community (Ploog, 1970).

It seems that nature is asking a high price from its creatures for the ability to communicate: the higher they are grouped in the vertebrate order, the more sophisticated are the peripheral structures releasing a diversity of emotional expressions and transmitting information. Facial expressions, reaching their development peak in higher primates, are a perfect example of the evolution of communication and emotionality. The complexity of the peripheral apparatus increases in correspondence with that of the central nervous system which sets this apparatus in motion, governs and controls it. Using facial expressions as an example of nonverbal communication, I have tried to give a sketchy outline of the peripheral system and its complicated cerebral control and have described those parts of the system that generate emotions. A much more detailed description of the voice has been given elsewhere. Under this ethological aspect, emotions are subjective correlates of innate facial expressions which, in the course of evolution, came step by step under volitional control. Clinical examples showed that volitionally controlled and emotional facial expressions can be impaired dissociatively and that facial expressions and affect experience can be disconnected. This supports the assumption that emotions are the subjective correlates of innate behaviour.

The neurological explanation of the disturbance of affect expression may serve as a model for affective disorders. It is very probable that the affective disorder of a depressive or manic psychosis originates in the same cerebral system we know from studies dealing with the anatomy and physiology of emotions. The analysis of nonverbal expressive behaviour in the course of affective disorders permits an insight into this system and may be a useful tool in the differential diagnosis and treatment of depressive disorders.

# References

AVARELLO, M. (1983) *Nonverbales Verhalten in klinischdiagnostischen Gesprächssituationen. Eine Eindrucksstudie*. Dissertation. Innsbruck: Leopold-Franzens-Universität.

BEAR, D. M. (1983) Hemispheric specialization and the neurology of emotion. *Archives of Neurology*, **40**, 195–202.

CHEVALIER-SKOLNIKOFF, S. (1973) Facial expression of emotion in nonhuman primates. In *Darwin and Facial Expression* (ed. P. Ekman). New York: Academic Press.

COURVILLE, J. (1966a) Rubrobulbar fibres to the facial nucleus and the lateral reticular nucleus. *Brain Research*, **1**, 317–337.

—— (1966b) The nucleus of the facial nerve: The relation between cellular groups and peripheral branches of the nerve. *Brain Research*, **1**, 338–354.

DARWIN, C. (1872) *The Expression of Emotions in Man and Animals*. London: Murray, p. 66.

EIBL-EIBESFELDT, I. (1979) Ritual and ritualization from a biological perspective. In *Human Ethology. Claims and Limits of a New Discipline* (eds M. v. Cranach, K. Foppa, W. Lepenies & D. Ploog). Cambridge: Cambridge University Press, p. 26.

—— (1984) *Die Biologie des menschlichen Verhaltens. Grundriß der Humanethologie*. München: Piper.

EKMAN, P. (1979) About brows: emotional and conversational signals. In *Human Ethology. Claims and Limits of a New Discipline* (eds M. v. Cranach, K. Foppa, W. Lepenies & D. Ploog). Cambridge: Cambridge University Press.

—— & FRIESEN, W. V. (1978) *The Facial Action Coding System*. Palo Alto: Consultant Psychiatrist Press.

ELLGRING, H. (1981) Nonverbal communication. A review of research in Germany. *German Journal of Psychology*, **5**, 59–84.

—— (1984) *Nonverbal Communication in Depression*. Cambridge: Cambridge University Press.

—— & PLOOG, D. (1985) Sozialkommunikatives Verhalten in klinischer Perspektive. In *Hirnorganische Psychosyndrome im Alter II* (eds D. Bente, H. Coper & S. Kanowski). Berlin: Springer.

GREDEN, J. F., GENERO, N. & PRICE, H. L. (1985) Agitation-increased electromyogram activity in the corrugator muscle region: A possible explanation of the "Omega sign"? *American Journal of Psychiatry*, **142**, 348–351.

——, PRICE, L., GENERO, H., FEINBERG, M. & LEVINE, S. (1984) Facial EMG activity levels predict treatment outcome in depression. *Psychiatry Research*, **13**, 345–352.

GRUHLE, H. (1948) *Verstehende Psychologie (Erlebnislehre)*. Stuttgart: Thieme.

HEIMANN, H. & SPOERRI, Th. (1957) Das Ausdruckssyndrom der mimischen Desintegrierung bei chronischen Schizophrenen. *Schweizerische Medizinische Wochenschrift*, 1126.

HJORTSJÖ, Ch. (1970) *Man's face and mimic language*. Malmoe: Nordens Boktryckeri.

HOOFF VAN, J. A. R. A. M. (1971) *Aspects of the Social Behaviour and Communication in Human and Higher Non-human Primates*. Rotterdam: Author.

JASPERS, K. (1913) *Allgemeine Psychopathologie*, 1st edn Heidelberg; Engl. translation (1963) *General Psychopathology*, by J. Hoenig & M. W. Hamilton. Manchester: Manchester University Press.

JÜRGENS, U. (1979) Neural control of vocalization in nonhuman primates. In *Neurobiology of Social Communication in Primates* (eds H. D. Steklis & M. J. Raleigh). New York: Academic Press.

—— (1986) The squirrel monkey as an experimental model in the study of cerebral organization of emotional vocal utterances. *European Archives of Psychiatry and Neurological Sciences*, **236**, 40–43.

—— & CRAMON D. v. (1982) On the role of the anterior cingulate cortex in phonation: a case report. *Brain and Language*, **15**, 234–248.

—— & PLOOG, D. (1985) On the neural control of mammalian vocalization. In *The Motor System in Neurobiology* (eds E. V. Evarts, S. P. Wise & D. Bousfield). Amsterdam: Elsevier.

KRAEPELIN, E. (1920) Die Erscheinungsformen des Irreseins. *Zeitschrift für Neurologie*, **62**, 1–29.

LAWICK-GOODALL VAN, J. A. (1968a) A preliminary report on expressive movements and communication in the Gombe Stream chimpanzees. In *Primates: Studies in Adaption and Variability* (ed. P. C. Jay). New York: Holt.

—— (1968b) The behaviour of free-living chimpanzees in the Gombe Stream Reserve. *Animal Behaviour Monographs*, **1**, 161–311.

LEYHAUSEN, P. (1973) *Verhaltensstudien an Katzen*. 3. Aufl. Berlin: Parey.

LORENZ, K. (1937) Über die Bildung des Instinktbegriffes. *Naturwissenschaften*, **25**, 289–300; 307–318; 324–331.

—— (1953) Über angeborene Instinktformeln beim Menschen. *Deutsche Medizinishe Wochenschrift*, **78**, 1566–1569; 1600–1604.

—— (1965) *Evolution and Modification of Behavior*. Chicago: Chicago Press.

PATTAY, S. (1982) *Stimmungsbeeinflussung und Stimmausdruck*. Diplomarbeit. München: Universität.

PLOOG, D. (1964) Verhaltensforschung und Psychiatrie. In *Psychiatrie der Gegenwart*, Bd.I/1B (eds H. W. Gruhle, R. Jung, W. Mayer-Gross & M. Müller). Berlin: Springer.

—— (1970) Social communication among animals. In *The Neurosciences* (ed. F. O. Schmitt). New York: The Rockefeller University Press.

—— (1976) Similarities and differences of behaviour as a function of cerebral evolution and dissolution. In *Methods of Inference from Animal to Human Behaviour* (ed. M. v. Cranach). Chicago: Aldaline Publishing.

—— (1977) Sozialverhalten und Hirnfunktion beim Menschen und seinen Verwandten. *Klinische Wochenschrift*, **57**, 857–867.

—— (1980) Soziobiologie der Primaten. In *Psychiatrie der Gegenwart*, 2. Aufl., Bd. I/2 (eds K. P. Kisker, J. E. Meyer, C. Müller & E. Strömgren). Berlin: Springer.

—— (1981) Neurobiology of primate audio-vocal behavior. *Brain Research Reviews*, **3**, 35–61.

—— (1986) Biological foundations of the vocal expressions of emotions. In *Emotion: Theory, Research and Experience, Vol. III, Biological Foundations of Emotion* (eds R. Plutchik & H. Kellerman). New York: Academic Press.

—— (1987) Neuroethology. In *Encyclopedia of Neuroscience*, Vol. II (ed. G. Adelman). Boston: Birkhäuser.

POECK, K. (1969) Pathophysiology of emotional disorders associated with brain damage. In *Handbook of Clinical Neurology, Vol. 3, Disorders of higher nervous activity* (eds P. J. Vinken & G. W. Bruyn). New York: Wiley.

RINN, W. E. (1984) The neuropsychology of facial expression: a review of the neurological and psychological mechanisms for producing facial expressions. *Psychological Bulletin*, **95**, 52–77.

ROTH, M. (1977) The borderlands of anxiety and depressive states and their bearing on new and old models for the classification of depression. In *Neuro-transmission and Disturbed Behaviour* (eds H. M. van Praag & J. Bruinvels). Utrecht: Scheltema Holkema.

—— (1978) Studies in the classification of affective disorder I: proposals towards a synthesis of new and old concepts. *Proceedings of the Adolph Meyer Symposium on Psychobiology*. Centennial of Johns Hopkins University, 15 March, 1976.

—— (1978) The classification of affective disorders. *Pharmakopsychiatry*, **11**, 27–42.

——, GURNEY, C., GARSIDE, R. F. & KERR, T. A. (1972) Studies in classification of affective disorders. *British Journal of Psychiatry*, **121**, 147–161.

SCHENKEL, R. (1947) Ausdrucksstudien an Wölfen. *Behaviour*, **1**, 81–129.

SCHWARTZ, G. E., FAIR, P. L., SALT, P., MANDEL, M. R. & KLERMAN, G. L. (1976) Facial expression and imagery in depression: An electromyographic study. *Psychosomatic Medicine*, **38**, 337–347.

# 45 The effect of social stress on the behaviour and physiology of monkeys

## JOHN S. PRICE

Various endocrine changes associated with submissive behaviour have been shown to occur in monkeys forced into a subordinate role, similar to previous findings with rodents. In the male vervet monkey submissive behaviour is associated with a change from blue to white in the colour of the scrotal skin, due to an alteration in the optical properties of the dermal collagen. This paper summarises a study carried out to determine whether the change is mediated by any of the hormonal changes known to be associated with the social stress of acute submission.

Shortly before I joined the Newcastle Department in 1971, as a direct result of a theoretical paper comparing some aspects of human psychopathology with the behavioural correlates of social submission in baboons (Price, 1967), my attention was drawn to a monkey which, in addition to manifesting baboon-like behavioural correlates of submission, also underwent a conspicuous physiological change in the form of a change in the colour of its scrotal skin. This monkey, a guenon usually called the vervet monkey, was, and as far as I know still is, the only primate, and probably the only mammal, to undergo an observable physiological change during social submission. It seemed, therefore, a suitable experimental animal to study the physiology of submission in animals as a model of some forms of psychopathology (such as depression and anxiety) in man. In this paper I shall review some relevant studies on the vervet monkey, and then summarise some work carried out with colleagues at Newcastle and subsequently at the Clinical Research Centre. But first I would like to make a provisional classification of submission, as it is obvious that, in human beings at least, submission is only occasionally associated with psychopathology.

### Classification of submission

Submission may be acute or chronic. Acute submission following defeat in an agonistic encounter I shall call *acute catathetic submission*, using the term catathetic (Price, in press) to indicate that the submitting individual has been "put down" by another individual (the winner). *Acute adulatory submission* is associated with positive affect on the part of the submitting individual and often with over-valuation of the individual submitted to. *Acute benign submission* may be said to occur when an individual submits without either fight or adulation.

Chronic submission takes the form of subordinate rank in group-living species and exclusion from territory in territorial species. Chronic submission may be *catathetic* (maintained by repeated catathetic or 'putting down' signals), *adulatory* or *benign*. We should also recognise a further category of *chronic reluctant submission*, characterised by envy of the privileges enjoyed by those of higher rank, and actual or potential challenge of the rank order; the manifestation of this state is likely to elicit an aggressive (catathetic) response from the dominant individual who is challenged, so that there is a blurring between catathetic and reluctant submission, when it is difficult to tell, or in systemic terms impossible to tell, whether the catathetic behaviour of the dominant individual is spontaneous or a response to reluctance manifested by the subordinate.

### Submission and psychopathology

Here I am concerned only with acute and chronic catathetic submission and with chronic reluctant submission. These are the states in which human experience can recognise at least two potentially pathogenic aspects of submission: the sight of others enjoying privileges which are denied one, and the receipt of punishment (catathetic signals) from a dominant person. These were identified by Galen as the two "passions of the soul": he recognised them in his own behaviour, both his envy of physicians who paraded the streets in carriages finer than his own, and his tendency to throw his quill at his slave when he was irritated.

## *The vervet monkey*

Vervet monkeys live in groups of about 20 animals, and except in the arid fringes of their East African habitat the groups contain more than one adult male. Brain (1965) reported as follows on the social structure of the group:

> "The day-to-day pattern of life of any individual monkey in the troop is determined by its position in the social order and by the temperament of any monkeys to which it is subordinate. A casual observer of the captive troop, or of a free-ranging one, might conclude that aggression between individuals is random and unpredictable; this is in fact far from the case and, as soon as the observer is sufficiently familiar with the individual monkeys to be able to recognise them, the existing order of social dominance will immediately become apparent to him."
>
> "It is abundantly clear that initial establishment of dominance of one monkey over another is not a matter of physical strength nor of size, but rather by a recognition of specific attributes . . . Among vervets the most important attributes are most probably confidence and imperturbability; these characteristics make possible the steady, level gaze of a dominant primate . . .. This steadiness of gaze is a well-marked characteristic of the most dominant monkeys in the troop, but is noticeably lacking in those individuals near the bottom of the social order."
>
> "Adult male vervets are characterised by the almost luminous blueness of their scrotal sacs; this colour has clear social significance and could probably be described as a status symbol; the intensity of the blueness is certainly variable and may well be related to the general state of well-being of the animal and its level of dominance."

The most marked changes in scrotal colour occur when a male falls in the dominance hierarchy. In such a case the scrotum may change from a brilliant blue to a "putty-white colour" over the course of seven to fourteen days. The colour change is associated with a behavioural change which the authors describe as "demoralisation" and "loss of self-confidence", and there is a marked inhibition of aggressive behaviour. For instance, when a monkey named Robert fell from the third position in Brain's captive group, "after a week he had lost all social status and did not retaliate when attacked singly by any of the lowest-ranking monkeys."

Normally, aggressive behaviour among vervets takes the form of threat or pursuit without biting (Gartlan & Brain, 1968). When biting does occur it is usually on the tail, or takes the form of nips around the knees and ankles which usually do not penetrate the skin. The animals are very sensitive to these attacks and may die after them, even though no real injury has been received. In captivity the biting may be more severe, particularly when a stranger is introduced into the troop. Brain (1965) describes the introduction of a stranger as follows:

> "On coming into contact with the new individual, the first reaction of the other male members of the troop was to examine the blue scrotum with the greatest diligence. Eventually, this prolonged scrutiny annoyed the new monkey who became aggressive. Had he been allowed to fight one member of the troop at a time, he would probably soon have achieved a high ranking position, as he showed clear attributes of a dominant individual. This never occurred, however, and the first signs of aggression precipitated a full-scale attack by the whole troop. Within a few days he was completely demoralised and shortly after removal from the cage, died of the injuries he had received. It was particularly noticeable that when this monkey was first placed with the troop, its scrotum was the most brilliant blue colour. As the animal lost confidence as a result of repeated attacks by the troop, the colour faded away to a pale powder-blue hue."

It is not yet known whether the colour change is reversible. Brain (1969) writes: "Concerning the relationship of the colour change to dominance: I was able to observe that the brightness of the colour faded as the male lost status, but I was never able to re-instate a male in the hierarchy, so was not able to demonstrate that the brilliance could be restored. Once a vervet becomes subordinate, it seems extremely difficult to restore its confidence".

Subsequent work on the social behaviour of the vervet monkey has confirmed the observations of Brain & Gartlan, but unfortunately the St Kitts vervet, on which most of the work has been done (McGuire *et al*, 1983) lacks the blue scrotal skin characteristic of the species.

The vervet monkey is a member of a genus which is remarkable for its multicoloured facial and perineal displays (Kingdon, 1980) and apart from the talapoin monkey it is the only member of the genus which lives in multi-male groups (Melnick & Pearl, 1987). It is also the only multi-male-group-living monkey of the cercopithecine family in which the female shows no perineal swelling or colour change at oestrus (Melnick & Pearl, 1987). Therefore it is possible that the genital skin hydration reaction, which in many cercopithecines mediates sexual change in the female, has in this monkey come to mediate social rank change in the male; and that, as in the other monkeys oestrogen prepares both the brain for sexual behaviour and the body for signals of sexual receptivity, in the vervet monkey some hormonal agent prepares both the brain for submissive behaviour and the body for submissive signalling. It was this possibility which provided the motivation for the work which I will now describe.

## The blue skin

Three male and two female vervet monkeys (*Cercopithecus aethiops pygerythrus*) were purchased from Animal Suppliers Ltd and the skin was examined by colleagues from the dermatology department of the University of Newcastle upon Tyne (Price *et al*, 1976).

The scrotal skin of the males was a vivid blue colour. The skin of the abdominal wall had a pale blue colour and this extended along the medial aspects of the upper arms and legs. The adult female showed a blue colouration which was most marked on the outer surfaces of the labia majora. In this area the colour was a dark blue without the vivid quality of the scrotal skin. A female infant born in captivity showed a similar dark blue colouration of the labia majora.

The bright blue colouration of the male scrotum was clearly visible from the front and side whether the male was sitting or standing. By contrast, the blue colouration of the female genitalia was not observed in any of the usual postures of the animal. The scrotal colouration was thus a very conspicuous feature of the male, which accords with the suggestion that it acts as a signal to other members of the species (Struhsaker, 1967). Apart from the scrotum which has little hair, the blue colour of the skin elsewhere was largely obscured by fur.

### Transillumination

It seemed possible that, as in other species, the blue colour would be due to the preferential scattering of short wave-lengths (Tyndall effect) above a layer of pigment (Fox & Vevers, 1960). This was supported by the findings on transillumination: when a bright light was shone through a fold of scrotal skin a reticulate pattern of brown patches (similar to the colour of melanin) was seen against a homogeneous red background.

### Histological examination

Both epidermis and upper dermis were free of pigment, but in the mid and lower dermis there were dense deposits of melanin, situated in cells which had the histological and electron microscopical appearances of melanocytes.

## The white skin

### The effect of tissue fluid on skin colour

Intradermal injection of saline and other colourless fluids immediately blanched the skin at the site of the bleb, the colour returning as the bleb was absorbed.

Removing tissue fluid by compressing the skin with an artery forceps for a few seconds gave a consistent response, the skin under the forceps taking on a deep blue colour. It was noticeable that this colour had none of the vivid quality of the normal scrotum; it was like the normal colour of the female labia but more intense. On each side of the deep blue colour under the forceps there were lines of pallor due to the tissue fluid which had been expressed sideways by the forceps.

These experiments suggested that colour change could be mediated *artificially* by altering the distribution of tissue fluid in the dermis above the melanin. However, it was not yet clear whether the *natural* occurrence of pallor was also associated with change in interstitial fluid. During the nine months of observation the intensity of the scrotal colour varied spontaneously from a dark blue to a bright blue to a vivid turquoise blue to a pale whitish colour. The whitish colour was always most marked in the upper anterior scrotum above the penis. Regardless of the degree of whiteness, the same intense dark blue could always be restored by compression of the scrotal skin applied for a few seconds with forceps. The pallor returned as the tissue fluid diffused back. The idea that the pallor was due to masking of the blue colour by accumulation of tissue fluid and was not due to a change in melanin was confirmed by histological and electron microscopic examination; the normal pale and blue scrotal skins and the deep blue skin elicited from the former by fluid expression showed no obvious difference in the number of melanocytes nor in the number of pigment granules and their dispersal. The only difference noted concerned the extracellular compartment; in the deep blue skin the melanocytes appeared closer to each other whereas in the pale skin they were separated by wide gaps.

## Electrical stimulation *in vitro*

Application of electrical current to male or female blue skin (placed on blotting paper and soaked in physiological saline) abolished the blue colour and left the dermis translucent except for the melanin network. The female skin returned to its normal blue colour in about 30 minutes, but in the bright blue male skin the affected areas turned white in roughly the same time.

A cathode was applied to the skin (anodal stimulation was ineffective) and pulses of 3 milliseconds duration at a rate of 100 per second were applied at an intensity of 5–10 milliwatts for durations of ½ to 4 minutes. After 30 seconds brown circular areas appeared under the electrode and these increased in number until the whole area was brown. *By transmitted light* the affected area was seen as a white circular patch against the usual pink background; in other words, the dermis (apart from the melanin network) had become translucent. In the female skin the pink colour (complementary to the Tyndall blue) returned in about 30 minutes, but in the male the affected area became opaque.

## The effect of ionic environment

Pieces of excised scrotal skin kept in physiological saline solution maintained their blue colour. Transferred to normal hydrochloric acid or sodium hydroxide for one minute the pieces of skin became black (translucent except for the melanin deposits). Transfer from the acid solution to a saturated salt solution caused an instantaneous change to white; further transfer to the alkaline solution caused a return of the black colour. Transfer of the black skin from the alkaline solution to a saturated salt solution caused a deep blue colour to develop over the course of one minute. This colour was stable in physiological saline, but the skin can be turned black again by immersion in either acid or alkaline solution.

These manipulations demonstrate that the vervet scrotal skin has the capacity to exist in states which render it blue or white or black to the human eye, and that it can be changed from one state to another by simple changes in the ionic environment.

## *The colour change*

Changes in interstitial fluid content of the skin could be due to hormonal, neural or mechanical mechanisms. A dependent oedema due to inertia or other mechanical causes seemed unlikely because it was the superior aspects of the scrotum which showed the greatest spontaneous fluctuations of fluid content during the months of observation. A neural mechanism could not be excluded, but seemed unlikely due to the time course of the colour change (a matter of days). Of the various hormonal possibilities, the most likely were androgens and corticosteroids which are known to be reduced and increased, respectively, during social stress (Bernstein *et al*, 1983), and oestrogens, which are already known to cause hydration of genital skin in the female of some primate species (Hrdy & Whitten, 1987).

### Androgenic hormones

Two males with somewhat pale scrotal sacs were given extra androgen to see if the blue colour could be enhanced. One was given methyltestosterone 5 mg orally daily for three weeks, the other testosterone propionate 2 mg i.m. daily for two weeks; neither showed any change in colour. One male was subjected to bilateral orchidectomy, followed four months later by bilateral adrenalectomy, in the expectation that the removal of androgen might induce hydration. However, the reverse occurred, and the genital skin became a darker blue with less apparent interstitial fluid, tending towards the condition of the adult female skin. This suggests that the hydration of male genital skin occurs in two stages: first, at puberty, there is a slight hydration mediated by androgenic hormones which switches the colour from dark blue to the turquoise blue characteristic of the adult male; then, associated with catathetic submission, and mediated by another hormone, there is the potential for a quantitatively greater (and perhaps qualitatively different) hydration which switches the colour from turquoise blue to pale blue and white.

## *Stress hormones*

In other species the physiological changes associated with acute catathetic submission, apart from reduction of androgenic secretion and increase in prolactin, are almost entirely due to increased activity of the pituitary/adrenocortical axis.

It seemed very likely that the skin colour change would also turn out to be secondary to an increase in circulating glucocorticoids. However, administration of the ACTH analogue Synachthen Depot 0.5 mg i.m. daily for 12 days in one animal, and dexamethasone 0.5 mg orally daily for three weeks in another, were without definite influence on skin colour. If anything, the skin was bluer after the steroid. Prolactin in a dosage of 3 mg i.m. daily for three weeks and the mineralocorticoid aldosterone 0.25 mg by intraperitoneal injection daily for four weeks were also without effect.

In some states of social stress there is chronic adrenomedullary overactivity but unfortunately we were not able to reproduce this condition artificially. Single injections of adrenaline, sufficient to cause marked tachycardia, were without effect on scrotal colour.

### Female sex hormones

Apart from the induction of inflammation by locally acting agents, the only hormones known to cause skin hydration are oestrogens. These sometimes cause a generalised dermal oedema in women during pregnancy, and they are responsible for the enormous genital skin swellings of some primate species during oestrus (Hrdy & Whitten, 1987). It seemed likely that the vervet scrotal skin would be sensitive to oestrogen, either because oestrogens might be important in the physiology of the male of this species (as they are, for instance, in the stallion), or because, even after the evolution of another hormonal trigger, the tissue might retain an atavistic sensitivity to oestrogen. However, ethinyloestradiol in a dosage range from 0.1 mg orally to 50 mg i.m. daily for four weeks, with or without the addition of the progestogen norethisterone acetate (5 mg daily), had no effect. The sex skin of the female was also insensitive to administered oestrogen.

## Discussion

The vervet scrotal skin is a remarkable organ. The optical properties of its dermal collagen can be rapidly and reversibly altered between three conditions:
  (a) all light is reflected giving a white colour
  (b) no light is reflected, giving a black colour
  (c) only short wavelengths are reflected, giving a blue colour
Only a small proportion of this capacity for signalling is actually used in nature. The black colour does not occur at all. The change from blue to white can be rapid or slow, but only the slow change occurs. The change from white to blue has not been observed. Nevertheless, even with this modest use of its potential, this piece of skin is unique as the only instance in which a signal depends on a change in the optical properties of the particles responsible for a Tyndall blue. Tyndall blues are widespread among fish, amphibia and reptiles, and it is an odd coincidence that loss of blue colouration is often a sign of social submission, as in the rainbow lizard (Greenberg & Crews, 1983). But the mechanism is quite different: the reptilian loss of blue is due to a migration of melanin-containing cells over the layer of guanine crystals responsible for the differential refraction (Fox & Vevers, 1960), and therefore the change in lizards is always from blue to brown rather than blue to white. Tyndall blues are rare in mammals, occurring

in the blue of blue eyes, the Mongolian spot, in certain pathological pigmentations of the dermis and in discrete patches on the skin of Old World monkeys. The vervet scrotal skin is the only instance in which loss of the blue colour constitutes a signal.

Further uniqueness lies in the fact that this is the only primate submission signal (except possibly blushing) which involves a physiological change. Other submission signals consist of posture, movement or vocalisation which are under higher nervous control and may be used for deception. Therefore the vervet is not only a model which offers a lead into the physiology of submission, but also an example of theoretical interest in the behavioural ecology of signalling.

## Acknowledgements

I am grateful to Professor Sir Martin Roth for his support while I worked in his department, to Professor Sam Shuster and Dr John Burton for their collaboration over the examination of the skin, to Dr Larry Evans for his help with the *in vitro* work and to Dr Peter Berry for his help with the hormonal studies.

## References

BERNSTEIN, I. S., GORDON, T. P. & ROSE, R. M. (1983) The interaction of hormones, behavior and social context in non-human primates. In *Hormones and Aggressive Behavior* (ed. B. B. Svare). New York: Plenum Press.

BRAIN, C. K. (1965) Observations on the behaviour of vervet monkeys, *Cercopithecus aethiops. Zoologica Africana*, **1**, 13–27.

—— (1969) Personal communication.

FOX, H. M. & VEVERS, G. (1960) *The Nature of Animal Colours*. London: Sidgwick & Jackson.

GARTLAN, J. S. & BRAIN, C. K. (1968) Ecology and social variability in *Cercopithecus aethiops* and *C. mitis*. In *Primates* (ed. P. C. Jay). New York: Holt, Reinhart & Winston.

GREENBERG, N. & CREWS, D. (1983) Physiological ethology of aggression in amphibians and reptiles. In *Hormones and Aggressive Behavior* (ed. B. B. Svare). New York: Plenum Press.

HRDY, S. B. & WHITTEN, P. L. (1987) Patterning of sexual activity. In *Primate Societies* (eds B. B. Smuts, D. L. Cheney, R. M. Seyfarth, R. W. Wrangham & T. T. Struhsaker). Chicago: University of Chicago Press.

KINGDON, J. S. (1980) The role of visual signals and face patterns in African Forest monkeys (guenons) of the genus *Cercopithecus. Transactions of the Zoological Society of London*, **35**, 431–475.

McGUIRE, M. T., RALEIGH, M. J. & JOHNSON. C. (1983) Social dominance in adult male vervet monkeys: general considerations. *Social Science Information*, **22**, 89–123.

MELNICK, D. J. & PEARL, M. C. (1987) Cercopithecines in multimale groups: genetic diversity and population structure. In *Primate Societies* (eds B. B. Smuts, D. L. Cheney, R. M. Seyfarth, R. W. Wrangham & T. T. Struhsaker). Chicago: University of Chicago Press.

PRICE, J. S. (1967) The dominance hierarchy and the evolution of mental illness. *Lancet, iii*, 243–246.

—— (in press) Alternative channels for negotiating asymmetry in social relationships. In *Social Fabrics of the Mind* (ed. M. R. A. Chance). Hove: Erlbaum.

——, BURTON, J. L., SHUSTER, S. & WOLFF, K. (1976) Control of scrotal colour in the vervet monkey. *Journal of Medical Primatology*, **5**, 296–304.

STRUHSAKER, T. T. (1967) Behavior of vervet monkeys and other Cercopithecines. *Science*, **156**, 1197–1203.

# VII. Miscellaneous

# 46 Psychiatric morbidity following cardiac surgery: A review

## PAMELA J. SHAW and DAVID A. SHAW, CBE

In 1949 Martin Roth published a paper in Brain entitled 'Disorders of the Body Image Caused by Lesions of the Right Parietal Lobe'. It was a scholarly dissertation based on detailed accounts of two patients whom he had studied while Medical Registrar at the Maida Vale Hospital for Nervous Diseases. The originality of his clinical observations and of their interpretation illuminated a subject that had excited the interest of many of the leading neurologists of the first half of the century. Towards the end of his paper, Sir Martin speculated on the possibility of a common patho-physiological mechanism underlying the phenomena of anosognosia and depersonalisation and his final sentence referred to "that fascinating borderland between neurology and psychiatry, the exploration of which will probably shed light on important problems of both subjects".

Over the years Sir Martin has continued to visit that borderland where, in company with fellow neuroscientists, he has conducted many important and fruitful explorations. The subject which is reviewed in this article dwells in the common territory shared by psychiatry and neurology and it is offered as a tribute to Sir Martin on behalf of those many neurologists who have so greatly enjoyed his company and learned from his wisdom.

Psychiatric disturbances occur more commonly after cardiac operations than after other surgical procedures. A study of the postoperative complications of coronary bypass surgery has shown that 1.2% (4/312) of patients undergoing this procedure developed a paranoid-hallucinatory psychosis in the early postoperative period.

Delirium or an organic psychosis are the most common post-surgical psychiatric complications although the reported incidence shows wide variation due largely to the lack of a consistent nosology. The aetiology appears to be multifactorial; factors of possible relevance have been considered under four headings: organic cerebral injury; preoperative psychological predisposition; postoperative cardiac or metabolic abnormality; the postoperative environment.

Recommended preventive and therapeutic measures include preoperative psychiatric intervention, environmental modification, correction of metabolic disturbances and the judicious use of major tranquillisers.

Other early postoperative psychiatric complications have received less attention and include hysteria and other neurotic and depressive reactions.

Long-term follow-up studies have frequently reported a favourable psychiatric outcome after cardiac surgery. However, psychological problems may detract from the overall benefit of cardiac surgical repair, particularly in patients with poor psychological adjustment prior to operation.

It has been known for many years that psychiatric disturbances may occur after surgical operations (Lipowski, 1967). Postoperative psychosis has been reported to occur in less than 0.1% of general surgical patients (Knox, 1961; Lewis, 1955). The incidence of psychiatric disorders after cardiac surgery is greater than that following other major operations and rates of psychosis or delirium as high as 40–57% have been described (Blachly & Starr, 1964; Egerton & Kay, 1964).

We have recently completed a study concerning the neurological (Shaw *et al*, 1985; Shaw *et al*, 1986b) and neuropsychological (Shaw *et al*, 1986a; Shaw *et al*, 1987) morbidity occurring after coronary bypass surgery. During the early postoperative period we noted overt psychiatric complications in a proportion of patients.

We present here the psychiatric findings of the Newcastle coronary bypass study and the literature review which it prompted. We aim to describe the spectrum of postoperative psychiatric disorders which may be encountered and to draw conclusions from the large volume of information available on possible aetiological factors and methods of prevention and treatment.

## Results of the Newcastle coronary bypass study

In this study we prospectively assessed a cohort of 312 patients undergoing elective coronary bypass surgery, using clinical neurological and neuropsychological methods. Postoperative psychosis was observed in four patients (1.2%). This consisted of a florid paranoid-hallucinatory state which in two patients was present immediately after anaesthesia and in the other two developed after a lucid interval of two to three days. Two patients had other abnormalities of the central nervous system and all four showed cognitive impairment on postoperative psychometric testing. The mental state returned to normal within 48 hours in two patients, but the other two were still mildly disturbed at the time of discharge from hospital.

A typical example of the postoperative psychotic disorder is illustrated by the case history of one of the four patients. She was a 60-year-old, recently retired, teacher of German who had suffered from angina pectoris of grade IIb severity for almost two years. There was no previous history of neurological or psychiatric illness and preoperative examination of the nervous system and mental state was entirely normal. Five coronary bypass grafts were undertaken in a routine, uneventful operation. She was discharged from the ITU (Intensive Therapy Unit) within 24 hours and for the first three days her recovery was uncomplicated.

During the night of the fourth day she had three episodes of extreme behaviour disturbance during which she ran through the ward shouting that the staff were trying to kill her and crying for help. On one occasion she rushed into the bathroom and locked herself in with another patient. She was physically violent towards the nurses who tried to coax her back to bed. She was sedated with chlorpromazine and the following day she remained paranoid, tense and disorientated in time. Psychiatric advice was sought and continuation of phenothiazine therapy was recommended. By the seventh postoperative day her mental state had recovered. She had insight into her previously disturbed condition and was able to describe some of her experiences during the previous 48 hours. Vivid visual hallucinations were described in terms of a net floating down from the ceiling to envelop her, or coloured, ill-defined objects swirling around the room. In addition she was aware of strange auditory perceptions. Everyone who talked to her seemed to have an aggressive German accent. Footsteps around the room sounded like someone wearing army boots. She felt that the other patients and attending medical and nursing staff were trying to harm her.

The patient attributed what she called this "period of madness" to several factors including sleeplessness, dependence on others in contrast to former independence, and the fact that the operation had been much more stressful than she had anticipated.

No postoperative neurological abnormalities were observed, but psychometric scores showed significant worsening on two of a battery of ten tests (Shaw *et al*, 1986a). During the follow-up for six months after surgery she remained neurologically and psychologically well.

The study having been set up primarily with neurological objectives, only the most overt psychiatric disturbances were recorded. We were impressed, however, at the frequency with which patients in the early postoperative period mentioned transient hallucinatory experiences and vivid nightmares, often with a combative theme. Affective changes including euphoria and depression were also frequently encountered.

## *Review of the literature on psychiatric morbidity following cardiac surgery*

### Early psychiatric complications

*Delirium/psychosis*

Postoperative psychiatric disturbances were described in the early accounts of the complications of heart surgery (Priest *et al*, 1957; Fox *et al*, 1954; Bliss *et al*, 1955). A variety of disorders were alluded to, including hysterical amnesia (Fox *et al*, 1954), catastophic reactions causing apathy and immobility (Meyer *et al*, 1961) and schizophrenic reactions (Bliss *et al*, 1955). In 1964 Blachly & Starr coined the term postcardiotomy delirium. This was defined as a psychosis occurring three to four days after surgery and comprising confusion and disorientation, with visual, auditory and perceptual illusions or hallucinations. Heller and co-workers (1970) differentiated between postcardiotomy delirium, which occurred three to five days after operation, and an early postoperative 'organic brain syndrome' which was characterised by disorientation without perceptual aberrations and which was apparent as soon as the patient awakened from anaesthesia.

*Incidence* As emphasised by Dubin and colleagues (1979) there has been a lack of agreement on diagnostic terms and the definition of delirium in different studies has not been uniform. A clear distinction has not always been made between mild subjective phenomena and overt psychosis. This lack of consistent nosology is reflected in the wide variation in the reported incidence of postcardiotomy delirium, ranging from 3% (Morin & Coupal, 1982) to 57% (Blachly & Starr, 1964). Blacher (1972) studied 12 apparently normal patients after cardiac surgery and found that eight had suffered major psychiatric upheaval which they had managed to conceal from their medical attendants. He suggested that psychosis after open heart surgery may be almost universal, but may only be revealed by careful interviewing. Henrichs *et al* (1972) reviewed 13 studies and found a mean incidence of 23% for postoperative psychiatric complications.

Several authors have reported that the incidence of postoperative psychosis is reduced in children and adults under 25 years (Kornfeld *et al*, 1965; Egerton & Kay, 1964; Kaplan *et al*, 1974). Other workers have recorded a lower incidence in patients undergoing coronary bypass compared with those having valve surgery (Rabiner *et al*, 1975; Willner *et al*, 1976). Recent estimates suggest that the incidence of psychosis/delirium is gradually decreasing (Heller *et al*, 1970; Kimball, 1969; Sveinsson, 1975).

*Clinical picture* Postoperative delirium/psychosis often presents as clouding of consciousness, incoherence, confusion and motor restlessness, together with perceptual distortions which may have a paranoid quality. There is often a disturbance of the sleep-wake cycle and marked fluctuation in the psychiatric state over the course of a day. The condition may present immediately after operation or may develop after a lucid interval of several days (Kornfeld *et al*, 1974; Layne & Yudofsky, 1971; Rubinstein & Thomas, 1969). Several possible explanations of the lucid interval have been proffered. Sensory monotony, sleep deprivation and anxiety engendered in intensive care, have been considered important post-operative factors causing progressive psychological stress and culminating in psychosis after several days (Blacher *et al*, 1972; Kornfeld *et al*, 1965; Vasquez & Chitwood, 1975). It is also known that various intra-operative factors may produce cerebral hypoxia, the clinical manifestations of which may be considerably delayed (Plum *et al*, 1962). Furthermore it is a fact that the EEG following cardiac surgery may take several days to become maximally abnormal (Sachdev *et al*, 1967).

Postoperative delirium/psychosis is generally a self-limiting condition. According to Vasquez & Chitwood (1975) the average duration of delirium is five days, with a range of two to 21 days. Nocturnal confusion and altered perception are usually the last symptoms to abate.

*Aetiology* Numerous hypotheses have been advanced to explain the postoperative psychosis associated with cardiac surgery. The initial reports singled out emotional disturbances as the most important cause (Fox *et al*, 1954). Later, as the relationship between organic brain damage and an abnormal psychological state was recognised, organic cerebral injury was thought to be the principal underlying factor (Zaks, 1959). Most authors would now agree that the aetiology of postoperative delirium is multifactorial. Several underlying mechanisms have been suggested.

*Organic cerebral injury*

Neurological studies have shown that many patients with postoperative behaviour disorders have definite focal neurological signs (Gilman, 1965; Javid *et al*, 1969;

Tufo *et al*, 1970). Gilman (1965) has stressed that parieto-occipital cerebral damage may superficially resemble psychiatric derangement. Freyhan and co-workers (1971) noted that mnestic and gnostic neurological disturbances were frequently associated with psychiatric abnormalities. In their study 23% of patients with postoperative psychiatric disorders had abnormal neurological signs.

Further support for the organic hypothesis comes from the observed correlation between postoperative psychosis and both EEG abnormality (Sachdev *et al*, 1967; Scheld *et al*, 1982; Freyhan *et al*, 1971) and cognitive change (Juolasmaa *et al*, 1981). Scheld and associates (1982) found minor EEG abnormalities in two thirds of patients with delirious symptoms. Replacement of the normal alpha rhythm by slower frequencies is the most constant EEG change observed (Sachdev *et al*, 1967). Factors, to be discussed later, that are thought to predispose to brain injury during cardiac operations appear no less important in the genesis of postoperative delirium and psychosis (Vasquez & Chitwood, 1975). Finally, autopsies of patients with postoperative psychiatric disorders have shown definite structural changes in the brain, particularly areas of infarction and anoxic lesions in the hippocampus (Vasquez & Chitwood, 1975; Tufo *et al*, 1970).

*Preoperative and intraoperative organic factors*
(a)   *Age* As noted above, age is an important determinant of postoperative psychiatric outcome, older patients being at greater risk of psychiatric morbidity (Blachly & Starr, 1964; Javid *et al*, 1969; Lee *et al*, 1971). Youth appears to be a protective factor, most authors reporting a negligible incidence of delirium in patients of less than 25 years (Egerton & Kay, 1964; Heller *et al*, 1970).
(b)   *Severity of the preoperative illness* A clear-cut association has been shown between the incidence of postcardiotomy delirium and the severity of the preoperative illness (Lee *et al*, 1971; Heller *et al*, 1970). Using the New York Heart Association system these authors reported an incidence of delirium of 0–29% in patients with class I disease and 40–100% in patients in class IV.
(c)   *Type of heart disease* The incidence of delirium is lower in patients with congenital heart lesions than in those with acquired disease (Heller *et al*, 1970). Coronary bypass patients appear to have less psychiatric morbidity than patients operated on for valvular lesions (Rabiner *et al*, 1975; Willner *et al*, 1976). In the study of Layne & Yudofsky (1971) aortic valve replacement was associated with a greater incidence of delirium (27%) than mitral valve replacement (4%). However, Egerton & Kay (1964) reached the opposite conclusion. Multiple valve replacements are particularly likely to be associated with delirium. Blachly & Starr (1966) estimated that delirium occurs in some 90% of middle aged males undergoing aortic and mitral valve replacement.
(d)   *Pre-operative organic brain disease* Patients with preoperative organic brain disease are at greater risk of developing postoperative confusion (Lipowski, 1967). Using the conceptual level analogy test to identify preoperative organic brain damage, Willner and associates (1976) were able to predict which patients would have postoperative psychiatric symptoms. Egerton & Kay (1964) found that 36% of patients with postoperative delirium had pre-existing brain damage; the prevalence of brain damage in the remainder was 8%
(e)   *Intra-operative hypotension* The literature contains conflicting evidence regarding the importance of low arterial blood pressure during surgery in the pathogenesis of cerebral injury. Several studies have shown that sustained mean

arterial pressure levels of less than 50 mmHg are significantly correlated with postoperative cerebral dysfunction (Lee *et al*, 1969; Tufo *et al*, 1970; Stockard *et al*, 1973). Other workers have argued that mean arterial pressure during bypass is not a major determinant of brain injury (Kolkka & Hilberman, 1980; Ellis *et al*, 1980).

(f)    *Duration of cardio-pulmonary bypass* The duration of extracorporeal perfusion seems to be one of the most clearly defined determinants of postoperative cerebral outcome. Several authors (Javid *et al*, 1969; Tufo *et al*, 1970) have reported that bypass times of longer than two hours significantly increase the risk of postoperative delirium.

## Preoperative psychological factors

(a)    *The sense of awe pertaining to the heart* The heart is not only a vital organ; it is viewed as the symbolic seat of love, courage, loyalty, and other strong emotions. The average patient resists the idea of physical handling of the heart. Blacher (1972) regarded the prospect of having one's heart incised as a prominent factor leading to postoperative psychosis.

(b)    *Preoperative personality and psychopathology* Patients with a preoperative history of psychiatric disorder have a raised incidence of delirium after cardiac surgery (Rubinstein & Thomas, 1969; Blachly & Starr, 1964). Excessive anxiety prior to surgery may predispose to psychiatric complications (Abram & Gill, 1961; Layne & Yudofsky, 1971). Those who have difficulty in expressing anxiety prior to surgery and who rely on the defence mechanism of denial, may also be at increased risk (Layne & Yudofsky, 1971). Denial as a coping mechanism tends to break down after the severe physical assault of cardiac surgery and exposure to the unfamiliar atmosphere of ITU. Egerton & Kay (1964) found that patients with pressing personal problems or marital difficulties were more likely to develop postoperative psychological disturbances.

Some authors have suggested that certain personality types are more prone to psychiatric complications than others but their conclusions have been inconsistent. Kornfeld and associates (1974) and Heller *et al* (1974) thought that active, dominant, self-confident types were more likely to experience delirium. It was postulated that the passive, immobilised confinement in the recovery room might be more stressful for individuals with this personality type. Other authors have suggested, however, that psychiatric complications occur more commonly in passive, dependent personalities (Rabiner *et al*, 1975). Several groups have found that acute psychotic reactions cannot be predicted from the patient's preoperative psychological profile (Lee *et al*, 1971; Knox, 1963). Kimball (1969) has undertaken one of the most comprehensive studies of the relationship between preoperative personality and postcardiotomy delirium. He divided patients into four groups based on preoperative assessment. Group 1 were well adjusted patients whose approach to life was purposeful and realistic; Group 2 were symbiotic patients who maintained a role of illness from which they derived secondary gain; Group 3 were anxious patients who were characterised by a determined adequacy in coping with life and who relied heavily on the defence mechanism of denial; Group 4 were depressed patients who felt hopeless about the future. Kimball found the highest postoperative mortality in the depressed group, the greatest psychiatric morbidity in the symbiotic and anxious groups and the best outcome in the adjusted group.

## Postoperative cardiac and metabolic status

Decreased cardiac output after operation has been found to be a factor in the causation of postcardiotomy delirium (Blachly & Kloster, 1966; Heller *et al*, 1979). Other predisposing factors include acute renal failure (Blachly & Starr, 1964); cardiac dysrhythmias (Blachly, 1967) and hypoxia and acidosis (Lee *et al*, 1969). Several authors have suggested that catecholamine levels may be important in the pathogenesis of postoperative delirium (Dubin *et al*, 1979; Lee *et al*, 1969) but this remains to be confirmed. Summers (1979) suggested that the use of certain drugs including anticholinergics, digitalis, barbiturates and narcotics may predispose to delirium. Egerton & Kay (1964) found that dehydration and hyponatraemia were important precipitating factors.

## Post-operative environmental factors

The sensory monotony, immobilisation and sleep deprivation that can occur during postoperative care in ITU have been cited as important factors underlying psychiatric disturbances and their cumulative effect may account for the lucid postoperative interval that is often observed (Kornfeld *et al*, 1974; Sveinsson, 1975). In support of this hypothesis, it has been shown experimentally that sleep deprivation and sensory monotony can produce perceptual aberrations (West *et al*, 1962; Ziskind *et al*, 1960). Other authors have refuted this hypothesis on the basis that they have found no significant difference in the number of days spent in ITU between delirious and non-delirious patients (Layne & Yudofsky, 1971).

In summary, it seems likely that delirium or psychosis after open-heart surgery is a final common outcome for various pathogenic factors including organic central nervous system injury, functional psychological factors and environmental stresses.

### Treatment and prevention

(a)   *Preventive measures* Preoperative psychiatric evaluation of patients has been recommended to identify those most at risk of postoperative delirium. Abramson & Block (1973) developed a method of intervention which appeared to be of therapeutic benefit with a relatively brief period of contact. They recommended a seven point ego-supportive care approach. Several other authors have suggested that preoperative interviews may reduce the incidence of postoperative delirium. In studies utilising control groups the incidence was reduced by 50% by single preoperative interviews (Layne & Yudofsky, 1971; Lazarus & Hagens, 1968). Surman and associates (1974) failed to replicate these findings, but showed that multiple preoperative psychiatric interviews tended to reduce the incidence of postoperative psychological disturbances. Preoperative psychiatric evaluation of cardiac surgical patients is unlikely to be practicable on a routine basis, but it has been recommended that patients who have a history of mental disorder or who display severe anxiety prior to surgery should be referred for psychiatric advice (Sveinsson, 1975).

Other preventive measures considered beneficial have included: familiarisation of patients with postoperative procedures prior to surgery; allowing periods of uninterrupted sleep after surgery (Dubin *et al*, 1979); shortening the time in ITU as much as possible and modification of the ITU environment to reduce monotony. Patients should also be warned about the possibility of postoperative perceptual disturbances and confusion and asked to report these so that early action can be taken.

(b)    *Correction of any contributory metabolic factors* In patients with postoperative delirium any metabolic disturbances that are detected, for example respiratory failure, reduced cardiac output, electrolyte imbalance or drug toxicity, should obviously be corrected as far as possible.

(c)    *Drug therapy* Phenothiazines or butyrophenones in small doses have been recommended as the drugs of choice for the treatment of postoperative delirium (Nadelson, 1976; Blachly & Starr, 1966). Hypnotics, preferably those that do not suppress rapid eye movement sleep, should be administered as required (Sveinsson, 1975).

### (b)    *Other psychiatric disturbances in the early postoperative period*

The attention of most authors has been focused on postcardiotomy delirium and there is much less information on other postoperative psychiatric disturbances.

(a)    *Hysteria* Knox (1963) described hysterical symptoms in 14% of patients after mitral valvotomy. Egerton & Kay (1964) found symptoms of conversion hysteria in five of 90 patients prior to open-heart surgery. These symptoms subsided in the early postoperative period, but recurred in two patients after discharge from hospital.

(b)    *Neurotic reaction* Egerton & Kay (1964) described two cases of neurotic reaction following inadequate anaesthesia during cardiac surgery. One patient showed features of the phobic anxiety-depersonalisation syndrome described by Roth (1959) who emphasised that this neurotic disorder often follows upon a calamity or acute physical illness. The second patient suffered from migraine and nightmares for three months after surgery.

Sveinsson (1975) described the occurrence of frequent vivid nightmares in the early postoperative period in 10% of his cohort of patients.

(c)    *Depression* Egerton & Kay (1964) found that depression was common towards the end of the first postoperative week, occurring in 6/60 (10%) of postcardiotomy patients. In one third the depression persisted for at least three months. In only one patient was the depression of psychotic intensity. Morgan (1971) found that 28/57 (49%) patients suffered a depressive reaction following cardiac surgery and there appeared to be three well defined patterns. Eleven had a brief 24–48 hour spell of feeling depressed or apathetic on the fourth or fifth day. Fifteen patients had a more prolonged depressive spell with irritability, fitful sleep and undue complaints of aches and pains. Two patients became depressed when postoperative complications developed. The incidence of depression was higher in those identified as overanxious prior to surgery.

Several authors have made the interesting observation that patients who were depressed prior to operation had a significantly greater perioperative mortality (Morgan, 1971; Kimball, 1969). It was suggested that patients with this affective state may be incapable of mounting the necessary physiological responses to cope with the stress of surgery.

## Late psychiatric complications

Several studies have reported a favourable long-term psychiatric outcome after cardiac surgery. Lucia & McGuire (1970) found that patients who had undergone valve surgery maintained and frequently improved their pre-surgical vocational, social and emotional status three or more years after operation. Jenkins and co-workers (1983) reviewed 318 patients before and six months after coronary bypass surgery. They found that measures of anxiety, depression and fatigue fell significantly, whereas levels of hostility remained essentially unchanged. These authors concluded that by six months after surgery most patients had experienced resolution of physical and related psychological symptoms and enjoyed enhancement of their quality of life. Bass (1984) also failed to find any evidence that heart surgery produced long-term psychiatric morbidity. He found that psychiatric dysfunction one year after surgery was related to preoperative psychological and social maladjustment, neurotic personality traits, type A behaviour and a previous history of psychiatric illness. Ramshaw & Stanley (1984) claimed that patients predisposed to a poor long-term psychiatric outcome can be identified before surgery. Those with a previous history of inability to cope with stressful events and those with neurotic personality traits were most likely to have a poor psychological outcome. Rabiner & Willner (1976) found that 7/46 (15%) patients studied 18 months after coronary bypass surgery had significant psychiatric symptoms within the diagnostic categories of depression alone, depression plus organic brain syndrome, chronic brain syndrome alone. A similar incidence (16%) of early postoperative psychiatric complications was found by this group (Rabiner *et al*, 1975). However, the patients with early and late complications comprised two almost entirely separate groups. Patients with psychiatric symptoms in the early postoperative period were not predisposed to late psychiatric morbidity. There was, however, a significant relationship between preoperative psychiatric illness and problems in the follow-up period. Mayou & Bryant (1987) found overall improvement in mental state, leisure activity and satisfaction in family life following cardiac surgery, but few benefits in terms of employment and sexual relations. They observed that mixed anxiety/depression was the commonest long-term postoperative psychiatric disturbance and that 6% of patients required psychiatric care during the first year after surgery.

Several other studies have reported somewhat less optimistic long-term results. Frank and colleagues (1972) in a retrospective questionnaire survey of 800 patients after cardiac surgery, found that psychological problems interfered with optimal long-term benefit in a substantial number. Similarly Heller and associates (1974) in a study of 70 patients one year after valve surgery, reported that in 38% of cases there were psychological hindrances to recovery, which in 21% were judged severe. This subgroup showed anxiety, depression, poor self-esteem, passive dependency, somatic preoccupation, paranoid tendency and withdrawal. There were often difficulties in sexual and marital relationships. Burgess *et al* (1967) found that 12 months after cardiac surgery 27% of their patients demonstrated an unfavourable psychological outcome. Horgan and co-workers (1984) reported that abnormally high scores on measures of anxiety and depression were present in 50% of 77 patients prior to coronary bypass surgery and in about 30% after operation. Various abnormal personality characteristics were reported after surgery which could not be attributed either to poor surgical outcome or to persistence of preoperative psychological symptoms. These authors also reported postoperative sexual dysfunction in 29% of patients. Gundle *et al* (1980) likewise reported a high incidence of sexual impairment after coronary bypass surgery, 57% of 30 continuing to complain one to two years after operation. The psychological state of these patients in relation to their sexual disorders was not clear. However, there was a high correlation with features of damaged self-image. Patients who had suffered cardiac symptoms for more than eight months prior to operation fared particularly badly and their diminished self-concept seemed to be reinforced rather than repaired by the experience of surgery. Reviewing postoperative changes in various quality of life measures such as general happiness, reduction in anxiety and depression, subjective improvement in job and family role, Kornfeld *et al* (1982) found least improvement in sexual adjustment.

An operation on the heart is a formidable proposition for both surgeon and patient. The pre-occupation of the surgeon must be the accomplishment of a complex technical procedure, inevitably carrying some risk to life, which, if successful, improves cardiac function and alleviates distress or disability. For the patient, prolongation of life and relief of symptoms are the rewards against which the risk, the discomfort and the fear of the ordeal have been measured. These primary concerns of both surgeon and patient, not forgetting the patient's family, are of such weight that it is understandable if psychological accompaniments or sequelae of the operation are either overlooked or accepted as a price worth paying. Yet they are of sufficient magnitude to warrant continued study and the concentration of scientific effort towards their elimination.

## References

ABRAM, H. S. & GILL, B. F. (1961) Predictions of postoperative psychiatric complications. *New England Journal of Medicine*, **265**, 1123–1128.

ABRAMSON, R. & BLOCK, B. (1973) Ego-supportive care in open-heart surgery. *International Journal of Psychiatry in Medicine*, **4**, 427–437.

BASS, C. (1984) Psychosocial outcome after coronary artery bypass surgery. *British Journal of Psychiatry*, **145**, 526–532.

BLACHER, R. S. (1972) The hidden psychosis of open-heart surgery with a note on the sense of awe. *Journal of the American Medical Association*, **222**, 305–308.

BLACHLY, P. H. (1967) Open-heart surgery. Physiological variables of mental functioning. *International Psychiatric Clinics*, **4**, 133–155.

—— & STARR, A. (1964) Post-cardiotomy delirium. *American Journal of Psychiatry*, **121**, 371–375.

—— & KLOSTER, F. E. (1966) Relation of cardiac output to post-cardiotomy delirium. *Journal of Thoracic and Cardiovascular Surgery*, **52**, 422–427.

—— & STARR, A. (1966) Treatment of delirium with phenothiazine drugs following open-heart surgery. *Diseases of the Nervous System*, **27**, 107–110.

BLISS, E. L., RUMEL, W. R. & BRANCH, C. H. H. (1955) Psychiatric complications of mitral surgery. *Archives of Neurology and Psychiatry*, **74**, 249–252.

BURGESS, G. N., KIRKLIN, J. W. & STEINHILBER R. M. (1967) Some psychiatric aspects of intracardiac surgery. *Proceedings of the Mayo Clinic*, **42**, 1–12.

DUBIN, W. R., FIELD, H. L. & GASTFRIEND D. R. (1979) Postcardiotomy delirium: a critical review. *Journal of Thoracic and Cardiovascular Surgery*, **77**, 586–594.

EGERTON, N. & KAY, J. H. (1964) Psychological disturbances associated with open-heart surgery. *British Journal of Psychiatry*, **110**, 433–439.

ELLIS, R. J., WISNIEWSKI, A., POTTS, R., CALHOUN, C., LOUCKS, P. & WELLS, M. R. (1980) Reduction of flow rate and arterial pressure at moderate hypothermia does not result in cerebral dysfunction. *Journal of Thoracic and Cardiovascular Surgery*, **79**, 173–180.

FOX, H. M., RIZZO, N. D. & GIFFORD, S. (1954) Psychological observations of patients undergoing mitral surgery. *Psychosomatic Medicine*, **16**, 186–208.

FRANK, K. A., HELLER, S. & KORNFELD, D. (1972) A survey of adjustment to cardiac surgery. *Archives of Internal Medicine*, **130**, 735–738.

FREYHAN, F. A., GIANNELLI, S., O'CONNELL, R. A. & MAYO, J. A. (1971) Psychiatric complications following open-heart surgery. *Comprehensive Psychiatry*, **12**, 181–195.

GILMAN, S. (1965) Cerebral disorders after open-heart operations. *New England Journal of Medicine*, **272**, 489–498.

GUNDLE, M. J., REEVES, B. R., TATE, S., RAFT, D. & MCLAURIN, L. P. (1980) Psychological outcome after coronary artery surgery. *American Journal of Psychiatry*, **137**, 1591–1594.

HELLER, S. S., FRANK, K. A., MALM, J. R., BOWMAN, F. O., HARRIS, P. D., CHARLTON, M. H. & KORNFELD, D. S. (1970) Psychiatric complications of open-heart surgery: a re-examination. *New England Journal of Medicine*, **283**, 1015–1020.

——, ——, KORNFELD, D. S., MALM, J. R. & BOWMAN, F. O. (1974) Psychological outcome following open-heart surgery. *Archives of Internal Medicine*, **134**, 908–914.

——, KORNFELD, D. S., FRANK, K. A. & HOAR, P. F. (1979) Postcardiotomy delirium and cardiac output. *American Journal of Psychiatry*, **136**, 337–339.

HENRICHS, T. F., MACKENZIE, J. W. & ALMOND, C. H. (1972) Psychological adjustment and psychiatric complications following open heart surgery. *Journal of Nervous and Mental Disease*, **152**, 332–345.

HORGAN, D., DAVIES, B., HUNT, D., WESTLAKE, G. W. & MULLERWORTH, M. (1984) Psychiatric aspects of coronary artery surgery. A prospective study. *Medical Journal of Australia*, **141**, 587–590.

JAVID, H., TUFO, H. M., NAJAFI, H., DYE, W. S., HUNTER, J. A. & JULIAN, O. C. (1969) Neurological abnormalities following open-heart surgery. *Journal of Thoracic and Cardiovascular Surgery*, **58**, 502–509.

JENKINS, C. D., STANTON, B. A., SAVAGEAU, J. A., DENLINGER, P. & KLEIN, M. D. (1983) Coronary artery bypass surgery. Physical, psychological, social and economic outcomes six months later. *Journal of the American Medical Association*, **250**, 782–788.

JUOLASMAA, A., OUTAKOSKI, J., HIRVENOJA, R., TIENARI, P., SOTANIEMI, K. & TAKKUNEN, J. (1981) Effect of open-heart surgery on intellectual performance. *Journal of Clinical Neuropsychology*, **3**, 181–197.

KAPLAN, S., ACHTEL, R. A. & CALLISON, C. B. (1974) Psychiatric complications following open-heart surgery. *Heart Lung*, **3**, 423–428.

KIMBALL, C. P. (1969) Psychiatric complications of surgical procedures. *American Journal of Psychiatry*, **126**, 348–359.

KNOX, S. J. (1961) Severe psychiatric disturbances in the postoperative period: a five year survey of Belfast hospitals. *Journal of Mental Science*, **107**, 1078–1096.

—— (1963) Psychiatric aspects of mitral valvotomy. *British Journal of Psychiatry*, **109**, 656–668.

KOLKKA, R. & HILBERMAN, M. (1980) Neurologic dysfunction following cardiac operation with low-flow, low-pressure cardiopulmonary bypass. *Journal of Thoracic and Cardiovascular Surgery*, **79**, 432–437.

KORNFELD, D. S., ZIMBERG, S. & MALM, J. R. (1965) Psychiatric complications of open-heart surgery. *New England Journal of Medicine*, **273**, 288–292.

——, HELLER, S. S., FRANK, K. A. & MOSKOWITZ, R. (1974) Personality and psychological factors in postcardiotomy delirium. *Archives of General Psychiatry*, **31**, 249–253.

——, ——, ——, WILSON, S. N. & MALM, J. R. (1982) Psychological and behavioural responses after coronary artery bypass surgery. *Circulation*, **66** (suppl. III), 24–28.

LAYNE, O. L. & YUDOFSKY, S. C. (1971) Postoperative psychosis in cardiotomy patients. The role of organic and psychiatric factors. *New England Journal of Medicine*, **284**, 518–520.

LAZARUS, H. R. & HAGENS, J. H. (1968) Prevention of psychosis following open-heart surgery. *American Journal of Psychiatry*, **124**, 1190–1195.

LEE, W. H., MILLER, W., ROWE, J., HAIRSTON, P. & BRADY, M. P. (1969) Effects of extracorporeal circulation on personality and cerebration. *Annals of Thoracic Surgery*, **7**, 562–569.

——, BRADY, M. P., ROWE, J. M. & MILLER, W. C. (1971) Effects of extracorporeal circulation upon behaviour, personality and brain function: Part II, hemodynamic, metabolic, and psychometric correlations. *Annals of Surgery*, **173**, 1013–1023.

LEWIS, A. (1955) The relation between operative risk and the patient's general condition: alcohol, other habits of addiction and psychogenic factors. *Bulletin de la Societé Internationale de Chirugie*, **14**, 421–430.

LIPOWSKI, Z. J. (1967) Delirium, clouding of consciousness and confusion. *Journal of Nervous and Mental Disease*, **145**, 227–255.

LUCIA, W. & MCGUIRE, L. B. (1970) Rehabilitation and functional status after surgery for valvular heart disease. *Archives of Internal Medicine*, **126**, 995–999.

MAYOU, R. & BRYANT, B. (1987) Quality of life after coronary artery surgery. *Quarterly Journal of Medicine*, **62**, 239–248.

MEYER, B. C., BLACHER, R. S. & BROWN, F. (1961) A clinical study of psychiatric and psychological aspects of mitral surgery. *Psychosomatic Medicine*, **23**, 194–218.

MORGAN, D. H. (1971) Neuropsychiatric problems of cardiac surgery. *Journal of Psychosomatic Research*, **15**, 41–46.

MORIN, P. & COUPAL, P. (1982) Délirium post-chirurgie cardiaque avec circulation extra-corporelle: aspects cliniques et observations dans un centre spécialisé. *Canadian Journal of Psychiatry*, **27**, 31–39.

NADELSON, T. (1976) The psychiatrist in the surgical intensive care unit. *Archives of Surgery*, **111**, 113–119.

PLUM, F., POSNER, J. B. & HAIN, R. F. (1962) Delayed neurological deterioration after anoxia. *Archives of Internal Medicine*, **110**, 18–25.

PRIEST, W. S., ZAKS, M. S., YACORZYNSKI, G. K. & BOSHES, B. (1957) The neurologic, psychiatric and psychologic aspects of cardiac surgery. *Medical Clinics of North America*, **41**, 155–169.

RABINER, C. J., WILLNER, A. E. & FISHMAN, J. (1975) Psychiatric complications following coronary bypass surgery. *Journal of Nervous and Mental Disease*, **160**, 342–348.

—— & —— (1976) Psychopathology observed on follow-up after coronary bypass surgery. *Journal of Nervous and Mental Disease*, **163**, 295–301.

RAMSHAW, J. E. & STANLEY, G. (1984) Psychological adjustment to coronary artery surgery. *British Journal of Clinical Psychology*, **23**, 101–108.

ROTH, M. (1959) The phobic anxiety-depersonalization syndrome. *Proceedings of the Royal Society of Medicine*, **52**, 587–595.

RUBINSTEIN, D. & THOMAS, J. K. (1969) Psychiatric findings in cardiotomy patients. *American Journal of Psychiatry*, **126**, 360–368.

SACHDEV, N. S., CARTER, C. C., SWANK, R. L. & BLACHLY P. H. (1967) Relationship between post-cardiotomy delirium, clinical neurological changes, and EEG abnormalities. *Journal of Thoracic and Cardiovascular Surgery*, **54**, 557–563.

SCHELD H. H., DAVIES-OSTERKAMP, S., MOHLEN, K., KALBHENN, U., KRAMER, M. & HEHRLEIN, F. W. (1982) Psychotic reactions in patients after open-heart surgery. In *Psychopathological and Neurological Dysfunctions following Open-Heart Surgery* (eds. R. Becker, J. Katz, M. J. Polonius, H. Speidel), pp. 32–38. Berlin Heidelberg: Springer-Verlag.

SHAW, P. J., BATES, D., CARTLIDGE, N. E. F., HEAVISIDE, D., JULIAN D. G. & SHAW, D. A. (1985) Early neurological complications of coronary artery bypass surgery. *British Medical Journal*, **291**, 1384–1386.

——, ——, ——, FRENCH, J. M., HEAVISIDE, D., JULIAN, D. G. & SHAW, D. A. (1986a) Early intellectual dysfunction following coronary bypass surgery. *Quarterly Journal of Medicine*, **255**, 59–68.

——, ——, ——, ——, —— & —— (1986b) Natural history of neurological complications of coronary artery bypass graft surgery: a six month follow-up study. *British Medical Journal*, **293**, 165–167.

——, ——, ——, ——, —— & —— (1987) Long term intellectual dysfunction following coronary artery bypass graft surgery: a six month follow-up study. *Quarterly Journal of Medicine*, **239**, 259–268.

STOCKARD, J. J., BICKFORD, R. G. & SCHAUBLE, J. F. (1973) Pressure dependent cerebral ischemia during cardiopulmonary bypass. *Neurology*, **23**, 521–529.

SUMMERS, W. K. (1979) Psychiatric sequelae to cardiotomy. *Journal of Cardiovascular Surgery*, **20**, 471–476.

SURMAN, O. S., HACKETT, T. P., SILVERBERG, E. L. & BEHRENDT, D. M. (1974) Usefulness of psychiatric intervention in patients undergoing cardiac surgery. *Archives of General Psychiatry*, **30**, 830–835.

SVEINSSON, I. S. (1975) Postoperative psychosis after heart surgery. *Journal of Thoracic and Cardiovascular Surgery*, **70**, 717–725.

TUFO, H. M., OSTFELD, A. M., SHEKELLE, R. (1970) Central nervous system dysfunction following open-heart surgery. *Journal of the American Medical Association*, **212**, 1333–1340.

VASQUEZ, E. & CHITWOOD, W. R. (1975) Postcardiotomy delirium: an overview. *International Journal of Psychiatry in Medicine*, **6**, 373–383.

WEST, L. J., JANSZEN, H. H., LESTER, B. K. & CORNELISOON, F. S. (1962) The psychosis of sleep deprivation. *Annals of the New York Academy of Science*, **96**, 66–70.

WILLNER, A. E., RABINER, C. J., WISOFF, B. G., HARTSTEIN, M., STRUVE, F. A. & KLEIN, D. F. (1976) Analogical reasoning and postoperative outcome. Predictions for patients scheduled for open-heart surgery. *Archives of General Psychiatry*, **33**, 255–259.

ZAKS, M. S. (1959) Disturbances in psychological functions and neuropsychiatric complications in heart surgery—a four year follow-up study. In *Cardiology: An Encyclopedia of the Cardiovascular System, Volume 3* (ed. A. A. Luisado), pp. 162–171. New York: McGraw Hill.

ZISKIND, E., JONES, H., FILANTE, W. & GOLDBERG, J. (1960) Observations on mental symptoms in eye patched patients: hypnogogic symptoms in sensory deprivation. *American Journal of Psychiatry*, **116**, 893–900.

# 47 Through the looking glass: a glimpse into the world of the anorexic

## KURT SCHAPIRA and FUAD HASSANYEH

It is almost 300 years since Dr Richard Morton published the first medical account of anorexia nervosa, the case history of "Mr Duke's daughter, who in her 18th year fell into a total suppression of her monthly courses for a multitude of cares and passions of her mind". There is also a description of a 16 year old male anorexic patient "the son of the Reverend Steele, my very good friend". These two cases were isolated rarities among the many causes of wasting diseases which Morton described in his book. The precise nature of "the multitude of cares and passions of the mind" which, Morton felt, caused or at least contributed to the illness, remains a subject of interest and study.

The syndrome of anorexia nervosa has seen a striking increase in its prevalence over the past 15 years. Prior to that it was somewhat in limbo with no specialty within medicine appearing to be comfortable with it. The emergence of "psychosomatic disorders" however, has provided it with at least a temporary refuge, allowing it to become the concern of a number of disciplines. This has fostered invaluable co-operation between psychiatrist, physician, psychologist and sociologist in trying to elucidate its mysterious and fascinating nature.

## The problem of diagnosis

Anorexia nervosa has been defined as a condition of "self inflicted starvation, without recognisable organic disease and in the midst of ample food" (Bruch, 1965). It was Hilde Bruch who first recognised distortion of body image as a central feature of the condition and also drew attention to the importance of "a paralysing sense of ineffectiveness" which at the same time is accompanied by an implacable resistance to change. She considered these features as characteristic of the primary syndrome of anorexia nervosa and noted their absence when weight loss was secondary to other psychiatric disorders. Moreover, the distinction carries important implications for management.

In an attempt to define more sharply diagnostic criteria suitable primarily for research purposes, Feighner et al (1972) proposed the following as being essential for the diagnosis of anorexia nervosa (AN):

  (a) age of onset prior to 25
  (b) anorexia with accompanying weight loss of at least 25% of original weight

(c) a distorted implacable attitude towards eating, food or weight, that overrides hunger, admonition, reassurance and threats

(d) no known medical illness that could account for the anorexia and weight loss

(e) no known psychiatric disorder, with particular reference to primary affective disorders, schizophrenia, obsessive compulsive and phobic neurosis

(f) At least two of the following manifestations:
   (i) amenorrhoea
   (ii) lanugo
   (iii) bradycardia (resting pulse of 60 or less)
   (iv) periods of over-activity
   (v) episodes of bulimia
   (vi) vomiting (may be self-induced)

In the *Diagnostic and Statistical Manual of Mental Disorders* (DSM–III, 1980) of the five criteria required for a diagnosis of AN four are similar to those of Feighner's criteria, but the fifth refers to the presence of weight phobia, i.e. "an intense fear of becoming obese, which does not diminish as weight loss progresses". Russell's diagnostic criteria for anorexia nervosa (Russell, 1970) comprise in our view the essential elements necessary for the diagnosis since they do not include two criteria which we also do not consider necessary: an age of onset of less than 25 years, and a loss of weight of 25% or more. As regards the former, we have seen a number of patients with classical features of the condition in whom the onset of the illness occurred after the age of 25; and indeed such cases have been reported throughout the literature. As for weight loss, an increasing awareness of anorexia nervosa has resulted in the referral of patients in the early stages of the illness when weight loss had not yet reached the 25% level. Furthermore, few clinicians would exclude the small number of patients in whom amenorrhoea precedes weight loss but who show the other classical features of the condition. We therefore favour Russell's criteria for anorexia nervosa which comprise three essential features:

(a) self-induced loss of weight (resulting mainly from the studious avoidance of foods considered by the patient to be fattening)

(b) a characteristic psychopathology consisting of an overvalued idea that fatness is a dreadful state

(c) a specific endocrine disorder which in the post-pubertal girl causes the cessation of menstruation, or a delay of events of puberty in the pre-pubertal or early pubertal female

## Understanding anorexia nervosa

In his seminal report, Gull (1874) regarded the condition as being due to a "morbid mental state" occurring at a time when the patient was prone to "mental adversity"—an astute recognition of the role of psychological factors in the aetiology of the condition. Moreover, almost 200 years previously Richard Morton (1684), who gave the first clinical description of anorexia nervosa, in both a female and a male patient, also had little doubt in attributing the illness to "Cares and Passions". His observation of the studious nature of Mr Duke's daughter who was "continually poring upon Books", highlights a phenomenon which continues to characterise many of today's patients.

It is quite remarkable, therefore, as Russell (1985) has pointed out in his interesting paper that not until 23 years ago (Bruch, 1965) has there been any mention of the presence of weight phobia or distortion of body image, both striking and singular features of the condition. This does raise the possibility that these features may only recently have been incorporated into the syndrome, reflecting perhaps the pathoplastic effect of social and cultural influences.

Farquharson & Hyland (1938) saw anorexia nervosa as developing in people of neurotic constitution, a view supported by Kay & Leigh (1954). In a later study from Newcastle which compared anorexic subjects with a matched group of non-anorexic neurotic patients, both similarities and differences were revealed (Kay *et al*, 1967).

Bruch (1965), from her psychotherapeutic experience with anorexic patients, came to regard the illness as a manifestation of the patient's struggle for control in the face of insoluble conflict, occurring after a childhood of "robot-like obedience".

The illness, occurring as it does most commonly in adolescence, has naturally focused attention upon the role of developmental problems peculiar to that period of life. Thus Crisp (1965) came to regard anorexia nervosa as a response to post-pubertal conflict, manifesting as a phobic avoidance of normal adult expectations (Crisp & Toms, 1972).

Garner & Garfinkel (1980) consider that pressure for thinness combined with expectations of high performance provided the conditions for the development of anorexia nervosa in vulnerable adolescents. The high rate of anorexia nervosa among ballet dancers, in whom thinness is of particular concern, would lend support to this idea. The importance of fashion and of the media in generating pressure on women to be slim is evidenced by the inordinate amount of space occupied by this topic and by diets to achieve slimness in women's magazines.

## Hypothesis

In a society where slimness is positively reinforced, it may become, for women, a powerful conditioned drive. Such has so far not been the case for men, but, if similar social pressures were to operate, then one might expect a parallel rise to occur in the prevalence of anorexia in males. In our current culture the incentive for young men has been to be fit; as women are encouraged to focus upon their figure and in particular upon body fat, males are exhorted to focus upon fitness and muscle mass. It is of interest, therefore, that physical activities in the form of excessive exercise, and in particular jogging, are prominent features of anorexia nervosa in males (Crisp *et al*, 1986; Schapira & Oyebode, in press). Indeed, it has been suggested that jogging in males is an equivalent of anorexic behaviour in females (Yates *et al*, 1983).

The acutely felt need for self-control in adolescence arises primarily from the young person's uncertainty about herself and her ability to cope with life's relationships and challenges. The psychosexual aspect, which is reflected by the adolescent's deep awareness of her developing femininity and its inherent challenges, is an important factor in the psychosexual regression which accompanies anorexia nervosa. The girl looks towards signposts indicating society's ideas of maturity and independence and finds society pointing towards control via slimness. Studies of the true prevalence of anorexia have proved difficult since it became recognised that the majority of girls and young women adhere to some form of dieting regime from time to time, with only a few taking the anorexic path. The increase of vegetarianism among young people may be seen as another manifestation of a preoccupation with food, asserting an identity in moral and ethical terms.

The anorexic patient, in addition to showing a gross distortion of body image, shows an equally severe misreading of her own personality. She sees herself as unloveable and ineffective. Apart from her ability to control her hunger and to maintain rigid anorexic behaviour in the face of all opposition and criticism, she sees her other personality attributes negatively. The anorexic shorthand for all of these negative attributes is 'fat'.

The patient, uncertain about herself or as to how she can cope with the challenges of maturation, turns to controlling her body size and shape, the only aspect of herself she feels able to change. Furthermore, supported in this by social pressure for slimness, she is 'succeeding' where thousands of other women are failing. She takes pride in enduring and resisting the pangs of hunger. Yet beneath the surface there is the realisation that her skeletal appearance is admired neither by her family nor by society at large. Indeed, because of it, she often has to face censure and rejection by the very people to whom she looks for acceptance and admiration.

By achieving the anorexic goal the patient is trapped in a prison of her making, Bruch's *Golden Cage* (Bruch, 1978), from which she is terrified to escape. The hope that thinness will have proved to be the path to salvation has not been fulfilled. It is replaced by the fear of losing control, which in many is confirmed by the appearance of bulimic episodes.

## Clinical profile

As Gull (1874) has pointed out, anorexia nervosa is an illness of the young. In the majority of cases the onset occurs in the teens or adolescence, rarely before the age of 10, or in middle age.

In virtually all cases anorexia nervosa starts as any other attempt at dieting, designed to lose a few pounds in weight. In anorexic subjects, however, slimness is not achieved by such limited weight loss. They, unlike the normal dieter, are spurred on by a profound insecurity in their self-image and by a dual obsession: to lose weight and to avoid the dread prospect of obesity.

As part of our research programme on eating disorders, we have recently reviewed data on 56 consecutive referrals of whom 53 were female; 50 of these were single and 26 were students, at school, college or university. The mean age of this cohort at referral was 19 years ($s.d. = 4$) with onset of illness at 17.3 years ($s.d. = 3.2$). There was an interval of 1.7 years ($s.d. = 1.8$) from the onset of the illness to medical referral. Before the onset of anorexia nervosa the average weight of the cohort was 57.2 kilogrammes ($s.d. = 11.2$). The lowest weight reached during the illness was 38 kilogrammes ($s.d. = 6$), representing a weight loss of 32.6% ($s.d. = 8$).

Of the 53 female patients, 46 developed amenorrhoea after significant weight loss, but in five amenorrhoea was the presenting symptom of the illness. When weight loss preceded amenorrhoea the latter occurred after an average reduction in weight of 7.9 kilogrammes (*s.d.* = 5.3).

Only 23 of the 56 patients were objectively overweight before the onset of the illness, although 31 claimed to have been teased about being fat. Seven patients described themselves as having been either "faddy" or "difficult eaters" before the onset of the illness. This finding is in agreement with that reported in an earlier study (Kay *et al*, 1967).

In addition to reducing their food intake drastically, 26 patients also induced vomiting, and a further 26 abused laxatives; 44 patients exercised vigorously in order to burn up calories. Thus more than half of the anorexic patients also employed methods other than starvation to achieve their desired goal. A similar proportion (32 patients) experienced bulimic episodes during their illness which were often, but not invariably, followed by episodes of self-induced vomiting.

In their social relationships, 13 of the anorexic patients described a detached or hostile relationship with their father, as compared to only two with mother. Nineteen of the patients, a third, described a disturbed mother-father relationship, eight of these ending in separation or divorce. Twenty-one patients experienced considerable social adjustment difficulties at school.

On the Eysenck Personality Questionnaire (Eysenck & Eysenck, 1975), the mean score for neuroticism ($n$) for the total group was 17.3 (*s.d.* = 4.1) (normative mean for a female group aged 16–19 years being 13.2 (*s.d.* = 5.2)). The mean extraversion (E) score was 9.4 (*s.d.* = 5.9) (normative mean for a female age group 16–19 years being 13.3 (*s.d.* = 4.6)).

## Distortion of body image

Halmi (1978) defines body image distortion in anorexia as a conviction on the part of the patient that she looks normal and even overweight in the face of cachexia or emaciation. However, distortion of body image may occur in females of normal weight without a history of anorexia nervosa (Halmi *et al*, 1977), as well as in pregnant women (Slade, 1977).

We have reviewed the data on our series of 56 patients, of whom 53 were female and three male. All the patients, including the three males, had a distortion of general body image. In 25 the distortion was also localised, affecting most commonly the abdomen (19 cases), waist (19 cases), hips (nine cases), and thighs (nine cases). In four cases only was perceptual distortion related to the chest, breasts or face. Patients in whom weight loss was secondary to other disorders showed no such distortion (Schapira & Hassanyeh, unpublished data).

## Treatment

Although recognising the importance of psychological factors, the earliest treatment regimes concentrated entirely upon the refeeding of the patient. The unwillingness of the patient to co-operate made it imperative for some control to be taken by the doctor. Thus William Gull (1874) stressed the importance of exercising "moral control" over the patient. His approach to treatment was to concentrate on getting the patient to eat in order to correct her emaciation. In addition to regular small meals, which he considered should contain "immunising doses" of carbohydrates, Gull also suggested a two hourly dessertspoonful of brandy, more expensive but perhaps as effective as chlorpromazine! Bed rest, in Gull's regime, was absolute until emaciation was relieved.

Charcot (1889), sensitive to family pressures which were evident in many of his patients, recommended separating the patient from her family and placing her treatment in the hands of someone who would take on the role of carer. The desirable attributes of such a person, he felt, were "a kind but firm hand, a calm demeanour, and much patience"; characteristics which are as desirable today as they were then. However, Charcot's specific preference for nuns in this context is more controversial!

The importance of separating the refeeding stage from that of psychotherapy has now become almost universal practice, and was strongly advocated by Bruch (1978) based on her experience in treating girls on both an in-patient and out-patient basis. She readily recognised the impossibility of carrying out appropriate psychotherapy in the face of progressive emaciation with all its physical complications, particularly that of electrolyte imbalance so readily produced by laxative abuse and/or vomiting. Psychotherapy can only be practised with some equanimity when a safe level of weight is attained, which, in our view, may be as much as 10–15% below the ideal weight.

We do not use psychotropic drugs during the refeeding phase for the majority of our patients, except that when psychiatric symptoms such as anxiety, restlessness or depression are prominent and interfere markedly with the management of the patient we consider their use for a limited period of time as justified. Dally *et al* (1979) thought that 30% of their in-patients required chlorpromazine.

Based on our experience of treating patients with anorexia nervosa, we have come to recognise the substantial commitment by the doctor to the patient, both in the short and long term. Above all, the therapist must take into account the natural history of the illness, which is one of slow change with periods when it seems that nothing is happening, or worse still, of clear setbacks which may be occasioned by the patient's own difficulty or by the reaction of the family and others to the patient's illness. The establishment of a trusting and caring relationship, as in all psychotherapy, is the corner-stone of successful management, with the overall aim of allowing the patient to find in herself a greater degree of self-confidence in her emotional development, as well as in her ability to control her eating more satisfactorily.

As regards in-patient treatment, the role of the nursing staff is crucial. It is they who spend most of the time with the patient, supervising her meal-times and encouraging her to eat. Being kind and firm are important, though not enough: an awareness of the weight phobia and of the reality to the patient of the body image distortion which constitute such obstacles to improvement, are essential.

The role of the dietician is also important but in our experience it often comprises a dialogue between experts. We have yet to see a patient whose knowledge of carbohydrates and calories in particular would not gain her full marks on any exam paper on human nutrition. The dietician, however, can be most helpful in drawing up a satisfactory and diverse dietary regime since anorexics do not only restrict their calories but often are markedly limited in the kinds of food that they are prepared to eat. An acceptable diet for the patient is one that emerges from a discussion with the dietician and is based on the patient's pre-illness food choices.

Following admission, the patient is initially confined to bed and her food intake gradually increased from 1000 calories a day to approximately 2500 calories over a period of a week. Although invariably complaining of feelings of fullness and abdominal distention even after the smallest amount of food, the patient is encouraged to persist with her meals, initially irrespective of the time this takes. She is reassured that this feeling of fullness will pass.

We have two main 'targets' as regards weight gain. The first is the weight at which the patient is mobilised and in our experience this should be after a modest increase, usually to within 15–20% of average weight. The second is the target set for discharge. With regard to the latter, the patient is strongly reassured that an 'upper safety net' weight is a component of the treatment programme, so that the aim of physical refeeding is not the restoration of an ideal body weight, but that we consider it satisfactory if before discharge she reaches a level of about 5 kg below that weight. The fear of losing control, i.e. that weight gain will continue relentlessly, is never far from the patient's mind. Hence, a rapid increase in weight which was, and is still favoured in some centres, would seem to us to be counter-productive if for no reason other than such rapid gains in weight are not conducive to the development by the patient of confidence in gradual weight control.

Since we believe both in the physical and psychological approach to management, it has been our practice to implement this in a practical way. Thus, over the last 20 years, we have, with the collaboration of our medical colleagues, treated almost all our in-patients on medical wards. Although initially this was a matter of necessity in some patients, it has become, we consider, the in-patient treatment of choice. It has brought in its wake many advantages, not least of which is a closer liaison work with our physician colleagues, as well as with general nursing staff, who have become both sensitive and skilful in the management of these patients. Furthermore, admission to a general medical ward may be more acceptable in the first instance both to the patient and her family. In an illness such as this where it is important to instigate treatment as early as possible, such a facility has much to recommend it.

It is often recommended that hospital visits by family and friends should be 'earned' and be part of a treatment programme. We do not feel that in the majority of cases this is either necessary or desirable. Furthermore, unless severely underweight, anorexic patients on bed rest should be afforded reasonable toilet privileges. We are, however, aware of the possibility of induced vomiting and disposal of food; this can be effectively dealt with by the stipulation that patients must remain at bed rest for two hours after meals.

Very rarely, when a patient's physical state is such as to endanger her life, her refusal to come into hospital is in our view justifiably met with by compulsory admission under Section 3 of the Mental Health Act (1983).

In general we take the view expressed by Hilde Bruch, whose contribution to our understanding of anorexia is unique: "the correction of the weight problem must be part of an integrated treatment approach. The patient needs to be instructed and also the family, that in spite of outer appearances, this is not an illness of weight and appetite—the essential problem relates to inner doubts and lack of self-confidence. However, in order to get help with these underlying problems the body needs to be in a better condition''.

## *Outcome*

The first reported case of Mr Duke's daughter (Morton, 1684) had a fatal outcome, but his male case survived, although Morton shrewdly observed that ''what will be the Event of this method, does not yet plainly appear'', which, in modern parlance, suggests a guarded prognosis. Although single cases, they do illustrate an interesting point: in females a fatal outcome does occur, whereas in males, in whom the prognosis is not as good (Oyebode *et al*, 1988), no death has yet been reported.

Gull's case report (Gull, 1874), illustrated by fascinating photographs, shows a recovery at the end of three months' treatment. Long term follow-up, nowadays regarded to be important, was not commented upon. Lasègue (1873) took a peculiarly optimistic view based on the fact that in none of his eight cases did the illness last for more than two years. He considered cure to have been permanent.

Ryle (1936) made the interesting observation that amenorrhoea was often the last symptom to resolve, a finding which, with some exceptions, continues to receive support from later studies. Of his 37 cases traced, 21 had recovered, six were improved, six remained unchanged and four had died.

Kay (1953), in his series from the Maudsley, found that of 25 patients, at follow-up only four had recovered. The majority of the cohort had only made a partial recovery, and all exhibited neurotic symptoms. Six of the patients had died during the follow-up period.

Crisp (1965) found normal weights at follow-up in 17 of 21 patients; the follow-up period was 2½ years; 13 (62%) showed normal eating behaviour, and 11 patients had normal menstruation.

In our own follow-up study (mean follow-up period of 2½ years) 23 of 56 patients (41%) had recovered, with seven patients much improved; 26 patients continued to show gross eating abnormalities.

Thirty of the 52 female patients (57%) had resumed menstruation, and although the majority were well in every other respect, some still showed abnormal food attitudes and behaviour. The average duration of amenorrhoea on the return of menstruation was three years. Thirty-nine of the 56 patients (70%) required one or more hospital admission for treatment of low weight.

The criteria for recovery used in our study were:
 (a) stable weight 90% or more of normal average weight for age and height
 (b) no evidence of bulimia, vomiting or laxative abuse
 (c) regular hunger sensation and normal eating habits
 (d) menstruation in females
 (e) no psychiatric disorder

The importance of long term follow-up studies in anorexia nervosa has been stressed by Theander (1985). In this interesting paper he makes the important point that in spite of all the follow-up studies and the criteria for good and bad prognosis, the view of Russell (1977), that one of the mysteries of anorexia nervosa is "the unpredictability in respect of course and outcome in an individual patient", has very much been the experience. We are still delighted and encouraged by the occasional patient we see in whom the illness takes an extremely benign course and results in a cure when a protracted and stormy course might have been anticipated.

In recent years family therapy has become much in vogue. Although in practice it may be difficult to obtain satisfactory co-operation from the whole family, the importance of the illness to the family in many ways cannot be over-emphasised. Commenting on this aspect Lasègue (1873) observes "the family has but two methods at its service which it always exhausts—entreaties and menaces. The delicacies of the table are multiplied in the hope of stimulating the appetite; but the more the solicitude increases, the more the appetite diminishes. The patient disdainfully tastes the new viands, and after having shown willingness holds herself absolved from any obligation to do more. She is besought, as a favour, and as a sovereign proof of affection, to consent to add even an additional mouthful to what she has taken: but this excess of insistence begets an excess of resistance".

We have chosen this quotation to end our contribution to this Festschrift, as much for its astute clinical perception as for its elegant style, both attributes of Sir Martin Roth, which we, his students and colleagues, have come to admire over the years.

## References

AMERICAN PSYCHIATRIC ASSOCIATION (1980) *Diagnostic and Statistical Manual of Mental Disorders*, (3rd edn) (DSM–III). Washington, DC: American Psychiatric Association.

BRUCH, H. (1965) Anorexia nervosa and its differential diagnosis. *Journal of Nervous and Mental Disease*, **141**, 55–66.

—— (1978) *The Golden Cage: The enigma of anorexia nervosa*. London: Open Books.

CHARCOT, J. M. (1889) *Diseases of the Nervous System, 111*. London: The New Sydenham Society.

CRISP, A. H. (1965) Some aspects of the evolution, presentation and follow-up of anorexia nervosa. *Proceedings of the Royal Society of Medicine*, **58**, 814–820.

—— & TOMS, D. A. (1972) Primary anorexia nervosa or weight phobia in the male: report on 13 cases. *British Medical Journal*, i, 334–338.

——, BURNS, T. & BHAT, A. V. (1986) Primary anorexia nervosa in the male and female: a comparison of clinical features and prognosis. *British Journal of Medical Psychology*, **59**, 123–132.

DALLY, P., GOMEZ, J. & ISAACS, A. J. (1979) *Anorexia Nervosa*. London: Heinemann Books.

EYSENCK, H. & EYSENCK, S. B. G. (1975) *Manual of the Eysenck Personality Questionnaire*. London: Hodder & Stoughton.

FARQUHARSON, R. F. & HYLAND, H. H. (1938) Anorexia nervosa. A metabolic disorder of psychological origin. *Journal of the American Medical Association*, **111**, 1085–1092.

FEIGHNER, J. P., ROBINS, E., GUZE, S., WOODRUFF, R. A., WINOKUR, G. & MUNOZ, R. (1972) Diagnostic criteria for use in psychiatric research. *Archives of General Psychiatry*, **26**, 57–63.

GARNER, D. M. & GARFINKEL, P. E. (1980) Socio-cultural factors in the development of anorexia nervosa. *Psychological Medicine*, **10**, 647–656.

GULL, W. W. (1874) Anorexia nervosa. *Transactions of the Clinical Society of London*, **7**, 22–28.

HALMI, K. A., GOLDBERG, S. C. & CUNNINGHAM, S. (1977) Perceptual distortion of body image in adolescent girls. *Psychological Medicine*, **7**, 253–257.

—— (1978) Anorexia nervosa: recent investigations. *Annual Review of Medicine*, **29**, 137–148.

KAY, D. W. K. (1953) Anorexia nervosa: a study in prognosis. *Proceedings of the Royal Society of Medicine*, **46**, 669–674.

—— & LEIGH, D. (1954) The natural history, treatment and prognosis of anorexia nervosa based on a study of 38 patients. *Journal of Mental Science*, **100**, 411–418.

——, SCHAPIRA, K. & BRANDON, S. (1967) Early factors in anorexia nervosa compared with non-anorexic groups. A preliminary report with discussion of methodology. *Journal of Psychosomatic Research*, **11**, 133–139.

LASÈGUE, E. C. (1873) De l'anorexie hystérique. *Archives of General Medicine*, **21**, 385–403.

MORTON, R. (1694) *Phthisiologia: Or a Treatise of Consumptions*. London: Smith & Walford.

OYEBODE, F., BOODHOO, J. A. & SCHAPIRA, K. (1988) Anorexia nervosa in males: clinical features and outcome. *International Journal of Eating Disorders*, **7**, 121–124.

RUSSELL, G. F. M. (1970) Anorexia nervosa: its identity as an illness and its treatment. In *Modern Trends in Psychological Medicine* (ed. J. H. Price). London: Butterworth.

—— (1985) The changing nature of anorexia nervosa. *Journal of Psychiatric Research*, **19**, 101–109.

RYLE, J. A. (1936) Anorexia nervosa. *Lancet*, *ii*, 893–899.

SCHAPIRA, K. & OYEBODE, F. (1988) Anorexia nervosa in the male. In *Eating Disorders in Adolescents and Young Adults* (eds D. Hardoff & E. Chigier), pp. 205–211. Israel: Freund Publishing House.

SLADE, P. D. (1977) Awareness of body dimensions during pregnancy: an analogue study. *Psychological Medicine*, **7**, 245–252.

THEANDER, S. (1985) Outcome and prognosis in anorexia nervosa and bulimia: some results of previous investigations, compared with those of a Swedish study. *Journal of Psychiatric Research*, **19**, 493–508.

YATES, A., LEEHEY, R. & SHISSLAK, C. M. (1983) Running—an analogue of anorexia? *New England Journal of Medicine*, **308**, 251–255.

# 48 Psychosurgery and deviance

## J. SYDNEY SMITH and LESLIE G. KILOH

On 11 November 1935 the first frontal leucotomy was performed by the Portuguese surgeon Almeida Lima under the direction of the neurologist Egas Moniz.

In 1949 Moniz shared with Hess the Nobel Prize for Physiology and Medicine. Although Moniz was also responsible for the development of cerebral angiography, it was for the introduction of psychosurgery that he received this award, the citation stating:

> "Frontal leucotomy, despite certain limitations of the operative method must be considered one of the most important discoveries ever made in psychiatric therapy, because through its use a great number of suffering people and total invalids have recovered and have been socially rehabilitated."

In 1954 Moniz wrote, prophetically:

> "We do not doubt that what we have undertaken here will provoke a great deal of lively discussion, in the fields of medicine, psychiatry, psychology, philosophy and sociology alike. This we expect, but we continue to hope that any such discussion will contribute to the progress of science, and above all, to the welfare of mental patients."

There can be no doubt that it was the American psychiatrist Walter Freeman who popularised the use of psychosurgical techniques. Propelled by a somewhat hypomanic zeal that was punctuated by one serious episode of depression and perhaps tempered by his habituation to barbiturates (Valenstein, 1986), Freeman cut a swathe through the frontal lobes of an American population pre-occupied at the time with fighting the Second World War.

In 1945 the Board of Control (England and Wales), reflecting public concern, instituted an investigation into the first 1000 psychosurgical operations performed in England and Wales. In her report to the Government, Wilson (1947) concluded:

> "Prefrontal leucotomy is usually a simple operation for the patient, if not always easy for the surgeon. Complications are infrequent and the death rate cannot be said to be high when the seriousness of established mental disorder is taken into account.

Reversible improvement in behaviour follows in a large percentage of cases who have had severe symptoms with poor prognosis and have failed to respond to other methods of treatment. Many are discharged from hospital and others, while unfit to leave, become much more placid and easier to nurse.

The question as to whether or not these results are achieved at the cost of the loss of some finer mental qualities is not yet answered and further study is needed on this important point.

We are of the opinion that the operation should be carried out only after careful consideration of each individual case by experienced psychiatrists.''

In the 1950s the controversy was quietened when the introduction of psychotherapeutic drugs resulted in a reduction in the number of psychosurgical operations. Some concern was expressed by churchmen—although not by the Roman Catholic Church—that the soul was damaged by psychosurgery, but the issue was perhaps laid to rest in 1952 by the sobering comment in the *British Medical Journal* that "if the soul can survive death it can surely survive leucotomy". In a further report to the British Government, Tooth & Newton (1961) reviewed 10 364 cases and noted that psychosurgery was safe and was effective especially in states of depression and anxiety.

With the introduction of the major tranquillising and antidepressant drugs, psychosurgery came to be reserved for the occasional patient whose illness was refractory to other treatments. Although there is no evidence that this conservative approach was ever rejected, except by the occasional eccentric practitioner, considerable opposition suddenly arose in the 1970s to the use, not only of psychosurgery, but also of ECT and other physical therapies. Valenstein (1980) had indicated that there was no significant increase in the number of operations performed in this period, but there was a renewed professional interest in the topic evidenced by the fact that whilst the first International Congress of Psychosurgery was convened in 1948, the second was not held until 1970, this being followed by meetings in 1972, 1975 and 1978, so creating the impression of a "resurgence in psychosurgery". Another very important reason for the opposition was that by the 1970s it was realised that some psychosurgeons had, in the preceding decade, begun to delve into the field of social deviance; this interest was not confined to the surgeons.

The book *Violence and the Brain* by Mark & Ervin (1970) had a dramatic impact. It demonstrated that rage and consequent violent behaviour could be elicited or inhibited through electrical stimulation in the region of the amygdaloid nuclei or permanently ameliorated by lesions of these structures; it also drew attention to the fact that violence sometimes arose from temporal lobe pathology. In the foreword Dr Sweet indicated that whilst violent patients were usually either denied hospitalisation and medical care, or incarcerated in gaol or in an institution for the criminally insane, they might in future be better cared for in a special institute, where the staff had been trained in the management of violent behaviours and where "tests may be developed to spot at an early stage the person with poor control of dangerous impulses".

In 1967 Mark, Sweet & Ervin, in a letter to the *Journal of the American Medical Association*, questioned the role that brain disease might play in riots and urban violence. Whilst their intention appears to have been to draw attention to the rare individual whose rage and violence were secondary to brain pathology and to the need to provide more enlightened facilities for the management of the psychiatrically disturbed violent patients, many interpreted their publications as suggesting that psychosurgery should be applied on a widespread basis to control socially dissident groups. The fault was the authors. Had they concentrated on the uncommon state of pathological rage, rather than the global issue of violent behaviour, the message might have been better understood and treated.

At that time a not insignificant force in the Western World was a group calling itself 'The Citizens' Commission for Human Rights' which was an affiliate of the controversial 'Church of Scientology'. This group, whilst espousing its own form of therapy for mental disturbances, expressed considerable antipathy towards all forms of physical treatment in psychiatry, and particularly to psychosurgery. It found an ally in Peter Breggin, a Washington doctor and student of Thomas Szaz, who in 1972 launched what has been described as "a one-man crusade against psychosurgery". In that year two lengthy articles by Breggin that expressed alarm about the 'holocaust' of psychosurgery were inserted into the Congressional Record. Breggin (1973) equated psychiatrists with the Nazis and stated:

> "In fact psychiatry was the primary instigator and the first practitioner of the final solution . . . even Hitler lacked enthusiasm but the psychiatrists were so devoted to the cause of destroying . . . they risked going on with it even after the war's end . . . it is time for the public to take direct action to stop current psychiatric atrocities and to prevent a recurrence of the Final Solution. A frontal assault upon lobotomy and psychosurgery is one of the most important skirmishes in this larger war. Action must be taken against psychosurgeons and their institutions, in the courts, state legislatures and the United States Congress.

The public distrust engendered by Breggin's sensational claims was fuelled by the novels *One Flew Over the Cuckoo's Nest*, *Clockwork Orange*, *The Terminal Man*, and more particularly by the films based upon them.

Unfortunately, in at least one case, the fiction was not too far removed from reality. It became publicly known that individuals within three Californian institutes—at Vacaville and Atascodero—had received 'Anectine Therapy'. In this Anectine (succinylcholine) had been injected so as to suspend the respiration of conscious individuals. It was used, sometimes without consent, to discourage violent behaviour, deviant sexual behaviour, drug addiction and lack of co-operation in the ward treatment programmes.

Subsequently it was reported in the *Washington Post* that within the Vacaville facility three prisoners with episodic violence had received amygdaloid surgery (Aarons, 1972). In each case consent had been obtained from the prisoner and members of the family. One was thought to have been markedly improved, one had a fair result and one showed little or no change. Whilst the surgery may have been performed with due regard to ethical considerations, alarm arose as it was only revealed during a press investigation into a request, in 1971, by the Californian Department of Corrections for the funding of an "expanded programme of brain surgery for inmates with organically caused aggressive seizures".

In 1972 two doctors at the Lafayette Clinic, Michigan, obtained funding from the State Legislature for a study of the treatment of uncontrollable aggression.

Two treatment modalities—amygdaloidotomy and giving cyproterone acetate—were to be compared. In November a man had been charged with murder and sexual violation of a woman and was committed without trial to hospital as a "criminal sexual psychopath". He signed an 'informed consent' form to participate in the study as a surgical subject. His parents also signed consent forms. Two committees which reviewed the scientific worthiness of the study and the validity of the consent approved the procedure.

Before the operation could be performed, Gabe Kaimowitz of the Medical Committee for Human Rights and the Michigan Legal Services expressed his concern to the lay press and filed a complaint for a writ of habeas corpus with the Circuit Court. Because of the publicity, the research team terminated the study. In March 1973 the court held that the patient's detention in hospital had been unconstitutional and ordered his release. Although the experimental programme had been terminated, the court considered that it might one day be resurrected and so proceeded to consider the case so as to determine "whether legally adequate consent could be obtained from adults, involuntarily confined in the State Mental Health System, for experimental or innovative procedures on the brain to ameliorate behaviour, and if it could be, whether the State should allow such experimentation on human subjects to proceed."

During the course of the deliberations, the patient withdrew his consent for surgery. Shuman (1974) indicates that Counsel for the plaintiff called Dr Peter Breggin and a neurosurgeon whose speciality was cerebrovascular disease and head injuries but did not call any witness qualified in neurology or with experience of EEGs. Shuman, who appeared on behalf of the defendants, categorised the neurosurgeon as a "competent medical scientist, who I believe was conscientious even if wrong, struggling to make sense to scientifically untrained judges of conceptual material which is not scientific". The court concluded that "there is no scientific basis for establishing that the removal or destruction of an area of the limbic brain would have any direct therapeutic effect in controlling aggressivity or improving tormenting personal behaviour absent in the showing of a well defined clinical syndrome such as epilepsy". It further stated that "psychosurgery flattens emotional responses, leads to lack of abstract reasoning ability, leads to a loss of capacity for new learning and causes general sedation and apathy". Finally, it decided that an involuntarily confined psychiatric patient could not give valid consent. Their decisions, while startling, have gained little subsequent acceptance.

Apparently at the urging of Dr Breggin, a United States Congressman subsequently proposed that a bill establishing the National Commission for the Protection of Human Subjects of Biomedical & Behavioural Research be amended to ban all psychosurgery in the United States. In the 1973 Senate debate he finally accepted a provision that mandated the Commission to conduct an investigation of psychosurgery in the United States. During the debate an amendment which provided for a two-year moratorium on the performance of psychosurgery in federally funded facilities was rejected on the grounds that Congress had insufficient information to justify such a measure.

The report of the National Commission was forwarded to the Secretary of the Department of Health, Education and Welfare (HEW) in March 1977. Although several, if not most, of the 11 members of the Commission had approached the study with a negative bias, all concluded, after an examination of the data, that some patients could benefit. It was recommended that psychosurgery should be allowed to continue, even in children, prisoners and involuntarily confined mental patients, provided certain safeguards were adopted.

In the meantime, laws had been passed in Oregon, California and Alabama that effectively stopped all psychosurgery in these states.

In 1978 the Secretary of HEW published recommendations that essentially over-ruled those of the National Commission and outlawed psychosurgery in children, prisoners, incompetents and the involuntarily committed.

Antagonism towards psychosurgery in the 1970s was not confined to the United States. Hirose (1979) reported that in Japan "radical psychiatrists" and "student radicals" who feared that the operation might be used against "political activists with undesirable ideas" were instrumental in causing the Japanese Society of Psychiatry and Neurology to oppose the use of psychosurgery. Hirose, one of the leading Japanese psychosurgeons, ceased operating in 1973.

In Australia, the disquiet about psychosurgery initially centred on the activities of one psychiatrist in private practice, Dr Harry Bailey. Through him Australia achieved, at the time, the dubious distinction of having the highest per capita rate of psychosurgery in the world (Valenstein, 1980). In a review of 150 patients who had frontal psychosurgery procedures it was claimed that this operation was "probably the treatment of choice for psychosexual exhibitionism and compulsive anti-social behaviour" and "in patients who have had the operation because of recurrent compulsive behavioural disturbances associated with depression, abolition of the anti-social behaviour with marked improvement in the patient's capacity for interpersonal relationships is seen in almost every case" (Bailey *et al*, 1973). In 1974 an Australian Broadcasting Commission programme revealed that two men, one an habitual criminal and the other a homosexual company director charged with indecently assaulting schoolboys, had received psychosurgery whilst on remand at this doctor's instigation. The newspaper headline in the following day of "Gaol's Slice up Brains" certainly captured the imagination of the public. Subsequently the medical profession, in conjunction with the Government, sought ways to curb the activities of this team.

In 1977, a Sydney television station published some sensational allegations by a woman who subsequently made public her affiliation with the local Citizens' Commission for Human Rights. Psychosurgical procedures using implanted electrodes at a Government-funded institute were likened to the experiments performed by the Nazis in the Belsen concentration camp. Newspaper headlines such as "Human Guinea Pig Storm" followed. The allegations led to the State Government placing a ban on psychosurgical procedures pending the outcome of a public enquiry. The four-man Committee of Enquiry found all of the allegations to be false. It stated that frontal leucotomy was a "safe, effective, simple and worthwhile procedure" but any surgical approach on the amygdaloid area was "essentially investigative". Nevertheless, it considered that amygdaloid surgery could properly be offered to patients suffering an "intractable affective disorder associated with epilepsy". Three members of the committee, at the encouragement of the State Attorney General, then produced the draft of a Bill that provided that all psychosurgery within the state be subject to review by a seven-member multi-disciplinary board that would consider the issues of informed consent, the reasonableness of the surgery and competence of the surgeons. They considered that psychosurgery should not be withheld from prisoners but that if the leucotomy committee considered surgery to be meritorious the capacity of the prisoner to consent to the procedure should be assessed by a Judge of the Supreme Court. These recommendations were incorporated into the NSW Mental Health Act that became law in 1984; they were implemented in 1987.

In Britain, the debate over the merits and application of various physical treatments in psychiatry centred in Parliament where the Government struggled to construct a new Mental Health Act. Sensationalism by the lay press fuelled the debate. Bridges & Bartlett (1976) commented on the presentation on commercial television of an unfavourable programme showing a patient who had psychosurgery for abnormally aggressive behaviour. In 1981 the *Bristol Journal*, under the headline "Human Guinea Pigs Used in Horror Op" asserted that "Mental patients are being used as human guinea pigs in Nazi-style operations at a Bristol hospital" (Johnstone, 1981). Not surprisingly the allegations were made by the Citizens' Commission for Human Rights. These claims were refuted in other lay publications (Lawrence, 1981; Michael, 1981). The Mental Health (Amendment) Act 1982 received Royal Assent on 28 October, 1982. Its provisions, for the most part, took effect from 30 September, 1983. It stipulates that psychosurgery cannot be performed unless the patient can and does give informed consent. The consent must be attested to by an independent doctor and two non-medical persons all nominated by the Mental Health Act Commission. The independent doctor must also certify that the treatment is appropriate but only after consulting with two persons who have been professionally concerned with the patient's treatment; one of the two must be a nurse and the other neither a nurse nor a doctor.

Repeated public enquiries in the Western World have thus attested to the value of psychosurgery in certain conditions, and those concerned with the rights of prisoners have asserted that they should not be denied any reasonable treatments. But what evidence is there that psychosurgical procedures can benefit those suffering deviant behaviours and what price do they have to pay?

There is a move afoot to replace the term 'Psychosurgery' with that of 'Limbic surgery' as the target area has always been the limbic or emotional brain. Such surgery acts, in the main, by reducing the emotional component of an illness. Behavioural change is a secondary phenomenon.

The major targets of surgery have been the projections from the orbital surface of the frontal lobe and the cingulate gyrus, the amygdala and the hypothalamus.

The surgical approaches over the years have been dramatically refined, the morbidity and mortality have diminished greatly. A review of the literature published since 1960 (Kiloh *et al*, 1987) reveals the following:

Surgery directed at the orbital surface of the frontal lobe or the cingulate gyrus is now very safe, stereotactic lesions being associated with a mortality rate of 0.1%, a risk of adverse personality change of 0.4% and a risk of epilepsy of 0.4%.

With amygdaloid and hypothalamic surgery the risks are, not surprisingly, appreciably higher, the mortality rate being about 2% and some 1–2% suffering persistent neurological complications such as hemiparesis.

Frontal and cingulate surgery appears to be of considerable value in alleviating severe and intractable states of depression and anxiety, some 50–60% being markedly improved and a further 25–30% having lesser degrees of improvement. It is equally effective in cases of severe obsessive-compulsive neurosis and it would appear that it was for this reason that Bailey *et al* (1973) promoted the operation for a variety of anti-social behaviours, erroneously believing such problems as psychosexual exhibitionism to be manifestations of an obsessional illness. In 1977 Bailey *et al* listed six obsessive-compulsive exhibitionists; one manic-depressive exhibitionist; one manic-depressive compulsive antisocial pederast; and two manic depressive personality disordered 'compulsive' thieves, claiming that all were markedly improved when last seen. Such a claim is hard to believe.

All other attempts to influence sexual deviance appear to have been made in West Germany. In 1966 Roeder from Gottingen introduced the procedure of ventro-medial hypothalamotomy for the treatment of sexual deviation. The rationale for the treatment is not entirely clear. He considered that the hypersexual behaviour of male cats produced by lesions of their amygdala and piriform cortex resembled 'human perversions'. Destruction of the two ventro-medial nuclei of the hypothalamus prevented this behaviour, although it made them more aggressive. On this basis he decided to test the effectiveness of hypothalamic lesions in patients he regarded as sexually deviant, hoping in the main for "a dampening effect on sexual function as a whole". The operative procedure was subsequently taken up by Dieckman and his associates in Homberg and Müller and his associates in Hamburg.

Public concern in West Germany led to the appointment in 1977 of a commission to review this surgery. Its final report was submitted in 1978 (Fülgraff & Barbey, 1978). From 1962 to 1976, 75 people had undergone surgery of whom 74 were men. Almost two thirds were imprisoned or involuntarily committed to a mental institution at the time of selection. Although the surgeons emphasised that the patients had all volunteered, the nature of the consent is questionable, especially as Dieckman *et al* in 1979 wrote "since 1969 we have received 30 requests from patients who were confined for deviant sexuality asking for a stereotactic hypothalamotomy instead of castration. From these 30 requests 11 patients were chosen for a stereotactic procedure. This was performed upon the request of the patients during their detention". The most frequent deviation leading to surgery was homosexual contacts with boys or adolescents (24 cases), while 11 had committed heterosexual rape and 9 were exhibitionists. The surgeons claimed a successful short-term outcome in 65 cases (86.7%) and 43 regained their freedom after the operation. One of the measures of success was the reported frequency of weekly orgasms and the accumulated data suggested that this decreased dramatically from a mean of 29 to a mean of 3 and one patient claimed no sexual activity at all. It was not clear whether any changes in sexual orientation occurred.

A long-term follow-up study of more than three years has only been reported by the Hamburg group (see Fülgraff & Barbey, 1978) but of the original 27 no more than six cases were seen. Of these, three were said to be "normal in every respect". Two were failures and underwent subsequent castration and one of these subsequently committed suicide. A further case, a paedophile with sadomasochistic fantasies was subsequently accused of murdering a 10-year-old boy.

The Commission concluded that "hypothalamotomy in the case of deviant sexual behaviour is still at the clinical experimental stage". In 1981, Schmidt & Schorsch reported that the surgery on sexually deviant patients had been abandoned by the surgeons themselves.

Rage and its expression in assaultive behaviour have rarely been considered indications for frontal leucotomy. However, three studies reporting a total of 25 patients have claimed marked improvement in 15 (60%) (Kiloh *et al*, 1987).

The major surgical targets for the control of aggressive behaviour have been the amygdaloid nuclei and their connections with the hypothalamic nucleus. Nine papers reporting the long-term results of amygdaloid ablations in 401 patients reveal a consolidated figure for marked improvement of 21%, whilst 22% were said to be moderately improved, 25% mildly improved and 3% worse (Kiloh *et al*, 1987).

Examination of these data suggests that little improvement can be expected unless the aggressive behaviour is generated by pathological rage. The cold blooded 'hit man' and the schizophrenic whose voices tell him to kill are not likely to benefit.

It would also appear that the surgery is predominantly effective in epileptic patients. In some of these the rapid onset of unprovoked feelings of rage of one to two minutes' duration with abrupt cessation and partial or total amnesia for the event, strongly suggest that the rage is an expression of an epileptic discharge. Nowadays, telemetric and depth EEG techniques and PET scanning often allow a discrete epileptic focus to be isolated. In these it is more rational to remove the epileptogenic focus rather than to treat the rage that is only one of its manifestations. If this is not possible, and the patient is incapacitated by frequent disabling outbursts or rage, then a procedure such as amygdaloidotomy is indicated.

Thus, whilst it is important that prisoners not be denied access to any reasonable treatment for what is clearly an illness, the evidence suggests that as far as psychosurgery is concerned, it is only likely to be of benefit to those who suffer epilepsy with consequent pathological rage that is expressed in violent behaviour and perhaps to the few cases with limbic lesions who have been spared the development of epilepsy. Whether such operations can benefit those individuals experiencing dangerous rage attacks with relatively minimal provocation whose behaviour is currently regarded as a socially defined deviation from the norm remains uncertain. But it seems unlikely in view of current State laws that in the foreseeable future this interesting and perhaps important problem can be solved.

# References

AARONS, L. F. (1972) Brain surgery is tested on three Californian convicts. *Washington Post*, 25 February, p 1.

BAILEY, H. R., DOWLING, J. L. & DAVIES, E. (1973) Studies in depression III, the control of affective illness by cingulotractotomy: A Review of 150 cases. *Medical Journal of Australia*, 2, 366–371.

——, —— & —— (1977) Cingulotractotomy and related procedures for severe depressive illness (Studies in Depression IV). In *Neurosurgical Treatment in Psychiatry, Pain and Epilepsy* (eds W. H. Sweet, S. Obrador & J. D. Martin-Rodriguez), pp. 229–251. Baltimore: University Park Press.

BRIDGES, P. K. & BARTLETT, J. R. (1976). Psychosurgery on television. *British Medical Journal*, i, 1018.

BREGGIN, P. R. (1973) The killing of mental patients. *Freedom*, September, 6–7.

BRITISH MEDICAL JOURNAL (1952) The ethics of leucotomy, *British Medical Journal*, i, 909.

DIECKMANN, G., HORN, H. J. & SCHNEIDER, H. (1979). Long term results of anterior hypothalamotomy in sexual offences. In *Modern Concepts in Psychiatric Surgery* (eds E. R. Hitchcock, H. T. Ballantine Jnr & B. A. Meyerson), pp. 187–195. Amsterdam: Elsevier.

FÜLGRAFF, G. & BARBEY, I. (1978) *Stereotaktische Hirnoperationen bei adweichenden Sexualverhalten. Abschlussbericht der Kommission beim Bundesgesundheitsamt.* Berlin: Reimer.

HIROSE, S. (1979). Past and present trends of psychiatric surgery in Japan. In *Modern Concepts in Psychiatric Surgery* (eds E. R. Hitchcock, H. T. Ballantine Jnr. & B. A. Meyerson), pp. 349–359. Amsterdam: Elsevier.

JOHNSTONE, M. (1981) Human guinea pigs in horror operation. *Bristol Journal,* **173,** 1.

KILOH, L. G., SMITH, J. S. & JOHNSON, G. (1987) *Physical Treatments in Psychiatry.* Melbourne: Blackwell Scientific.

LAWRENCE, S. (1981). Doctors probe brain's secrets. *Evening Post,* 10 November, 19.

MARK, V. H. & ERVIN, F. R. (1970) *Violence and the Brain.* New York: Harper & Row.

MARK, V. H., SWEET, W. H. & ERVIN, F. R. (1967) The role of brain disease in riots and urban violence. *Journal of the American Medical Association,* **201,** 895.

MICHAEL, J. (1981) A heavy burden. *Out West,* **27,** 8–9.

MONIZ, E. (1954) How I succeeded in performing the prefrontal leucotomy. *Journal of Clinical and Experimental Psychopathology,* **15,** 373–379.

ROEDER, F. D. (1966) Stereotactic lesions of the tuber cinereum in sexual deviation. *Confinia Neurologica,* **27,** 162–163.

SCHMIDT, G. & SCHORSCH, E. (1981) Psychosurgery of sexually deviant patients: a review and analysis of new empirical findings. *Archives of Sexual Behaviour,* **10,** 301–321.

SHUMAN, S. I. (1974) The emotional, medical and legal reasons for the special concern about psychosurgery. In *Medical, Moral and Legal Issues in Mental Health Care* (ed. Frank J. Ayd), pp. 48–79. Baltimore: Williams & Wilkins.

TOOTH, G. C. & NEWTON, M. P. (1961) *Leucotomy in England and Wales 1942–54. Ministry of Health. Reports on Public Health and Medical Subjects No. 104.* London:HMSO.

VALENSTEIN, E. S. (1980) Rationale and surgical procedures. In *The Psychosurgery Debate* (ed. E. S. Valenstein), pp. 55–86. San Francisco: W. H. Freeman.

—— (1986) *Great and Desperate Cures: The Rise and Decline of Psychosurgery and other Radical Treatments for Mental Illness.* New York: Basic Books.

WILSON, I. (1947) *Pre-Frontal Leucotomy in 1,000 Cases.* London: HMSO.

# 49 Dream life: C. G. Jung and neurophysiology

**NATHANIEL D. MINTON**

I became a senior registrar in Martin Roth's Department in Newcastle in 1970, with the qualifications of a Diploma in Psychological Medicine (DPM) and a training analysis in depth psychotherapy at the Zurich C. G. Jung Institute. Roth suggested to me that I should think through the concepts of Jung's analytical psychology to ascertain in which way they might have a relevance to contemporary psychiatry. At about the same time, he emphasised during case discussions the role of the temporal lobe as the watershed of the brain.

The core of my own training analysis had been the detailed recordings of many of my own dreams with my associations, and imaginative writing as well as selected reading in anthropology, mythology and comparative religion.

To a great extent, to think through and be rational about Jung's concepts is to develop a cognitive understanding of dream contents, together with and developing further ideas of Freud. Jung moved into analysis from his association experiments with Bleuler and then his psychological partnership with Freud, who wrote in *Interpretations of Dreams*, "We may expect that the analysis of dreams will lead us to a knowledge of man's archaic heritage, of what is psychically innate in him". In this sentence, Freud has anticipated Jung's later concept of the collective unconscious and its archetypal structure.

The experience of dreams while asleep correlates with certain neuro-physiological events, especially in the temporal lobe and other brain structures. My initial conversations with Roth have led me to an exploration of the inter-relationship between the psychic manifestation of the dream and the simultaneous activity of the immense number of neurones and their axones within the human brain. To aid me in my attempt to understand this inter-relationship, I have turned to the work and ideas of Sherrington, Penfield and Adrian rather than Crick and Mitchison, whose theory of reverse learning in dreaming, although worthy of consideration as one possible mechanism, rests on unproven speculation which over-simplifies brain function.

It is Adrian's attitude that has allowed a bridge to be created between the two apparent incompatibles of subjective inner experience and objective 'brain events'. Adrian wrote in 1966, "the physiologist is not forced to reject the old fashioned picture of himself as a conscious individual with a will of his own, for the position allows some kind of validity to the introspective as well as the physiological account".

Penfield, in his remarkable book *The Mystery of the Mind* (1975), comes to the conclusion that there are two fundamental elements, mind and brain. This was also the view of his original teacher, Sherrington. This dichotomy was not for Penfield an *a priori* belief, but an inescapable conclusion after reviewing and interpreting the data from his decades of experimental research, in which he stimulated different areas of the human cortex in conscious subjects with electrodes giving two or three volts. From his work which included a comprehension of the different forms of epilepsy, he derived the concept of the highest brain mechanism and the mind's mechanism.

Penfield wrote, "when a local discharge occurs in prefrontal or temporal areas of the cortex, it may spread directly to the highest brain-mechanism by bombardment (the mind's mechanism). When it does this, it produces automatism. On the other hand, the sensory and motor convolutions of the cortex, when overcharged electrically, bombard the automatic sensory-motor mechanism (the computer's mechanism) in the higher brain stem. One may surmise then that there must be a mind's mechanism that has direct access to prefrontal and temporal cortex, but has only indirect access to sensory and motor mechanisms of the cerebral cortex".

Penfield states clearly that the action of the highest brain mechanism is essential to the existence of consciousness, and also, "it is the mind (not the brain) that watches and at the same time directs". "Mind comes into action and goes out of action with the highest brain-mechanism, it is true, but the mind has energy. The form of that energy is different from that of neuronal potentials that travel the axone pathways. There I must leave it".

For Penfield, a leading neuro-surgeon and neurophysiologist, the mind's energy is a reality. For Freud 'excitation' and the movement of 'excitation' is of paramount importance. For Jung, psychic energy is a central concept. Possibly these three investigators are describing in different words the same phenomenon.

In the chapter on regression in Freud's *Interpretation of Dreams* he writes, "The only way in which we can describe what happens in hallucinatory dreams is by saying that the excitation moves in a backward direction. Instead of being transmitted towards the motor end of the apparatus, it moves towards the sensory end and finally reaches the perceptual system. If we describe as progressive the direction taken by psychical processes arising from the unconscious during waking life, then we may speak of dreams as having a regressive character". And further, "In the waking state, however, this backward movement never extends beyond the mnemic images; it does not succeed in producing a hallucinatory revival of the perceptual images". As if taking this idea further, Jung wrote in 1946 in his paper 'On The Nature of the Psyche', "In spite of the non-measurability of psychic processes, the perceptual changes effected by the psyche cannot possibly be understood except as a phenomenon of energy".

Rycroft in his interesting book *Innocence Of Dreams* (1979), although acknowledging the considerable contributions of both Freud and Jung to depth psychology, is dismissive of Freud's concept of mental energy and Jung's concept of the collective unconscious. The activity of the Imagination, as described by Coleridge, underlies dreaming according to Rycroft. This view is not new because Freud included a paper by Rank on 'Dream and Poetry' in the earlier editions of his *Interpretation of Dreams*. However, by negating the concepts of mental energy and the collective unconscious in dream studies, the connection is lost between science and art; the value of Penfield's conclusions are obscured and the images contained in universal myths not understood as emanating from unseen principles or archetypes. As Jung demonstrated, fragments and parts of these collective myths can be dreamt, as a result, so he postulated, of a regressive flow of psychic energy into the most phylogenetically ancient psychoid part of our being.

Before considering recent research on REM (rapid eye movement, an accompaniment of certain EEG changes during vivid dreams) sleep which correlates probably with most, but not all, dreaming, it might be illuminating to reflect on the content of two dreams, one of Freud's and one of Jung's. Aniela Jaffé, who edited Jung's *Memories, Dreams, Reflections*, and who introduced Jung to cabalistic symbolism (personal communication), has written a remarkable paper, 'The Creative Phases in Jung's Life' in her book, *Jung's Last Years* (1984). In Freud's own nightmare recollected from his seventh or eighth year and recorded in his *Interpretation Of Dreams*, he saw "his beloved mother, dead, carried into a room by two or three persons with birds' beaks. The bird people remind him of an Egyptian tomb relief, the pall-bearers are related to the bird-headed Horus, and because of the solar quality of this God, they must be governed by the realm of daylight, by logos and reason". Jung's childhood dream in his fourth or fifth year was very different. "The boy discovers a hole in the ground with steps leading downward into the depths . . . he finds a wonderful golden throne at the end of a long room. On the throne sits a gigantic thing like a tree trunk . . . On its skull is a single eye that gazes steadily upwards. Around its head is a glow of light that illuminates the entire room". He then hears his mother's voice, "Yes, just look at him. That is the man-eater". At this point, Jung records years later, he became even more terrified. It is a pity that there is not a sleep EEG for this dream, which Aniela Jaffé thinks anticipated Jung's life's work. It was probably an REM dream, but it could have been from a light stage of S sleep or even a night terror, which classically is not usually remembered. Aneila Jaffé comments that "he always remembered that vision of light in the darkness which he saw for the first time in his childhood dream. Jung wanted to illuminate the dark, unknown, rejected side of the psyche. In the imagery of a different culture, one could say that he was drawn to the core of light in Yin and the core of darkness in Yang".

As is now well known, Dement and Kleitman described REM sleep in the mid-1950s. This is also referred to as D sleep, as the EEG is desynchronised. REM sleep is also characterised by low voltage EEG activity, variation in pulse, respiration, blood pressure, penile erection, loss of muscle tone and muscular twitching of the face and hands. During a normal person's sleep, periods of non-REM and REM alternate. REM recurs at regular intervals five to seven times each night. Young adults have 20–25% on REM sleep time. Most dream research in the laboratory has concentrated on REM sleep. However, some dream researchers claim that although much more dream material occurs in REM sleep, similar dreams occur in non-REM periods. Perhaps more dream laboratory research needs to be done on the dream content of non-REM sleep.

Hobson's and McCarley's research from North America in the 1970s, which can be seen as a development of Jouvet's neurophysiological research in the area of the cat's pontine brainstem, assumes that all dreaming occurs in REM sleep. Their conclusions that REM dreaming depends on periodic activation of the forebrain during sleep may be correct, but their hypothesis "that the activated forebrain synthesises the dreams by fitting experiential data to information endogenously and automatically generated by reticular, vestibular and oculomotor neurons in the pontine brainstem'', has been strongly criticised by Vogel in his erudite paper 'An Alternative View Of The Neurobiology Of Dreaming', in which he writes, "Contrary to the activation-synthesis hypothesis of Hobson and McCarley, in the intact animal, the forebrain has a crucial role in the instigation, timing, maintenance and activation pattern of most episodes of D sleep".

Burns (1968), in his book *The Uncertain Nervous System*, writes, "In general, it is changes in the environment rather than steady environmental states that determine reaction of the nervous system. It is not surprising, therefore, to find that in many cortical districts, units are most excited by alterations of sensory input and appear to disregard steady states''. This principle of Burns perhaps explains the biological and neuropsychological necessity of activating the forebrain at the beginning of REM sleep with monophasic electrical bursts, referred to as pontine-geniculate occipital spikes and occurring synchronously with the eye movements. Perhaps during non-REM sleep the forebrain is slowly returning to a steady state.

Both classes of sleep, as Crisp (1977) points out in his paper on 'Sleep: Normal and Abnormal', are associated with widespread and characteristic metabolic activities as well as restorative and synthetic processes as outlined by Oswald. Crisp thinks, "It may be that what we detect as dreams comprises an active process of inspecting previous experience not normally available to consciousness—especially in symbolic form—in the light of the experience of the past day''.

In dreaming, when the main perceptions are visual and less acoustic, the occipital psychic areas and their close interpretative cortex, of the temporal lobe, are of necessity activated. Probably this activation passes to the hippocampi. As Penfield described it, "The hippocampi seem to store keys-of-access to the record of the stream of consciousness. With the interpretative cortex, they make possible the scanning and the recall of experiential memory''. During REM dreaming, when there is hypotonia due to blocking of motor output, the forebrain activation presumably passes from the hippocampi into the limbic system and hypothalamus. Davison points out that during the cortical arousal of REM sleep, "electrical activity in the cortex, diencephalon, and mesencephalon and particularly the hippocampus is similar to that found in the waking state, nevertheless, the subject is behaviourally deeply asleep" (Davison & Bagley, 1969).

A neo-Freudian, Altman, in his book *The Dream In Psychoanalysis* (1975), also links the concept of mental energy with neurophysiological processes. He writes with insight, "The neurophysiological changes which take place during REM periods suggest that activation of the limbic area of the brain—an area associated with primitive functioning of drives and affects, is involved. Such neurophysiological retrogression supports Freud's theory of the dream as a regressive phenomenon which returns us to primitive states of infancy. So far as we know, dreams are produced by bursts of psychic activity which, because sleep cuts off the possibility of voluntary motor action, seek sensory release''.

Attention has not been focused on Freud's early emphasis on instinctual wishes or drives in dreams, being disguised by the censor or super-ego through condensation of images and displacement. This dream work theory of Freud described how thoughts changed to visual images during a regressive flow of psychic energy. It distinguished manifest from latent content. For Jung, the more profound the regression of 'mind's energy' during dreaming, the more meaningful manifest content might be, as it approached a pure symbolic expression, on a supra-personal level for the dreamer. The regression was seen as travelling beyond the infancy of the individual into the infancy of human tribal life, when symbolic form derived from nature gave meaning, morality and religion to our ancestors.

A relative re-programming of previous learnt behaviour patterns and a degree of emotional re-integration may occur in dreams never recalled, which are the majority. Unconscious dream experiences of compensation and conflict dramatically expressed, may be part of the homeostatic mechanisms of the limbic system and hypothalamus, consistent with preservation and survival. However, Meier *et al*'s (1968) sleep and dream laboratory research on forgetting of dreams indicated that in remembered dreams there was an apparent upward gradient of consciousness similar to an attention engram and that the dream experienced and remembered itself engenders consciousness.

Jung maintained that the maturation and integration of the personality can be aided by a psychological process he called individuation, during which a certain sequence of symbolic images occur in dreams. A relative individuation usually occurs in older people when self-awareness or consciousness is increased. Roth's scientific work with the elderly supports this view in so far as he has observed that judgement improves with age and some visual artists continue to paint into great old age.

Penfield wrote after a lifetime in neurophysiology and neurosurgery, "Likewise, if the mind of man communicates with the mind of God directly, that also suggests that energy, in some form, passes from spirit to spirit". Perhaps if this phenomenon is true, it can occur in certain kinds of dreams.

*References*

ADRIAN, E. D. (1966) Consciousness. In *Brain and Conscious Experience* (ed. J. C. Eccles), pp. 238–248. New York: Springer-Verlag.

ALTMAN, L. L. (1975) *The Dream in Psychoanalysis.* New York: International Universities Press.

BURNS, B. (1968) *The Uncertain Nervous System.* London: Edward Arnold.

CRICK, F. & MITCHISON, G. (1983) The function of dream sleep. *Nature*, **304**, 111–114.

CRISP, A. (1977) Sleep: normal and abnormal. *Hexagon* (Roche), **5**, 9–14.

DAVISON, K. & BAGLEY, C. B. (1969) Part II *Current Problems in Neuro-psychiatry* (ed. R. N. Herrington) Royal Medico-Psychological Association. Ashford Kent: Headley Brothers.

DEMENT, W. & KLEITMAN, N. (1957) Cyclic variations in EEG during sleep and their relation to eye movement, body motility, and dreaming. *Electroencephalography and Clinical Neurophysiology*, **9**, 673–690.

FREUD, S. (1961) *The Interpretation of Dreams.* London: George Allen & Unwin.

HARTMAN, E. L. (1965) The D-state. A review and discussion of studies on the physiologic state concomitant with dreaming. *New England Journal of Medicine*, **273**, 30–35 and 87–92.

HOBSON, J. A. & McCARLEY, R. W. (1977) The brain as a dream state generator: An activation-synthesis hypothesis of the dream process. *American Journal of Psychiatry*, **134**, 1335–1348.

JACOBI, J. (1959) Complex archetype symbol. In *The psychology of C. G. Jung* (Bollingen Foundation). London: Routledge & Kegan Paul.

JAFFÉ, A. (1984) *Jung's Last Years.* Dallas, Texas: Spring Publications.

JUNG, C. G. (1973) *Experimental Researches* (Vol. 2 Collected Works). London: Routledge & Kegan Paul.

—— (1960) On the nature of the psyche. In *The Structure and Dynamics of the Psyche* (Vol. 8 Collected Works). London: Routledge & Kegan Paul.

McGUIRE, W. (1974) *The Freud/Jung Letters*. London: The Hogarth Press and Routledge & Kegan Paul.

MEIER, C. A., RUEF, H., ZIEGLER, A. & HALL, C. S. (1968) *Forgetting of Dreams in the Laboratory, Perceptual and Motor Skills*, vol. 26, pp. 551–557, California: Southern University Press.

OSWALD, I. (1970) Sleep, The great restorer. *New Scientist*, **46**, 170–172.

PENFIELD, WILDER. (1975) *The Mystery of The Mind*. Princeton University Press.

RANK, O. (1919) Traum und Dichtung. In *Die Traum Deuting* (S. Freud). Leipzig and Vienna: Franz Deuticke.

ROTH, M. (1969) Chapter X: Ageing and the mental diseases of the aged. *Clinical Psychiatry* (W. Mayer-Gross, E. Slater & M. Roth, third edition). Eastbourne: Baillière, Tindall & Cassell.

RYCROFT, C. (1979) *Innocence of Dreams*. London: The Hogarth Press.

VOGEL, Gerald, W. (1978) An alternative view of the neurobiology of dreaming. *American Journal of Psychiatry*, **135**, 1531–1535.

# Index

## Compiled by STANLEY THORLEY

Abbreviations: App. = Appendix. Fig. = Figure. Tab. = Table. Other abbreviations given in the Index.